METHODS IN MOLECULAR BIOLOGY

Series Editor
John M. Walker
School of Life and Medical Sciences,
University of Hertfordshire, Hatfield,
Hertfordshire AL10 9AB, UK

For further volumes:
http://www.springer.com/series/7651

Comparative Genomics

Methods and Protocols

Edited by

João C. Setubal

Department of Biochemistry, Institute of Chemistry, University of São Paulo, São Paulo, SP, Brazil

Jens Stoye

Faculty of Technology and Center for Biotechnology (CeBiTec), Bielefeld University, Bielefeld, Germany

Peter F. Stadler

Bioinformatics Group, Department of Computer Science, Interdisciplinary Center for Bioinformatics, University of Leipzig, Leipzig, Germany

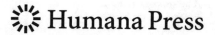 Humana Press

Editors
João C. Setubal
Department of Biochemistry
Institute of Chemistry
University of São Paulo
São Paulo, SP, Brazil

Jens Stoye
Faculty of Technology and Center
for Biotechnology (CeBiTec)
Bielefeld University
Bielefeld, Germany

Peter F. Stadler
Bioinformatics Group
Department of Computer Science
Interdisciplinary Center for Bioinformatics
University of Leipzig
Leipzig, Germany

ISSN 1064-3745   ISSN 1940-6029   (electronic)
Methods in Molecular Biology
ISBN 978-1-4939-8493-0   ISBN 978-1-4939-7463-4   (eBook)
https://doi.org/10.1007/978-1-4939-7463-4

Cover image: Cover image design by Georges Hattab

Printed on acid-free paper

This Humana Press imprint is published by Springer Nature
The registered company is Springer Science+Business Media, LLC
The registered company address is: 233 Spring St, New York, NY 10013, U.S.A.

Preface

Since the rise of genetics and molecular biology during the twentieth century, a high potential was seen in the benefits of a better understanding of the molecular mechanisms underlying life, including more efficient food production and improved health care. More recently, other goals have been added, such as higher energy efficiency, DNA forensics, improved disease diagnostics, personalized medicine, and environmentally related aims, such as sustainable agricultural production. Because information coded in the DNA underlies essentially all molecular activity in cells, this motivated the continuous development of DNA sequencing technology. This development in turn created a new research field called genomics, whose subject of study is the genomes of every organism on Earth. Collecting, analyzing, and understanding genes and genomes became a major effort in molecular biology, a general effort that achieved a significant milestone with the sequencing of the human genome in 2001.

Genomes, however, just like the organisms to which they belong, are not isolated entities, and many additional insights can be gained by looking at more than one genome at a time. Studies comparing several genomes use the observation that functionally relevant regions of a genome are conserved over time due to selection pressures, while other regions are free to mutate. This led to the important field of comparative genomics, a more functionally oriented successor to the classical fields of taxonomy and phylogenetics, where mainly the evolutionary interrelationships between species are of interest.

Today it is possible to obtain and study the genomes of large numbers of individuals from a population, or even multiple samples from each individual. One pioneer large-scale human population genome sequencing project is the 1000 Genomes Project (now International Genome Sample Resource, IGSR, http://www.internationalgenome.org/), initiated with the goal of sequencing the genomes of more than one thousand human individuals to identify 95% of all genomic variants in the population with allele frequency of at least 1% (down to 0.1% in coding regions). Other initiatives followed, such as Genomics England, which aims at sequencing 100,000 whole genomes from patients and their families, focusing on rare diseases, some common types of cancer, and infectious diseases (https://www.genomicsengland.co.uk/). In the United States, the Federal Precision Medicine Initiative (the All of Us research program) aims to analyze genetic information from more than one million American volunteers (https://www.nih.gov/research-training/allofus-research-program/). The day is not far off when every human being on earth will have the choice of having his or her genome sequenced at the cost of a simple blood group test.

Not only humans have had their genomes sequenced, of course. Classic model organisms, such as the fly Drosophila, have genomes available for several different species, with *D. melanogaster* currently having five genomes available. Bacteria, which have smaller genomes, have hundreds of thousands of genomes available. The champion organism in terms of number of genomes available is *E. coli*, which, as of this writing, has close to 6,000. The recent popularization of metagenomics, which allows DNA sequencing of basically all organisms living in any small environmental niche (such as human saliva), is leading us to the point where every life form on Earth will have its genome sequenced.

Even more recent is the technique of single-cell genomics, which seeks to provide genome sequences for single cells, as opposed to the traditional "bulk DNA" sequencing, in which the DNA of many cells is pooled and sequenced, leading therefore to the loss of inter-cell genetic variation information.

In spite of all these developments, it is still true that the understanding of the genetic and genomic basis of organism phenotypes, and its relationship with other factors such as the particular environment in which an organism finds itself, is far from complete. Comparative genomics is a powerful way of providing insights into these questions and is therefore the motivation for this volume.

While DNA sequencing is the technology that made all of this possible, the hard part of making sense of all this data falls by and large on the shoulders of bioinformatics. Hence, all of the chapters in this volume deal with various algorithmic and computational techniques related to comparative genomics, as well as analyses made possible by these techniques.

In parallel with the flood of genome sequences, the literature on comparative genomics is vast and continually growing; therefore this volume can only offer a glimpse of what is currently being done in this rapidly evolving discipline. Nevertheless, by covering a broad spectrum of topics, we hope that the chapters included in this volume will be useful to students and researchers alike for many years to come.

São Paulo, SP, Brazil   *João C. Setubal*
Bielefeld, Germany   *Jens Stoye*
Leipzig, Germany   *Peter F. Stadler*

Contents

Contributors

NALVO F. ALMEIDA • *School of Computing, Federal University of Mato Grosso do Sul, Campo Grande, MS, Brazil*

DANILLO OLIVEIRA ALVARENGA • *Departamento de Tecnologia, Faculdade de Ciências Agrárias e Veterinárias, Universidade Estadual Paulista "Júlio de Mesquita Filho"–UNESP, Jaboticabal, SP, Brazil*

DEYVID AMGARTEN • *Department of Biochemistry, Institute of Chemistry, University of São Paulo, São Paulo, SP, Brazil*

YOANN ANSELMETTI • *Institut des Sciences de l'Évolution, Université Montpellier 2, Montpellier, France*

SÈVERINE BÉRARD • *Institut des Sciences de l'Évolution, Université Montpellier 2, Montpellier, France*

ROLF BACKOFEN • *Bioinformatics Group, Department of Computer Science, University of Freiburg, Freiburg, Germany; Center for Non-coding RNA in Technology and Health, University of Copenhagen, Frederiksberg, Denmark*

MATTHIAS BERNT • *Swarm Intelligence and Complex Systems Group, Institute of Computer Science, University Leipzig, Leipzig, Germany*

THOMAS BRETTIN • *Computation Institute, University of Chicago, Chicago, IL, USA; Computing, Environment and Life Sciences, Argonne National Laboratory, Argonne, IL, USA*

MICK CHANDLER • *Laboratoire de Microbiologie et Génétique Moléculaires, Toulouse Cedex, France*

CEDRIC CHAUVE • *Department of Mathematics, Simon Fraser University, Burnaby, BC, Canada*

JAMES J. DAVIS • *Computation Institute, University of Chicago, Chicago, IL, USA; Computing, Environment and Life Sciences, Argonne National Laboratory, Argonne, IL, USA*

DANIEL DOERR • *School of Computer and Communication Sciences, EPFL, Lausanne, Switzerland*

PEDRO FEIJÃO • *Faculty of Technology, Bielefeld University, Bielefeld, Germany; Center for Biotechnology (CeBiTec), Bielefeld University, Bielefeld, Germany*

SVETLANA GERDES • *Computing, Environment and Life Sciences, Argonne National Laboratory, Argonne, IL, USA; Fellowship for Interpretation of Genomes, Burr Ridge, IL, USA*

JAN GORODKIN • *Department of Veterinary and Animal Sciences, Center for Non-coding RNA in Technology and Health, University of Copenhagen, Frederiksberg, Denmark*

TOM HARTMANN • *Swarm Intelligence and Complex Systems Group, Institute of Computer Science, University Leipzig, Leipzig, Germany*

IVO L. HOFACKER • *Institute for Theoretical Chemistry, University of Vienna, Wien, Austria; Bioinformatics and Computational Biology Research Group, University of Vienna, Vienna, Austria; Center for Non-coding RNA in Technology and Health, University of Copenhagen, Frederiksberg, Denmark*

GUILLAUME HOLLEY • *Faculty of Technology, Bielefeld University, Bielefeld, Germany; Center for Biotechnology (CeBiTec), Bielefeld University, Bielefeld, Germany; International Research Training Group 1906, Bielefeld University, Bielefeld, Germany*

STEFANIE KÖNIG • *Institut für Mathematik und Informatik, Ernst Moritz Arndt Universität Greifswald, Greifswald, Germany*

RONALD KENYON • *Biocomplexity Institute, Virginia Tech, Blacksburg, VA, USA*

FELIPE PRATA LIMA • *Department of Biochemistry, Institute of Chemistry, University of São Paulo, São Paulo, SP, Brazil; Instituto Federal de Alagoas, Maceió, Alagoas, Brazil*

NINA LUHMANN • *Faculty of Technology, Bielefeld University, Bielefeld, Germany; Center for Biotechnology (CeBiTec), Bielefeld University, Bielefeld, Germany; International Research Training Group 1906, Bielefeld University, Bielefeld, Germany*

DUSTIN MACHI • *Biocomplexity Institute, Virginia Tech, Blacksburg, VA, USA*

CHUNHONG MAO • *Biocomplexity Institute, Virginia Tech, Blacksburg, VA, USA*

JOAQUIM MARTINS JR. • *Department of Biochemistry, Institute of Chemistry, University of São Paulo, São Paulo, SP, Brazil*

MARTIN MIDDENDORF • *Swarm Intelligence and Complex Systems Group, Institute of Computer Science, University Leipzig, Leipzig, Germany*

LEANDRO M. MOREIRA • *Departamento de Ciências Biológicas–Núcleo de Pesquisas em Ciências Biológicas-NUPEB, Universidade Federal de Ouro Preto, Ouro Preto, Minas Gerais, Brazil*

BERNARD M. E. MORET • *School of Computer and Communication Sciences, EPFL, Lausanne, Switzerland*

LIVIA MARIA SILVA MOURA • *Department of Biochemistry, Institute of Chemistry, University of São Paulo, São Paulo, SP, Brazil*

EMMANUEL DIAS-NETO • *Medical Genomics Laboratory, CIPE/A.C. Camargo Cancer Center, São Paulo, SP, Brazil; Laboratory of Neurosciences (LIM-27) Alzira Denise Hertzog Silva, Institute of Psychiatry, Faculdade de Medicina, Universidade de São Paulo (USP), São Paulo, SP, Brazil*

ROBERT OLSON • *Computation Institute, University of Chicago, Chicago, IL, USA; Mathematics and Computer Science Division, Argonne National Laboratory, Argonne, IL, USA*

MARTIN OTI • *Institute of Biophysics Carlos Chagas Filho (IBCCF), Federal University of Rio de Janeiro (UFRJ), Rio de Janeiro, RJ, Brazil*

ROSS OVERBEEK • *Computing, Environment and Life Sciences, Argonne National Laboratory, Argonne, IL, USA; Fellowship for Interpretation of Genomes, Burr Ridge, IL, USA*

ATTILIO PANE • *Institute of Biomedical Sciences (ICB), Federal University of Rio de Janeiro (UFRJ), Rio de Janeiro, RJ, Brazil*

JOSÉ S. L. PATANÉ • *Department of Biochemistry, Institute of Chemistry, University of São Paulo, São Paulo, SP, Brazil*

GORDON D. PUSCH • *Computing, Environment and Life Sciences, Argonne National Laboratory, Argonne, IL, USA; Fellowship for Interpretation of Genomes, Burr Ridge, IL, USA*

CHRISTIAN RÖDELSPERGER • *Department for Evolutionary Biology, Max Planck Institute for Developmental Biology, Tübingen, Germany*

LARS ROMOTH • *Institut für Mathematik und Informatik, Ernst Moritz Arndt Universität Greifswald, Greifswald, Germany*

MICHAEL SAMMETH • *Institute of Biophysics Carlos Chagas Filho (IBCCF), Federal University of Rio de Janeiro (UFRJ), Rio de Janeiro, RJ, Brazil*

DAVID SANKOFF • *Department of Mathematics and Statistics, University of Ottawa, Ottawa, ON, Canada*

JOÃO C. SETUBAL • *Department of Biochemistry, Institute of Chemistry, University of São Paulo, São Paulo, SP, Brazil*

MAULIK P. SHUKLA • *Computation Institute, University of Chicago, Chicago, IL, USA; Computing, Environment and Life Sciences, Argonne National Laboratory, Argonne, IL, USA*

ALINE MARIA DA SILVA • *Department of Biochemistry, Institute of Chemistry, University of São Paulo, São Paulo, SP, Brazil*

PETER F. STADLER • *Bioinformatics Group, Department of Computer Science, Interdisciplinary Center for Bioinformatics, University of Leipzig, Leipzig, Germany; Max Planck Institute for Mathematics in the Sciences, Leipzig, Germany; Fraunhofer Institute for Cell Therapy and Immunology, Leipzig, Germany; Institute for Theoretical Chemistry, University of Vienna, Wien, Austria; Center for Non-coding RNA in Technology and Health, University of Copenhagen, Frederiksberg, Denmark; Santa Fe Institute, Santa Fe, NM, USA*

MARIO STANKE • *Institut für Mathematik und Informatik, Ernst Moritz Arndt Universität Greifswald, Greifswald, Germany*

RICK STEVENS • *Computation Institute, University of Chicago, Chicago, IL, USA; Computing, Environment and Life Sciences, Argonne National Laboratory, Argonne, IL, USA; Department of Computer Science, University of Chicago, Chicago, IL, USA*

JENS STOYE • *Faculty of Technology, Bielefeld University, Bielefeld, Germany; Center for Biotechnology, Bielefeld University, Bielefeld, Germany*

ERIC TANNIER • *UMR CNRS 5558 - LBBE "Biométrie et Biologie Évolutive", Inria Grenoble Rhône-Alpes and University of Lyon, Lyon, France*

ANDREW MALTEZ THOMAS • *Department of Biochemistry, Institute of Chemistry, University of São Paulo, São Paulo, SP, Brazil; Medical Genomics Laboratory, CIPE/A.C. Camargo Cancer Center, São Paulo, SP, Brazil*

CHRIS UPTON • *Department of Biochemistry and Microbiology, University of Victoria, Victoria, BC, Canada*

ALESSANDRO M. VARANI • *Departamento de Tecnologia, Faculdade de Ciências Agrárias e Veterinárias, Universidade Estadual Paulista "Júlio de Mesquita Filho"–UNESP, Jaboticabal, SP, Brazil*

VERONIKA VONSTEIN • *Computing, Environment and Life Sciences, Argonne National Laboratory, Argonne, IL, USA; Fellowship for Interpretation of Genomes, Burr Ridge, IL, USA*

ANDREW WARREN • *Biocomplexity Institute, Virginia Tech, Blacksburg, VA, USA*

ALICE R. WATTAM • *Biocomplexity Institute, Virginia Tech, Blacksburg, VA, USA*

FANGFANG XIA • *Computation Institute, University of Chicago, Chicago, IL, USA; Mathematics and Computer Science Division, Argonne National Laboratory, Argonne, IL, USA*

HYUNSEUNG YOO • *Computation Institute, University of Chicago, Chicago, IL, USA; Computing, Environment and Life Sciences, Argonne National Laboratory, Argonne, IL, USA*

TINA ZEKIC • *Faculty of Technology, Bielefeld University, Bielefeld, Germany; Center for Biotechnology (CeBiTec), Bielefeld University, Bielefeld, Germany; International Research Training Group 1906, Bielefeld University, Bielefeld, Germany*

CHUNFANG ZHENG • *Department of Mathematics and Statistics, University of Ottawa, Ottawa, ON, Canada*

Chapter 1

Gene Phylogenies and Orthologous Groups

João C. Setubal and Peter F. Stadler

Abstract

This chapter covers the theory and practice of ortholog gene set computation. In the theoretical part we give detailed and formal descriptions of the relevant concepts. We also cover the topic of graph-based clustering as a tool to compute ortholog gene sets. In the second part we provide an overview of practical considerations intended for researchers who need to determine orthologous genes from a collection of annotated genomes, briefly describing some of the most popular programs and resources currently available for this task.

Key words Orthologs, Paralogs, Gene family, Protein family, Phylogeny

1 Fitch's Definition

The concepts of orthology and paralogy were introduced in a clear and concise manner by Walter Fitch in 1970 [1]:

> Where the homology is the result of gene duplication so that both copies have descended side by side during the history of an organism, (for example, alpha and beta hemoglobin) the genes should be called paralogous (para = in parallel). Where the homology is the result of speciation so that the history of the gene reflects the history of the species (for example alpha hemoglobin in man and mouse) the genes should be called orthologous (ortho = exact).

Although the distinction between orthologous and paralogous genes as defined above seems simple enough, a controversy about their proper usage and their consequence in the context of gene function ensued at the turn of the millennium [2–4]. In this contribution we adopt the point of view that homology and therefore also orthology and paralogy refer only to the evolutionary history of a collection of genes. A *gene family* thus comprises all genes (in the set of genomes under consideration) that share a common evolutionary origin. Our usage of the terms homology and gene family deliberately avoids any reference to gene function, distinguishing homologous genes (those that share a common descent and thus belong to same gene family) and analogous genes (those

João C. Setubal et al. (eds.), *Comparative Genomics: Methods and Protocols*, Methods in Molecular Biology, vol. 1704, https://doi.org/10.1007/978-1-4939-7463-4_1, © Springer Science+Business Media LLC 2018

that have similar functions but are evolutionarily unrelated). As a consequence, orthology and paralogy can be understood completely in terms of (i) a species tree of the species under consideration, (ii) the gene tree of a particular gene family, and (iii) the mutual relation of these two trees.

The usefulness of the notions of orthology and paralogy is of course linked to their tight correlation with gene function [5]: While functional similarity is not a defining feature of orthology, it is of course true that orthologous genes in closely related genomes *usually* and *approximately* have the same function. More strictly, one-to-one orthologs are in most cases functionally equivalent. Paralogs, in contrast, often have related, but clearly distinct functions [6–8] (but *see* also [9]). Since orthologs usually evolve in a clock-like fashion, that is, with an approximately constant rate of evolution (at least as long as there are no duplications), they are the characters of choice in molecular phylogenetics [10]. If one gene per species is selected at random from groups of paralogs, furthermore, the resulting gene tree will in general not be congruent with the species tree. Thus molecular phylogenetics applications strive to restrict their input data to one-to-one orthologs. Beyond its important role in phylogenetics, the reliable identification of orthologs also plays a key role in comparative genomic analyses [11]: Orthologs serve as anchors for chromosome alignments and thus are an important basis for synteny-based methods. The reconstruction of ancestral proteomes also depends crucially on high-quality ortholog data sets.

2 Theory

2.1 Phylogenetic Trees

A *phylogenetic tree* T is a rooted tree $T = (V, E)$ with a set of directed edges E, a set of leaves $L \subseteq V$, and a set of interior vertices $V^0 = V \setminus L$ that does not contain any vertices with in- and outdegree one and whose root $\rho_T \in V$ in the only node that indegree zero. In order to avoid uninteresting trivial cases, we will usually assume that T has at least three leaves. For our purposes it will be most convenient to slightly modify this standard notion of a phylogenetic tree by a single extra node 0 and an edge "preceding" the original root. From now on we will call this "dummy node" the root of T.

The ancestor relation $\preceq$ on V is the partial order defined, for all $x, y \in V$, by $x \preceq_T y$ whenever y lies on the (unique) path from the root to x. For any subset $W \subseteq V$ we define $\mathrm{lca}_T(W)$ as the *last common ancestor* of W, i.e., the $\preceq_T$-smallest node $u \in V$ so that $w \preceq_T u$ for all $w \in T$. The subtree $T[x]$ of T rooted at $x \in V$ consists of all vertices $y \preceq x$ and the edges of T connecting them.

A *refinement* of a phylogenetic tree T is a phylogenetic tree T' on the same leaf set such that T can be obtained from T' by collapsing edges. The *restriction* $T|_{L'}$ of T to L' is the phylogenetic

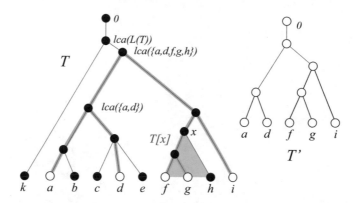

Fig. 1 The phylogenetic tree is augmented by an artificial root 0 above the last common ancestor lca($L(T)$) of all leaves. The tree T' on the leaf set {a, d, f, g, i} is displayed by T. The gray outline shows how T' is embedded in T. The subtree $T[x]$ rooted at the inner node x is shown by a blue shading

tree with leaf set L' obtained from $T\backslash(L\backslash L')$, the tree obtained from T by deleting all vertices in $L\backslash L'$ and their incident edges, by additionally suppressing all vertices of degree two with the exception of ρ_T if ρ_T is a node retained in $T\backslash(L\backslash L')$. A phylogenetic tree T' on some subset $L' \subseteq L$ is said to be *displayed* by T (or equivalently that T *displays* T') if T' is equivalent with $T|_{L'}$. See Fig. 1.

A set $\mathscr{T}$ of phylogenetic trees T each with leaf set L_T is called *consistent* if $\mathscr{T} = \emptyset$ or there is a phylogenetic tree T on $L = \bigcup_{T\in\mathscr{T}} L_T$ that *displays* $\mathscr{T}$, that is, T displays every tree contained in $\mathscr{T}$.

2.2 Reconciliation of Gene Trees and Species Trees

A collection of ancestrally related genes G can be assumed to have evolved in a tree-like manner. The true gene tree $\widehat{T}$ represents all extant as well as all extinct genes, and all duplication and all speciation events. It also accounts for horizontal transfer or retroposition. Extinct genes, however, are not observable from extant gene data. The observable part $T = T(V, E)$ of $\widehat{T}$ is simply the restriction of $\widehat{T}$ to the set G of extant genes, which of course form the leaves of T, i.e., $T = \widehat{T}|_G$. The evolutionary relationships between the species is also encoded by a phylogenetic tree S, known as the *species tree*. With the exception of a metagenomics setting, furthermore, it is safe to assume that we know for each gene from which species it has been isolated. Formally, this relationship is described by a map $\sigma: G \to L(S)$. The observable part of $\widehat{S}$ is therefore the restriction of S to the species for which we actually have sequence data, i.e., $S = \widehat{S}|_{\sigma(G)}$. The best we can hope for is of course to understand the relation of the observable trees T and S.

In the absence of horizontal gene transfer (and other "weird" effects such as incomplete lineage sorting) the gene tree T must "follow" the species tree S as indicated in Fig. 2 [12].

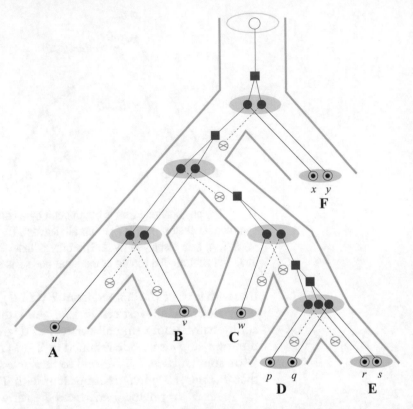

Fig. 2 Illustration of a gene history embedded in a phylogenetic tree of six species. Interior nodes of the species tree correspond to speciation events. These directly translate to interior nodes of the gene tree, here marked as red filled circles. The other event types in the gene tree are gene duplications (blue filled square) and gene losses (green crossed circle). The extant genes (one in species *A*, *B*, *C* and two in species *D*, *E*, and *F*) are indicated by circled dots

The true evolutionary history of a single ancestral gene has four components: (1) a true gene tree $\widehat{T}$, (2) a true species tree $\hat{S}$, (3) a *reconciliation map* μ assigning every node of $\widehat{T}$ to a node or edge of $\hat{S}$, and (4) an assignment of an event type to each node of $\widehat{T}$.

The basic idea is that inner nodes of the gene tree are mapped to inner nodes of the species tree (in the case of speciations) or to the edges of the species tree (in the case of duplications). Strictly speaking, the following formal conditions must hold only if both *S* and *T* are fully resolved. The complications arising from multi-furcations are numerous and have not been fully disentangled in the literature (but see, e.g., [13]). For example, multifurcations in the species tree might correspond to a mix of speciation and duplication events, violating the condition that μ is a map; we will disregard such cases here.

The reconciliation map $\mu\colon V(T) \to E(S) \cup V(S)$ satisfies the following set of natural axioms:

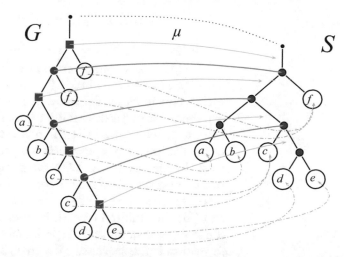

Fig. 3 Example of the mapping μ of some vertices of the gene tree T to the species tree S. Speciation nodes in the gene tree are mapped to nodes in the species tree, duplication nodes to edges in the species tree, and leaves in the gene tree to leaves in the species tree. Leaves in the gene tree are labeled with the corresponding species name

(0) $\mu(0_T) = 0_S$.

(i) If $x \in L(T)$, then $\mu(x) = \sigma(x)$.

(ii) Suppose $x \prec_T y$. Then

    (a) If $\mu(x) \in V(S)$ or $\mu(y) \in V(S)$, then $\mu(x) \prec_S \mu(y)$

    (b) If $\mu(x) \in E(S)$ and $\mu(y) \in E(S)$, then $\mu(x) \preceq_S \mu(y)$

The first two conditions constrain the mapping μ with respect to the known assignment σ of genes $L(T)$ to species $L(S)$ and to the mapping of the (dummy) roots of the trees onto each other. Conditions (ii.a) and (ii.b) together are known as the *Ancestor Consistency Constraint*. An example is shown in Fig. 3.

In most of the literature an additional condition is introduced that explicitly links μ to the so-called Last Common Ancestor (LCA) map, which is defined as $\lambda(u) := \mathrm{lca}_S(\sigma(L(T_u)))$. The map λ maps every node of the gene tree to the last common ancestor of the set of species in which the gene set $L(u)$ is found. It is computable in linear time [14].

We waive this LCA condition and instead investigate the reconciliation map μ defined above a bit further. As shown in [15, Lemma 3], μ satisfies

$$\mathrm{lca}_S(\mu(x), \mu(y)) \preceq_S \mu\left(\mathrm{lca}_T(x, y)\right) \tag{1}$$

for all $x, y \in V(T)$. A simple consequence of Eq. 1 is the following condition

$$\text{lca}_S(\mu(L(T_u))) \preceq_S \mu(u) \quad \text{for all } u \in V(T) \tag{2}$$

which specializes to $\lambda(u) \preceq_S \mu(u)$ for all $u \in V(T)$.

In [16], a stronger condition is postulated, requiring that equality, $\mu(u) = \lambda(u)$ holds for all u with $\mu(u) \in V(S)$. We call such reconciliations *LCA-like*. We note, finally, that different formal frameworks for describing reconciliation have been used in the literature, see, e.g., [17] for a recent overview. Instead of the reconciliation map μ, a *minimum reconciled tree* $R(G, S)$ can be used. In analogy to the LCA mapping it is defined as the smallest tree that satisfies (i) G is a homomorphic subtree of $R(G, S)$, (ii) the sets of species labels of all subtrees coincide between $R(G, S)$ and S, and (iii) the children of each interior node of $R(G, S)$ have either the same or disjoint sets of species labels [18, 19]. A closely related formalism is the so-called DLS tree [20].

2.3 Event Labels and Optimal Reconciliations

The mapping μ defines the type of events associated with the vertices of the gene tree T:

(i) $t(u) = \bullet$, a speciation, if $\mu(u)$ is a proper interior node of the species tree, i.e., iff $\mu(u) \in V(S) \backslash (L(S) \cup \{0_S\})$.

(ii) $t(u) = \bullet$, a duplication, if $\mu(u) \in E(S)$.

(iii) $t(u) = \odot$ if $u \in L(T)$ and hence $\mu(u) \in L(S)$.

(iv) $t(u) = \bigcirc$ if $u = 0_T$ and hence $\mu(u) = 0_S$.

A duplication event implicitly also defines losses since all genes present at a certain point in time are propagated through all subsequent speciation events unless they are lost again along a particular edge. Hence, the descendants of a gene u must appear in all species in $L(\mu(T_u))$ unless they have been deleted. This realization suggests we should associate a cost with μ that discourages superfluous duplication and loss events. The most natural cost function thus is the total number of duplication and gene loss events implied by μ [21, 22].

The assignment of event labels defined by μ also highlights a conceptual problem with the LCA-reconciliation λ. It maps $u \in V(T)$ to $V(S)$, hence there are no duplication nodes. This is obviously problematic when our aim is to disentangle speciations and duplications.

For *some* nodes of the gene tree we know directly from T that they logically must be duplication nodes:

(c) If $u \in V(T)$ and u', u'' are two distinct children of u with $\sigma(L(u')) \cap \sigma(L(u'')) \neq \emptyset$, then $t(u) = \square$.

Condition (c) states that for u to be a speciation node the gene sets of the children of u must be disjoint. It imposes a further restriction on μ by partially specifying the event labeling t.

For larger gene trees additional obstructions may appear. A recent study [15] shows that these can be characterized in terms of triplets in the following manner. We write $uv \mid w$ for the rooted tree on three leaves in which the path connecting u and v does not intersect the path from the root r of the triplet to w. Colloquially, this means that u and v are more closely related than uw and vw. Now let $uv \mid w$ be a gene triplet so that (i) $\sigma(u)$, $\sigma(v)$, and $\sigma(w)$ are pairwise disjoint, and (ii) the root r is a speciation, i.e. $t(r) = \bullet$, and denote by $\mathfrak{S}$ the set of all corresponding species triplets $\sigma(u)\sigma(v) \mid \sigma(w)$.

Theorem 1 ([15]). Let t be an event labeling on T. Then there is a reconciliation map $\mu: \mathrm{T} \to \mathrm{S}$ if and only if all triplets in $\mathfrak{S}$ are displayed by $\mathfrak{S}$.

A similar condition is derived in [23], using the converse of (c) to define speciation nodes consistent with a given species tree S.

2.4 Back to Orthology

We now can rephrase Fitch's notion of orthology in terms of an event-labeled gene tree.

Definition 1. Given a gene tree T and an event labeling $t: V(T) \to \{\bullet, \square, \odot, \circ\}$ we say that two genes $x, y \in L(T)$ are *orthologs*[1] if their last common ancestor in the gene tree was a speciation event, i.e., $\mathrm{lca}_T(x,y) = \bullet$. If their last common ancestor in T is a duplication event, $\mathrm{lca}_T(x,y) = \square$, and we say that x and y are *paralogs*.

It is trivial to check that any two distinct genes are either orthologs or paralogs in our setting, which, as we recall, explicitly excludes horizontal gene transfer, lineage sorting, and similar effects. A quite useful subclassification of paralogs distinguishes between *in-paralogs* and *out-paralogs* [25]. Consider two genes x, y in species A and a third gene z in a different species B. Then x and y are in-paralogs relative to z if $\mathrm{lca}(x,y) \prec \mathrm{lca}(x, z) = \mathrm{lca}(y, z)$, i.e., in-paralogs are genes that diverged by a duplication that occurred after a speciation event separating A and B. Conversely, out-paralogs diverged before the speciation of A and B, i.e., $\mathrm{lca}(x, z) \prec \mathrm{lca}(x, y) = \mathrm{lca}(y, z)$ or $\mathrm{lca}(y, z) \prec \mathrm{lca}(x, y) = \mathrm{lca}(x, z)$ (Fig. 4).

It is important to note that orthology explicitly depends on the reconciliation map. Of course, there is a particular reconciliation map μ^* that corresponds to the true evolutionary history. One has to keep in mind, however, that μ^*, just like the true gene tree G^* and the true species tree S^*, can only be approximated on any given dataset. A systematic investigation into the space of possible reconciliations can be found, e.g., in [26]. While earlier methods aimed

---

[1] Certain papers in the literature use the term *co-ortholog* instead of simply *ortholog*, to emphasize that this is not always a one-to-one relation. However, the literature also records the usage of *co-orthologs* in the sense of paralogs [24]. To avoid confusion, we use the simpler term.

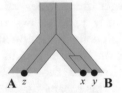 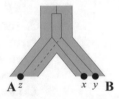

Fig. 4 Definition of in-paralogs and out-paralogs. On the left: *x* and *y* are in-paralogs w.r.t. *z* since the gene duplication temporally follows the speciation of *A* and *B*. On the right: *x* and *y* are out-paralogs w.r.t. *z* since the gene duplication temporally precedes the speciation of *A* and *B*

at finding a most parsimonious reconciliation [27, 28], there are nowadays also fully probabilistic models of reconciliation [29–31].

Irrespective of the exact choice of reconciliation map, however, we can derive general properties of orthology and paralogy. Surprisingly this aspect of the theory has been developed only very recently, although key ingredients have been available for quite some time with equivalence of "symmetric dating maps" and "symbolic ultrametrics" [32] (see also [33]):

Theorem 2. Let Θ be an irreflexive, symmetric, binary relation on X. Then there is a rooted tree T and an event labelling t on the interior vertices of T with $t(u) \neq t(v)$ for any two adjacent vertices u, v and $t(\mathrm{lca}(x,y)) = \Theta(x,y)$ for all x $\neq$ y if and only if there are no four pairwise disjoint genes {x, y, p, q} $\subseteq$ X such that

$$\Theta(x,y) = \Theta(y,p) = \Theta(p,q) \neq \Theta(y,q) = \Theta(x,q) = \Theta(x,p)$$

The latter condition means that the graph representation of Θ does not contain an induced path P_4 on four vertices. This condition characterizes an important and well-known class of graphs, the so-called co-graphs. Hence

Corollary 3 ([33]).: Both the orthology and the paralogy relation form a co-graph.

The importance of the latter statement lies in contrasting orthology relations with clustering. While all clusterings, i.e., partitions into complete graphs, are co-graphs, the converse is not true. The problem of correcting an orthology relation to a co-graph that is consistent with a gene tree is considered directly in [23, 34, 35].

2.5 Direct Orthology Estimation from Data

Orthology can be estimated from data in two fundamentally different ways: First, one may start from a gene-tree/species-tree pair (G, S), compute a reconciliation μ and a corresponding event labeling t, and finally convert this into an orthology relation. A plethora of algorithms and software tools have been developed for this indirect approach [36–40]. The alternative is to estimate Θ directly from data. There is also a large number of tools implementing this paradigm, some of which we will consider in Subheading 3.

For now, we are concerned only with the theoretical justification of the latter approach.

Our task is to find the orthologs in a species B for a query gene x taken from species $A = \sigma(x)$. For convenience we write, abusing the notation, $x \in A$ instead of $\sigma(x) = A$. If we knew the true divergence times $d_t(x, y)$ for any pair of genes, this would be easy: for any pair of genes $x \in A$ and $y \in B$ we know that their divergence time cannot be smaller than the divergence time $d_T(A, B)$ of the two species. In fact it equals the $d_T(A, B)$ if and only if x and y are orthologs; otherwise, x and y would have arisen before the divergence of A and B, thus coexisted in the ancestor $lca_S(A, B)$ and thus must have originated by a duplication. Orthology therefore is equivalent to $d_t(x, y) = d_T(A, B)$. In the absence of losses, furthermore, for every $x \in A$ there is an ortholog $y \in B$, whence $d_t(A, B) = \min_{z \in B} d(x, z)$ for all $x \in A$. The set of orthologs of $x \in A$ in species B is therefore

$$O(x, B) := \{y \in B | d_t(x, y) = \min_{z \in B} d_t(z, x)\} \qquad (3)$$

By definition, membership in the ortholog sets is reciprocal, i.e., for all $x \in A$ and $y \in B$, $y \in O(x, B)$ holds if and only if $x \in O(y, A)$. Of course, the divergence times are usually not known and can be measured only indirectly. Under the assumption of a molecular clock that runs with the same rate (possibly time- and lineage-dependent) for all members of a given gene family within a given lineage, the divergence time $d_t(x, y)$ can be replaced in Eq. 3 by any measure of $d_g(x, y)$ of genetic distance. This provides a justification for the reciprocal best hit (RBH) methods [41, 42].

For real-life data, however, neither assumption will be strictly satisfied. To accommodate variations in evolutionary rates within a gene family, a relaxed definition

$$O^\varepsilon(x, B) := \{y \in B | d_g(x, y) \leq (1 + \varepsilon) \min_{z \in B} d_g(z, x)\} \qquad (4)$$

has been proposed [43]. Candidate orthologs are then the pairs $\{x, y\}$ with $x \in A$, $y \in B$, $y \in O^\varepsilon(x, B)$ and/or $x \in O^\varepsilon(y, A)$.

As a consequence of gene losses, the true set of orthologs may be empty. The simplest (well-known) example of this type is shown in Fig. 5. Such cases lead to an overprediction of pairs in the orthology relation. Additional information can be used to filter orthology assignments. Among such techniques is the explicit recognition of one-to-one orthologs, the distinction of in- and out-paralogs, and the use of synteny as an additional criterion.

A good estimate for one-to-one orthologs is obtained by identifying pairs of genes that are unique reciprocal best matches, i.e., that satisfy for $x \in A$ and $y \in B$ the inequalities

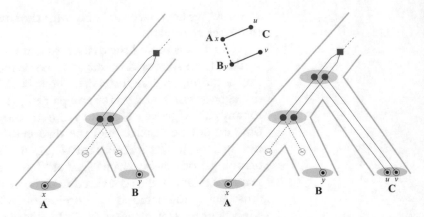

Fig. 5 Undetectable paralogy (left). A reciprocal best hit method erroneously classifies $x \in A$ and $y \in B$ as candidate orthologs since there is no direct evidence in a comparison of only species A and B for the duplication and loss events. Including a third species C in which both paralogs survived (on the right) leads to a non-co-graph, in this case a P_4, which can be edited to the co-graph $K_2 \,\dot{\cup}\, K_2$ by removing the spurious orthology edge between x and y

$$x \sim y \quad \Leftrightarrow \quad \begin{aligned} &d_e(x,y) < d_e(x,z) - \varepsilon \quad \forall\, z \in B \backslash \{y\} \; and \\ &d_e(x,y) < d_e(z,y) - \varepsilon \quad \forall\, z \in A \backslash \{x\} \end{aligned} \quad (5)$$

for $x \in A$ and $y \in B$.

A version of this estimate with ε derived from the variances of the evolutionary distances is used, for example, in OMA [44] as "stable pair." The definition of in- and out-paralogs immediately implies that z is orthologous to all in-paralogs w.r.t. z, but to at most one gene in any pair of out-paralogs (Fig. 4). Incorrect assignments of orthology in the situation of Fig. 5 can often be identified using a third genome C that has retained both paralogs as a "witness of non-orthology" [45]. In this case additive evolutionary distances support only the quadruple $xu \mid yv$, i.e., $d_e(x, u) + d_e(x, v) \ll d(x, v) + d(y, u)$, $d(x, y) + d(u, v)$, i.e., the initially inserted edge $x \sim y$ can be removed again.

The mathematical structure of the orthology relation also imposes rather strong constraints. It appears natural, therefore, to correct the candidate ortholog set to the edge set of a co-graph with the minimal number of edge-insertions and deletions. Although this so-called co-graph editing problem is NP-complete in general [46], it remains tractable if the input graph is not too far away from a co-graph. Furthermore, useful heuristics have been developed [47]. For comparison, one should keep in mind that most of the methods used in the indirect, phylogeny-based approach also need to tackle NP-hard problems, including the multiple sequence alignment problem and tree inference with parsimony or maximum likelihood as a cost function.

2.6 Orthology and Clustering

Orthologs are often summarized as *clusters of orthologous groups* (COGs) [41]. Since the orthology relation is not transitive in general, COGs only represent an approximation. Within the OMA framework, COGs are obtained from the graph G_{1-1} of estimated one-to-one orthologs, i.e., stable pairs, only. The one-to-one orthology relation is transitive by construction and comprises exactly the cliques of G_{1-1} [44]. The OMA-COGs [44] therefore are subsets of the true orthology relation. It is worth noting in this context that both clique-finding and the partitioning of a graph into vertex disjoint cliques that maximize the total number of included edges (the min-edge clique partition) are NP-hard problems in general. Both become very easy, however, when G is a co-graph [48], i.e., when the input graph is a mathematically correct orthology relation.

Other frameworks allow COGs to include many-to-many relations and thus include orthologs and paralogs within the same group [41]. Informally, the rules for building COGs (*see* Subheading 3.1.2) result in genes from different species being predominantly orthologs. COGs are then identified using a wide array of clustering techniques. As a consequence, the definition of such COGs necessarily depends on stringency parameters that gauge the tradeoff between size and stringency of COGs. From a theoretical point of view the transitivity clustering [49] is interesting because of its conceptual similarity to co-graph editing: here the initial orthology estimate is edited by insertion and deletion of edges to a transitive graph, i.e., a partitioning into COGs. In [50] instead of cliques, maximal Túran (complete multipartite) graphs, which form a special class of co-graphs, are computed to account for the fact that two genes residing in the same species are never orthologous.

2.7 Horizontal Gene Transfer and Retrogenes

More elaborate models of gene tree/species tree reconciliation explicitly account for horizontal gene transfer. Two genes that are related by a horizontal transfer event are called *xenologs*. Often the term xenolog is in addition restricted to pairs of homologs whose last common ancestor underwent a speciation event. Horizontal gene transfer introduces two additional technical complications: (1) Each node of the gene tree is mapped not to a single node of the gene tree but rather to a sequence of nodes and/or edges. The reason is that for a single horizontal transfer event both the donor and the acceptor position in the species tree must be specified. (2) An explicit timing function θ_S on (the nodes and edges of) the species tree needs to be defined. The donor and acceptor of a horizontal transfer event by definition are synchronous. In the species tree, however, donor and acceptor are by definition located in disjoint subtrees and thus incomparable. The horizontal transfer events therefore imply an additional restriction of the partial order on the species tree. For a concise formal presentation, we refer the

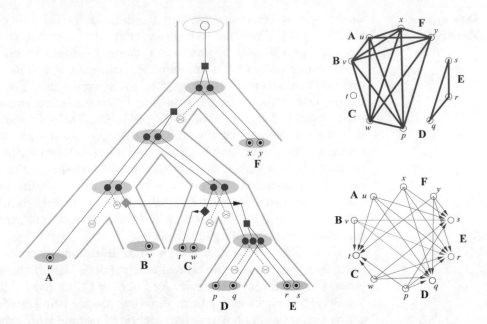

Fig. 6 A scenario with a horizontal transfer and a retroposition event. The definitions of the orthology (red) and paralogy (blue) relations are naturally restricted to subtrees of the gene tree without directed edges (upper right). Antisymmetric relations encapsulate useful information on the directionality of transfer events (lower right). These can either be ortholog-like (with the descendent genes winding up in two distinct genomes) or paralog-like (with both descendants in the same genome. In either case, the asymmetry arises from the fact that original and copy can be distinguished. Note that the gene $t \in \mathbf{C}$ is not connected to either of $q \in \mathbf{D}$, r, $s \in \mathbf{E}$ since all such paths contain directed edges in both directions

reader to [51]. Given a timing on the species tree, maximum parsimony versions of the reconciliation problem can still be solved in polynomial time by means of dynamic programming [52–54]. In the absence of timing information, however, the problem is NP-hard [55].

Horizontal gene transfer is intimately related to the concept of *xenology*. A formal definition of xenology is less well established and by no means consistent in the biological literature. First we note that horizontal transfer is intrinsically a directional event, i.e., there is a clear distinction of the donor and acceptor. As a consequence, an additional annotation is attached to the *edges* that connect the vertices in the gene tree that correspond to the horizontal transfer event (diamonds in Fig. 6) with their horizontally transferred offspring. Since the gene tree is rooted, this is equivalent to give the edge an explicit direction (Fig. 6). Similarly, the formation of a new paralog by retroposition (retrogenes) [56] is a directional process that can be viewed as a within-genome version of horizontal transfer. Mathematically, this idea connects to directed co-graphs and so-called uniformly non-prime 2-structures, *see* [57] for details. The most commonly used definition calls a pair of genes *xenologs* if the history since their common ancestor involves horizontal transfer of at least one of them [58, 59]. In our terminology, x and y are xenologs if and only if the unique path in T connecting x and y contains at least one directed edge.

The presence of horizontal transfer events also can be associated with a modified definition of orthology. In this setting the HGT event itself is usually treated as gene duplication event. Every homolog is then still either an ortholog or a paralog. Both orthologs and paralogs may have been xenologs at some point in their evolutionary histories [59]. Alternatively, the definition of orthologs and paralogs may be modified to accommodate HGT events as different event types. Hence x and y are orthologs (paralogs) if their last common ancestor is a speciation (duplication) node, *and* the path from x to y does not contain a directed edge in T. By construction this restricts both orthology and paralogy to the subtrees of T obtained by removing all directed edges. The union of orthology and paralogy relations then covers exactly the edges of the corresponding leaf (gene) sets; both the orthology and paralogy relations therefore retain the co-graph property. As a detailed mathematical characterization of xenology is still an open problem, it remains to be seen which of these alternatives turns out to be more fruitful.

2.8 Gene (Sub)-Families and Clustering	In the introduction we have colloquially introduced a gene family as collection of homologous genes. In practical applications we are usually interested in gene families w.r.t. a given set G of annotated genes in a given set S of species. First, we observe that G can be partitioned into maximal disjoint subsets G_i of homologs. For each family G_i, therefore, there is an evolutionary tree T_i whose leaf set is G_i.

A (proper) subfamily H of G_i is the leaf set of a subtree of T_i. The key property of subfamilies is that for a particular gene $x \in H$ and a given genome (species) $s \in S$, H will contain either all orthologs $y \in s$ of x, or no genes from s at all. The subfamilies of G therefore form a hierarchy.

We say that a subfamily H is *complete* if for every $x \in H$ and every species $s \in S$ that has a gene in H, there is an ortholog $y \in s$ of x contained in H. A complete subfamily therefore corresponds to a subtree of T_i that is rooted in a speciation event. As a consequence, there is a coarsest partition of G_i into complete subfamilies whose elements are exactly the (leaf sets of) the maximal subtrees whose roots are speciation events. These maximal complete subfamilies correspond exactly to paralog groups whose origin predates the last common ancestor of the species set S. Alternatively, the maximal complete subfamilies are exactly the connected components of the orthology relation.

Continuing the discussion of Subheading 2.5 one can define a *similarity graph* Γ whose vertices are the genes. Edges are inserted between any two genes if they exhibit a "significant" level of sequence similarity. The edges of Γ are typically labelled by a similarity value $s(x, y)$ between genes. We will briefly return to the details of measuring similarity and its significance in the following section. Since similarity and the genetic distance d_t in Subheading 2.5 are interconvertible, one can extract the candidate orthologs set and related constructs directly from Γ.

The problem of determining "interesting" subfamilies of G therefore corresponds to finding clusters in the similarity graph Γ. Unless our data are extremely noisy and we make way too many false homology statements, a simple vertex clustering algorithm should therefore be able to identify the maximal sets of homologs G_i as well as the maximal complete subfamilies.

3   Practice

In this section we will cover the topic of computation of protein families from a practical point of view. There are basically two ways this can be done: (a) build your own protein families from scratch; (b) use existing protein-family resources.

There are two general methods for computing gene families from scratch [60]: (1) determine similarity relationships among the genes being considered, and then try to separate orthologs from paralogs by mapping these relationships onto gene and species trees (which is the method outlined theoretically in Subheading 2.4); and (2) obtain vertex clusters from the similarity graph Γ (*see* Subheading 2.8). Because implementations of this second approach are much faster in practice than those based on the first method, in this part we will present details for this method only. Readers interested in the first method can look up references provided in the bibliography [36–40].

3.1 Gene Families and Clustering

The starting point for clustering-based orthology tools for large data sets is the similarity graph Γ. In order to build it the first step is an all-against-all similarity computation carried out for all genes in the input set. The result is processed to create Γ, whose vertices are the genes in the input. An edge is created between two vertices u and v if and only if the similarity between the corresponding gene sequences satisfies some pre-defined, usually empirically derived, constraints. Typically, empirically derived thresholds for the minimum score, maximum e-value, and/or minimum length of the alignment relative to the length of the two input sequences are invoked. Once the graph is created a vertex clustering algorithm is employed to extract clusters from Γ. We refer the reader to reference [61] for additional details. The available software tools differ mostly in their clustering strategies. In the following we outline the most important examples.

When using any of the tools described below, it is important to keep in mind the possible errors that may be present in the results. The most important ones are false negatives and false positives. In this context, a false negative is a gene that should have been assigned to family X but was not; and a false positive is a gene that was wrongly considered as belonging to family X. In principle, different tools could be evaluated in terms of these errors against a "gold standard benchmark"; unfortunately, no general (valid for both eukaryotes and prokaryotes) benchmark exists. For eukaryotes one such benchmark has been developed [62], consisting of 70 manually curated families. The reader is referred to that publication for a more extensive discussion of the pitfalls and challenges of ortholog computation. An ongoing project to offer an orthology set benchmark to the community can be found at http://orthology. benchmarkservice.org, and its associated publication [63]; other relevant publications are [7, 64].

In discussing methods for computing gene families de novo it is important to note that the all-against-all sequence comparison step may be a computational bottleneck in the whole process, depending on the number of genomes being compared. For example, for bacterial genomes containing about 4000 genes, computing gene families for 100 or more genomes would already require powerful computers, parallel computation, or both. Note that in addition to the computation itself, the storage and the downstream analysis of the matrix of similarity scores are also quite demanding in terms of computational resources.

3.1.1 OrthoMCL

OrthoMCL [65] is among the most popular programs for determining gene families from scratch. The all-against-all step is done by BLAST [66]. Clustering of the similarity graph uses the Markov Cluster (MCL) algorithm [67, 68]. It simulates random walks within the graph by alternating expansion (forming a power w.r.t. normal matrix multiplication) and inflation (forming a component-wise power and subsequent rescaling). This increases within-cluster and decreases between-cluster weights and thus converges to clusters in an unsupervised manner.

OrthoMCL seeks to distinguish in-paralogs from out-paralogs using a simple rule. Two genes from the same species will be included in the same orthologous group only if their reciprocal BLAST similarity is larger than the similarity to any gene not belonging to that species. Those genes are considered "recent paralogs."

OrthoMCL is not a simple program to run; one way to deal with this difficulty is to run it through the convenient Get_Homologues package [69].

3.1.2 The COG Algorithm

An important resource for pre-computed gene families is the Clusters of Orthologous Groups (COGs) resource [41, 70], to be covered in more detail below (Subheading 3.2.1). Here we sketch the COGtriangles algorithm it uses to determine ortholog relationships [41].

COG uses the reciprocal best match strategy to construct the similarity graph. Two vertices are connected by an edge whenever the corresponding sequences have each other as best hits in a BLAST search. This makes it possible to dispense with e-value or alignment coverage requirements. The clustering strategy proceeds in a greedy manner from triangles. A triangle is a set of three vertices, each belonging to a different species, all connected to each other. Families are seeded by triangles; additional members of the family are determined by merging triangles if they share an edge. This merging process continues (merging triangles or previously merged triangles) until no more mergings can be done. The resulting subgraph constitutes a COG. The algorithm has a pre-processing step in which all in-paralogs are determined and converted to single vertices.

The COGtriangles algorithm was improved in terms of computational complexity by the EdgeSearch algorithm [60]. EdgeSearch is also one of the options of the Get_Homologues package [69]. It is worth noting that the COG building algorithms allow a gene to belong to more than one COG, whereas OrthoMCL generates a strict partition of the input genes. The reason for this difference can be explained as follows. COGs are intended primarily as a gene annotation tool and therefore are associated with functional descriptions. Some genes may have more than one function, and therefore should be annotated with more than one COG. OrthoMCL, on the other hand, is a gene family computation method. Assignment of functions to families is seen as a separate task, independent of OrthoMCL, to be carried out by other tools. A gene g with more than one function would be grouped by OrthoMCL in just one family, along with other sufficiently similar genes that (presumably) also have the same multiple functions as g.

3.1.3 ProteinOrtho and POFF

ProteinOrtho [43] was designed with large data sets in mind. Its similarity search step also uses BLAST [66]. To overcome the problem that reciprocal best matches underpredict orthologs, it uses a set of nearly optimal matches as introduced in Subheading 2.5 and inserts an edge between $v \in A$ and $u \in B$ into the similarity graph Γ if both $v \in O^\varepsilon(u, B)$ and $u \in O^\varepsilon(v, A)$. Since the resulting similarity graph is very sparse, the stringency of determining the sets of almost best hits can be varied by the user. In an extension called POFF [71] the edge set of Γ is then filtered by synteny information. For this purpose, it makes use of the heuristic FFAdj-MCS [72], which assesses gene order similarity with a measure related to the breakpoint distance.

`ProteinOrtho` and `POFF` use spectral clustering. The so-called Fiedler vector, i.e., the second eigenvalue of the Laplacian matrix of Γ, is used to determine a bipartition of the vertex set. Together with removal of tree-like appendages from Γ, the spectral partitioning step is used recursively to subdivide the gene set G into families.

A practical advantage of `ProteinOrtho` and `POFF` is that much care has been taken to make the tool memory-efficient and allow easy parallelization of the similarity computation. Such careful coding avoids the memoization of a complete pairwise scoring matrix and constructs an approximate orthology graph stepwise from pairwise genome or proteome comparisons. At comparable accuracies it runs more than an order of magnitude faster than other tools and can be run on modern desktop computers for data sets comprising several thousand prokaryote genomes. Recent versions of `POFF` can export the similarity graph to make it available for third-party analysis methods. This facility was used in [73], for instance, to obtain a pairwise orthology relation via co-graph editing instead of a clustering result.

3.2 Gene Family Resources

In this section we briefly describe a few resources that offer pre-computed gene families. Given the book's topic, we want to examine these resources from a comparative genomics perspective. However, we must note that the intention of most or all of these resources is not primarily to facilitate genomic comparison. Generally speaking, these resources seek to determine what are the gene families that exist in nature, and what are the molecular functions associated with each one. This means that one primary objective of these resources is to facilitate *genome annotation*, that is: to help determine the functions coded by genes present on any given genome using a computational method (as opposed to an experimental approach). This is done basically as follows: given a protein family resource (the *database*), a protein sequence (the *query*), and a method or program that can search the database with the query, use that program to determine to which family the query belongs. Once this is achieved, the query is annotated with the function associated with the family found by the program. An excellent reference for protein family resources in general and a few in-depth descriptions of specific protein families is the book by Orengo and Bateman [74].

How can pre-computed families help in genomic comparisons? The general principle is as follows. First, it is necessary that the genes in the genomes to be compared have been annotated with the pre-computed families that exist in the chosen resource. Once this is done, the following questions can be easily answered:

1. For a given family, which genomes have genes that have been assigned to that family? The answer to this question allows the

definition of the *shared gene* concept. In this context, the word *gene* is overloaded with two meanings. The first, and concrete, meaning is the individual gene present in a specific genome. The second, and abstract, meaning is the family to which it belongs. We say that a certain gene (second meaning) is *shared* between two genomes A and B if both A and B have genes (first meaning) belonging to the same family. Let us give a concrete example. Consider the family (or the gene [second meaning]) *dnaA*, which is described as the gene for a chromosomal replication initiator protein in bacteria. In the genome of *Escherichia coli* strain K-12 substrain MG1655 it can be found in locus tag b3702, given by the GenBank accession number NP_418157. But a gene (first meaning) belonging to the same family (which in this example happens to be COG0593; more on this further on) can also be found in the *Bacillus subtilis* subsp. *subtilis* strain 168 genome, in locus tag BSU00010, given by accession number NP_387882. Therefore, we can say the genomes of these strains of *E. coli* and *B. subtilis* share the *dnaA* gene.

2. How do genomes compare in terms of shared genes? This can be done by simply counting protein families in which the genomes being compared have representatives (the answer to the previous question, for all families). The shared genes are typically represented using Venn diagrams (when the number of genomes being compared is small) or tables (when large). A Venn diagram will also have regions corresponding to *specific* or *unique* genes: these are the genes that are present in one genome but are not shared by any other genome in the set. The term *pangenome* refers to the union of all genes found across different strains. The intersection of the strains' gene sets is usually referred to as the *core genome*.

3. Assuming families can be grouped by category (and some gene-family resources already provide this categorization, as will be seen), then for a given category, how many genes in that category each genome has? The results are typically visualized as pie charts.

4. How do genomes compare in terms of these categories?

For a gene family resource to be really useful in genome comparisons, its **coverage** of the universe of possible protein products is an important consideration. Coverage in this context simply means the number of different families in the resource. Another important consideration is the **quality** of the gene family resource. Quality here means two things: first, that the molecular function (and other attributes) associated with that family is correct and as precise as possible; and second, that the genes listed as belonging to that family are indeed true members of that family. Quality generally depends on the amount of manual curation that has been invested on the resource. Generally speaking, there exists a trade-off between coverage and manual curation. Resources that are well curated tend to have low coverage; and resources that have high coverage tend to have little or no manual curation.

The coverage issue is crucial in whole-genome comparisons. In particular, a genome comparison approach based on pre-computed families will fail to classify genes that do not belong to any family included in the resource. Because new genomes almost always have genes that belong to families that have not yet been characterized on any resource (even simply as conserved hypothetical genes), this approach is not recommended for whole-genome comparisons that need a thorough clustering of gene sequences; the methods presented in Subheading 3.1 should be used instead.

Because pre-computed gene families generally seek to associate function with each family, it should be the case that any gene family with an associated function must have at least one member for which the gene family function has been demonstrated experimentally. Ideally, this member should be annotated as the *seed* for that family, so that users can easily determine which one it is, and easily track down the associated publication. The best source of potential seeds for gene families is provided by the Swiss-Prot database [75]. All entries in this database have been curated, and for each entry the database contains links to papers in the literature that report on the function of that protein. When running BLAST within the Uniprotkb website, the reported hits that are part of Swiss-Prot (if there are any) are clearly marked.

Finally, one must take into account the reliability of the association that can be obtained between a pre-computed gene family and a new gene sequence. This is also known as the *orthology detection problem* [11]. This will depend on the association (or assignment) method to be used. Sometimes, this method is ad-hoc, such as a BLAST comparison with some user-defined e-value threshold. Preferably, each gene-family resource should provide its own association method, with well-defined guidelines and parameter values for creating these associations.

3.2.1 The COG Resource

The COG resource is a collection of annotated prokaryotic protein families, known as Clusters of Orthologous Groups, or COGs. We have already covered the clustering algorithm underlying the COG resource (Subheading 3.1.2); please refer to that section for the algorithmic definition of a COG. The COG resource was first introduced in 2003 [41]; an update was made available in 2015 [70].

The COG resource is intended as a tool for prokaryote protein product annotation. In its most recent release, it is based on COGs created from 711 genomes, of which 83 are archaea and 628 are bacteria.

In the COG resource most protein families (or COGs) are associated with a protein function, manually assigned and curated by COG resource curators. Some COGs do not have defined functions; they simply represent families of conserved coding sequences for which the function is unknown.

COGs are organized in a two-level hierarchy. At the base of the hierarchy there are the individual COGs. At the next level there are functional categories, of which there are a total of 26 (example: category A, *RNA processing and modification*). At the top level categories are grouped into four high-level functional descriptions: information storage and processing (includes five categories), cellular processes and signaling (10), metabolism (8), and poorly characterized (2). The two categories in the last group are: category R, "general function prediction only," and category S, "function unknown." Examples of COGs in category R are: COG0110 *Acetyltransferase (isoleucine patch superfamily)*; and COG0388 *Predicted amidohydrolase*. One perhaps confusing feature of COGs is that a COG can belong to category R as well as to another category. For example, COG0477, *MFS family permease*, belongs to categories G, E, and P, in addition to R. A typical description of a COG in category S is: *Uncharacterized membrane protein YbhN, UPF0104 family* (COG0392). A new category was introduced in 2014: X, for phage-derived proteins, transposons, and other mobilome components. The authors warn [70] that this category also includes poorly or uncharacterized COGs.

In the most recent release there are 4631 COGs. Given that each COG has been manually curated, this number is reasonably high, but it still falls far short of the diversity of prokaryotic protein families that exist in nature. Evidence for this is that most bacterial genomes available from the RefSeq resource at NCBI [76] have between 20% and 30% of protein-coding genes for which no existing COG can be assigned. A typical example is the bacterium *Xanthomonas citri* str. 306. Its RefSeq annotation has 4312 protein-coding genes. Of those, only 3379 have a COG annotation (78%). Nevertheless, COGs are an excellent resource for comparative genomics of prokaryotes; and one hopes the resource will continue to be updated on a regular basis in the coming years, thereby providing increasingly better coverage.

An important extension or offshoot of the COG resource is eggNOG [77]. As of 2016 it is in version 4.5, and includes more than 190,000 orthologous groups (OGs), covering nearly 3700 organisms, including both prokaryotes and eukaryotes. Thus, a simple comparison of numbers (4361 versus more than 190,000) shows that eggNOG has far greater coverage than the COG resource. However, the OGs are all automatically generated, as are the functions and other data associated with each group.

The OGs in eggNOG can be used to annotate genes by way of predefined Hidden Markov Models, or HMMs, made available for download in the resource. We provide more details on HMM-based protein family resources in Subheading 3.2.5. eggNOG provides much more information than just a set of OGs, and is overall an excellent resource for comparative genomics.

3.2.2   KEGG Orthologs

The Kyoto Encyclopedia of Genes and Genomes (KEGG) [78] offers an ortholog resource similar to COGs, which is called KEGG Orthologs, or KOs. With each KO a number is associated, the *K number*, and a function description. One major difference between KOs and COGs is that KOs are used as the central hub for the KEGG general resource, which includes many other resources besides ortholog families. For example, KEGG includes an extensive collection of metabolic pathways, and the enzymes that play roles in each pathway all have *K* numbers. KOs are manually curated, and include references to the literature reporting experimental functional characterization of at least one member in the family. The number of KOs is more than 19,000 [78]. That would be a coverage substantially higher than COGs, but KOs also include eukaryotes.

The KEGG resource provides three methods for assigning gene sequences to KOs: these are called KOALA (for internal annotation, using a Smith-Waterman implementation), BlastKOALA (for genome annotation by KEGG users), andGhostKOALA (for metagenome annotation by KEGG users). Details about these methods have been published [79–81].

3.2.3   OrthoMCL Database

For eukaryotes, a good source of pre-computed ortholog groups is the orthoMCL database, which is based on the orthoMCL program [65] (*see* Subheading 3.1.1). The website http://www. orthomcl.org offers pre-computed orthologous groups for 150 species (version 5), of which most (99) are eukaryotes; the remaining are archaea (15) and bacteria (36).

The orthoMCL database is different from COGs and KOs in the sense that they do not provide manually curated functions for each family. They are simply pre-computed clusters of genes. Each group is annotated automatically with EC numbers and/or PFAM domains; no manual functional curation is done.

3.2.4   OrthoDB

The OrthoDB resource [24] is a rich resource with excellent coverage (version 9.1 as of January 2017) of both prokaryotes (3663 bacterial genomes) and eukaryotes (588 genomes). Similarly to COG and KO, it provides functional annotations for its orthologous families, derived from automated procedures. A distinctive feature of OrthoDB is that it also provides evolutionary information for orthologous groups, such as rate of sequence divergence.

The number of orthologous groups in the resource seems tricky to determine. The file with orthologous group IDs that can be downloaded from the site has 4,277,560 entries. This would be a far larger dataset than any other currently existing resource. This huge number likely reflects some amount of redundancy and/or orthologous groups existing at different phylogenetic levels (i.e., the authors have also counted orthologs that are inferred to exist at internal nodes of reconstructed phylogenetic trees); it certainly reflects lack of human curation.

3.2.5 Protein Families Based on Hidden Markov Models

In order to create orthologous groups, the resources described so far (except for eggNOG) rely on direct similarity between coding sequences. Another way to create a set of orthologous families is to use a technique called Hidden Markov Models, or HMMs.

A detailed description of the theory behind HMMs and their implementation is beyond the scope of this chapter. Briefly, an HMM is a way of encapsulating a multiple sequence alignment, encoding in the model the pattern of conservation in conserved sections of the alignment and the variations in spacing between conserved sections. When properly done, it is a much more sensitive way of determining whether a given gene sequence belongs or not to a family for which an HMM model already exists. A more detailed description of HMMs can be found in the short primer by Eddy [82].

Another attractive feature of HMMs is that there exists an excellent software package with various programs for HMM computation. The package is called HMMER [83]. In that package one finds program `phmmer`, which allows the search of an HMM database using a protein sequence as query. This would be the method that one would employ to determine to which family a given protein sequence possibly belongs, if the HMM database is a database of gene families.

Among protein family resources that are based on HMMs, we mention three (in addition to eggNOG, described in Subheading 3.2.1): PFAM, TIGRFAMs, and Panther. We also mention here a nonHMM but related resource called HAMAP. We briefly describe each of these in turn.

PFAM [84] is a database of protein families, each represented by a multiple sequence alignment and an HMM. The criterion for creating a family is the presence of shared protein domains. Because a given protein may contain several domains, that protein may belong to several different PFAM families. In this chapter our concern is with full-length proteins, rather than families based on single domains, as is the case with PFAM. In this sense, PFAM is a resource that is more relevant for protein domain studies and protein annotation, but not as much in comparative genomics.

TIGRFams [85] is a resource that presents HMMs that do consider the full length of proteins. It is a resource that covers primarily prokaryotes. Each family has been manually curated, and mainly for this reason the coverage is somewhat limited. As of TIGRFams release 15, there are 4488 models. TIGRFams have two features that are worth pointing out. One is that each family includes manually determined cutoff scores for determining family membership. The other is a classification of models in terms of the adequacy of the model for genome annotation. The most adequate models are termed *equivalogs*, meaning that such families can be readily used for annotation. Models that are not equivalogs represent more complex families, and their use in automated annotation might generate incorrect annotations. Out of the current 4488 models, 2366 are equivalogs.

Panther families [86–89] and their classifications "are the result of human curation as well as sophisticated bioinformatics algorithms" (quoted from the Panther website). Currently (version 10.0) the resource offers 11,928 families and 83,190 subfamilies. Both eukaryotes and prokaryotes are included (104 genomes are represented, a third of which are prokaryotes). Each family and subfamily is represented by its own HMM. HMMs are annotated with terms from the Gene Ontology [90]. In order to speed up the comparison between a query protein sequence and the HMM library, the resource offers a script that selects which HMMs to compare to based on BLAST scores against HMM consensus sequences. Query function assignment is left to the user, under the following guidelines based on e-value range: any hit with an e-value equal to or better than 10^{-23} is considered "closely related"; e-values between 10^{-23} and 10^{-11} are deemed "related"; and between 10^{-11} and 10^{-3} as "distantly related."

HAMAP [91] is another manually curated protein family resource, covering primarily prokaryote families. Instead of HMMs, HAMAP offers its own specific multiple-sequence-alignment-derived profiles. Each family has a "seed member" manually chosen based on literature curation. Among the resources covered here HAMAP is perhaps the best curated and the one that offers the most careful method for determining whether a new sequence belongs or not to a family, and thereby whether it can properly inherit its properties. These "annotation rules" take into account, for example, the valid taxonomic scope for that family and the presence or absence of key protein residues necessary for annotation propagation. Probably because of the carefulness with which the resource is built its coverage is relatively small: currently the resource contains only 2071 families.

4 Perspectives

Orthology computation is an interesting theoretical problem and an extremely important practical problem in comparative genomics. To our knowledge this chapter is the first text that attempts to provide a linked overview of these two important facets of the problem.

One issue of concern from both theoretical and practical standpoints is the continued superexponential increase in the amount of genomic data. Most of the algorithms and programs for orthology computation do not scale well; the never ending and rapid increase in data also makes many ortholog resources difficult to maintain.

One clearly needed improvement in currently existing resources and software is in the quality of the results, that is, accuracy and completeness of resulting gene families. The scalability pressure seems to be taking its toll, and quality is now more of a problem than it already was a few years ago, in particular for large gene families (for example, G-protein-coupled receptors and kinases). Based on our survey, this seems to be much more of an issue for large eukaryotic genomes than for prokaryotes. We can expect that improvements will be obtained by basing orthology assignments not only on sequence similarity and even on phylogenetic placement, but also on information such as synteny and exon/intron structure.

A wide open issue that cannot be addressed with current techniques is orthology of repetitive elements, including multi-copy genes such as tRNAs and rRNAs, as well as some other gene families that have high levels of concerted evolution. In such cases gene trees as well as pairwise best hit strategies yield no information at all.

Acknowledgements

This work was funded in part by the *Deutsche Forschungsgemeinschaft* (Proj. No. MI439/14-1) (to PFS) and a CNPq fellowship (to JCS).

References

1. Fitch WM (1970) Distinguishing homologous from analogous proteins. Syst Zool 19:99–113

2. Petsko GA (2001) Homologuephobia. Genome Biol 2:comment1002

3. Koonin EV (2001) An apology for orthologs – or brave new memes. Genome Biol 2:comment1005

4. Gerlt JA, Babbitt PC (2000) Can sequence determine function? Genome Biol 1:R5

5. Koonin E (2005) Orthologs, paralogs, and evolutionary genomics. Ann Rev Genet 39:309–338

6. Innan H, Kondrashov F (2010) The evolution of gene duplications: classifying and

distinguishing between models. Nat Rev Genet 11:97–108

7. Altenhoff AM, Studer RA, Robinson-Rechavi M, Dessimoz C (2012) Resolving the ortholog conjecture: orthologs tend to be weakly, but significantly, more similar in function than paralogs. PLoS Comput Biol 8:e1002514

8. Studer RA, Robinson-Rechavi M (2009) How confident can we be that orthologs are similar, but paralogs differ? Trends Genet 25:210–216

9. Nehrt NL, Clark WT, Radivojac P, Hahn MW (2011) Testing the ortholog conjecture with comparative functional genomic data from mammals. PLoS Comput Biol 7:e1002073

10. Gabaldon T, Koonin EV (2013) Functional and evolutionary implications of gene orthology. Nat Rev Genet 14:360–366

11. Sonnhammer EL, Gabaldón T, Sousa da Silva AW, Martin M, Robinson-Rechavi M, Boeckmann B, Thomas P, Dessimoz C, and the Quest for Orthologs consortium (2014) Big data and other challenges in the quest for orthologs. Bioinformatics 30(21):2993–2998

12. Maddison WP (1997) Gene trees in species trees. Syst Biol 46:523–536

13. Vernot B, Stolzer M, Goldman A, Durand D (2008) Reconciliation with non-binary species trees. J Comput Biol 15:981–1006

14. Zhang L (1997) On a Mirkin-Muchnik-Smith conjecture for comparing molecular phylogenies. J Comput Biol 4:177–187

15. Hernandez-Rosales M, Hellmuth M, Wieseke N, Huber KT, Moulton V, Stadler PF (2012) From event-labeled gene trees to species trees. BMC Bioinf 13(Suppl. 19):S6

16. Doyon J-P, Chauve C, Hamel S (2008) Algorithms for exploring the space of gene tree/species tree reconciliations. In: Nelson CE, Vialette S (eds) Comparative genomics; international workshop, RECOMB-CG 2008. Lecture notes in computer science, vol 5267. Springer, New York, pp 1–13

17. Doyon J-P, Ranwez V, Daubin V, Berry V (2011) Models, algorithms and programs for phylogeny reconciliation. Brief Bioinform 12:392–400

18. Page R (1994) Maps between trees and cladistic analysis of historical associations among genes. Syst Biol 43:58–77

19. Bonizzoni P, Della Vedova G, Dondi R (2005) Reconciling a gene tree to a species tree under the duplication cost model. Theor Comput Sci 347:36–53

20. Górecki P, Tiuryn J (2006) DLS-trees: a model of evolutionary scenarios. Theor Comput Sci 359:378–399

21. Guigó R, Muchnik I, Smith TF (1996) Reconstruction of ancient molecular phylogeny. Mol Phylogenet Evol 6:189–213

22. Page RDM, Charleston MA (1997) From gene to organismal phylogeny: reconciled trees and the gene tree/species tree problem. Mol Phylogenet Evol 7:231–240

23. Lafond M, Semeria M, Swenson KM, Tannier E, El-Mabrouk N (2013) Gene tree correction guided by orthology. BMC Bioinf 14(S15):S5

24. Kriventseva EV, Tegenfeldt F, Petty TJ, Waterhouse RM, Sim ao FA, Pozdnyakov IA, Zdobnov EM (2015) Orthodb v8: update of the hierarchical catalog of orthologs and the underlying free software. Nucleic Acids Res 43:D250–D256, Database issue

25. Sonnhammer ELL, Koonin EV (2002) Orthology, paralogy and proposed classification for paralog subtypes. Trends Genet 18:619–620

26. Doyon JP, Chauve C, Hamel S (2009) Space of gene/species trees reconciliations and parsimonious models. J Comput Biol 16:1399–1418

27. Page RDM (2000) Extracting species trees from complex gene trees: reconciled trees and vertebrate phylogeny. Mol Phylogenet Evol 14:89–106

28. Ma B, Li M, Zhang L (2000) From gene trees to species trees. SIAM J Comput 30:729–752

29. Arvestad L, Berglund AC, Lagergren J, Sennblad B (2003) Bayesian gene/species tree reconciliation and orthology analysis using MCMC. Bioinformatics 19:i7–i15

30. Arvestad L, Lagergren L, Sennblad B (2009) The gene evolution model and computing its associated probabilities. J ACM 56:1–44

31. Górecki P, Burleigh GJ, Eulenstein O (2011) Maximum likelihood models and algorithms for gene tree evolution with duplications and losses. BMC Bioinf 12:S15

32. Böcker S, Dress AWM (1998) Recovering symbolically dated, rooted trees from symbolic ultrametrics. Adv Math 138:105–125

33. Hellmuth M, Hernandez-Rosales M, Huber KT, Moulton V, Stadler PF, Wieseke N (2013) Orthology relations, symbolic ultrametrics, and cographs. J Math Biol 66:399–420

34. Lafond M, El-Mabrouk N (2014) Orthology and paralogy constraints: satisfiability and consistency. BMC Genomics 15(S6):S12

35. Lafond M, Dondi R, El-Mabrouk N (2016) The link between orthology relations and gene trees: a correction perspective. Algorithms Mol Biol 11:4

36. Krishnamurthy N, Brown D, Kirshner D, Sjö-lander K (2006) Phylofacts: an online structural phylogenomic encyclopedia for protein functional and structural classification. Genome Biol 7:R83

37. Sjölander K, Datta R, Shen Y, Shoffner G (2011) Ortholog identification in the presence of domain architecture rearrangement. Brief Bioinform 12(5):413–422

38. Pryszcz LP, Huerta-Cepas J, Gabaldon T (2011) MetaPhOrs: orthology and paralogy predictions from multiple phylogenetic evidence using a consistency-based confidence score. Nucleic Acids Res 17(39):e32

39. Afrasiabi C, Samad B, Dineen D, Meacham C, Sjölander C (2013) Phylofacts fat-cat webserver: ortholog identification and function prediction using fast approximate tree classification. Nucleic Acids Res 41(W1): W242–W248

40. Huerta-Cepas J, Capella-Gutierrez S, Pryszcz LP, Marcet-Houben M, Gabaldon T (2014) PhylomeDB v4: zooming into the plurality of evolutionary histories of a genome. Nucleic Acids Res 18(42):897–902

41. Tatusov RL, Koonin EV, Lipman DJ (1997) A genomic perspective on protein families. Science 278:631–637

42. Wolf YI, Koonin EV (2012) A tight link between orthologs and bidirectional best hits in bacterial and archaeal genomes. Genome Biol Evol 4:1286–1294

43. Lechner M, Findeiß S, Steiner L, Marz M, Stadler PF, Prohaska SJ (2011) Proteinortho: detection of (co-)orthologs in large-scale analysis. BMC Bioinf 12:124

44. Roth ACJ, Gonnet GH, Dessimoz C (2008) Algorithm of OMA for large-scale orthology inference. BMC Bioinf 9:518

45. Dessimoz C, Boeckmann B, Roth ACJ, Gonnet GH (2006) Detecting non-orthology in the COGs database and other approaches grouping orthologs using genome-specific best hits. Nucleic Acids Res 34:3309–3316

46. Liu Y, Wang J, Guo J, Chen J (2012) Complexity and parameterized algorithms for cograph editing. Theor Comput Sci 461:45–54

47. Hellmuth M, Fritz A, Wieseke N, Stadler PF (2015) Techniques for the cograph editing problem: module merge is equivalent to edit P_4's (submitted). arXiv 1509.06983v2

48. Gao Y, Hare DR, Nastos J (2013) The cluster deletion problem for cographs. Discret Math 313:2763–2771

49. Rahmann S, Wittkop T, Baumbach J, Martin M, Truß A, Böcker S (2007) Exact and heuristic algorithms for weighted cluster editing. In: Proceedings of the 6th LSS conference on computational systems bioinformatics (CSB2007). Life Sciences Society, pp 391–401

50. Falls C, Powell B, Snœyink J (2008) Computing high-stringency COGs using Turán-type graphs. Technical Report, University of North Carolina

51. Nguyen TH, Ranwez V, Pointet S, Chifolleau AMA, Doyon J-P, Berry V (2013) Reconciliation and local gene tree rearrangement can be of mutual profit. Algorithms Mol Biol 8:12

52. Doyon J-P, Scornavacca C, Gorbunov KY, Szöllősi G, Ranwez V, Berry V (2010) An efficient algorithm for gene/species trees parsimonious reconciliation with losses, duplications and transfers. In: Tannier E (ed) Comparative genomics. Lecture notes in computer science, vol 6398. Springer, Heidelberg, pp 93–108

53. Wieseke N, Bernt M, Middendorf M (2013) Unifying parsimonious tree reconciliation. In: Darling A, Stoye J (eds) Algorithms in bioinformatics WABI 2013. Lecture notes in computer science, vol 8126. Springer, Heidelberg, pp 200–214

54. Donati B, Baudet C, Sinaimeri B, Crescenzi B, Sagot M-F (2015) EUCALYPT: efficient tree reconciliation enumerator. Algorithms Mol Biol 10:3

55. Hallett MT, Lagergren J (2001) Efficient algorithms for lateral gene transfer problems. In Lengauer T (ed) Proceedings of the fifth annual international conference on computational biology (RECOMB). ACM, New York, pp 149–156

56. Fablet M, Bueno M, Potrzebowski L, Kaessmann H (2009) Evolutionary origin and functions of retrogene introns. Mol Biol Evol 26:2147–2156

57. Hellmuth M, Stadler PF, Wieseke N (2017) The mathematics of xenology: di-cographs, symbolic ultrametrics, 2-structures and tree-representable systems of binary relations. J Math Biol 75:199–237

58. Fitch WM (2000) Homology a personal view on some of the problems. Trends Genet 16:227–231

59. Jensen RA (2001) Orthologs and paralogs – we need to get it right. Genome Biol 2:8

60. Kristensen DM, Kannan L, Coleman MK, Wolf YI, Sorokin A, Koonin EV, Mushegian A (2010) A low-polynomial algorithm for assembling clusters of orthologous groups from intergenomic symmetric best matches. Bioinformatics 26:1481–1487

61. Holm L, Heger A (2014) Automated sequence-based approaches for identifying

domain families. In: Orengo CA, Bateman A (eds) Protein Families: relating protein sequence, structure, and function. Wiley series in peptide and protein science. Wiley, New York, pp 3–24

62. Trachana K, Larsson TA, Powell S, Chen W-H, Doerks T, Muller T, Bork P (2011) Orthology prediction methods: a quality assessment using curated protein families. Bioessays 33 (10):769–780

63. Altenhoff AM, Boeckmann B, Capella-Gutierrez S, Dalquen DA, DeLuca T, Forslund K, Huerta-Cepas J, Linard B, Pereira C, Pryszcz LP, Schreiber F, da Silva F, Szklarczyk D, Train CM, Bork P, Lecompte O, von Mering C, Xenarios I, Sjölander K, Jensen LJ, Martin MJ, Muffato M, Gabaldón T, Lewis SE, Thomas PD, Sonnhammer E, Dessimoz C (2016) Standardized benchmarking in the quest for orthologs. Nat Methods 13 (5):425–430

64. Trachana K, Forslund K, Larsson T, Powell S, Doerks T, Mering C, Bork P (2014) A phylogeny-based benchmarking test for orthology inference reveals the limitations of function-based validation. PLoS One 9: e111122

65. Li L, Stoeckert CJ Jr, Roos DS (2003) OrthoMCL: identification of ortholog groups for eukaryotic genomes. Genome Res 13:2178–2189

66. Altschul SF, Madden TL, Schaffer AA, Zhang J, Zhang Z, Miller W, Lipman DJ (1997) Gapped BLAST and PSI-BLAST: a new generation of protein database search programs. Nucleic Acids Res 25:3389–3402

67. van Dongen S (2000) Graph clustering by flow simulation. PhD Thesis, University of Utrecht, Utrecht

68. Enright AJ, Van Dongen S, Ouzounis CA (2002) An efficient algorithm for large-scale detection of protein families. Nucleic Acids Res 30:1575–1584

69. Contreras-Moreira B, Vinuesa P (2013) GET_HOMOLOGUES, a versatile software package for scalable and robust microbial pan-genome analysis. Appl Environ Microbiol 79:7696–7701

70. Galperin MY, Makarova KS, Wolf YI, Koonin EV (2015) Expanded microbial genome coverage and improved protein family annotation in the COG database. Nucleic Acid Res 43: D261–D269

71. Lechner M, Hernandez-Rosales M, Doerr D, Wieseke N, Thévenin A, Stoye J, Hartmann RK, Prohaska SJ, Stadler PF (2014) Orthology

detection combining clustering and synteny for very large datasets. PLoS ONE 9:e105015

72. Doerr D, Thévenin A, Stoye J (2012) Gene family assignment-free comparative genomics. BMC Bioinf 13(Suppl 19):S3

73. Hellmuth M, Wieseke N, Lechner M, Lenhof H-P, Middendorf M, Stadler PF (2015) Phylogenetics from paralogs. Proc Natl Acad Sci USA 112:2058–2063

74. Orengo CA, Bateman A (eds) (2014) Protein Families: relating protein sequence, structure, and function. Wiley series in peptide and protein science. Wiley, New York

75. The UniProt Consortium (2015) UniProt: a hub for protein information. Nucleic Acids Res 43:D204–D212

76. Pruitt KD, Tatusova T, Maglott DR (2005) NCBI reference sequence (RefSeq): a curated non-redundant sequence database of genomes, transcripts and proteins. Nucleic Acids Res 33 (Suppl. 1):D501–D504

77. Huerta-Cepas J, Szklarczyk D, Forslund K, Cook H, Heller D, Walter MC, Rattei T, Mende DR, Sunagawa S, Kuhn M, Jensen LJ, von Mering C, Bork P (2016) eggNOG 4.5: a hierarchical orthology framework with improved functional annotations for eukaryotic, prokaryotic and viral sequences. Nucleic Acids Res 44(D1):D286–D293

78. Kanehisa M, Sato Y, Kawashima M, Furumichi M, Tanabe M (2016) KEGG as a reference resource for gene and protein annotation. Nucleic Acids Res 44:D457–D462

79. Kanehisa M, Goto S, Sato Y, Kawashima M, Furumichi M, Tanabe M (2014) Data, information, knowledge and principle: back to metabolism in KEGG. Nucleic Acids Res 42: D199–D205

80. Moriya Y, Itoh M, Okuda S, Yoshizawa AC, Kanehisa M (2007) KAAS: an automatic genome annotation and pathway reconstruction server. Nucleic Acids Res 35:W182–W185

81. Suzuki S, Kakuta M, Ishida T, Akiyama Y (2014) GHOSTX: an improved sequence homology search algorithm using a query suffix array and a database suffix array. PLoS ONE 9 (8):e103833

82. Eddy SR (2004) What is a hidden Markov model? Nat Biotechnol 22:1315–1316

83. Eddy SR (2011) Accelerated profile HMM searches. PLoS Comput Biol 7:e1002195

84. Finn RD, Coggill P, Eberhardt RY, Eddy SR, Mistry J, Mitchell AL, Potter SC, Punta M, Qureshi M, Sangrador-Vegas A, Salazar GA, Tate J, Bateman A (2016) The Pfam protein families database: towards a more sustainable future. Nucleic Acids Res 44:D279–D285

85. Haft DH, Selengut JD, Richter RA, Harkins D, Basu MK, Beck E (2013) TIGRFAMs and genome properties in 2013. Nucleic Acids Res 41:D387–D395; Database issue

86. Thomas PD, Campbell MJ, Kejariwal A, Mi H, Karlak B, Daverman R, Diemer K, Muruganujan A, Narechania A (2003) PANTHER: a library of protein families and subfamilies indexed by function. Genome Res 13:2129–2141

87. Mi H, Lazareva-Ulitsky B, Loo R, Kejariwal A, Vandergriff J, Rabkin S, Guo N, Muruganujan A, Doremieux O, Campbell MJ, Kitano H, Thomas PD (2005) The panther database of protein families, subfamilies, functions and pathways. Nucleic Acids Res 33: D284–D288; Database issue

88. Mi H, Guo N, Kejariwal A, Thomas PD (2007) PANTHER version 6: protein sequence and function evolution data with expanded representation of biological pathways. Nucleic Acids Res 16(35):D247–D252

89. Mi H, Muruganujan A, Casagrande JT, Thomas PD (2013) Large-scale gene function analysis with the panther classification system. Nat Protoc 8(8):1754–2189

90. Ashburner M, Ball CA, Blake JA, Botstein D, Butler H, Cherry, JM, Davis AP, Dolinski K, Dwight SS, Eppig JT, Harris MA, Hill DP, Issel-Tarver L, Kasarskis A, Lewis S, Matese JC, Richardson JE, Ringwald M, Rubin GM, Sherlock G (2000) Gene ontology: tool for the unification of biology. Nat Genet 25(1):25–29

91. Pedruzzi I, Rivoire C, Auchincloss AH, Coudert E, Keller G, de Castro E, Baratin D, Cuche BA, Bougueleret L, Poux S, Redaschi N, Xenarios I, Bridge A (2015) HAMAP in 2015: updates to the protein family classification and annotation system. Nucleic Acid Res 43: D1064–D1070

Chapter 2

Pan-Genome Storage and Analysis Techniques

Tina Zekic, Guillaume Holley, and Jens Stoye

Abstract

Computational pan-genome analysis has emerged from the rapid increase of available genome sequencing data. Starting from a microbial pan-genome, the concept has spread to a variety of species, such as plants or viruses. Characterizing a pan-genome provides insights into intra-species evolution, functions, and diversity. However, researchers face challenges such as processing and maintaining large datasets while providing accurate and efficient analysis approaches. Comparative genomics methods are required for detecting conserved and unique regions between a set of genomes. This chapter gives an overview of tools available for indexing pan-genomes, identifying the sub-regions of a pan-genome and offering a variety of downstream analysis methods. These tools are categorized into two groups, gene-based and sequence-based, according to the pan-genome identification method. We highlight the differences, advantages, and disadvantages between the tools, and provide information about the general workflow, methodology of pan-genome identification, covered functionalities, usability and availability of the tools.

Key words Comparative genomics, Pan-genomics, Core genome, Accessory genome

1 Introduction

As the advances in DNA sequencing technologies lead to a decrease in sequencing time and costs, the number of completely sequenced genomes continues to grow. The availability of different genomes originating from related organisms initiated comparative analysis methods, confronting new questions on a higher species level [1]. Tettelin et al. first introduced the term *pan-genome*, referring to the complete gene content of a microbial species. Initially, two parts have been distinguished within a pan-genome, a *core* genome, representing the set of genes shared among all strains and the *dispensable* genome, composed of strain-specific or genes shared among a subset of strains. However, the commonly used partitioning of a pan-genome (*see* Fig. 1) differentiates three main parts: the core genome, the dispensable or *accessory* genome, and the *singleton* genome.

The core genome provides the genomic basis of the phylogeny of a species and is thought to be representative at various taxonomic

João C. Setubal et al. (eds.), *Comparative Genomics: Methods and Protocols*, Methods in Molecular Biology, vol. 1704,
https://doi.org/10.1007/978-1-4939-7463-4_2, © Springer Science+Business Media LLC 2018

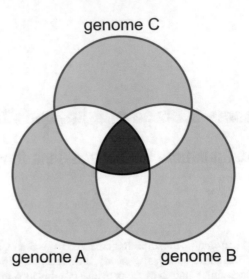

Fig. 1 Pan-genome of three genomes *A*, *B*, and *C*. The core genome is shown in black, the white intersections represent the dispensable genome and the grey sections the singleton genome

levels [2]. The accessory genome may contain supplementary biochemical pathways, providing some selective advantages such as environmental adaptation, specific virulences, or antibiotic resistance [3, 4]. As the genomes of different strains are available, research may target questions related to the species' evolution, elucidating the genomic diversity of a species through comparative analysis. Essential genes present in all strains of a pathogenic species could be used as potential antibiotic targets [5].

In the last 10 years, after establishing the pan-genome concept, several projects were attempted, some of them focusing on taxonomic levels higher than species. In their review, Vernikos et al. [4] provide a short overview of projects realized so far. Initially, a pan-genome referred to the full gene pool of a microbial species. However, the usage spread and the pan-genome concept was proposed for other organisms like plants [6]. Pan-genome analysis projects have been conducted for different plants like *Zea mays* [7] and *Arabidopsis thaliana* [8], and even for viruses such as *Synechococcus* infecting podoviruses [9].

Given a limited number of sequenced strains, it is of interest to estimate the approximate pan-genome size in order to identify the required number of genome sequences needed to characterize the gene repertoire of a species [10]. For pan-genome size estimation different mathematical models have been proposed, such as the *Streptococcus agalactiae* pan-genome model [1], Heaps law model [10], binomial mixture model [11], etc. With the pan-genome size, the openness/closeness [12] can be inferred: A *closed* pan-genome has a finite size, meaning that after a certain number of genomes added, the pan-genome of the species can be fully characterized. An *open* pan-genome is unbounded and continues to grow as the number of genomes increases. During a sequencing project, the estimation of a closed pan-genome can be useful to predict the number of genomes still required to be sequenced in order to characterize the species.

Pan-genome analysis is specially interesting in cases of studying pathogenic strains. A large-scale analysis of *Pseudomonas aeruginosa* was performed [13], a pathogen that revealed high resistance to attempted treatments. The study showed a high genomic variability across the species, including those proteins used as targets for developed vaccines, partially explaining the resistance towards treatments. In another study on *Acinetobacter baumannii* [14] first a pan-genome was constructed. In the following steps the detected conserved regions were then analyzed on protein level from which potential vaccine targets were detected.

Sophisticated tools for the analysis and storage of pan-genomes are needed, maintaining large-scale datasets and providing automatized pan-genome construction as well as further downstream analysis options.

In this chapter we give an overview of established tools related to pan-genome analysis. The chapter is structured as follows: Subheading 2 contains information about tools in which the pan-genome computation is purely gene-based. Another list of tools identify the pan-genome based on genome sequences and are presented in Subheadings 3 and 4. The chapter finishes with concluding remarks in Subheading 5.

2 Gene-Based Tools

A pan-genome of a set of genomes can be identified based on the gene-content. This is a common approach, established in the majority of pan-genome analysis tools. Therefore, the gene content of a genome must be known, i.e. an annotation must be available. For newly sequenced strains or the ones lacking an annotation, gene prediction tools such as Prodigal [15], Glimmer [16], or genome annotation systems like GenDB [17] may be used for preprocessing.

This section is organized in two parts. It starts with a description of the general workflow of tools for pan-genome analysis in Subheading 2.1, followed by Subheading 2.2 providing information about the functionality and properties of tools established so far.

2.1 General Strategy

The general workflow of gene-based pan-genome analysis tools can be divided into three main stages:

1. orthologous gene assignment,

2. pan-genome identification,

3. downstream analysis.

Genes in two different species are *orthologous* to each other if they originate from a single common gene in the last common ancestor of these species [18]. In contrast, *paralogous* genes are genes evolved by a duplication event from a single gene within a genome. (For a more detailed discussion of this topic, *see* Chapter 5 of this volume.) Orthologous genes have mostly retained the same biological function, whereas paralogs tend to diverge functionally.

The problem of identifying orthologous genes has been studied thoroughly in the last years, resulting in many different proposed approaches [19–23]. All tools presented in Subheading 2.2 use graph-based methods for orthology assignment (see the review of Kuzniar et al. [24] for detailed description of orthology assignment categories). The predicted protein sequences represent nodes in the graph. For this set, all pairwise sequence similarities are computed and the derived values used to weight the edges of the graph. Some methods apply a clustering step on the pairwise similarities in order to retrieve multi-species groups of orthologs [24]. The sensitivity and specificity of the estimation highly depends on the chosen sequence comparison algorithm and the scoring scheme. Commonly, BLAST [25] is used to align the sequences. The chosen clustering techniques and orthology criteria such as similarity cut-offs or overlap criteria highly impact the orthology assignment and consequently the derived pan-genome structure. Hence, the main focus of research in the gene-based tool family was concerning the orthology estimation.

Using the information obtained with the orthology assignment, the pan-genome structure can be retrieved. Downstream analysis methods include multiple sequence alignment of the core genes, construction of phylogenetic trees, estimation of the pan-genome size, visualizations, etc.

2.2 Analysis Tools

EDGAR [26, 27] is a precomputed database containing information about bacterial pan-genomes. Using the software in open access mode, only the pre-processed strains available in the database can be used for analysis. For orthology estimation, EDGAR applies the *bidirectional best hits* (BBH) approach using BLAST. The concept of BBH is widespread and defines a pair of orthologs such that both genes are found as the best match of the opposite. For orthology estimation, EDGAR estimates a threshold based on the *BLAST Score Ratio* (BSR). The BSR of a gene a against a gene b is defined as follows: $BSR(a, b) = S_{a,b}/S_{a,a}$, where $S_{a,b}$ refers to the BLAST alignment bit score, in which a is the query and b the reference/database sequence. The threshold is derived using cutoff values for each genome pair and applying a heuristic approach. Based on the derived ortholog estimation, the core genome is identified. EDGAR supports several downstream analysis options such as multiple sequence alignment of the core genes. The content of orthologous genes can be analyzed using the incorporated

comparative view or creating synteny plots. Furthermore, phylogenetic trees can be created for the core genome and Venn diagrams
of the gene content for up to five genomes. The EDGAR database
contains 2160 genomes from 167 genera a user can choose from.

The Prokaryotic-genome Analysis Tool (PGAT) [28] is a
web-based database application. To create the database, first all
gene sequences of the input genomes are aligned using BLASTP
in order to identify gene families. For each gene family one gene is
chosen as a reference. The reference gene sequences are aligned
against all ORFs (all six-frame translations) of each genome
sequence. Genes having a sequence identity percentage greater
than 91–92% and including more than 80% of the gene length in
the sequence alignment are considered as orthologs. The set of
reference genes is expanded by novel genes identified using Glimmer. After selecting one of the nine available organisms on the
PGAT website, some analysis steps can be performed. Selecting to
list orthologs of all genomes corresponds to computing the set of
genes building the pan-genome. The option presence/absence of
genes allows to identify genes present or absent in a chosen subset
of genomes. Therefore, by selecting all genomes the list of core
genes can be identified. For each gene information about identified
SNPs are available, which are derived by computing the multiple
sequence alignment of orthologs using Muscle [29]. PGAT is also
linked to KEGG, such that the presence of genes in different
metabolic pathways can be studied. A main disadvantage of PGAT
is the lack of an option for uploading own data, making PGATs
analysis opportunities limited. After the first publication in 2011,
there are no new versions of the software released. Only the database has been slightly increased (from stated four genomes in [28]
up to nine currently available at the website).

The Pan-genome Analysis Pipeline (PGAP) [30] is a stand-
alone application, composed of a bundle of Perl scripts and is one of
the most established tools so far. The application provides five
functional analysis modules. The first module, *cluster analysis for
functional genes*, corresponds to the identification of a pan-genome
from the input data. For this, two methods have been integrated
into PGAP, the MultiParanoid (**MP**) method and the Gene Family
(**GF**) method. In the MP method, InParanoid [22] is used to find
orthologs between each pair of strains. The InParanoid algorithm
performs an all-against-all BLAST comparison among all protein
sequences and then applies a set of orthology rules to group orthologs including a pairwise alignment score cut-off and overlap criteria. In the next step MultiParanoid [23] is used in order to group
the orthologs into multi-strain clusters. The GF method generates
a dataset in which for each strain the protein sequences are mixed
with the genes of the given strain. A BLASTALL search is performed among the dataset, and the results are then clustered with
the Markov Cluster (MCL) algorithm [31]. The relation between

the pan-genome size and the number of genomes can be derived with the second module, *pan-genome profile analysis*. Furthermore, PGAP offers a module for *detection of genetic variations* in a cluster by computing a multiple alignment of all protein sequences in the cluster. Reported mutations include indels, synonymous and non-synonymous mutations. PGAP also computes the dN/dS ratio of divergence at non-synonymous and synonymous sites. The fourth module, *species evolution analysis*, enables the construction of phylogenetic trees based on two datasets. One input is a gene distance matrix, whose entries are filled based on derived gene cluster profiles for each strain, and the second dataset is based on detected variations in the core gene clusters. Phylogenetic trees are computed using the PHYLIP package. Finally in the fifth module, *function enrichment analysis*, PGAP annotates each gene cluster with the most frequent function description and COG classification of its members. All analysis steps are invoked from a single run. So far, PGAP is only available under Linux.

PanOCT [32] is a tool for clustering orthologous genes among a set of bacterial strains or closely related species. The all-against-all comparison of protein sequences with BLASTP needs to be performed separately and is required as an input for PanOCT. In order to cluster orthologs and more accurately exclude paralogs, PanOCT combines information from conserved gene neighborhood (CGN) together with pairwise sequence identity using BSR. After the pairwise scores of potential orthologous pairs are computed, potential frame-shifted genes are detected. The CGN scores are computed for all pairs, considering homology scores of n genes upstream and downstream of the target and the query protein in a potential orthologous pair (*see* Fig. 3 in [32] for a detailed description of the score). By using the derived CGN scores of the protein pairs as the underlying metric, complete linkage clustering is performed in order to retrieve orthologous clusters. PanOCT only covers the step 1 of the general workflow described in Subheading 2.1.

GET_HOMOLOGUES [33] is an open-source software package for the analysis of microbial pan-genomes. The tool offers three different algorithms for clustering orthologs to choose between, i.e. OrthoMCL [19], COGtriangles [21], and another version of the bidirectional best hit algorithm developed by the authors. All three methods are based on the BBH using BLAST. The sequences are scanned against the Pfam database [34] in order to retrieve the protein domain content. This information is used to filter out clusters containing sequences with different domain architectures. The tool provides a set of scripts supporting downstream analysis. An option is available to compute the intersection between the three cluster groups, referred to as *consensus clusters*. An estimation for the size of the core and pan-genome can be computed under the exponential [10] or binomial mixture model. From clusters of orthologs, pan-genome matrices can be generated and then used to create phylogenetic trees. Different sets of genes can be identified and used for pan-genome analysis. However, it must be noted that a new partitioning of a pan-genome's gene pool is introduced. Besides the core genome, which remains the same, the authors differentiate the *soft core*, composed of genes shared among 95% of the genomes, the *cloud*, bundling genes present only in few genomes and the *shell*, containing the remaining genes, present in several genomes. If a dataset contains a draft genome with some missing or fragmented genes, using the soft core's definition should avoid an underestimation of the core size. GET_HOMOLOGUES is a command line tool available for Linux and MacOSX. The package provides a well-documented manual, including example scenarios of how to use some analysis scripts. However, for smooth usage some basic programming skills are advantageous.

PanFunPro [35] is a pan-genome analysis tool available as a stand-alone application or as a web server. For pan-genome computation, only the predicted protein sequences of the input genomes are used. If no annotations are available, the gene prediction tool Prodigal is applied to the genome sequence to identify potential ORFs. In the next step, the potential coding sequences are scanned against three protein databases: Pfam-A, TIGRFAM [36], and Superfamily [37] in order to retrieve the functional domain content. Based on this content, protein families are defined in order to group homologous proteins. All sequences having no match in any of the databases are collected and clustered using CD-HIT [38] with a minimal sequence identity of 60%. The resulting clusters are considered as protein families and are combined with the HMM-based families. The protein families are used to generate a whole genome protein profile for each genome. The pan-genome is then computed based on the derived protein families, so the pan-genome is composed of all unique functional profiles observed in the input genomes. In order to compare shared protein content, a pan-matrix is generated and visualized, where each entry contains the ratio of non-shared sequences. All proteins contained in the core or pan-genome are listed and Gene Ontology (GO) information can be extracted for the pan-genome. PanFunPro is available as a web-server or can be used by downloading the source code.

The Integrated Toolkit for Exploration of Microbial Pangenomes (ITEP) is a bundle of scripts with a backend database introduced by Benedict et al. [39]. At first, ITEP generates a SQLite database by performing an all-against-all comparison between the sequences using BLASTP and BLASTN. The results are clustered using the Markov Cluster (MCL) algorithm, for which different metrics can be used, i.e. clustering by maximal *minbit* or *maxbit*. According to the tool's manual, the alignment bit score is either normalized by the minimum or maximum of the self bit scores. Hence *maxbit* will emphasize stronger hits whereas in *minbit* also shorter fragmented hits will be considered. However, results from any other orthologous prediction tools can be used as well. After the database is built, different analysis steps can be conducted, for which ITEP provides interfaces, i.e. wrapper scripts to external software performing the analysis. Options for studying predicted protein families are provided, such as generation of multiple alignments, phylogenetic trees or the possibility of appending gene neighborhood information. Different gene sets can be extracted, such as conserved genes (core genes), unique genes, and *present genes* (corresponding to genes of the accessory genome). Some other options are provided within ITEP such as the possibility of annotation curation, identification of gene presence or absence of genes within a phylogeny, or the generation of draft metabolic networks. For each analysis step a different script must be used. Therefore, some basic programming skills are advantageous. However, well-documented tutorials are available on the tool's GitHub as well as separate manuals for each script, facilitating its usage.

PanGP [40] is a tool for pan-genome profile analysis. In order to maintain profile analysis of large-scale datasets, two sampling algorithms are proposed, *totally random* and *distance guided*. The two algorithms sample s combinations consisting of n strains, in order to avoid computing all $\binom{N}{n}$ combinations, for $1 \leq n \leq N$, where N is the total number of strains. Profiling is performed by a series of proposed mathematical models (*see* Supplementary Material of [40] for more details). PanGP provides a graphical user interface (GUI) and is available for several platforms.

The Large Scale BSR method (LS-BSR) [41] is a tool for comparing the gene content between a large set of bacterial genomes. Each gene sequence is aligned against all input genomes and itself in order to retrieve the BSR value. As an output the tool generates a matrix that contains for each gene the BSR value in each genome. The tool includes a script for filtering the gene sequences based on user-defined thresholds, which can be used to identify gene sets of interest. Besides that, the output matrix can be transformed into a PanGP compatible format, allowing to derive statistics about gene distribution and conservation at different genome depths. Other downstream analysis steps are not covered. However, the authors refer to several tools for which the BSR matrix can be used as input. The main advantage of LS-BSR is its parallel nature facilitating a modest runtime for large datasets and outperforming PGAP, GET_HOMOLOGUES, and ITEP in terms of runtime (*see* Table 1 in [41]).

Targeting the inefficient runtime of all-against-all comparisons with BLAST, **Roary** [42] reduces the dataset by preclustering and filtering the protein sequences. After some basic filtering steps (e.g., excluding sequences with less than 120 nucleotides), CD-HIT is used to precluster similar sequences. Performing in an iterative fashion, CD-HIT finds core sequences which are then removed from the dataset. An all-against-all comparison with BLASTP is performed on the reduced dataset and later clustered with MCL. The results of this clustering step are then combined with the pre-computed CD-HIT clusters. In order to separate true orthologs from paralogs which are possibly contained in the results, information about conserved gene neighborhood is used (*see* Supplementary Material in [42]). Roary provides options for computing gene intersections and unions, which can be used to identify the core and the pan-genome. A nice feature is that Roary's output can be used as input for interactive visualization tools referenced from the tool's site. It offers several other options such as providing a relative order of the clusters by creating a graph or clustering the input genomes based on gene presence/absence.

micropan [5] is an R package offering different functionalities for analyzing microbial pan-genomes. Two approaches for deriving gene clusters are incorporated. The first method uses BLAST to perform an all-against-all search between the set of protein sequences of each genome. Gene clusters are then identified using a hierarchical clustering approach. The second method is searching for protein domains in the genes using HMMER3 against the Pfam-A database. All sequences having the same protein domain content in the same non-overlapping order are clustered together. The protein domain based method should facilitate analysis for larger datasets, as the all-against-all search runtime scales quadratically with the number of input genomes. From the derived clustering, a *pan-matrix* is computed, in which rows represent genomes, columns represent gene clusters, and each entry is the number of times a gene cluster is found in a genome. The pan-matrix is the basis for all further analysis functions provided in the package, such as pan-genome size estimation, principal component analysis or the construction of a phylogenetic tree. Similar to GET_HOMOLO-GUES, micropan defines new gene types being part of a pan-genome, i.e. *core genes* that are present in (almost) all input genomes, *shell genes* that are present in a large subset of the genomes, and *cloud genes* that are present in only few genomes. A main advantage of micropan is its easy-to-use nature. All functions needed for analysis, including external software can be invoked directly from the R environment. Therefore, standard R options may also be used.

PanCoreGen [43] is a standalone software with a basic graphic user interface (GUI). The method for pan-genome identification is another BLAST based approach slightly different from the ones presented before. The pan-genome computation is performed in an iterative fashion, where in each iteration another genome serves as a reference. The annotated genes of the reference are compared to the other genomes using BLASTN. In the next iteration, the reference is replaced by another genome and only those genes that did not have matching orthologs in previous iterations are used as queries. In each iteration step, genes unique to the current reference are identified, whereby the core and accessory (here called *mosaic*) gene sets are expanded by new hits relative to the new reference. Like this, the number of found orthologs might be overestimated for genes duplicated in one genome. As a result, PanCoreGen provides the list of all gene groups (core, mosaic, and strain-specific) in an Excel file and a FASTA file containing nucleotide sequences of all genes constituting the pan-genome. For each gene, another FASTA file is generated containing the sequences of all matching orthologs. An option is available for downloading genomes directly from NCBI, as well as (re)annotation of input draft genome sequences. So far PanCoreGen is only available for Windows, and with the described functions it provides only limited options for performing analysis steps.

The Bacterial Pan Genome Analysis (BPGA) tool [44] is a recently published package for pan-genome downstream analysis. At first, orthologous gene or protein clusters are identified, for which the three clustering tools USEARCH [45], CD-HIT, and OrthoMCL are included. A user can choose between the tools and adapt the cut-off value. After detecting orthologs, pan-genome analysis steps can be conducted, for which BPGA offers seven analysis modules. The *pan-genome profile analysis* generates plots for pan- and core genome size, gene family frequencies within the genomes and number of genes added by each genome to the pan-genome. Within this module, the size of the pan- and core genome can be computed. The second module identifies the different gene sets of the pan-genome based on the derived orthologous families and extracts a representative sequence from each. The *exclusive gene family analysis* module can be used to identify orthologous gene families containing genes from all but not a single specified genome or only containing genes of a single genome. Gene sequences which show a deviating (higher or lower) GC content compared to their average genome GC content can be extracted with the *atypical GC content* module. Pan-genome functional analysis is performed by comparing the representative protein sequences found by the second module, against COG and KEGG databases using BLASTP. Using the *phylogenetic analysis* module, phylogenetic trees can be generated for the core genome using a concatenation of core gene alignments, using a computed binary pan-matrix or user-selected housekeeping genes. The latter option enables selection of specific subsets of the input genomes on which the analysis steps will be conducted. BPGA is written in Perl and the code is freely available. Moreover, the tool provides executable (Windows and Linux) files for download, maintaining easy installation.

2.3 Related Tools

In order to compare a set of genomes, the available annotations need to be clean and error-free. However, inconsistencies in annotations are not rare, e.g. presence of false positive identified genes. The bias of individual annotation, i.e. annotation performed by different methodology, may be crucial [46]. Since these discrepancies could have a non-negligible impact on the pan-genome structure, several tools have been proposed for cleaning the input data. **Pannotator** [47] is a pipeline computing the annotation of closely related genomes from scratch, whereas **eCAMBer** [46] and **Mugsy-Annotator** [48] are tools for improving and correcting available annotations.

Hennig et al. [49] introduced **Pan-Tetris**, an interactive visualization tool for pan-genomes. Within Pan-Tetris, an alternative alignment-based method for pan-genome computation is used. In order to compute the pan-genome, first the *SuperGenome* is constructed, a concept proposed and used in the software GenomeRing [50]. First, a whole genome multiple alignment of the input organisms is constructed using progressiveMauve [51]. By the nature of the progressive alignment approach, the multiple alignment is composed of a set of local alignments, also called *blocks*. All blocks are concatenated in the order given by the reference genome of the alignment. Based on the alignment coordinates of the concatenation, the SuperGenome coordinate system is built. For each genome, a bidirectional mapping between its blocks and the SuperGenome coordinate system is derived. The second step is the pan-genome computation based on the derived SuperGenome. Further computations rely on the assumption that orthologous genes should be aligned in a multiple alignment and therefore will overlap in the coordinate system of the SuperGenome. The genes are mapped into the SuperGenome, and overlapping ones are then clustered into groups of orthologous genes called *pan genes*. The set of all pan genes are visualized in Pan-Tetris. However, the main focus of the work was not in developing another algorithm for pan-genome computation, but more developing an interactive visualization tool, which can be helpful for detection of possible erroneous annotations. Options such as extraction of core or accessory genes are not provided but are planned for future releases.

3 Sequence-Based Tools

Along the years, the definition of pan-genome has acquired a broader meaning than its original definition [12]. It nowadays also refers to a collection of sequences from different genomes [52]. Such a collection can be analyzed naively by indexing separately each sequence it is composed of. This representation is however wasteful in memory since core genome and accessory genome need to be stored as many times as they occur in the strains.

Furthermore, such a representation would require analyzing each genome separately, leading to time inefficient methods. If a pan-genome is composed of similar genomes, it is naturally more efficient to index variants of a collection of genomes with respect to a reference. Such methods will be reviewed in Subheading 3.1. Yet, computing similarities or variants is a complex task achieved by aligning sequences of the pan-genome. As a consequence, much attention has been paid to methods that either provide scalable sequence alignments for many similar genomes or extract directly from a sequence alignment the shared and unique regions of the pan-genome (Subheading 3.2). This exercise is not trivial and is the reason for the design of graph-based methods (Subheading 3.3) that take advantage of the similarity and difference not only with a reference but also with other indexed genomes. A special case of graph-based methods are the de Bruijn graph methods (Subheading 3.4) which are alignment-free and reference-free. Other methods reviewed in Subheading 4 enable large scale k-mer indexing and querying of genomes. Note that the following sections focus only on sequence-based data structures and methods for pan-genome indexing and querying at the DNA level in contrast to database oriented tools. Other tools for computational pan-genomics are reviewed in [52].

3.1 Reference-Based Methods

The **Referentially Compressed Search Index** (RCSI) [53] uses referential indexing to index a pan-genome and to search for exact or inexact matches. The reference is first indexed using a Compressed Suffix Tree (CST) [54–57] and the other genomes are then encoded as ordered lists of subsequence matches to the reference, called *referential match entries*. The index is built with respect to a maximum query length and a parameter representing the maximum number of edit distance operations allowed during an inexact search. RCSI exploits the *seed-and-extend paradigm* [58] based on the pigeonhole principle stating that for a sequence S, a pattern P and at most M mismatches, there exists at least one matching substring, called *seed*, of length $\left\lfloor \frac{|P|}{M+1} \right\rfloor$ between S and P. When queried, the reference is first searched for matching seeds that are then extended. Matches found are transferred onto the referential match entries using a hashing structure to identify genomes in which matches are found with at most M mismatches.

Another approach of referential indexing is to index variants instead of similarities. The **Multiple Genome Index** (MuGI) [59] applies this approach by maintaining a database of variants. Additionally, the occurrence positions of k-mers in the genomes are stored in arrays, sorted by lexicographic order of k-mers. The seed-and-extend paradigm employs the k-mer arrays for the exact or inexact matching algorithms such that genomes can be searched without scanning the reference, hence offering faster queries than other state-of-the-art data structures while using less memory during the search. MuGI requires less memory than RCSI to build the index but its search algorithms can only handle mismatches while RCSI also supports insertions and deletions. Also, MuGI considers that variants are provided as input, which allows to keep the reference non-indexed while RCSI computes the subsequence matches itself by indexing the reference.

The **Journaled String Tree** (JST) [60] is another data structure for indexing similar genomes based on encoding genome variants with respect to a reference. The novelty of this work is that it can be "plugged-in" with existing sequential pattern matching algorithms instead of proposing a new search method. A JST is composed of a reference and an array of *branch-nodes* representing variants of one or multiple genomes forming branches with respect to the reference. Each genome is referentially compressed as a *journaled string* consisting of an insertion buffer and a binary search tree. The insertion buffer is a string which is the concatenation of genome subsequences not present in the reference (insertions). The binary search tree maintains positions and lengths of inserted or shared subsequences with respect to the reference. Pattern matching algorithms scanning a sequence in a left-to-right manner can be used in combination with the JST: as soon as a branch-node occurs in the reference, the state of the search algorithm is saved for later processing and the algorithm processes the occurring branch that is extracted from the corresponding journaled strings. Experiments with exact and inexact pattern matching algorithms show better running time and memory consumption compared to a naive scheme where sequences are processed in a sequential manner. However, MuGI shows better performance during the search, mainly due to its fully indexed search, while JST supports only sequential search.

Self-indexes, like the FM-Index [61] and the CST, are data structures that compress and index data while providing random access to the indexed data as well as pattern matching functionalities. Mäkinen et al. [62] introduced a new family of self-indexes [63] for storage, retrieval, and search of highly similar sequence collections. The central idea of this approach is that previous self-indexes could not capture the high similarity of multiple sequences that differ only by few variants. Hence, the newly proposed family extends existing self-indexes to achieve greater compression than the high-order entropy of the sequence collection. The approach is then used to introduce new basic structures, including an advanced suffix array sampling scheme, that are adapted afterwards to a CST. This representation of a collection of highly repetitive sequences uses $\mathcal{O}\big(n\log\frac{N}{n} + \omega\log^2 N\big)$ bits on average in which N is the total length of the collection, n is the length of the reference, and ω is the total number of mutations. Exact pattern matching of a pattern P is achieved in $\mathcal{O}(|P|\log N)$ time. The provided basic structures require each sequence to be pairwise aligned with the reference of the collection to provide basic query operations.

BWBBLE [64] builds an *augmented reference* by including all variants detected between a set of genomes to a reference. For this purpose, a linear augmented reference is built and its Burrows-Wheeler Transform (BWT) [65] is computed such that it can then be used by an aligner based on the FM-Index. SNPs are handled by making use of the International Union of Pure and Applied Chemistry (IUPAC) nucleotide code in which each symbol represents either one nucleotide or multiple possible nucleotides. More complex variants such as indels (insertions or deletions) are linearized: One of the indels is incorporated in the augmented reference and its surrounding characters in the augmented reference are padded to the extremities of the other indels. These other indels are then concatenated to the augmented reference using a special separation symbol. Exact and inexact matching algorithms with the augmented reference use an extension of the BWT-based backward search that handles IUPAC nucleotide symbols. As a IUPAC nucleotide symbol can represent multiple nucleotides, a query can match several different substrings in the augmented reference and, thus, different suffix array intervals. While being more accurate with the augmented reference than BWA with a single reference [66], the aligner is slower and uses significantly more memory.

The **Positional Burrows-Wheeler Transform** (PBWT) [67] is another data structure based on the BWT to represent a haplotype sequence collection with w binary allelic variable sites for efficient haplotype matching and compact storage. The proposed algorithms derive first a reverse prefix ordering of the sequences instead of the classical lexicographic ordering of suffixes in the suffix array. This new ordering ensures that locally maximal sequences are adjacent. Consequently, forward search of the sequences can be used to find all set-maximal matches from a new sequence or a sequence from the collection. Both matchings can be computed in linear time, $\mathcal{O}(w)$ time in the former case and $\mathcal{O}(wN)$ in the latter case with N being the total length of the sequence collection. The PBWT is highly compressible and uses the FM-Index for the forward search.

3.2 Alignment-Based Methods

Panseq [68] is an online tool for pan-genome analysis relying on Pairwise Sequence Alignment (PSA), Multiple Sequence Alignment (MSA), and Local Sequence Alignment (LSA) for its different modules described in the following. The *Novel Region Finder* module extracts novel regions out of a set of input sequences by iteratively adding them to a database if there are no PSA matches with sequences already in the database. The *Core and Accessory Genome Finder* module eliminates first the singleton genome of the input sequences by creating a pool of input sequence segments that match at least two genomes. Segments are then broken into fragments of user-specified length such that an LSA determines if they are part of the core or accessory genome. Core genome sequences are built for each input sequence by concatenating its core genome fragments. The core genome is provided as an MSA of the core genome sequences while the accessory genome is provided as a binary matrix indicating the presence of each fragment in the input sequences. Finally, the *Loci Selector* module constructs a locus set based on the unique number of fingerprints and the discriminatory power of the loci among the input sequences.

The **Harvest suite** [69] uses a variant of whole genome alignment for rapid core genome extraction of highly similar microbial genomes ($\geq 97\%$ average nucleotide similarity). The suite is composed of two tools: *Parsnp* for core genome MSA and *Gingr* for dynamic visualization of large scale MSA as well as core genome Single Nucleotide Polymorphism (SNP) tree exploration. The first tool relies on the fact that core genome MSA has a lower complexity than MSA because it focuses only on regions shared by all genomes. Parsnp starts by indexing an input genome using a CST which is then queried with the remaining genomes in order to identify in a first step multiple Maximum Unique Matches (multi-MUMs) present in all input genomes and in a second step Locally Collinear Blocks of multi-MUMs. Gaps between collinear multi-MUMs are then aligned. Additional post-processing steps are performed to filter out unreliable SNPs and build the core genome SNPs tree. Parsnp was compared to whole-genome alignment methods, k-mer based methods, and read mapping methods. Results show that its accuracy is a compromise between whole-genome alignment methods and read mapping methods but depends on the input data (draft or finished assemblies). However, Parsnp has the advantage to run in a small fraction of the other methods' running times.

Nguyen et al. [70] formulated the pan-genome construction problem as a genome rearrangement problem in which the arrangement and orientation of sequence alignment blocks for a set of genomes partitioned by homology must be optimized. Its complexity has been shown to be NP-hard and a heuristic using Cactus graphs [71] was provided.

3.3 Graph-Based Methods

The Variant-based Graph (VG) representation of a collection of genomes was introduced in the tool **GenomeMapper** [72] for sequence alignment against multiple genomes. This representation follows a similar principle as reference indexing methods with the exception that the underlying data structure does not index variants with respect to a reference but instead implements a fully indexed multi-genome reference in the form of a graph. GenomeMapper fragments each input genome into blocks of equal length maintained in a *block table*. Blocks corresponding to shared regions in the genomes are stored only once and each block is connected to its neighboring blocks, thus forming a graph in which bubbles are formed by blocks of divergent sequences. In addition, a k-mer hash-based index is built to map each k-mer occurring in the input genomes to a list of blocks and positions in the blocks. This index is used to identify *seeds* for the alignment.

The **Generalized Compressed Suffix Array** (GCSA) [73, 74] is a self-index data structure which indexes an MSA of genomes into a finite automaton. The latter is encoded using a generalization of the BWT to finite automata, achieving in the expected case for a constant-size alphabet $\mathcal{A}$ an $\mathcal{O}\left(n \cdot \left(1 + \frac{|\mathcal{A}|}{\omega} \right)^{\mathcal{O}(\log n)} \right)$ bits representation. Possible applications are read alignment, split-read alignment using splicing graphs, probe and primer design as well as alignment to assembly graphs. GCSA has been improved into GCSA2 [75] which is the core data structure of a VG toolkit, vg [76], providing sequence alignment and read mapping over a multi-genome reference using the seed-and-extend paradigm.

HISAT2 [77] is a VG alignment tool for populations of genomes based on HISAT [78]. It uses a *Hierarchical Graph FM-Index* (HGFM) composed of a main Graph FM-Index (GFM) based on GCSA to represent the general population of genomes and a large number of small GFMs, each representing a small genomic region.

PanCake [79] is an extension of string graphs, known from genome assembly [80], which achieves compression based on PSA. PanCake graph vertices represent a reference subsequence and a set of tuples called *feature instances*. Such a tuple contains a chromosome identifier, the position of a subsequence located in the identified chromosome and similar to the reference subsequence, as well as compressed information necessary to reconstruct the subsequence. Feature instances from the same chromosome are ordered in a doubly linked list, such that the entire chromosome can be reconstructed by iterating over the list and concatenating the reconstructed subsequences. New genomes to be inserted in the data structure are pair-wise aligned with the chromosomes already inserted in the graph. One application of PanCake graphs is core and singleton genomes extraction: Singleton regions are the vertices that contain a unique feature instance, while core regions are the vertices containing at least one feature instance from every genome stored in the graph.

3.4 de Bruijn Graph Based Methods

A *de Bruijn graph* (dBG) is a directed graph $G = (V, E)$ in which each vertex $v \in V$ represents a k-mer, a string of length k over an alphabet $\mathcal{A}$. A directed edge $e \in E$ from vertex v to vertex v' representing k-mers x and x', respectively, exists if and only if $x[2 \ldots k] = x'[1 \ldots k - 1]$. Each k-mer x has $|\mathcal{A}|$ possible *successors* $x[2 \ldots k] \odot a$ and $|\mathcal{A}|$ possible *predecessors* $a \odot x[1 \ldots k - 1]$ with $a \in \mathcal{A}$ and $\odot$ being the concatenation operator. Note that in the original definition of the dBG, all possible k-mers for an alphabet $\mathcal{A}$ are represented in the graph. However, the definition of dBG used in the computational biology literature is less strict and only a subset of all possible k-mers are represented in the graph. These k-mers are extracted from the sequences the dBG is built from. A usual step following the dBG construction is to *compact* it in order to decrease the memory requirements and simplify the graph for further analysis. Hence, a dBG is compact if all of its maximal non-branching paths of η vertices are merged into single vertices representing words of length $k + \eta - 1$. As building a compacted dBG requires to build the uncompacted dBG first, much attention has been focused on algorithms enabling the direct construction of the compacted dBG without its uncompacted counterpart.

SplitMEM [81] makes use of the dBG to extract shared regions of a set of similar genomes. The algorithm directly builds the compacted dBG in $\mathcal{O}(N\log g)$ time and $\mathcal{O}(N + |G|)$ space with g being the length of the longest genome and $|G|$ the size of the compacted dBG. To this end, SplitMEM exploits the relations between dBG and suffix tree [82] with the use of *suffix skips*, a generalization of *suffix links* that allow to connect internal vertices of a suffix tree by trimming multiple characters at the beginning of a suffix. The augmented suffix tree allows to identify first all *maximum exact matches* (MEMs, i.e. MUMs without the cardinality constraint) of length at least k in the genomes. As MEMs can overlap and be nested, they are split using suffix skips in order to build the set of *repeatNodes*, substrings occurring at least twice in the pan-genome. Then, *uniqueNodes*, unique substrings of the pan-genome that link repeatNodes, as well as outgoing edges for each vertex, are identified. Core or accessory genome extraction can be performed with core genome defined as subsequences of the pan-genome occurring in at least 70% of the indexed genomes.

Baier et al. [83] improved SplitMEM with two algorithms, one using the CST and the other using the BWT. The CST algorithm follows the same two steps as SplitMEM: first, identifying repeatNodes based on left and right maximality of repeats, then identifying uniqueNodes that link repeatNodes, as well as edges of the graph. It runs in $\mathcal{O}(N)$ instead of $\mathcal{O}(N\log g)$ time, as suffix skips are not required to identify repeatNodes and a non-comparison sorting algorithm is used to identify uniqueNodes and edges of the dBG. Instead, the BWT algorithm computes the complete compacted dBG in a single backward pass over the pan-genome and runs in $\mathcal{O}(N\log|\mathcal{A}|)$ for an alphabet $\mathcal{A}$.

TwoPaCo [84] is a highly parallel method to build the compacted dBG of many similar whole genome sequences. It reduces the problem of finding maximal non-branching paths in the dBG to finding in the input sequences the positions of *junctions*, k-mers that are branching and k-mers that start or finish an input sequence. For this purpose, the algorithm considers first a set of candidate junction positions in the input sequences. For each such position i, the two $(k + 1)$-mers starting at positions i and $i - 1$ are inserted into a data structure D. Then, each such position i is processed again by querying D for all possible successors and predecessors of the k-mer starting at position i. If the k-mer has an edge in-degree of 1 and an edge out-degree of 1, it is not a junction. TwoPaCo uses this method in a first pass with a Bloom filter (BF) [85] as data structure D to be memory efficient and select the candidate junction positions. Those positions are then used as input for the second pass with a hash table as data structure D to remove the false positive junctions generated by the BF. Because the two-pass method can still be memory intensive, k-mers are divided into partitions and the two-pass method deals with each partition once at a time. The expected running time is $\mathcal{O}(Nf + k \cdot (|G| + \sigma\phi\psi))$ with f being the number of hash functions used in the BF, σ being the number of non-junctions in G, ϕ being the probability of a non-junction to be a false positive and ψ being the average number of times a false positive junction occurs in an input sequence. The expected memory is $\mathcal{O}(\text{Max}(m, k \cdot (\delta + \sigma\phi)))$ with m being the number of bits in the BF and δ being the number of junctions.

BCALM [86] and by extension its highly parallel version BCALM 2 [87] are methods to compact efficiently the dBG from reads and whole genome sequences. The approach used is the inverse of the one of TwoPaCo: Instead of identifying junction k-mers, BCALM 2 progressively compacts the dBG such that junction k-mers naturally arise from it. In BCALM 2, k-mers are first partitioned in clusters with regard to their minimizer [88], the smallest of their p-mers with $p < k$. Each k-mer x is attributed to the cluster corresponding to the minimizer min_p of its prefix $x[1,k-1]$. It is also attributed to the cluster corresponding to the minimizer min_s of the suffix $x[2,k]$ if $min_p \neq min_s$. This ensures that k-mers with the same left or right minimizer are in the same cluster. Then, the clusters are compacted in parallel based on their respective $(k-1)$-length overlaps and minimizers. Each such compaction produces a set of strings with each string of length $k + \eta - 1$ being the compaction of η k-mers. Each compacted string of cluster min might have a left (reciprocally right) *lonely end*, a $(k-1)$-length prefix (reciprocally suffix) for which min is not the minimizer. These strings are candidates to merge with strings of other clusters in a reuniting step. Note that TwoPaCo and BCALM 2 build the compacted dBG of single or multiple genomes, but neither index the dBG nor store the dataset identity from which the k-mers originate.

The usage of colored de Bruijn graphs (cdBGs) in a pan-genome context was introduced by the de novo assembler **Cortex** [89]. A cdBG is a dBG $G = (V, E, C)$ in which C is a set of colors such that each vertex $v \in V$ maps to a subset of C. In a pan-genomic context, colors of the cdBG represent genomes in which the k-mers occur. Cortex can perform assembly of single genomes and populations of genomes that scale to eukaryotic genome sizes, and its algorithms can genotype simple and complex variants. Bubble calling and path divergence algorithms make extensive use of the colors to aggregate information from different samples and accurately identify the variant types. The cdBG data structure of Cortex is a hash table in which hashed k-mers are associated to various information such as colors and coverage.

The **Bloom Filter Trie** (BFT) [90] is an alignment-free, reference-free and incremental succinct data structure for large scale indexing and querying of a pan-genome represented with a cdBG. It allows to efficiently index, compress, and traverse a cdBG built from reads or whole genome sequences. The BFT is based on the *burst trie* [91] such that a path from the root to a leaf represents a k-mer associated with a set of colors. Vertices of the BFT store lists of containers that are of two types. Uncompressed containers index k-mer suffixes associated with their colors and have a limited capacity of suffixes. When the k-mer suffix capacity of such a container is exceeded during the insertion process, the container is *burst*: shared prefixes of the k-mer suffixes are indexed in a new compressed container that replaces the uncompressed one. The shared prefixes are linked to their corresponding suffixes and associated color sets stored in new uncompressed containers, themselves stored in new child vertices. Bloom filters enable an efficient navigation among the containers and optimize the cdBG traversal by grouping together k-mer neighbors. To the best of our knowledge, BFT is the only data structure among the dBG methods for pan-genome indexing that can be dynamically updated with new genomes without the need to rebuild partially or entirely the index. The BFT proposes additional features to cdBG traversal such as sequence querying, k-mer extraction and prefix matching over the set of indexed k-mers. Experimental results show better time and memory performance compared to another state-of-the-art data structure based on an approximate representation of k-mer sets [92]. The BFT is the core data structure of a dynamic read compression tool named DARRC [93] for pan-genome read storage.

Vari [94] is also a succinct data structure for indexing a pan-genome as a cdBG. It uses the BOSS representation [95] of succinct dBGs based on an adaptation of the FM-Index. The BOSS representation of a dBG G is defined by the edge-BWT of G and two bitvectors. The edge-BWT of G is the sequence of edge labels sorted according to the edges' co-lexicographic order of their starting nodes. The bitvectors register the positions of specific edges for each node. Vari builds the BOSS representation of the union of individual dBGs and stores additionally a two-dimensional binary array containing the colors of each edge. Vari was compared to Cortex on multiple sets of similar whole genome sequences by constructing the cdBG and performing a bubble calling algorithm. Results show that Vari outperforms Cortex regarding the memory efficiency while Cortex is the most time efficient algorithm.

4 *k*-Mer Based Methods

As q-gram indexes, also called k-mer indexes, require large amount of memory and are often used for sequence alignment purposes, Claude et al. [96] proposed two compressed q-gram indexes dedicated to highly repetitive sequence collections. The first method divides a sequence collection of total length N into blocks of length l and establishes an index that associates every occurring q-gram to a list of blocks in which it appears. The sequence collection is encoded using a grammar-based compressor that can efficiently encode long repetitions and provides linear time decompression. Lists of blocks are first delta-encoded to limit the size of each number in the list. Then, each number is encoded using a variable-length encoding technique that assigns a shorter encoding to smaller numbers. Finally, LZ-77 [97] compresses the previously encoded list to take advantage of its internal repetitions. Search time for a q-gram is in $\mathcal{O}\left(N \cdot \left(1 - \left(1 - \frac{l}{N}\right)^{occ}\right)\right)$ average time and $\mathcal{O}(\text{Min}(l \cdot occ, N))$ worst-case time, with occ being the occurrence number of a searched q-gram. The second proposed index is a grammar-compressed self-index based on a Straight-Line Program (SLP), a grammar generating a unique string. Indexing a collection of sequences based on SLPs of minimum size can achieve some compression, but computing it is an NP-complete problem. Instead, the authors proposed to use a grammar-based compressor that does not exactly generate an SLP but provides a good heuristic for this problem. This self-index requires $\gamma \cdot \left(\log r + \log \gamma + \frac{\log N}{|\mathcal{A}|}\right) + r \cdot (3\log r + \log N)$ bits where γ is the length of the final compressed stream, r is the number of rules, and $\mathcal{A}$ is the grammar used. Worst-case running time is in $\mathcal{O}((q \cdot (q + \log N) + occ)\log N \log r)$.

The **Sequence Bloom Tree** (SBT) [92] is a data structure for large scale querying of genomic experiments. It is designed as a binary tree with BFs as vertices. Leaves of the tree approximately represent genomic experiments: k-mers are extracted from each such experiment and inserted into the BF of the corresponding leaf. An internal vertex is the union of its two children BFs, i.e., a BF in which a bucket is set to 1 if the bucket at the same position in at least one of the two children is 1. As BFs generate false positives, leaves do not represent dBGs but approximations of k-mer pools instead. Although the BFs' size must be the same for all vertices of the tree, BFs are compressed using RRR [98] such that over-sized BFs have a higher compression ratio. An SBT is queried with a pattern P by decomposing it into k-mers which are in turn used to query the SBT in a top-down manner. For each vertex v of an SBT t traversed during the querying, the subset of k-mers that are present according to the vertex BF is determined. This subset is then used to query *children*(v, t). It enables to prune the search for branches that do not contain the queried k-mers. A match of pattern P in a genomic experiment represented by leaf v is reported if $\theta \cdot (\mid P \mid - k + 1)$ k-mers from P are reported present in v with $0 \leq \theta \leq 1$ being a user-defined threshold. Because of the false positives and the heuristics used for the pattern matching, the number of experiments in which P occurs is a subset of the ones reported by the SBT.

5 Conclusion

With the development of high-throughput sequencing technologies, pan-genome studies evolved towards analyzing large-scale datasets. This chapter gave an overview of a variety of pan-genome tools established so far. Based on the input, the tools can be separated into gene- and sequence-based. Relying on predicted coding sequences, gene based tools trigger pan-genome analysis by searching for orthologous genes between the set of genomes. While some tools introduce their own orthology criteria, others use established orthology prediction algorithms. Based on the assignment, the pan-genome's gene sets are derived, for which the tools offer several downstream analysis options. The other tool set is purely sequenced based, avoiding the requirement of available annotations and the choice of orthology criteria. In order to detect shared sequences, different approaches are conducted. While some tools use sequence alignment to find similar sequences, others build the pan-genome by choosing one reference and indexing the other genomes based on the reference. Graph-based tools use information of shared sequences with not only a reference but also more sequences. The last presented subset of tools use a de Bruijn graph to represent a pan-genome and are alignment-free and reference-free. All of these tools facilitate pan-genome analysis and cover different spectra of functionalities. While some focus more on reducing memory usage and runtime to maintain large datasets, others offer functional analysis modules allowing to gain biological knowledge of the dataset.

References

1. Tettelin H, Masignani V, Cieslewicz MJ, Donati C, Medini D et al (2005) Genome analysis of multiple pathogenic isolates of streptococcus agalactiae: implications for the microbial "pan-genome". Proc Natl Acad Sci USA 102(39):13950–13955

2. Ochman H, Lerat E, Daubin V (2005) Examining bacterial species under the specter of gene transfer and exchange. Proc Natl Acad Sci USA 102(Suppl 1):6595–6599

3. Read TD, Ussery DW (2006) Opening the pan-genomics box. Curr Opin Microbiol 9 (5).496–498

4. Vernikos G, Medini D, Riley DR, Tettelin H (2015) Ten years of pan-genome analyses. Curr Opin Microbiol 23:148–154

5. Mira A, Martín-Cuadrado AB, D'Auria G, Rodríguez-Valera F (2010) The bacterial pan-genome: a new paradigm in microbiology. Int Microbiol 13(2):45–57

6. Morgante M, De Paoli E, Radovic S (2007) Transposable elements and the plant pan-genomes. Curr Opin Plant Biol 10 (2):149–155

7. Hirsch CN, Foerster JM, Johnson JM, Sekhon RS, Muttoni G et al (2014) Insights into the maize pan-genome and pan-transcriptome. Plant Cell 26(1):121–135

8. Weigel D, Mott R (2009) The 1001 genomes project for Arabidopsis thaliana. Genome Biol 10(5):107

9. Huang S, Zhang S, Jiao N, Chen F (2015) Comparative genomic and phylogenomic analyses reveal a conserved core genome shared by estuarine and oceanic cyanopodoviruses. PloS One 10(11):e0142962

10. Tettelin H, Riley D, Cattuto C, Medini D (2008) Comparative genomics: the bacterial pan-genome. Curr Opin Microbiol 11 (5):472–477

11. Snipen L, Almøy T, Ussery DW (2009) Microbial comparative pan-genomics using binomial mixture models. BMC Genomics 10(1):385

12. Medini D, Donati C, Tettelin H, Masignani V, Rappuoli R (2005) The microbial pan-genome. Curr Opin Genet Dev 15 (6):589–594

13. Mosquera-Rendón J, Rada-Bravo AM, Cárdenas-Brito S, Corredor M, Restrepo-Pineda E, Benítez-Páez A (2016) Pangenome-wide and molecular evolution analyses of the pseudomonas aeruginosa species. BMC Genomics 17 (1):45

14. Hassan A, Naz A, Obaid A, Paracha RZ, Naz K, Awan FM, Muhmmad SA, Janjua HA, Ahmad J, Ali A (2016) Pangenome and immuno-proteomics analysis of Acinetobacter baumannii strains revealed the core peptide vaccine targets. BMC Genomics 17(1):732

15. Hyatt D, Chen G-L, LoCascio PF, Land ML, Larimer FW, Hauser LJ (2010) Prodigal: prokaryotic gene recognition and translation initiation site identification. BMC Bioinf 11 (1):119

16. Delcher AL, Harmon D, Kasif S, White O, Salzberg SL (1999) Improved microbial gene identification with glimmer. Nucleic Acids Res 27(23):4636–4641

17. Meyer F, Goesmann A, McHardy AC, Bartels D, Bekel T et al (2003) Gendb–an open source genome annotation system for prokaryote genomes. Nucleic Acids Res 31 (8):2187–2195

18. Fitch WM (1970) Distinguishing homologous from analogous proteins. Syst Biol 19 (2):99–113

19. Li L, Stoeckert CJ, Roos DS (2003) Orthomcl: identification of ortholog groups for eukaryotic genomes. Genome Res 13(9):2178–2189

20. Tatusov RL, Koonin EV, Lipman DJ (1997) A genomic perspective on protein families. Science 278(5338):631–637

21. Kristensen DM, Kannan L, Coleman MK, Wolf YI, Sorokin A, Koonin EV, Mushegian A (2010) A low-polynomial algorithm for assembling clusters of orthologous groups from intergenomic symmetric best matches. Bioinformatics 26(12):1481–1487

22. Sonnhammer ELL, Östlund G (2015) Inparanoid 8: orthology analysis between 273 proteomes, mostly eukaryotic. Nucleic Acids Res 43(D1):D234–D239

23. Alexeyenko A, Tamas I, Liu G, Sonnhammer ELL (2006) Automatic clustering of orthologs and inparalogs shared by multiple proteomes. Bioinformatics 22(14):e9–e15

24. Kuzniar A, van Ham RCHJ, Pongor S, Leunissen JAM (2008) The quest for orthologs: finding the corresponding gene across genomes. Trends Genet 24(11):539–551

25. Altschul SF, Gish W, Miller W, Myers EW, Lipman DJ (1990) Basic local alignment search tool. J Mol Biol 215(3):403–410

26. Blom J, Albaum S, Doppmeier D, Pühler A, Vorhölter FJ, Zakrzewski M, Goesmann A (2009) EDGAR: a software framework for the comparative analysis of prokaryotic genomes. BMC Bioinf 10:154

27. Blom J, Kreis J, Spänig S, Juhre T, Bertelli C, Ernst C, Goesmann A (2016) EDGAR 2.0: an enhanced software platform for comparative gene content analyses. Nucleic Acids Res 44 (W1):W22–W28

28. Brittnacher MJ, Fong C, Hayden HS, Jacobs MA, Radey M, Rohmer L (2011) PGAT: a multistrain analysis resource for microbial genomes. Bioinformatics 27(17):2429–2430

29. Edgar RC (2004) MUSCLE: multiple sequence alignment with high accuracy and high throughput. Nucleic Acids Res 32 (5):1792–1797

30. Zhao Y, Wu J, Yang J, Sun S, Xiao J, Yu J (2012) PGAP: pan-genomes analysis pipeline. Bioinformatics 28(3):416–418

31. Enright AJ, Van Dongen S, Ouzounis CA (2002) An efficient algorithm for large-scale detection of protein families. Nucleic Acids Res 30(7):1575–1584

32. Fouts DE, Brinkac L, Beck E, Inman J, Sutton G (2012) PanOCT: automated clustering of orthologs using conserved gene neighborhood for pan-genomic analysis of bacterial strains

and closely related species. Nucleic Acids Res 40(22):e172

33. Contreras-Moreira B, Vinuesa P (2013) GET_HOMOLOGUES, a versatile software package for scalable and robust microbial pan-genome analysis. Appl Environ Microbiol 79 (24):7696–7701

34. Finn RD, Coggill P, Eberhardt RY, Eddy SR, Mistry J et al (2016) The Pfam protein families database: towards a more sustainable future. Nucleic Acids Res 44(D1):D279–D285

35. Lukjancenko O, Thomsen MC, Larsen MV, Ussery DW (2013) PanFunPro: PAN-genome analysis based on FUNctional PROfiles. F1000Research, 2

36. Haft DH, Selengut JD, White O (2003) The TIGRFAMs database of protein families. Nucleic Acids Res 31(1):371–373

37. Gough J, Karplus K, Hughey R, Chothia C (2001) Assignment of homology to genome sequences using a library of hidden Markov models that represent all proteins of known structure. J Mol Biol 313(4):903–919

38. Fu L, Niu B, Zhu Z, Wu S, Li W (2012) CD-HIT: accelerated for clustering the next-generation sequencing data. Bioinformatics 28 (23):3150–3152

39. Benedict MN, Henriksen JR, Metcalf WW, Whitaker RJ, Price ND (2014) ITEP: an integrated toolkit for exploration of microbial pan-genomes. BMC Genomics 15(1):8

40. Zhao Y, Jia X, Yang J, Ling Y, Zhang Z, Yu J, Wu J, Xiao J (2014) PanGP: a tool for quickly analyzing bacterial pan-genome profile. Bioinformatics 30(9):1297–1299

41. Sahl JW, Gregory Caporaso J, Rasko DA, Keim P (2014) The large-scale blast score ratio (LS-BSR) pipeline: a method to rapidly compare genetic content between bacterial genomes. PeerJ 2:e332

42. Page AJ, Cummins CA, Hunt M, Wong VK, Reuter S et al (2015) Roary: rapid large-scale prokaryote pan genome analysis. Bioinformatics 31(22):3691–3693

43. Paul S, Bhardwaj A, Bag SK, Sokurenko EV, Chattopadhyay S (2015) PanCoreGen–Profiling, detecting, annotating protein-coding genes in microbial genomes. Genomics 106 (6):367–372

44. Chaudhari NM, Gupta VK, Dutta C (2016) BPGA-an ultra-fast pan-genome analysis pipeline. Sci Rep 6:24373

45. Edgar RC (2010) Search and clustering orders of magnitude faster than BLAST. Bioinformatics 26(19):2460–2461

46. Wozniak M, Wong L, Tiuryn J (2014) eCAMBer: efficient support for large-scale comparative analysis of multiple bacterial strains. BMC Bioinf 15(1):1

47. Santos AR, Barbosa E, Fiaux K, Zurita-Turk M, Chaitankar V et al (2013) PANNOTATOR: an automated tool for annotation of pan-genomes. Genet Mol Res 12:2982–2989

48. Angiuoli SV, Hotopp JCD, Salzberg SL, Tettelin H (2011) Improving pan-genome annotation using whole genome multiple alignment. BMC Bioinf 12(1):272

49. Hennig A, Bernhardt J, Nieselt K (2015) Pan-Tetris: an interactive visualisation for Pan-genomes. BMC Bioinf 16(Suppl 11):S3

50. Herbig A, Jäger G, Battke F, Nieselt K (2012) GenomeRing: alignment visualization based on SuperGenome coordinates. Bioinformatics 28(12):i7–i15

51. Darling AE, Mau B, Perna NT (2010) progressiveMauve: multiple genome alignment with gene gain, loss and rearrangement. PloS One 5(6):e11147

52. Computational Pan-Genomics Consortium (2016) Computational pan-genomics: status, promises and challenges. Brief Bioinform bbw089 https://doi.org/10.1093/bib/bbw089

53. Wandelt S, Starlinger J, Bux M, Leser U (2013) RCSI: scalable similarity search in thousand (s) of genomes. Proc VLDB Endowment 6 (13):1534–1545

54. Sadakane K (2007) Compressed suffix trees with full functionality. Theor Comput Syst 41 (4):589–607

55. Fischer J, Mäkinen V, Navarro G (2009) Faster entropy-bounded compressed suffix trees. Theor Comput Sci 410(51):5354–5364

56. Ohlebusch E, Fischer J, Gog S (2010) CST++. In: Proceedings of the international symposium on string processing and information retrieval (SPIRE'10), vol 6393, pp 322–333

57. Russo L, Navarro G, Oliveira AL (2011) Fully compressed suffix trees. ACM Trans Algorithms 7(4):53

58. Rasmussen KR, Stoye J, Myers EW (2006) Efficient q-gram filters for finding all ε-matches over a given length. J Comput Biol 13 (2):296–308

59. Danek A, Deorowicz S, Grabowski S (2014) Indexes of large genome collections on a PC. PloS One 9(10):e109384

60. Rahn R, Weese D, Reinert K (2014) Journaled string tree—a scalable data structure for analyz-

ing thousands of similar genomes on your laptop. Bioinformatics 30(24):3499–3505

61. Ferragina P, Manzini G (2000) Opportunistic data structures with applications. In: Proceedings of the 41st symposium on foundations of computer science (FOCS'00), pp 390–398

62. Mäkinen V, Navarro G, Sirén J, Välimäki N (2010) Storage and retrieval of highly repetitive sequence collections. J Comput Biol 17 (3):281–308

63. Navarro G (2012) Indexing highly repetitive collections. In: Proceedings of the 23rd international workshop on combinatorial algorithms (IWOCA'12), vol 7643, pp 274–279

64. Huang L, Popic V, Batzoglou S (2013) Short read alignment with populations of genomes. Bioinformatics 29(13):i361–i370

65. Burrows M, Wheeler M (1994) A block-sorting lossless data compression algorithm. Digital SRC Research Report 124

66. Li H, Durbin R (2009) Fast and accurate short read alignment with Burrows-Wheeler transform. Bioinformatics 25(14):1754–1760

67. Durbin R (2014) Efficient haplotype matching and storage using the positional Burrows–Wheeler transform (PBWT). Bioinformatics 30(9):1266–1272

68. Laing C, Buchanan C, Taboada EN, Zhang Y, Kropinski A, Villegas A, Thomas JE, Gannon VPJ (2010) Pan-genome sequence analysis using Panseq: an online tool for the rapid analysis of core and accessory genomic regions. BMC Bioinf 11(1):461

69. Treangen TJ, Ondov BD, Koren S, Phillippy AM (2014) The Harvest suite for rapid core-genome alignment and visualization of thousands of intraspecific microbial genomes. Genome Biol 15(11):524

70. Nguyen N, Hickey G, Zerbino DR, Raney B, Earl D, Armstrong J, Haussler D, Paten B (2015) Building a pangenome reference for a population. J Comput Biol 22(5):387–401

71. Paten B, Diekhans M, Earl D, John JS, Ma J, Suh B, Haussler D (2011) Cactus graphs for genome comparisons. J Comput Biol 18 (3):469–481

72. Schneeberger K, Hagmann J, Ossowski S, Warthmann N, Gesing S, Kohlbacher O, Weigel D (2009) Simultaneous alignment of short reads against multiple genomes. Genome Biol 10(9):R98

73. Sirén J, Välimäki N, Mäkinen V (2011) Indexing finite language representation of population genotypes. In: Proceedings of the 11th international workshop on algorithms in bioinformatics (WABI'11), vol 6833, pp 270–281

74. Sirén J, Välimäki N, Mäkinen V (2014) Indexing graphs for path queries with applications in genome research. IEEE/ACM Trans Comput Biol Bioinf 11(2):375–388

75. Sirén J (2017) Indexing variation graphs. In: Proceedings of the 19th workshop on algorithm engineering and experiments (ALENEX'17), pp 13–27

76. vg team (2015) vg implementation. https://github.com/vgteam/vg [Online; Accessed 23 Feb 2017]

77. Kim D, Langmead B, Salzberg SL (2016) HISAT2 implementation. https://github.com/infphilo/hisat2 [Online; Accessed 23 Feb 2017]

78. Kim D, Langmead B, Salzberg SL (2015) HISAT: a fast spliced aligner with low memory requirements. Nat Methods 12(4):357–360

79. Ernst C, Rahmann S (2013) PanCake: a data structure for pangenomes. In: Proceedings of the German conference on bioinformatics 2013 (GCB'13), vol 34, pp 35–45

80. Myers EW (2005) The fragment assembly string graph. Bioinformatics 21:ii79–ii85

81. Marcus S, Lee H, Schatz MC (2014) SplitMEM: a graphical algorithm for pan-genome analysis with suffix skips. Bioinformatics 30(24):3476–3483

82. Weiner P (1973) Linear pattern matching algorithms. In: Proceedings of the 14th annual symposium on switching and automata theory (SWAT'73)

83. Baier U, Beller T, Ohlebusch E (2016) Graphical pan-genome analysis with compressed suffix trees and the Burrows-Wheeler transform. Bioinformatics 32(4):497–504

84. Minkin I, Pham S, Medvedev P (2016) TwoPaCo: an efficient algorithm to build the compacted de Bruijn graph from many complete genomes. Bioinformatics btw609 https://doi.org/10.1093/bioinformatics/btw609

85. Bloom BH (1970) Space/time trade-offs in hash coding with allowable errors. Commun ACM 13(7):422–426

86. Chikhi R, Limasset A, Jackman S, Simpson JT, Medvedev P (2015) On the representation of de Bruijn graphs. J Comput Biol 22 (5):336–352

87. Chikhi R, Limasset A, Medvedev P (2016) Compacting de Bruijn graphs from sequencing data quickly and in low memory. Bioinformatics 32(12):i201–i208

88. Roberts M, Hayes W, Hunt BR, Mount SM, Yorke JA (2004) Reducing storage requirements for biological sequence comparison. Bioinformatics 20(18):3363–3369

89. Iqbal Z, Caccamo M, Turner I, Flicek P, McVean G (2012) De novo assembly and genotyping of variants using colored de Bruijn graphs. Nat Genet 44(2):226–232

90. Holley G, Wittler R, Stoye J (2016) Bloom Filter Trie: an alignment-free and reference-free data structure for pan-genome storage. Algorithms Mol Biol 11:3

91. Heinz S, Zobel J, Williams HE (2002) Burst tries: a fast, efficient data structure for string keys. ACM Trans Inf Syst 20(2):192–223

92. Solomon B, Kingsford C (2016) Fast search of thousands of short-read sequencing experiments. Nat Biotechnol 34(3):300–302

93. Holley G, Wittler R, Stoye J, Hach F (2017) Dynamic alignment-free and reference-free read compression. In: Proceedings of 21st international conference on research in computational molecular biology (RECOMB'17), vol 10229, pp 50–65

94. Belk K, Boucher C, Bowe A, Gagie T, Morley P, Muggli MD, Noyes NR, Puglisi SJ, Raymond R (2016) Succinct colored de Bruijn graphs. bioRxiv 040071

95. Bowe A, Onodera T, Sadakane K, Shibuya T (2012) Succinct de Bruijn graphs. In: Proceedings of 12th international workshop on algorithms in bioinformatics (WABI'12), vol 7534, pp 225–235

96. Claude F, Farina A, Martínez-Prieto MA, Navarro G (2010) Compressed q-gram indexing for highly repetitive biological sequences. In: Proceedings of the IEEE international conference on bioinformatics and bioengineering (BIBE'10)

97. Ziv J, Lempel A (1977) A universal algorithm for sequential data compression. IEEE Trans Inf Theory 23(3):337–343

98. Raman R, Raman V, Rao SS (2007) Succinct indexable dictionaries with applications to encoding k-ary trees, prefix sums and multisets. ACM Trans Algorithms 3(4):43

Chapter 3

Comparative Genomics for Prokaryotes

João C. Setubal, Nalvo F. Almeida, and Alice R. Wattam

Abstract

Bacteria and archaea, collectively known as prokaryotes, have in general genomes that are much smaller than those of eukaryotes. As a result, thousands of these genomes have been sequenced. In prokaryotes, gene architecture lacks the intron-exon structure of eukaryotic genes (with an occasional exception). These two facts mean that there is an abundance of data for prokaryotic genomes, and that they are easier to study than the more complex eukaryotic genomes. In this chapter, we provide an overview of genome comparison tools that have been developed primarily (sometimes exclusively) for prokaryotic genomes. We cover methods that use only the DNA sequences, methods that use only the gene content, and methods that use both data types.

Key words Prokaryotic genome, Pangenome analysis, Whole genome alignment

1 Introduction

This chapter addresses the following situation: a scientist is interested in studying the genomes of a group of bacteria and/or archaea (prokaryotes), usually several species in a genus or several strains of a single species. These genomes may have been recently sequenced, or the dataset may also include publicly available genomes. The scientist has phenotypic information about the strains of interest. Phenotype here means laboratory observations, for example results of various kinds of biochemical tests, behavior in growth media, or host-pathogen interactions. Usually, the researcher has selected the strains or species to study based on differences in these phenotypes, and she or he would like to know what is the genomic basis for the observed phenotypic differences. This chapter presents an overview of methods that allow researchers to determine what are the genomic differences between the genomes selected, so that this information can then be interpreted in light of what is known about the phenotypes of these organisms.

João C. Setubal et al. (eds.), *Comparative Genomics: Methods and Protocols*, Methods in Molecular Biology, vol. 1704,
https://doi.org/10.1007/978-1-4939-7463-4_3, © Springer Science+Business Media LLC 2018

In addition to the genome sequences, most methods to be described in this chapter require that genomes be *annotated*. We briefly describe the process of genome annotation.

We will assume that each genome to be studied is *complete*. This means that there are no gaps in the genome sequence, and that the overall quality of the sequence is very good, meaning that the probability of sequencing errors is less than 1 in 10,000 base pairs, and all bases have been called (no Ns). Nowadays, most prokaryote genome sequencing projects *do not* generate complete genomes; the norm has become the *draft sequence* (which typically contains dozens or hundreds of gaps, in addition to more sequencing errors than are normally expected in complete genomes). We discuss the implications of having draft genome sequences to the methods to be discussed in Subheading 8.

There are basically two steps to the genome annotation process: *gene finding* and *function assignment*. The gene finding process aims to predict the sections of the genome that contain genes. For the case of protein-coding genes, this typically means determining the *coding sequence* of the gene: where does it start (the translation start) and where does it end (the translation stop). Coding sequences are always Open Reading Frames (ORFs), but the converse is not necessarily true. Despite this asymmetry, it is common to find papers in the literature that describe a genome as having so many ORFs, when they in fact mean so many coding sequences, or more accurately, coding sequences of predicted protein-coding genes. There are many programs available that do a good job in predicting protein-coding genes in prokaryotic genomes; three of the most popular are prodigal [1], glimmer [2], and geneMark [3].

In addition to protein-coding genes, genomes include a variety of other kinds of genes. Among these are the ribosomal RNA genes (rRNA), transfer RNA genes (tRNA), and other noncoding RNA genes. In this chapter we focus on protein-coding genes. It should also be noted that the biological entity *gene* is not restricted to a coding sequence. A gene will have other components, such as a promoter region, a transcription start site, and transcribed but untranslated regions. However, the vast majority of comparisons (in the case of prokaryotes) focus on the coding sequences of genes.

Once coding sequences have been predicted, the function assignment step seeks to predict the function of the coded proteins. Typically, this is done by complex automated pipelines, which try to associate various kinds of information with a coding sequence, generally using the technique of sequence similarity across various sequence databases. If successful, the end result is that the coding sequence will be associated with a reasonably specific *protein product description* (e.g., chromosomal replication initiator protein) and with a short gene name or gene symbol (e.g., *dnaA*). Good pipelines store the provenance of these annotations (also known as *annotation evidence*) so that it can be verified by human curators, should the need arise.

For any given gene, the annotation pipeline may not succeed in assigning a function. This can happen for basically two reasons: (1) the gene sequence is similar to other gene sequences in the database, but none of these other sequences has a known function. In these cases the product description is typically given as *conserved hypothetical protein*. (2) The gene sequence is not sufficiently similar to any other known sequence in the databases used ("no-hits"). In this case, the product description is given as *hypothetical protein*. However, this nomenclature is not standard. The databases are full of hypothetical or conserved hypothetical protein-coding genes annotated as "unknown protein," "unnamed protein product," and other similar terms.

Annotation pipelines are available in two modes: by a locally installed program and in web platforms. A local annotation pipeline is a program or collection of programs that can be downloaded and run on local computers. In this category a popular package is Prokka [4]. A web platform is an annotation system available on the web, which requires users to upload their unannotated genomes to a given server, and request that it be annotated. Among web platforms we mention NCBI [5], IMG [6], and RAST [7]. For users intending to submit their annotated genomes to GenBank, the NCBI pipeline has the advantage that its annotations conform to NCBI standards (for obvious reasons), thus possibly speeding up the submission process.

With a set of annotated genomes, it is possible to determine their gene families. This means clustering the genes in the various genomes in groups that we call homolog or ortholog families. Having these families is an essential step for the methods to be described next.

2   Gene Content Comparison Based on Orthology

The simplest comparison that can be done for a set of genomes with their gene families in hand is to verify which genomes have genes in which families. This can be readily done putting together a *presence/absence gene matrix* (or *gene table*), as illustrated by Table 1.

It is straightforward to generate such a table from the output of a program that computes ortholog groups for a given set of genomes. A graphical representation of such tables is Venn diagrams. A *Venn diagram* is a graphic way to represent set relationships; an example is given in Fig. 1. Venn diagrams can be generated from presence/absence tables in packages such as R [8]. Even though Venn diagrams are easier to understand than a presence/absence matrix, they are only useful to represent gene content relationships for at most a handful of genomes. Above that, Venn diagrams

Table 1
Schematic representation of a presence/absence gene matrix. Genomes are represented in columns, and gene families are represented in rows

Gene	Genome						
	A	B	C	D	E	F	G
1	✓	✓			✓	✓	
2	✓		✓	✓	✓	✓	✓
3		✓		✓			
4		✓			✓		
5				✓			
6		✓			✓	✓	
7		✓		✓			✓

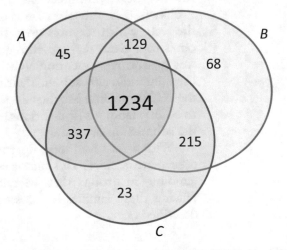

Fig. 1 Illustration of a gene content Venn diagram for three hypothetical genomes *A*, *B*, and *C*. The numbers inside each region indicate the number of genes contained in that region. For example, the region that represents the intersection of all three circles contains 1234 genes, meaning that the three genomes share these many genes. The region representing the intersection of genomes *B* and *C* contains 215 genes: these are the genes that *B* and *C* share that are absent from *A*. Genome *A* on the other hand has 45 genes that are specific to it with respect to the other two genomes

become progressively more complicated. The reason is that the number of regions in a Venn diagram grows exponentially with the number of participating sets: a Venn diagram of n sets has $2^n - 1$ regions. For example, if we want to display gene family relationships for 10 genomes (not a large number of genomes to compare), the corresponding Venn diagram would have to display $10^{10} - 1 = 1023$ regions.

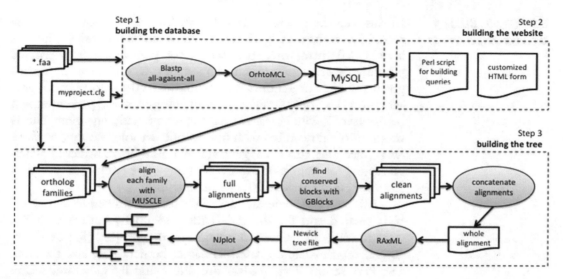

Fig. 2 OrthologSorter pipeline

For comparisons of a large number of genomes (above 10 or so) in terms of their gene families a specialized tool is needed. One such tool is described next.

2.1 OrthologSorter

OrthologSorter is an automatic pipeline to compare genomes in terms of their protein-coding gene content, created by the authors. It is based on a relational database coupled with a user-friendly graphical interface; it thus provides a powerful platform to determine presence/absence of genes in up to several dozen genomes.

As input, the user needs to provide a folder containing all predicted proteins of each genome (usually .faa files such as the ones provided by NCBI) and a configuration file (example shown below). The whole pipeline (Fig. 2), contains three main steps:

2.2 Step 1: Building the Database of Genes, Genomes and Families

This step first takes as input all .faa files and runs an all-against-all Blastp [9] comparison of protein sequences in all genomes. The result of the Blastp run is used as input to OrthoMCL [10] in order to find protein families.

With all predicted protein files, all families found by OrthoMCL, and the configuration file (provided by the user) in hand, OrthologSorter builds a simple MySQL database with three tables, namely *genome, gene*, and *family*. The first holds information about each genome, including a binary (0/1) column that tells whether the genome is to be considered an outgroup. The gene table keeps information about each predicted protein gene, including the protein sequence itself, its product, the genome where the protein came from and its family, if any.

2.3 Step 2: Building the Web Pages

In this step the pipeline reads the database and builds two customized files to be used by the user to make further queries. The first is an HTML form, where the user can compare genomes in terms of presence/absence of genes in the families. In this form the user is given a choice for genome representation in the output: no representation (i.e., only families without this genome represented will be displayed); with at least one gene; with exactly one gene (this is useful to obtain families with one-to-one orthologs only), or *don't care* (meaning that this genome will not be considered when searching for families). Figure 3 shows an example of the web form for eight species of the genus *Bacillus*.

This step also generates a Perl script, customized for the database created and for the data (title and URL) informed in the configuration file. Given the name of the project (for example, *myproject*), this name is used to name the database, and to name the Perl script. Two folders are automatically generated. One should be copied to the directory where the Apache server can run executable files and the other is where web pages are located (in most Linux machines they should be placed (assuming "myproject" as a name) in /usr/lib/cgi-bin/myproject/ and /var/www/myproject/, respectively).

The main goal of the Perl script is to create MySQL query statements to find families according to the choices made by the user in the web form. After deciding which families satisfy the criteria chosen by the user, a list of families is created and for each one of those families a query is called in order to get its information.

The query below shows the resulting SQL query to find family 228 in the *Bacillus* example (one of the families containing exactly one gene of each genome):

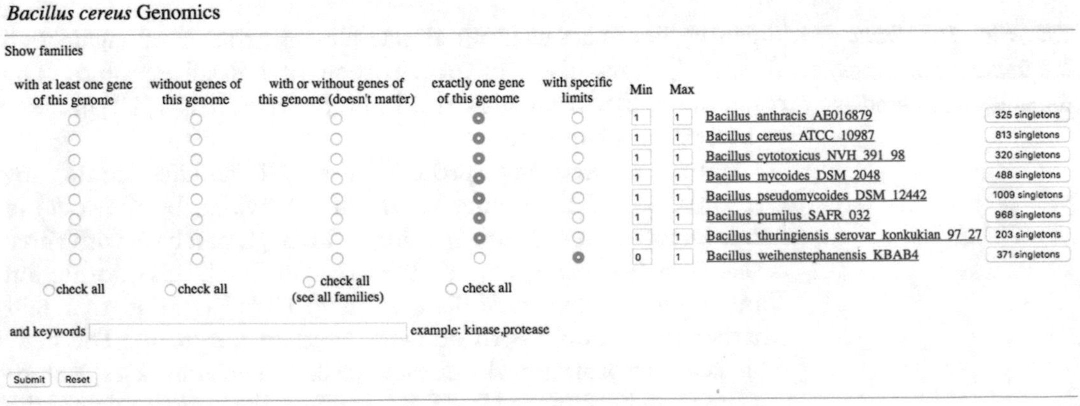

Fig. 3 Example of a web form built by the OrthologSorter pipeline

```
select gene_gi,gene_product,gene_sequence,gene_genome from
cereus.gene where gene_family=228 order by gene_genome.
```

Figure 4 shows some of the families found with this query.

2.4 Step 3: Building the Species Tree

Given the configuration file, the protein FASTA files, and the database built in **Step 1** (Subheading 2.2), OrthologSorter can automatically build a species tree using a supermatrix approach [11]. In this method it is necessary to avoid paralogs, so the pipeline selects gene families that contain exactly one gene from each ingroup genome, allowing zero or one gene from each outgroup genome. A multiple alignment of the proteins present in each family is generated using MUSCLE [12]. When there is no gene from a specific outgroup genome in the family, a row of spaces is used in the alignment to represent it. GBlocks [13] is then used to remove poorly aligned positions and divergent regions of each alignment. After this clean-up step, all alignments are concatenated and the concatenated alignment is fed as input to RAxML [14], which builds an unrooted phylogenetic tree, using by default the PROTCATJTT substitution model, with rapid bootstrapping (100 replicates) and subsequent Maximum Likelihood search. The tree is generated in Newick format. This Newick file is then given to NJplot [15] to generate a PDF file. Figure 5 shows the tree obtained for the set of eight *Bacillus* species, using *B. pumilus* SAFR 032 as an outgroup.

All the steps described above are easily managed by the user. Only two command-line calls are necessary. The first builds the

```
Result: 1580 families

========================================
>Family 228  -- Gblocks
30265505      nr  NP_847882.1 rnpA gene product [Bacillus anthracis str. Ames]
42784683      nr  NP_981930.1 rnpA gene product [Bacillus cereus ATCC 10987]
152977686     nr  YP_001377203.1 ribonuclease P [Bacillus cytotoxicus NVH 391-98]
229014653     nr  ZP_04171767.1 Ribonuclease P protein component [Bacillus mycoides DSM 2048]
228994206     nr  ZP_04154106.1 Ribonuclease P protein component [Bacillus pseudomycoides DSM 12442]
157694478     nr  YP_001488940.1 rnpA gene product [Bacillus pumilus SAFR-032]
49481129      nr  YP_039477.1 rnpA gene product [Bacillus thuringiensis serovar konkukian str. 97-27]
163943167     nr  YP_001648051.1 ribonuclease P [Bacillus weihenstephanensis KBAB4]
----------------------------------------
number of proteins = 8


========================================
>Family 229  -- Gblocks
30265504      nr  NP_847881.1 spoIIIJ-2 gene product [Bacillus anthracis str. Ames]
42784682      nr  NP_981929.1 spoIIIJ gene product [Bacillus cereus ATCC 10987]
152977685     nr  YP_001377202.1 OxaA-like protein precursor [Bacillus cytotoxicus NVH 391-98]
229014652     nr  ZP_04171766.1 Membrane protein oxaA 1 [Bacillus mycoides DSM 2048]
228994205     nr  ZP_04154105.1 Membrane protein oxaA 1 [Bacillus pseudomycoides DSM 12442]
157694477     nr  YP_001488939.1 spoIIIJ gene product [Bacillus pumilus SAFR-032]
49481123      nr  YP_039476.1 spoIIIJ gene product [Bacillus thuringiensis serovar konkukian str. 97-27]
163943166     nr  YP_001648050.1 OxaA-like protein precursor [Bacillus weihenstephanensis KBAB4]
----------------------------------------
number of proteins = 8


========================================
>Family 230  -- Gblocks
30265503      nr  NP_847880.1 jag gene product [Bacillus anthracis str. Ames]
42784681      nr  NP_981928.1 jag gene product [Bacillus cereus ATCC 10987]
152977684     nr  YP_001377201.1 single-stranded nucleic acid binding R3H domain-containing protein [Bacillus cytotoxicus NVH 391-98]
229014651     nr  ZP_04171765.1 hypothetical protein bmyco0001_50510 [Bacillus mycoides DSM 2048]
228994204     nr  ZP_04154104.1 hypothetical protein bpmyx0001_49270 [Bacillus pseudomycoides DSM 12442]
157694476     nr  YP_001488938.1 jag gene product [Bacillus pumilus SAFR-032]
49480476      nr  YP_039475.1 jag gene product [Bacillus thuringiensis serovar konkukian str. 97-27]
163943165     nr  YP_001648049.1 single-stranded nucleic acid binding R3H domain-containing protein [Bacillus weihenstephanensis KBAB4]
----------------------------------------
number of proteins = 8
```

Fig. 4 Example output of the tool OrthologSorter. In this example, 1580 families were found (for the same genomes shown in Fig. 3). Here we show descriptions for three families

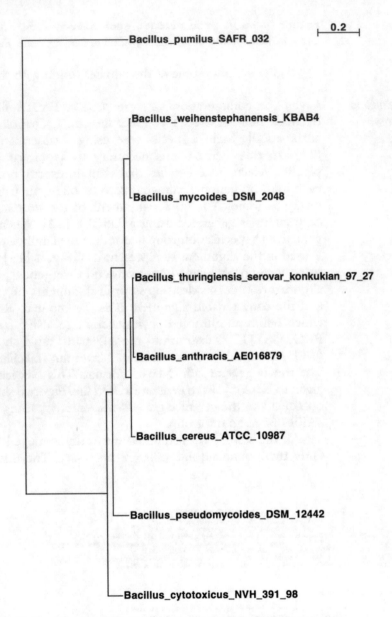

0.2

Bacillus_pumilus_SAFR_032

Bacillus_weihenstephanensis_KBAB4

Bacillus_mycoides_DSM_2048

Bacillus_thuringiensis_serovar_konkukian_97_27

Bacillus_anthracis_AE016879

Bacillus_cereus_ATCC_10987

Bacillus_pseudomycoides_DSM_12442

Bacillus_cytotoxicus_NVH_391_98

Fig. 5 Phylogenetic tree resulting from the final step in the OrthologSorter pipeline

database and the website; the second builds the tree. The user may skip some substeps. For instance, if the user provides the results of the all-against-all Blastp comparison (which is usually the computational bottleneck), OrthologSorter can start with the OrthoMCL step. The same applies to the OrthoMCL result itself; if provided, the tool starts the pipeline with the database building step. These bypassing tricks are automatic; the user only needs to place the Blastp and/or OrhtoMCL results in the right subfolders.

OrhtologSorter is available for download from http://git.facom.ufms.br/bioinfo/orthologsorter.git.

2.5 False Negatives and False Positives in Gene Content Comparisons

As noted in the Introduction, gene content comparison depends crucially on genome annotations. Because genome annotation is an imperfect process, regardless of the tool used, it is important to take into account two basic kinds of errors: missing (unannotated) genes (false negatives); and false predictions (false positives).

Missing genes are gene predictions that should have been made (because the corresponding genes do exist) but for some reason were not. This means that the content of a given cell in the presence/absence matrix is listed as *absent*, when in fact it should be listed as *present* (this error is particularly probable when there are draft genomes in the set under study; more on this in Subheading 8). False predictions are the opposite error: the gene is listed as *present*, when in fact it should be listed as *absent*. Both kinds of errors are inevitable, and one thing that can be done to minimize their occurrence is to ensure that the same automated pipeline is used to annotate all genomes of interest. This may be more difficult to implement than it may appear at first, especially if the genome set contains a mixture of publicly available genomes, and genomes that are not yet public. In these cases, it is likely that the publicly available genomes have been annotated with one pipeline, whereas the nonpublic genomes may have been annotated with another pipeline. We recommend that, whenever feasible, all genomes be annotated or reannotated with the same pipeline. In addition, it is good practice to examine manually "suspect" cases, such as presence or absence of genes that deviate from a given expectation or from some known pattern. For example, in Table 1 we see that genome *B* is the only one that does not have gene 2; this suggests that gene 2 may be a missing prediction in *B*. On the other hand, genome *D* is the only one to contain gene 5; this may be an indication that gene 5 is a false prediction. The evidence for the latter case would be weak, since we know from numerous genome reports over the years that it is still the case that almost every new genome will contain genes found in it and in no other genomes (so-called *orphan genes*). But it is also true that the majority of false predictions are found among such genes.

Note, finally, the following. Genome analysis papers usually refer to specific genes by their *locus tags*; these are gene identifiers and label specific physical locations in genomes. Every genome housed in GenBank has genes identified by locus tags. If one were to reannotate a public genome to ensure uniformity in annotation methods (as suggested above), then new locus tags would be generated, different from those publicly available. This may create some confusion. This can be mitigated by creating a correspondence table between newly generated locus tags and public ones.

3 Pan/Core Genome Analysis

Another kind of genome comparison that can be done with gene families is the pan and core genome analysis. The concept of pan genome analysis was introduced by Tettelin et al. [16], and it soon became an important tool in comparative genomics. A useful review of developments over 10 years after the introduction of the concept is given by Vernikos et al. [17] (but see also [18]).

Pan and core genomes are defined over a given set of genomes of interest, usually defined as strains of a species or species of a genus. A *pan genome* is defined as the set of distinct gene families that have been observed in *any* genome of the genomes being compared. The *core genome* is defined as the set of distinct gene families that have been observed in *all* genomes being compared. In other words, in order to belong to the core genome, a given gene family must be present in all genomes in the group.

These concepts can be easily understood by reference to a Venn diagram (Fig. 1). The pan genome is the union of all observed gene families (all regions in the Venn diagram); the core genome is the intersection of all observed gene families (the central region in the Venn diagram). In the case of the example of Fig. 1, we would have a core genome with 1234 genes, and a pan genome with $1234 + 129 + 337 + 215 + 45 + 68 + 23 = 2051$ genes.

There is a third related concept, which is known as the *variable* or *accessory genome*. This refers to gene families that do not belong to the core genome. For example, the region in Fig. 1 that represents the genes that are present in genomes *A* and *B*, but that are absent from genome *C* (containing 129 genes) would be part of the variable or accessory genome of these three genomes. The biological interpretation of these concepts is as follows. The core genome represents gene content that can be said to define members of the group under study: every member of the group must have these genes. The pan genome represents the universe of gene families that can be found in members of the group; and the variable genome represents those gene families that define subgroups within the large group, and potentially can be associated with phenotypic traits of interest that differentiate the members of a given subgroup from the rest.

The concepts of pan and core genomes seek to describe a given group of organisms, for which usually we have only a sample of individuals. It may be the case that the sample we have is not representative of the group, in which case the results may not be conclusive. Take for example the genus *Xanthomonas*. When we want to compute and describe its pan genome we will be restricted to available complete genomes in this genus, and this is just a small sample of the entire natural repertoire of species in this genus. Therefore, pan and core genomes are usually shown not by Venn

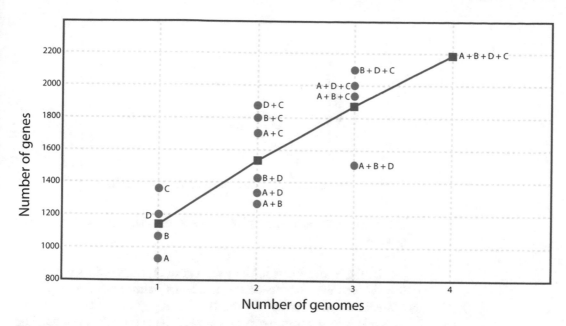

Fig. 6 Pan genome *curve* for four bacterial genomes, *A, B, C,* and *D.* Adapted from [37]

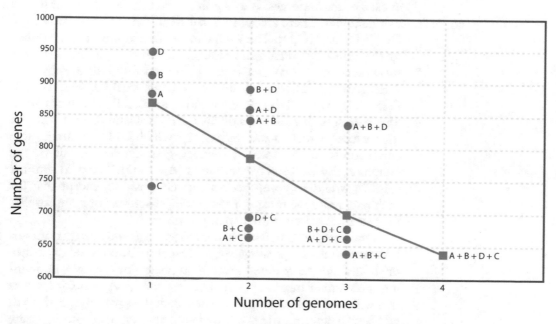

Fig. 7 Core genome *curve* for four bacterial genomes, *A, B, C,* and *D.* Adapted from [37]

diagrams or presence/absence tables, but by curves in graphs, which show the variation in pan and core genome size as more and more individual genomes are added to the computation (Figs. 6 and 7). We now describe the method to compute these curves. We will use a toy example with just four genomes: *A, B, C,* and *D,* and the computation of its pan genome.

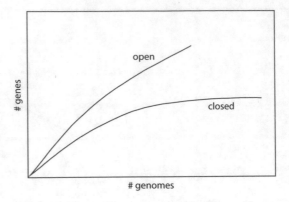

Fig. 8 Schematic representation of *curves* representing *open* and *closed* pan genomes

In Fig. 6 the *x* axis in the graph contains axis points representing the possible subsets of the genomes being considered. *X* axis point one corresponds to subsets of one genome. Because in our example we have four genomes, we will have four data points. The *y* value for each of those points corresponds to the number of genes in each of the genomes. *X* axis point two corresponds to subsets of two genomes. There are six such subsets: {A,B}, {A,C}, {A,D}, {B, C}, {B,D}, and {C,D}. The *y* value for each such subset corresponds to the sum of distinct gene families in the two genomes in that subset (the set union). *X* axis point three corresponds to subsets of three genomes. There are four such subsets: {A,B,C}, {A,B,D}, {A, C,D}, {B,C,D}, and the same reasoning applies. Finally, *x* axis point four corresponds to subsets of four genomes, and there is just one such subset, which is the entire set itself: {A,B,C,D}. Its *y* value corresponds to the sum of distinct gene families in all of the genomes, that is, the pan-genome of {A,B,C,D}. The core genome (Fig. 7) would be computed in a similar fashion, except that for each data point we must compute the *intersection* of gene families for the given subset, rather than the *union*.

One complicating issue in computing pan and core genomes is how to account for paralogs. Should paralogs be counted only once or should they be counted more than once? For example, in defining the number of genes contained in genome *A* alone, it appears that we should count all of its genes, including paralogs. But when we want to determine the union of genes present in *A* and *B*, we are faced with the following problem. A gene family in which both *A* and *B* have representatives should be counted only once, even if each genome has more than one representative in it (i.e., paralogs). What about a gene family with paralogs present only in *A*? Should we count it once or more than once?

Figure 8 represents schematically an example with an unspecified number of genomes (could be dozens, hundreds, or thousands). It allows us to introduce two other important concepts in pan genome analysis, which are the *open* and *closed* pan genomes. An *open pan genome* is one in which the addition of new genomes always increases the size of the pan genome (upper curve in Fig. 8); a *closed pan genome* is one in which the addition of any new genome, after a certain number, will not increase the size of its pan genome (lower curve in Fig. 8). In other words, for an open pan genome, every new genome sequenced will likely show the presence of genes not seen before in the group; whereas in a closed pan genome, if we have reached the upper limit, we will have seen all gene families that can possibly exist for that genome group. In order to determine whether a pan genome is closed or open we need to undertake a curve-fitting regression analysis on the pan genome data points (the medians for every computation point in the x-axis). If using a power law to do the regression, then the curve will have the general form $n = c\,N^{-\alpha}$, where n is the number of genes in the pan genome, N is the number of genomes being considered, c is a constant, and α is the exponent determined by the regression. If α is less than or equal to one, then the pan genome is open; otherwise it is closed. An example of an open pan genome is that of *Escherichia coli* (more than 16,000 genes [19]); an example of a closed pan genome is *Bacillus anthracis* (about 3000 genes [20]).

The computation of pan and core genome curves by the method described can become computationally prohibitive for a large number of genomes, because the number of subsets of n objects grows exponentially with the number of objects (2^n). Therefore, practical methods approximate this computation; we refer the reader to [17] for details.

A nice program for the computation of pan genomes is Get_Homologues [21]. Get_homologues uses 3rd party programs for computing orthologous groups. Once these have been computed, scripts in the package compute the pan and core genomes, as well as provide estimates for the core and pan genome sizes based on models given by Snipen et al. [22]. Another pan-genome analysis program is Roary [23]. Roary does not depend on 3rd party software, requires all input genomes to be from the same species, but is able to handle up to 1000 genomes even on a regular desktop.

4   Gene Content Comparison in Terms of Function

In the Introduction we mentioned that the second basic step of genome annotation is function assignment, and that one of the results is the association between a gene sequence and a protein product description together with a gene name or gene symbol. Given two or more annotated genomes, we describe here methods that allow comparison in terms of gene function.

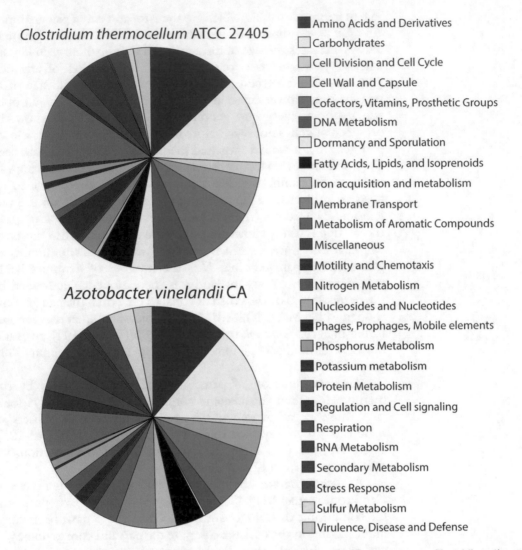

Fig. 9 Functional classification of two bacterial genomes based on RAST subsystems. *Clostridium thermocellum* (also known as *Ruminiclostridium thermocellum*) is a firmicutes bacterium first isolated in Yellowstone National Park, which is used as a model for studies in lignocellulose degradation [38]. *Azotobacter vinelandii* is a soil gammaproteobacterium capable of nitrogen fixation [39]. *C. thermocellum* is a sporulating bacterium, whereas *A. vinelandii* is not. This difference is evident from a comparison of the two pie charts, under category "Dormancy and sporulation"

A simple comparison can be readily achieved if some protein function description system, such as subsystems [7] or COG [24], has been used in gene annotation. For example, Fig. 9 illustrates two pie-charts giving subsystems functional annotations for two bacterial genomes. In this case the comparison is making use of *functional categories* available in subsystems. In general, functional comparisons can be made based on orthologous relationships as long as the resource that provides the ortholog families does include functional information associated with each family.

The actual implementation of this method can be seen as simple binning, i.e., for each genome in the set to be compared, count how many genes it has in category *A*, how many in category *B*, and so on. For this method to be correctly employed it is of course necessary that the same annotation pipeline be applied to all genomes being compared; note that it is not sufficient that all genomes be annotated with subsystems or COGs, because, for example, two different annotation pipelines might both be using the COG system, but assign COGs to protein sequences in not exactly the same way.

The method sketched above could also use the Gene Ontology (GO) [25]. The GO project is ambitious in scope, having as aim the "unification of biology" in terms of a controlled vocabulary (the GO terms) and relationships between the various terms. It is a hierarchical system, having at the top three terms: *molecular function*, *biological process*, and *cellular component*. All other terms in the system are the "children" or descendants of these three terms. Every term receives an identifier. For example, GO:0030254 denotes the term "protein secretion by the type III secretion system." Note however that COGs and GO are different entities. GO is an ontology; it does not prescribe how its terms should be associated with actual gene products, as is the case with COGs. In fact, GO has a long list of *evidence codes* that seek to cover all possible ways in which a GO term can be associated with a protein product, one of them being "Inferred from Direct Assay" (IDA) and another being "Inferred from Sequence or structural Similarity" (ISS). Over the years there have appeared in the literature several programs that seek to automatically associate protein sequences with GO terms; one of the most popular is the commercial program Blast2GO [26].

The reader should bear in mind that GO was initially developed having in mind eukaryotic model organisms, such as *Saccharomyces cerevisiae* (baker's yeast), *Caenorhabditis elegans* (a worm), *Drosophila melanogaster* (a fruit fly), and *Mus musculus* (the mouse). Even though more than 16 years have passed since GO was launched, it is still the case that COGs are a better system for the annotation of prokaryote genomes, for the simple reason that COG was initially developed as a functional classification system for prokaryote annotation.

Regardless of which system is used, genome comparison in terms of function may need to employ a *functional enrichment analysis tool*. These are tools that can do a statistical analysis of annotations as categorized by COGs or GO terms and determine whether certain functions or functional categories are statistically enriched in certain genomes compared to others. For GO, functional enrichment analysis is one of the tools provided by the program Blast2GO.

5   Whole Genome Alignments

Another important and useful way to compare genomes is to align them. Sequence comparison or alignment is a venerable subject in bioinformatics, and is arguably the problem that created this field. Here, we will briefly describe the problem in the context of whole genomes, and briefly describe tools to obtain whole genome alignments.

First, we need to define what we mean by whole genome. Because in this chapter we are dealing with prokaryotes only, we will adopt the simplifying assumption that a genome is a bacterial chromosome. A bacterial chromosome for the purposes of this section can be understood as a long (i.e., about 5 million bp) linear DNA sequence (the case of circular sequences is dealt with at the end of this Section).

Conceptually, whole genome alignment is also sequence alignment; thus in theory any sequence alignment algorithm could be used to compare whole genomes. However, the length of whole genomes, even when restricted to bacterial chromosomes, makes the use of certain sequence comparison algorithms impractical; under this category are all algorithms based on dynamic programming, of which the best known example is the Smith-Waterman algorithm (whose description can be found in textbooks, for example [27]). This means that, from a computational perspective, whole genome alignment and protein (or short DNA) sequence alignment are two different problems.

Another distinction that needs to be made is that between the pairwise alignment case and the multiple (three or more genomes) alignment case. The comparison of two sequences can be seen as a special case of the comparison of n sequences, meaning that an algorithm for the multiple case can be used to compare two sequences; however, such an approach would be highly undesirable, because it would not take into account the simplifications available for the case of $n = 2$, both in theory and in practice.

With these preliminaries covered, we can now describe the pairwise case, followed by the multiple case.

5.1 Pairwise Alignments

The goal in this case is to obtain the alignment of two whole genomes. The result is often displayed graphically, as shown in Fig. 10. However, any pairwise alignment tool should also generate a *coordinate file*, in which we can examine the alignment in much greater detail than would be possible in a low-resolution graphical display.

Whole genome alignment programs use a technique first pioneered by BLAST [9], and generally known as the seed-and-extend method. The idea is to determine short sequences (between, say, 10 and 30 bp) that are shared and identical by the two genomes in a

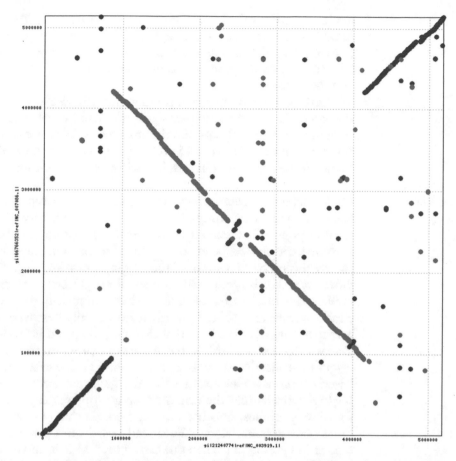

Fig. 10 Whole genome pairwise alignment between the chromosomes of *Xanthomonas citri* subsp. *citri* strain A306 (*x* axis) and *Xanthomonas campestris* pv. *campestris* strain 8004 (*y* axis). This alignment was obtained with the nucmer script of program MUMmer. Every *dot* in the diagram is a MUM. *Red* dots represent MUMs that match in the same strand on both genomes; whereas *blue* dots represent MUMs that match in opposite strands. The X-pattern seen in this figure means that one genome underwent a chromosomal inversion with respect to the other [40]

very efficient manner; the result of this step is a collection of short alignments, or *seed alignments*. In a second step the algorithm seeks to extend these seeds into longer alignments, perhaps connecting those that are close enough. Because the first step usually dramatically decreases the space of possible alignments, it is possible to use more refined (and therefore slower) techniques for this second step, such as running the Smith-Waterman algorithm on the two sequences that are between two previously found seed alignments.

Among the available programs for whole genome pairwise alignment, one of the most popular is MUMmer [28]. The seed alignments in MUMmer are called Maximal Unique Matches, or MUMs. The program finds them thanks to a very efficient implementation of the suffix tree data structure [29]. As a result, MUMmer is very fast, being capable of aligning two average-size (4 Mbp) bacterial chromosomes on a standard desktop computer in less than a minute. The alignment shown in Fig. 10 was created with MUMmer.

YOC [30] is a more recent program for pairwise whole genome alignment. It employs a simpler algorithm than that of other similar programs, and its authors claim that, as a result, YOC is easier to use and parameterize. However, YOC can only align genomes that are known to be basically collinear, i.e., without translocations.

5.1.1 How to Deal with Circularity

Most bacterial chromosomes are circular, but are represented as linear sequences in computer files. It is a convention that the starting point of a linear sequence representing a circular bacterial chromosome should be at the origin of replication, or close to it (when the precise location of the origin is not known). Because different research groups will in general use different strategies to predict the origin of replication, when comparing two circular chromosomes represented linearly it is generally best to execute a preprocessing step to ensure that their starting point is "the same." One way to deal with this is to run the same program to predict the origin of replication on both genomes, and re-linearize them both based on results. This assumes that the genomes are close enough phylogenetically that the origin of replication region is conserved for these genomes. Another strategy assumes that one of the genomes (say, genome A) was linearized based on a good origin of replication prediction. Then one can align A with B, and determine where in genome B is the alignment with base 1 from genome A; and then re-linearize B based on that information. This would be the strategy to linearize a newly assembled genome based on an alignment with a reference genome.

5.2 Multiple Alignments

In terms of computational requirements, whole genome multiple alignment is a much more complex problem than the pairwise case. This means that aligning ten bacterial genomes will in general require much more than simply five times more time and memory than aligning two genomes of the same length. Nevertheless, it can be done, again using variations of the seed-and-extend technique already mentioned. The program MAUVE [31] is currently perhaps the most powerful and versatile program for multiple whole genome alignment. One of its most popular features is a nice graphical interface. An example alignment obtained with MAUVE can be seen in Fig. 11.

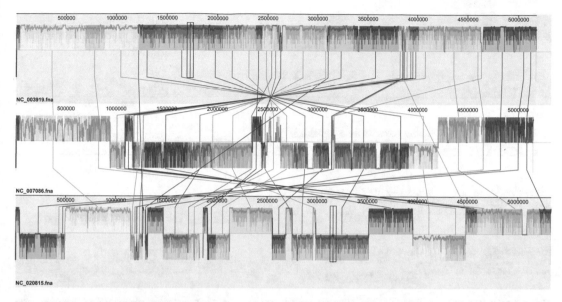

Fig. 11 Three-way chromosome alignment of *Xanthomonas citri* subsp. *citri* strain A306 (*first row*), *Xanthomonas campestris* pv. *campestris* strain 8004 (*second row*), and *Xanthomonas citri* subsp. *citri* strain Aw12879. The alignment was obtained with program MAUVE. The colored blocks are alignment regions, or *local collinear blocks* in the MAUVE terminology. The inversion noted in the pairwise alignment of Fig. 10 is clearly visible here as well, although in a different representation. The alignment also makes clear that the two citri strains have more rearrangements between them than either one has with the campestris strain, a fact, given the taxonomy, somewhat surprising

6   Ortholog Alignments and Synteny

An important concept in the comparison of whole genomes is *synteny*. In a genomic context, synteny means conservation of gene order. That is, we will say a genome region *g* in genome *A* is *syntenic* with a genome region *h* in genome *B*, if each gene present in region *g* has a corresponding ortholog in *h*, and all genes in *g* appear in the same order as the genes in *h*. We say that regions *g* and *h* form a *syntenic block*. When comparing one or more genomes, it is important to look for synteny, because syntenic blocks generally represent conserved blocks, that is, genome sections that have not undergone internal rearrangements since the most recent common ancestor of the genomes being compared; this conservation in turn may suggest functional evolutionary constraints that are worth knowing about.

The detection of synteny can be done with the whole genome alignment programs that we discussed in the previous section. Any aligned region containing more than one gene will very likely be a syntenic block. However certain syntenic blocks may be missed by these programs, as we now explain.

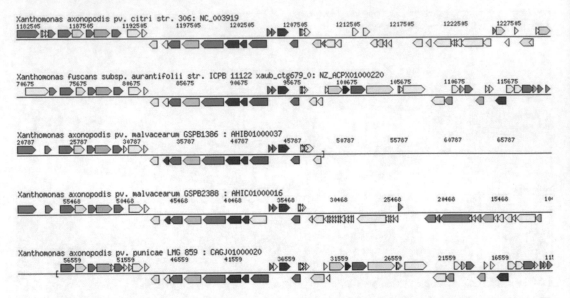

Fig. 12 An ortholog alignment between a small section (20 kbp) of five Xanthomonas genomes obtained with the IMG system [6]. Each *line* represents one genome, and the *arrows* represent genes. Orthologous genes are represented with the same *color*. It is clear that there is a syntenic block in the *central* region of this alignment. To the *left* and *right* of this region there is less conservation. The alignment was generated by requesting the genomic neighborhood of *Xanthomonas axonopodis* pv. *citri* str. 306 gene with locus tag XAC1046, which is annotated as an isocitrate dehydrogenase. The other genomes that appear in the alignment are chosen automatically by the IMG tool

The program MAUVE requires as input nucleotide sequences; it bases its comparison on nucleotide sequence similarity. If a pair of orthologs is sufficiently diverged, MAUVE will likely miss it (i.e., display their region as not aligned because it is not similar enough); a whole syntenic block may be missed if this divergence applies to all genes in the block. MUMmer is less susceptible to this problem because it provides a script called *promer* that allows for the comparison of translated nucleotide sequences.

An entirely different approach that can in principle deal with this problem is to compare the genomes not in terms of their nucleotide sequences, but in terms of orthology relationships. This can be done as follows (assuming a pairwise alignment). First, we have to determine the orthology relationships between the protein-coding gene sets in the two genomes. Then, treating each pair of orthologs as a *symbol*, and assigning each non-ortholog a separate and different symbol, we align the two genomes using a standard alignment algorithm (such as Smith-Waterman), treating each genome as a sequence of these symbols. Syntenic blocks will then be the resulting aligned regions. An example of such an alignment can be seen in Fig. 12.

To our knowledge there is no public tool that will accept user-provided genomes and generate ortholog alignments. But both the IMG platform [6] and PATRIC [32] offer the possibility of visualizing a pile-up of genomic neighborhoods, once a specific gene in a given genome present in their databases is chosen. Depending on how much conservation of order there is either downstream or upstream of the chosen gene, the neighborhood may contain a syntenic block.

7   Single-Value Whole Genome Comparison

Another useful way to compare whole genomes is by computing a value that summarizes their similarity or distance. The concept of sequence distance is in a certain mathematical sense the opposite of sequence similarity: two identical sequences have 100% identity and zero distance. Sequences that are not identical have similarity as measured by % identity that is less than 100%, and their distance will be greater than zero. A rigorous mathematical analysis of similarity and distance can be found in [27].

Single-value genomic comparisons are most useful when we want to obtain a simple and general picture of the relationships between several genomes, without resorting to full-blown alignments. Usually, this is done by computing all pairwise distances for the genomes of interest, thereby creating a *genome distance matrix*. Depending on the situation, this matrix by itself can already be quite informative. It can also be used to reconstruct a phylogeny, by feeding it to a distance-based phylogeny reconstruction algorithm such as neighbor-joining (as implemented, for example, by MEGA [33]).

Here, we describe two practical implementations of genomic distance. The reader should keep in mind that each of these methods adopts a different concept of genomic distance, and therefore they are not comparable.

The first method is called MUMi, or MUM index [34]. It is based on the concept of MUM (explained above) and the program MUMmer. The distance formula is simply

$$MUMi = 1 \cdot L_{mum} / L_{av},$$

where L_{mum} is the sum of the lengths of all nonoverlapping MUMs and L_{av} is the average length of the two genomes being compared. By this definition MUMi values are always in the interval [0,1], with values close to one meaning that the genomes are quite dissimilar. MUMi values are computed by a simple perl script provided in the supplementary information in the cited paper. The MUMi paper contains the result that most species within a genus are generally at a MUMi distance of 0.9–1 from each other; this indicates that MUMi is most effective when comparing different strains rather than different species, although this result will vary depending on genus.

The second method we mention is called Genome Blast Distance Phylogeny (GBDP), first proposed in a 2005 paper [35], and subsequently refined, most recently in [36]. GBDP is a much more sophisticated genome distance measure than MUMi, since it seeks to be a rigorous in silico replacement for DNA–DNA hybridization wet-lab experiments, and hence the basis for a genome-based taxonomy gold standard for bacteria and archaea. Among other features, GBDP in its latest incarnation allows the computation of confidence intervals on the computed values. It is possible to perform GBDP comparisons on the developers' website (http://ggdc.dsmz.de).

8   Draft Genomes: How Incompleteness Affects Comparisons

As stated in the introduction, we assumed that genomes being compared are complete. However, nowadays the vast majority of sequenced prokaryotic genomes are made available only in draft format. Usually, the deposited sequences of draft genomes are the result of automated assembly, without any curation, which may therefore contain incorrectly assembled contigs. Hence, when the genomes to be compared include some in draft format, care must be exercised. Here we outline a few precautions, considering the methods we have covered.

For gene-content comparison, the obvious caveat is that one needs to be very careful about statements pointing to the absence of genes in draft genomes, for the obvious reason that those apparently missing genes might be there, but were missed in the sequencing process. For precisely this same reason, draft genomes may be a particular concern when computing pan and core genomes. Unless draft genomes are in a "near finished" status, meaning that there is confidence that a small fraction (less than 1%) of the genome is missing, they should not be used in pan/core computations.

For whole genome alignments, draft genomes can be a problem, especially if the number of contigs is large. Some useful information can still be obtained by pairwise alignment of draft genomes; the program MUMmer for example can readily compare two draft genomes, and will provide detailed results on how contigs align to one another.

9   Conclusion

We currently live in the age of the genomic revolution. In the not too distant future there will be more than a million prokaryotic genomes available for study and comparison. Fortunately, there has been a parallel revolution in the development of computational tools to compare all these genomes. This chapter has presented a glimpse of what is available. The authors hope that this sample will provide students and researchers with an entry point into the exciting world of prokaryote genome comparisons.

Acknowledgments

This work was supported in part by a CNPq researcher fellowship (J.C.S. and N.F.A.); by CAPES grant 3385/2013 (BIGA project) (J.C.S. and N.F.A.); by Fundect-MS grants TO141/2016 and TO007/2015 (N.F.A); and by the National Institute of Allergy and Infectious Diseases, National Institutes of Health, Department of Health and HumanServices, under contract no. HHSN272201400027C (A.R.W.).

References

1. Hyatt D et al (2010) Prodigal: prokaryotic gene recognition and translation initiation site identification. BMC Bioinformatics 11:119

2. Delcher AL et al (1999) Improved microbial gene identification with GLIMMER. Nucleic Acids Res 27(23):4636–4641

3. Besemer J, Borodovsky M (2005) GeneMark: web software for gene finding in prokaryotes, eukaryotes and viruses. Nucleic Acids Res 33 (Web Server issue):W451–W454

4. Seemann T (2014) Prokka: rapid prokaryotic genome annotation. Bioinformatics 30 (14):2068–2069

5. Tatusova T et al (2016) NCBI prokaryotic genome annotation pipeline. Nucleic Acids Res 44(14):6614–6624

6. Markowitz VM et al (2012) IMG: the integrated microbial genomes database and comparative analysis system. Nucleic Acids Res 40(Database issue):D115–D122

7. Overbeek R et al (2014) The SEED and the rapid annotation of microbial genomes using subsystems technology (RAST). Nucleic Acids Res 42(Database issue):D206–D214

8. Chen H, Boutros PC (2011) VennDiagram: a package for the generation of highly-customizable Venn and Euler diagrams in R. BMC Bioinformatics 12:35

9. Altschul SF et al (1997) Gapped BLAST and PSI-BLAST: a new generation of protein database search programs. Nucleic Acids Res 25 (17):3389–3402

10. Li L, Stoeckert CJ Jr, Roos DS (2003) OrthoMCL: identification of ortholog groups for eukaryotic genomes. Genome Res 13 (9):2178–2189

11. Lang JM, Darling AE, Eisen JA (2013) Phylogeny of bacterial and archaeal genomes using conserved genes: supertrees and supermatrices. PLoS One 8(4):e62510

12. Edgar RC (2004) MUSCLE: a multiple sequence alignment method with reduced time and space complexity. BMC Bioinformatics 5:113

13. Castresana J (2000) Selection of conserved blocks from multiple alignments for their use in phylogenetic analysis. Mol Biol Evol 17 (4):540–552

14. Stamatakis A (2014) RAxML version 8: a tool for phylogenetic analysis and post-analysis of large phylogenies. Bioinformatics 30 (9):1312–1313

15. Perriere G, Thioulouse J (1996) On-line tools for sequence retrieval and multivariate statistics in molecular biology. Comput Appl Biosci 12 (1):63–69

16. Tettelin H et al (2005) Genome analysis of multiple pathogenic isolates of Streptococcus agalactiae: implications for the microbial "pan-genome". Proc Natl Acad Sci U S A 102 (39):13950–13955

17. Vernikos G et al (2015) Ten years of pan-genome analyses. Curr Opin Microbiol 23:148–154

18. Marschall T (2016) Computational pan-genomics: status, promises and challenges. Brief Bioinform bbw089

19. Kaas RS et al (2012) Estimating variation within the genes and inferring the phylogeny of 186 sequenced diverse Escherichia Coli genomes. BMC Genomics 13:577

20. Rouli L et al (2014) Genomic analysis of three African strains of bacillus anthracis demonstrates that they are part of the clonal expansion of an exclusively pathogenic bacterium. New Microbes New Infect 2(6):161–169

21. Contreras-Moreira B, Vinuesa P (2013) GET_HOMOLOGUES, a versatile software package for scalable and robust microbial pangenome analysis. Appl Environ Microbiol 79 (24):7696–7701

22. Snipen L, Almoy T, Ussery DW (2009) Microbial comparative pan-genomics using binomial mixture models. BMC Genomics 10:385

23. Page AJ et al (2015) Roary: rapid large-scale prokaryote pan genome analysis. Bioinformatics 31(22):3691–3693

24. Galperin MY et al (2015) Expanded microbial genome coverage and improved protein family annotation in the COG database. Nucleic Acids Res 43(Database issue):D261–D269

25. Ashburner M et al (2000) Gene ontology: tool for the unification of biology the gene ontology consortium. Nat Genet 25(1):25–29

26. Conesa A et al (2005) Blast2GO: a universal tool for annotation, visualization and analysis in functional genomics research. Bioinformatics 21(18):3674–3676

27. Setubal JC, Meidanis J (1997) Introduction to computational molecular biology. PWS, Boston, MA

28. Kurtz S et al (2004) Versatile and open software for comparing large genomes. Genome Biol 5(2):R12

29. Gusfield D (1997) Algorithms on strings, trees, and sequences. Cambridge University Press, New York

30. Uricaru R et al (2015) YOC, a new strategy for pairwise alignment of collinear genomes. BMC Bioinformatics 16:111

31. Darling AC et al (2004) Mauve: multiple alignment of conserved genomic sequence with rearrangements. Genome Res 14 (7):1394–1403

32. Wattam AR et al (2014) PATRIC, the bacterial bioinformatics database and analysis resource. Nucleic Acids Res 42(Database issue): D581–D591

33. Kumar S, Stecher G, Tamura K (2016) MEGA7: molecular evolutionary genetics analysis version 7.0 for bigger datasets. Mol Biol Evol 33(7):1870–1874

34. Deloger M, El Karoui M, Petit MA (2009) A genomic distance based on MUM indicates discontinuity between most bacterial species and genera. J Bacteriol 191(1):91–99

35. Henz SR et al (2005) Whole-genome prokaryotic phylogeny. Bioinformatics 21 (10):2329–2335

36. Meier-Kolthoff JP et al (2013) Genome sequence-based species delimitation with confidence intervals and improved distance functions. BMC Bioinformatics 14:60

37. Wulff NA et al (2014) The complete genome sequence of 'Candidatus Liberibacter americanus', associated with citrus huanglongbing. Mol Plant Microbe Interact 27(2):163–176

38. Akinosho H et al (2014) The emergence of clostridium thermocellum as a high utility candidate for consolidated bioprocessing applications. Front Chem 2:66

39. Setubal JC et al (2009) Genome sequence of Azotobacter vinelandii, an obligate aerobe specialized to support diverse anaerobic metabolic processes. J Bacteriol 191 (14):4534–4545

40. Eisen JA et al (2000) Evidence for symmetric chromosomal inversions around the replication origin in bacteria. Genome Biol 1(6): RESEARCH0011

Chapter 4

Assembly, Annotation, and Comparative Genomics in PATRIC, the All Bacterial Bioinformatics Resource Center

Alice R. Wattam, Thomas Brettin, James J. Davis, Svetlana Gerdes, Ronald Kenyon, Dustin Machi, Chunhong Mao, Robert Olson, Ross Overbeek, Gordon D. Pusch, Maulik P. Shukla, Rick Stevens, Veronika Vonstein, Andrew Warren, Fangfang Xia, and Hyunseung Yoo

Abstract

In the "big data" era, research biologists are faced with analyzing new types that usually require some level of computational expertise. A number of programs and pipelines exist, but acquiring the expertise to run them, and then understanding the output can be a challenge.

The Pathosystems Resource Integration Center (PATRIC, www.patricbrc.org) has created an end-to-end analysis platform that allows researchers to take their raw reads, assemble a genome, annotate it, and then use a suite of user-friendly tools to compare it to any public data that is available in the repository. With close to 113,000 bacterial and more than 1000 archaeal genomes, PATRIC creates a unique research experience with "virtual integration" of private and public data. PATRIC contains many diverse tools and functionalities to explore both genome-scale and gene expression data, but the main focus of this chapter is on assembly, annotation, and the downstream comparative analysis functionality that is freely available in the resource.

Key words Assembly, Annotation, Comparative genomics, Bacteria, Archaea, Bioinformatics

1 Introduction

The Pathosystems Resource Integration Center (PATRIC) is the all-bacterial Bioinformatics Resource Center (BRC) http://www.patricbrc.org [1]. Established by the National Institute of Allergy and Infectious Diseases (NIAID), PATRIC provides researchers with an online resource that stores and integrates a variety of data types [e.g., genomics, transcriptomics, protein–protein interactions (PPIs), three-dimensional protein structures, and sequence typing data] and associated metadata. The PATRIC website is primarily organism-centric, with various levels of genomic data and associated information related to each included organism. While the PATRIC homepage lists the 22 watch list genera for easy access to

João C. Setubal et al. (eds.), *Comparative Genomics: Methods and Protocols*, Methods in Molecular Biology, vol. 1704, https://doi.org/10.1007/978-1-4939-7463-4_4, © Springer Science+Business Media LLC 2018

data associated with many pathogenic species, compilation and organization of all relevant data for "All Bacteria" are standardized according to bacterial (NCBI) taxonomy, with options for viewing sets of genomes within the hierarchical bacterial tree.

With an emphasis on consistency in comparative genomic analysis, PATRIC has standardized annotation of all available bacterial genomes using the RAST (rapid annotation using subsystems technology) system [2, 3]. All of the 114,000+ genomes in PATRIC (March 2016) have been annotated using RAST [2, 3], which facilitates the ease of comparative analysis. In addition to the RAST-based annotations, PATRIC preserves and provides the historical annotations present at GenBank (RefSeq), allowing researchers to compare differences between the two. Summaries of the different data types (genes, RNAs, etc.) from both PATRIC and RefSeq annotations are available across different taxonomic levels, and also provided for both genomes and for individual genes.

PATRIC has expanded its research capabilities by now offering new services that include assembly and annotation pipelines, and allows researchers to compare their private data to all the public data currently available using a suite of analysis tools. PATRIC also provides pipelines for RNA-Seq, metabolic modeling, and a new variation service. The ability to take raw data, run it through appropriate pipelines, and then "virtually integrates" it with all the public data found in the resource provides PATRIC users with a powerful analysis experience.

Here, we describe two of the new PATRIC services that allow researchers to upload and assemble their raw reads, and then annotate them using the RASTtk pipeline. We then demonstrate how researchers can analyze their private genomic data with the analysis tools that PATRIC provides, including the Proteome Comparison and Protein Family Sorter comparative analysis tools.

2 Material

New services in PATRIC allow researchers to take their raw reads from a variety of sequencing machines and produce an annotated genome. The specific services include a variety of options for assembly of reads as well as a pipeline to annotate those reads. The newly annotated genome, which can only be seen by the researcher who submitted it, can be compared to up to nine genomes by BLASTP using PATRIC's Proteome Comparison tool, or up to 400 genomes using the Protein Family Sorter. This allows researchers to do a more fine-detailed analysis comparing a few genomes, or a broad reaching analysis that looks for patterns shared across hundreds of genomes.

3   Methods

3.1   Assembling a Genome at PATRIC

There are a variety of programs that can be used to assemble the reads that are produced from sequencing machines into contigs or chromosomes, but these can require an advanced programming ability that research biologists are sometimes lacking. To meet this need PATRIC allows researchers to assemble short reads that are single or paired (typically from Illumina machines), and also long reads from PacBio or Nanopore [4] machines. PATRIC provides several assembly tools and pipelines, the results of which are downloaded into a researcher's private workspace.

Below is the methodology showing the assembly for single reads using the default assembly method.

3.1.1   Locating the Assembly Service App

1. At the top of any PATRIC page, find the Services tab (Fig. 1).
2. Click on Genome Assembly.
3. This will open up the Assembly landing page where researchers can submit long reads, single or paired read files (Fig. 2).

3.1.2   Uploading Sequence Reads and Submitting a Paired-Read Assembly Job

Many paired read libraries are given as file pairs, with each file containing half of each read pair. Paired read files are expected to be sorted in such a way that each read in a pair occurs in the same Nth position as its mate in their respective files. These files are specified as READ FILE 1 and READ FILE 2. For a given file

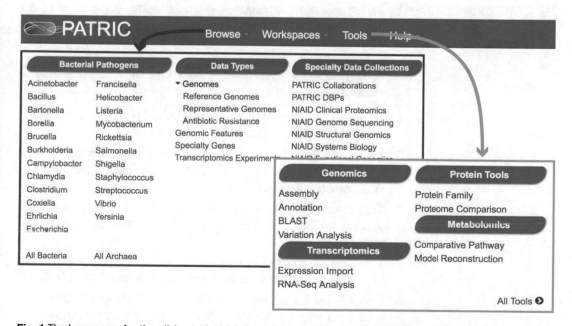

Fig. 1 The homepage for the all-bacterial bioinformatics resource center, PATRIC (www.patricbrc.org) with the Services and Tools tabs that provide access to pipelines and tools for data analysis

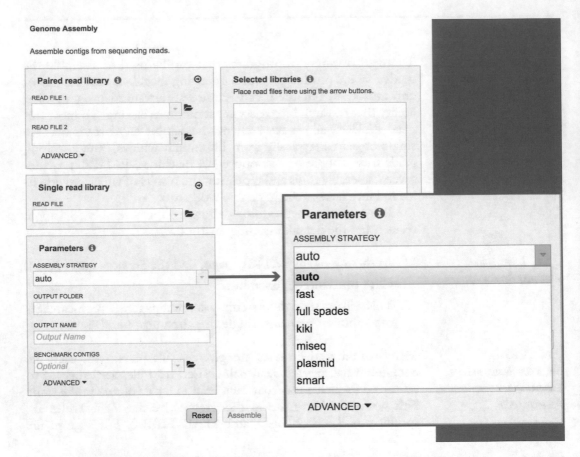

Fig. 2 PATRIC's genome assembly landing page where researchers can assemble either single- or paired-end short reads, or longer reads from PacBio or Nanopore, with an enlargement showing the different assembly strategies available

pair, the selection of which file is READ 1 and which is READ 2 does not matter.

1. To upload a fastq file that contains paired reads, locate the box called "Paired read library."

2. The reads must be located in the workspace. To initiate the upload, first click on the folder icon that follows the text box underneath READ FILE 1.

3. This opens up a window where the files for upload can be selected. Click on the upload icon that has an arrow pointing up.

4. This opens a new window where the file you want to upload can be selected. Click on the blue bar that is labeled "Select File."

5. This will open a window that allows you to choose files that are stored on your computer. Select the file where you stored the fastq file on your computer.

6. Once selected, the name of the file will be auto-filled under the words File Selected. You can see it in the screenshot below. Click on the Upload Files button that you will see at the bottom of the window.

7. This will auto-fill the name of the document into the text box below READ FILE 1 in the Paired read library box.

8. Repeat **steps 2–5** to upload the second pair of reads.

9. To finish the upload, click on the icon of an arrow within a circle that you will see in the upper right corner of the Paired read library box. This will move your file into the Selected libraries box that you will see in the adjacent panel.

3.1.3 Uploading Single Reads and Submitting an Assembly Job

1. To upload a fastq file that contains single reads, locate the box called "Single read library."

2. If the reads have previously been uploaded, click the down arrow next to the text box that occurs below the words "Read File."

3. This opens up a drop-down box that shows all the reads that have been previously uploaded into the user account. Click on the name of the reads of interest.

4. This will auto-fill the name of the document into the text box that occurs below the words "Read File."

5. To finish the upload, click on the icon of an arrow within a circle that you will see in the upper right corner of the Single read library box. This will move your file into the Selected libraries box that you will see in the adjacent panel, where it is ready to be assembled.

3.1.4 Selecting the Right Parameters for an Assembly Job

1. The last step of the assembly process is filling in the metadata parameters that define where the assembled contigs are placed in the workspace. PATRIC offers several different assembly strategies that can be viewed by clicking on the down-arrow following the text box under Assembly Strategy in the Parameters box.

   - The **auto** assembly strategy runs BayesHammer [5] on short reads, followed by three assembly strategies that include Velvet [6], IDBA [7], and Spades [8], each of which is given an assembly score by ARAST, an in-house script.

   - The **fast** assembly strategy runs MEGAHIT [9] and Velvet, with each assembly given a score determined by ARAST.

   - Users can also choose the **full spades** strategy, which runs BayesHammer followed by Spades.

   - Choosing **kiki** runs the Kiki assembler, an in-house script.

- Illumina MiSeq reads should be assembled using **miseq**, which runs Velvet with hash length 35, and then BayesHammer on reads and assembles with SPAdes with k up to 99, followed by a score using ARAST.

- The **smart** strategy can be used for long or short reads. The strategy for short reads when using **smart** involves running BayesHammer on reads, Kmergenie [10] to choose hashlength for Velvet, followed by the same assembly strategy using Velvet [6], IDBA [7], and Spades [8]. Assemblies are sorted with an ALE score [11] and the two best assemblies are merged using GAM-NGS [12].

- PacBio and Nanopore long reads only work with the auto and smart strategies. In either case, they are automatically assembled using MiniASM [13].

2. First time assembly users will have to create a folder to hold the assembly jobs. Click on the folder icon that is next to the text box under the words OUTPUT FOLDER.

3. In the window that pops up, click on the folder icon.

4. In the available text box, enter the name for the new folder, then click the OK button at the bottom right of the box.

5. This will auto-fill the name of folder that the assembly job will be stored in.

6. The next step is to assign the name of the assembly. Enter the name into the text box below OUTPUT NAME.

7. To compare the PATRIC assembly to a known assembly, click on the down-arrow next to the text box under BENCHMARK CONTIGS and follow the same upload instructions Subheadings 3.1.2 or 3.1.3 above.

3.1.5 Submitting the Assembly Job

1. To submit the job, click on the Assemble button that is in the bottom center of the window.

2. If the job was submitted successfully, a message that says "Assembly Job has been queued" will appear above the Assemble button.

3. To check the status of the assembly job, click on the Jobs indicator at the bottom right of the PATRIC page. This is to the right of a box that indicates the number of uploads.

4. Clicking on Jobs box opens the Jobs Status page, where researchers can see the progression of the assembly job as well as the status of all the previous service jobs that have been submitted.

3.2 Genome Annotation in PATRIC

The Genome Annotation Service uses the RAST tool kit (RASTtk) [3] to provide annotation of genomic features. All genomes in PATRIC have been annotated with this service, and researchers can submit their own private genome to the annotation service, where it will be deposited into their private workspace for their perusal.

3.2.1 Locating the Annotation Service App

1. At the top of any PATRIC page, find the Services tab.
2. Click on Genome Annotation.
3. This will open up the Annotation Service landing page (Fig. 3).

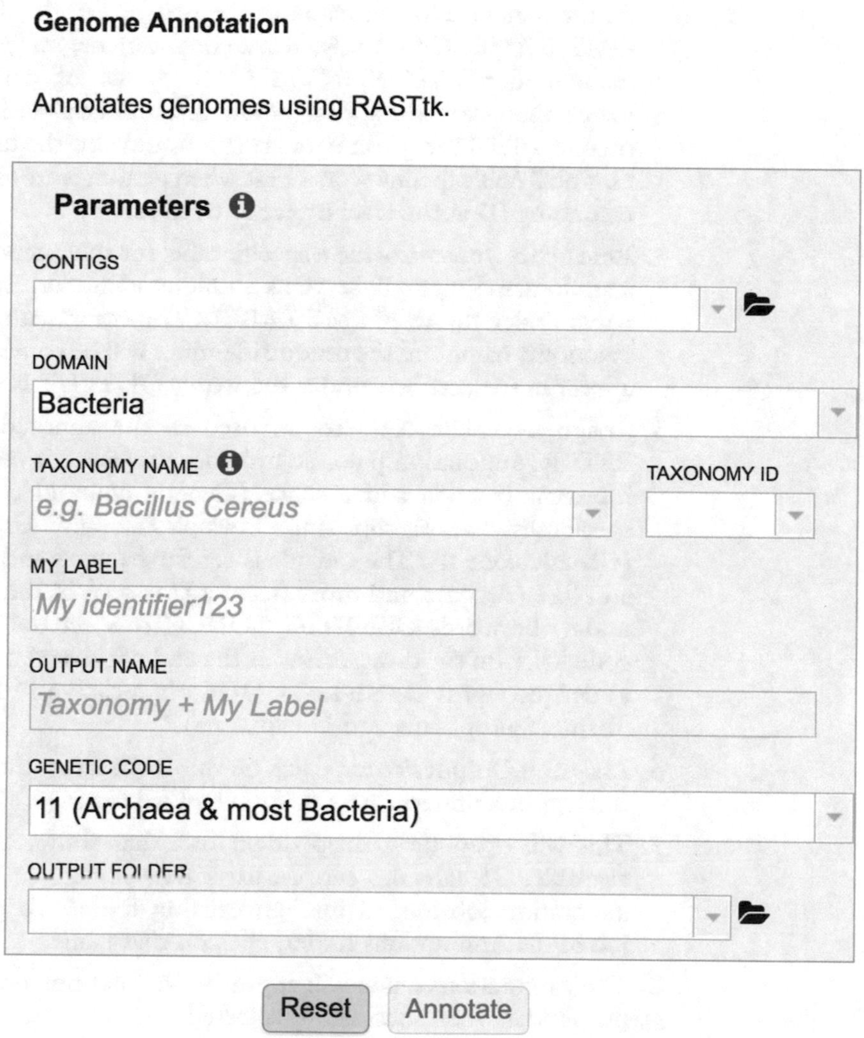

Genome Annotation

Annotates genomes using RASTtk.

Parameters ❶

CONTIGS

DOMAIN

Bacteria

TAXONOMY NAME ❶   TAXONOMY ID

e.g. Bacillus Cereus

MY LABEL

My identifier123

OUTPUT NAME

Taxonomy + My Label

GENETIC CODE

11 (Archaea & most Bacteria)

OUTPUT FOLDER

Reset   Annotate

Fig. 3 The genome annotation landing page where researchers can annotate assemblies they have generated in PATRIC, or that have been assembled elsewhere

3.2.2   Uploading Contigs
and Submitting an
Annotation Job

1. Researchers can upload contigs from an assembly job completed in PATRIC, or from an external source. To submit a PATRIC assembly for annotation click on the down arrow that follows the text box underneath the words CONTIGS.

2. This will open up a drop-down box that will show all the assemblies that are currently in the researcher's private workspace. Click on the one of interest to upload it. The name will then appear in the text box beneath the word CONTIGS.

3. Researchers must assign a taxonomy rank for their genome. They can either enter the NCBI taxonomy id (http://www.ncbi.nlm.nih.gov/taxonomy) for their organism, or begin typing the name. Entering the taxonomy id number in the box below TAXONOMY ID will show the id number, and will also fill the matching taxon name in the text box under TAXONOMY NAME. Conversely, researchers can begin typing the name under TAXONOMY NAME. A list of names that match the entry will appear below the text box, and clicking on one will fill the taxon name text box and also the taxonomy id. The RAST pipeline works best when genomes are assigned a taxonomy ID at the level of genus or lower.

4. Researchers must provide a specific label for their genome, like a strain name that will serve as a unique identifier. Enter that name under the words MY LABEL. The combination of the taxonomy name and the unique identifier will be combined and appear in the text box under the words OUTPUT NAME.

5. Assign a genetic code to be used in the annotation. The PATRIC annotation pipeline provides two genetic codes, one for most bacteria and archaea (Genetic code 11), and one specifically for Mycoplasma, Spiroplasma and Ureaplasma (Genetic code 4). The default is set for bacteria and archaea, and "11 (Archaea and most Bacteria)" is seen in the text box under the words GENETIC CODE. To select the alternate code, click on the down arrow at the end of the text box that is under the words GENETIC CODE, then click on "4 (Mycoplasma, Spiroplasma and Ureaplasma)."

6. Assign an Output Folder. Click on the down arrow that follows the text box underneath OUTPUT FOLDER.

7. This will open up a drop down box that shows all folders available. Researchers can create a new folder, or have the annotation job loaded into an existing folder. To place the job in the Annotations folder, click on that name.

8. The Annotations name will appear in the text box under Output Folder when successfully selected.

9. Start the annotation job by clicking on the Annotate button at the bottom center of the page.

10. A message will appear below the box to indicate that the job is now in the queue that says "Annotation Job has been queued."

3.2.3 Checking the Status of the Annotation Job

1. Click on the Jobs indicator at the bottom right on the PATRIC page.

2. This will open the Jobs Status page where researchers can see the status of their annotation job. The statuses of all the service jobs that have been submitted to PATRIC are also available.

3.3 Exploring Private Genomes in PATRIC

3.3.1 Locating a Privately Annotated Genome with Global Search

1. Enter the name of the private genome in the Global Search text box at the top left of any PATRIC page (under the words PATRIC) and hit return. This opens the Search Results page that is divided into Features, Genomes, Taxonomy, and Experiments. If named specifically, the private genome should be on the first page of the Search results.

2. Clicking on the genome name will open the landing page for that genome. The information on this page includes the size and number of genes as well as several tabs (Fig. 4a).

3.3.2 Genome Browser

Clicking on the Genome Browser tab will open up the genome browser (Fig. 4b). Private genomes show only the PATRIC annotation, but public genomes also display the RefSeq annotation. If the genome is in multiple contigs, the browser will load the first contig. To explore different contigs, researchers will need to click on the down arrow in the blue band at the top of the browser, which will open up a list of the available contigs . Scroll down that list to choose the contig of interest, and clicking on the name will reload the browser with that information.

3.3.3 Circular Viewer

PATRIC provides a circular viewer that will show all contigs together from an assembly (Fig. 4c). The closer a genome is to being closed, the better this image will look. The image, using Circos [14] technology, includes the coding sequences (CDS) on the forward and reverse strands, the RNA genes, GC content, and GC skew. Users can upload custom tracks or their own data, resize the image, and download it as a publication quality scaled vector graphic (svg).

3.3.4 Feature Table

1. The tab for Feature Table contains information about all the features annotated on a genome, from CDS to RNAs, pseudogenes and miscellaneous features. Most of the public genomes include RefSeq or alternate locus tags, but these are not seen in private genomes.

2. Filters on top of the table allow users to narrow down the table display by Feature Type (ex. tRNAs, CDS or pseudogenes) or Annotation (PATRIC or RefSeq). A Keyword search allows users to find specific genes. To do this, enter specific text

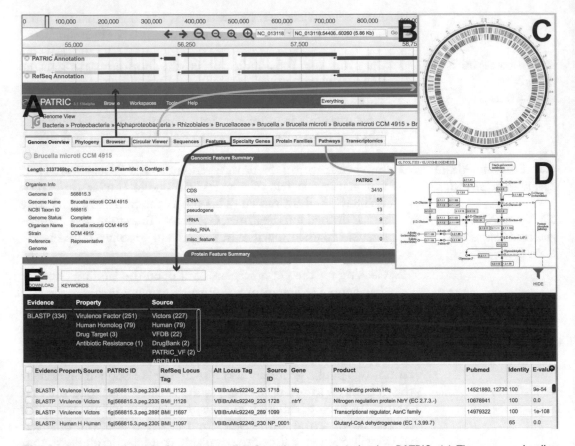

Fig. 4 Information available for genomes that have been annotated using PATRIC. (**a**) The genome landing page. (**b**) Genome browser. (**c**). Circular view of the genome. (**d**) Pathway summaries. (**e**) Specialty gene page where researchers can filter on genes in their genome that are associated with virulence, antibiotic resistance, drug targets, or human homologs

(names or locus tag) in the search box and click on the Filter Table button. This will filter the table to show genes that match the terms used.

3. The results of the filtering can be saved. Clicking on the box in front of the PATRIC ID (first column) auto-selects all the genes in the table. Users can use the check boxes to also select individual genes.

4. Click on the folder icon in front of Add Feature(s). This opens a pop-up window. To create a group, click on the down arrow that follows the word "None" in the text box. This will open up a drop down box that allows you to create a new group. To create a new group, click on the line that says "Create New Group." Then type in a name to identify the group in the text box below the words "Add to genome." To save that group, click on the Save to Workspace button at the bottom of the pop-up box.

3.3.5 Specialty Genes

The Specialty Genes tab shows all the features in a genome that have homology to genes previously identified as having specific properties (Fig. 4d). PATRIC BLASTs all the genes in the annotated genome against specific databases that contain genes identified as virulence factors (The Virulence Factor Database [15, 16], PATRIC virulence factors [17], and Victors, which is part of the Phidias database [18]), which are involved in antibiotic resistance (the Antibiotic Resistance Database [19] and the Comprehensive Antibiotic Resistance Database [20]), have been used as drug targets, or are human homologs. The left side of this page contains a filter to narrow the results, and a table listing the results on the right.

1. To see this specific evidence, use the filter. Click on the Virulence Factor property. There are three databases to choose from (Victors, PATRIC_VF, and the Virulence Factor Database [VFDB] [16]). Both PATRIC and Victors provide PubMed Ids that show direct links to the evidence. Click on Victors under Source.

2. This will resort the table to show all the genes in the genome that have homology to genes in the Victors database. To see more information about those individual genes, click on the PubMed link. This will open up a new page that shows the paper(s) that are the base of that evidence.

3.3.6 Pathways

1. PATRIC maps genes with functional evidence to the pathways they belong to. The source of pathway information comes from the Kyoto Encyclopedia of Genes and Genomes (KEGG) [21, 22], to which PATRIC maps protein data. To find the pathway data for a private genome, users should click on the Pathways tab.

2. The top of the Pathways table has a filter that allows researchers to filter the table on the Pathway Class, the Pathway Name, Enzyme Commission (EC) Number, or Annotation type (PATRIC or RefSeq annotation). Click on the down arrow in the box that follows the "Pathway Name" and this will open up a list of pathway names. Scroll down to find a pathway name of interest (ex. "Benzoate degradation via hydroxylation"). Click on that, and the table will show that single pathway. To see the pathway map, click on the name in the table that you can see in the second column with the header "Pathway Name."

3. This will open up a page that shows a list of the EC Numbers on the left side, and the KEGG pathway map on the right. Green boxes correspond to the EC numbers on the left side of the page. White boxes indicate EC numbers that are not present in this genome.

3.3.7 Protein Families

1. PATRIC has three types of protein families. The oldest, called FIGFams, contain isofunctional homologs. Two new sets of protein families, called PATtyFams [23], are assembled from the function-based groups into families by the use of k-mers and a Markov Cluster algorithm (MCL) [24, 25]. Click on the Protein Families tab. There is a filter on the left and a table on the right that lists the protein families, their IDs, Product Description, and statistics on the amino acids contained across your selection on the right. For individual genomes, these statistics will be limited.

2. As with the Feature Table mentioned above, use the filter to search for specific protein families. This will filter on the name of the family, which is not necessarily on the product description of the individual genes, so the results from the Feature Table and the Protein Family table will not match exactly. To find specific genes, enter a gene name or product description (NOT a locus tag) in the filter box in the left panel and then click the filter button at the bottom of the left panel. This will filter the results to show the protein families in the table on the right that match the search.

3.3.8 Literature

The literature tab opens up a page that shows a filter on the right, and on the left, a list of publications relevant to the taxonomic level. For privately annotated genomes, it assembles recent publications at the genus level.

1. Use the filters on the right side to refine the search by clicking on specific keywords that are available in the left panel under the heading "By Keyword." This will filter the publications to a list that matches the selection.

3.4   Protein Family Analysis: Creating Genome Groups

Once researchers have found genomes or data of interest, PATRIC allows them to create groups based upon their selections. User-specified groups of genomes are an important precursor to many of PATRIC's sophisticated analysis tools. To save these groups, PATRIC provides registered users with a private workspace that includes the ability to form and retain groups of genomes or proteins for later reference. This is especially useful as researchers sometimes must take considerable efforts to locate genomes or proteins that they are interested in comparing, and would like to be able to return to where they left off in the analysis without starting from scratch. These saved datasets are especially useful for researchers working on publications, or merely checking alignments or IDs of data of interest.

3.4.1 Creating a Group Using PATRIC's Global Search

1. Enter select text into the search box as seen in the screenshot below and hit return. This will open the Search Results page that is divided into Features, Genomes, Taxonomy, and Experiments. The results returned for Genomes are indicated.

2. To see all the results, click on the number that follows "Genomes" in the central panel. This will open up a page that contains all the genomes that were returned by the search parameters. Users will see a filter on the left side of the page, and a table with a list of genomes on the right side.

3. Find the genome that you want to save to a group and click on the box in front of it. You can click as many boxes as you want to include in the group. This will open a header on the top of the table that allows you to save a group of genomes. To create a group that contains the genomes, click on the Add Genomes button at the top left of the table.

4. This will open up a pop-up window. To create a group, click on the down arrow that follows the word "None" that you can see in the text box. This will open up a drop down box that allows users to create a new group, or to add genome to an existing group. To create a new group, click on the line that says "Create New Group" then type in a unique name for the group in the text box. To save that group, click on the Save to Workspace button at the bottom of the pop-up box.

3.4.2 Creating a Group with Public and Private Genomes by Taxonomy

1. Enter a genus, species, or taxon name in the global search box and return. This will open up the Search Results page that is divided into Features, Genomes, Taxonomy, and Experiments. Scroll down to the bottom of the page to find the results returned for Taxonomy and click on that taxonomic level of interest.

2. A landing page for that taxonomic designation will open. Across the top of the page there are a number of tabs. Click on the Genome List Table.

3. A page will open that contains a list of all the genomes within at that taxonomic level, and a filter on the left can be used to narrow the search. At the top of the filter users can select freely available in PATRIC (denoted as Public), or those they have annotated that are in their workspace (denoted as Private) by clicking on the box in front of the word. This will change the table to only show the genomes that meet that designation.

4. Researchers can select one or more of the genomes by clicking on the box in front of the name in the central table. To save the selection to a group, click on the Add Genomes button in the Workspace box immediately above the genome names at the top of the table.

5. This will open up a pop-up window. To create a group, follow the steps in Subheading 3.4.1, **step 4**.

6. Once saved, the table view will return to where more genomes can be selected. To select from the genomes that are freely available in PATRIC, click on the box in front of the word "Public." This will resort the table to show all the genomes that meet that criterion under the taxon level you have chosen.

7. To find complete genomes, click on the box in front of the word "Complete" (in the filter on the left side underneath the words "Genome Status") and this will resort the table to show all the complete genomes.

8. To select all the complete genomes click on the box in front of "Genome Name" at the top left of the table. This will select all the genomes in the table. To save those genomes to a group, click on the Add Genomes button at the top of the table.

9. To add these genomes to a group that has been previously created click on the down arrow that follows the word "None" that you can see in the text box. Scroll down the list of names until the group of interest is located and click on it. This will auto-fill the text box with the name of the genome group. To add the new genomes to this group, click on the Save to Workspace button at the bottom of the pop-up box.

10. To check the genomes included in the group, find the Workspace icon at the top of any PATRIC page that you can see in the blue header band. Click on that to open the private workspace.

11. Scroll down to find Genome Groups. Once located, double click on the icon in front of it and this opens a page with all the genome groups.

12. At the top right of the Genome Groups page is a column head named Created. To find the more recently created group, double click on that column head. The first click sorts the table from the oldest group to the most recent, and the second click reverses this to put the most recent group at the top. All of the column heads in PATRIC tables are sortable.

13. The most recently created group will appear in the top row. To see the genomes in that group, double click on the icon that is in front of the name you gave that group. This opens a page that shows specific for that group, and will show all the included genomes.

3.5 Protein Family Analysis: Protein Family Sorter

The Protein Family Sorter tool (Fig. 5) at PATRIC allows users to select a set of genomes of interest (maximum up to 500 genomes) and examine distribution of protein families across the genomes, commonly referred to as the "pan genome," which in this case

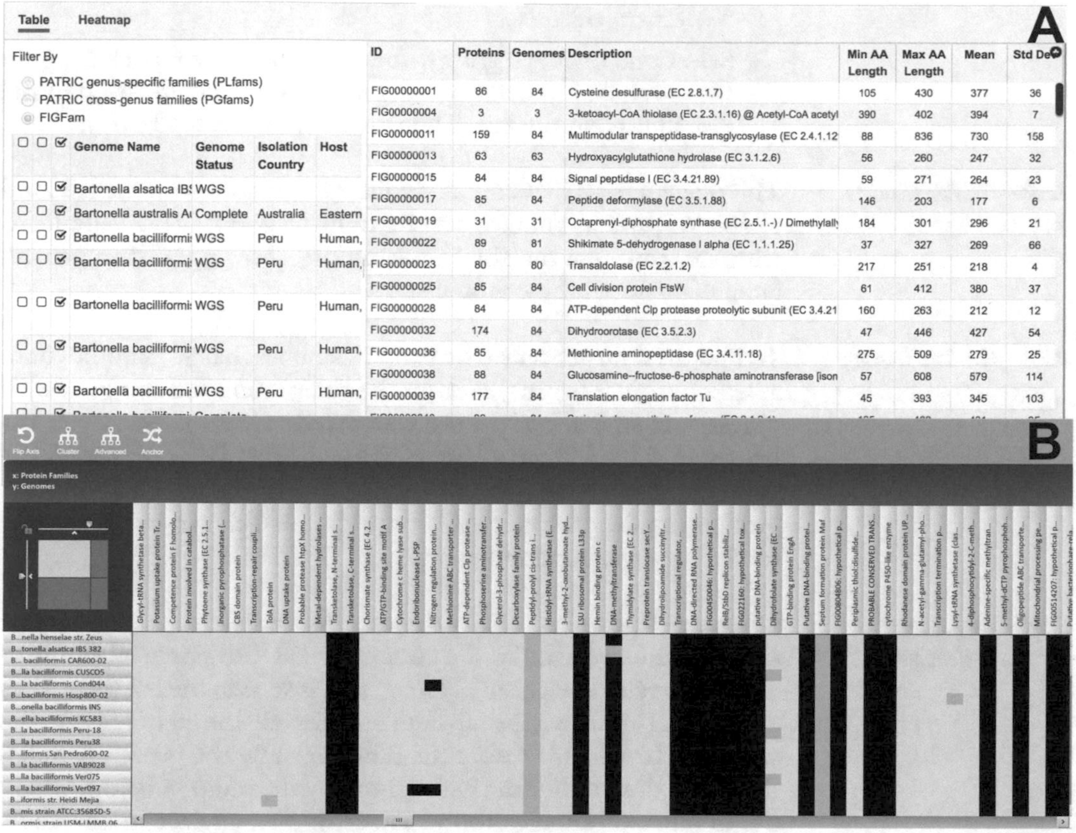

Fig. 5 PATRIC's Protein Family Sorter Tool. (**a**) Tabular results of all the data across all the selected genomes with a dynamic filter on the *left*. (**b**) Heatmap view of the same results that show genes that are missing (*black cells*) or present (*colored*) across all the selected genomes

refers to the superset of proteins found in all selected genomes. This tool provides various filtering options to quickly locate protein families that are conserved across all the genomes ("core genome"), conserved only in a subset of the selected genomes ("accessory genome") or that match a specified function. A tabular view shows protein families matching filtering criteria and an interactive heatmap viewer provides a bird's-eye ("pan genome") view of the distribution of the protein families across multiple genomes, with clustering and anchoring functions to show relative conservation of synteny and identify lateral transfers.

3.5.1 Finding the Tool

Go to the Tools tab across the top of any PATRIC page and click on it. This will open up a list of tools. Click on the Protein Family Sorter. This opens up a landing page for the tool, and users who are logged in will see the groups they have created in the box under

1. "Select organism(s)."

2. Select one or more groups for comparison by first clicking on the check box in front of the group name that are listed in the Search box on the left. Then click on the Search button.

3.5.2 The Pan Genome

This opens a page that contains a filter for genomes on the left, and a table of protein families on the right (Fig. 5a). This page loads with the pan genome for the selection, showing all the protein families across all the genomes.

3.5.3 The Core Genome

To find the core genome (the protein families that all genomes have at least one member in), click on the circle under the column called "Present in all families" in the row called "Genome Name" in the left panel. This will auto select "Present in all families" for all the genomes in your selection. It will also resort the table to show the protein families that meet this condition, which can be seen at the top left of the central table.

3.5.4 Individual Accessory Genome

Users can find the accessory genome for individual strains by first checking the circle under the column called "Absent in all families" in the row called "Genome Name" that is seen in the left filter. This auto selects "Absent in all families" for all the genomes in the selection. It will also resort the table to show the protein families that meet this condition (highlighted by the red box below, where the number of families found is zero). Next, select to the circle under the column called "Present in all families" for a single genome. This will show the protein families that are unique to just that genome. It will also resort the table to show the protein families that meet this condition.

3.5.5 Searching for Specific Protein Family Names

The text box near the bottom of the filter can be used to find specific protein families. This will filter on the name of the family, not necessarily on the product description of the individual genes, so the results from the Feature Table and the Protein Family table will not necessarily match. To find specific protein families, enter a name (NOT a locus tag) in the filter box on the left and then click the filter button at the bottom of the filter panel. This will filter the results to show the protein families that match the search.

3.5.6 Visualizing Protein Families

1. A visual representation of the presence or absence of protein families across particular genomes is available in a Heatmap view (Fig. 5b). Click on the Heatmap tab at the top of the table. This opens the heatmap view page. Protein families are listed on the x-axis across the top of this view, and genomes along the y-axis.

2. To see the names of the individual protein families and/or genomes, move the sliders to expand the view. The sliders are

found at the top left of the heatmap. Clicking on and moving the sliders to the right (x axis) or down (y axis) will expand the heatmap headers so that the names of the genomes and the protein families can be read.

3. Clicking on the legend at the top left, just outside of the heatmap, shows what the different colors of the cells mean. Yellow cells in the heatmap indicate a single protein that belongs to that protein family annotated in that genome. Mustard-colored cells indicate that there are two proteins belonging to that family in that genome. Orange cells indicate three or more proteins, and when there is a black cell it means that the genome does not have a protein annotated in that family.

3.5.7 Clustering Protein Families

Click on the word cluster, which is found in the top left under the number of families found, to resort to heatmap to show similar patterns in the presence or absence of protein families across all the genomes in the selection. The default settings for the clustering button are based on the Pearson Correlation Algorithm and a Pairwise Average-linkage Clustering Type.

3.5.8 Anchoring Protein Families

1. PATRIC also provides a function where the presence and absence of protein families across all the genomes can be compared in the order that the genes appear in a single genome. "Anchoring" is a good way to look for genomic islands. Click on the down arrow that is part of the text box following the words "Advanced Clustering" in the blue header directly above the heatmap. This opens a dropdown box that shows all the genomes in the group. Select one genome from that box by clicking on its name.

2. This resorts the protein families to show the order that they occur in the genes occurs on the reference genome. Using the scroll bar at the bottom of the heatmap allows users to follow along the genome.

3. Mousing over individual cells shows the names of both the genome and the protein family in the blue header box above the heatmap.

3.5.9 Downloading Data from Heatmap

1. To get the data and names on protein families, use the mouse to draw a box (select) around an area of interest in the heatmap. A pop-up window will appear that allows users to download the heatmap data in the selection, download the proteins from your selection, show the proteins from the selection, add the proteins to a group, or cancel the selection. To see the proteins, click on "Show Proteins."

2. A new window will load that shows the data behind the selection, including the name of the genome, accession number, PATRIC and RefSeq locus tags, the size of the protein, and the product description. Once in this view, users have a number of options that they can perform with these genes. These include saving them to a group, get the nucleotide or amino acid sequences, download the information, see if they were important in any metabolic pathways, generate a multiple sequence alignment for them, or find other identifiers that map to them from other resources.

3.5.10 Pathway Summary of Genes in the Selection

1. To find functionality that genes from the selection might share, click on the box in front of "Genome Name." This will select all the genes in the table. Then click on the Pathway Summary button at the top of the table toward the right side (next to Multiple Seq Alignment).

2. This will open a table that shows all the pathways that the genes selected are present in. To find the pathway that has the most of the selected genes present in it, double-click on the "# of Genes Selected" column header. This will reorder the pathways to show the one that has the most of the selected genes in it at the top. Click on that pathway name in the first column.

3. This will open up a page that contains a summary of the Enzyme Commission (EC) numbers present in this genome on the left, and the KEGG map for that pathway on the right.

4. Clicking on the legend opens it. Green boxes indicate that this genome has at least one gene annotated with that EC number. Blue boxes indicate those genes that were part of your selection from the heat map, and white boxes indicate that these genes are not annotated in this genome.

3.6 Proteome Comparison: Comparing Annotated Proteins Across Genomes

PATRIC's Proteome Comparison tool (Fig. 6) can be used to readily identify insertions and deletions in up to nine target genomes that are compared with one reference, which can be a researcher's private genome in PATRIC, a genome that has been annotated outside PATRIC, any of the publicly available genomes in PATRIC, or a set of proteins that you have saved in PATRIC as a feature group.

The Proteome Comparison tool is based on the original Sequence-based Comparison tool that was part of RAST [26]. This tool colors each gene based on protein similarity using BLASTP and marks each gene as either unique, a unidirectional best hit, or a bidirectional best hit when compared to the reference genome. The output includes a whole-genome schematic that is colored based on BLAST. A table that details all the results can be downloaded for further analysis, as can a scalable vector graphic (svg) diagram of the results that is publication quality.

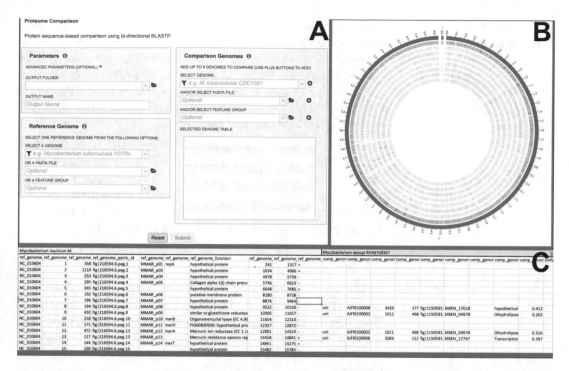

Fig. 6 PATRIC's Proteome Comparison Tool. (**a**) The landing page for the proteome comparison tool. (**b**) The SVG image that provides a visual representation of the shared identity across all the genes in the genomes that are compared against the selected reference genome. (**C**) The proteome comparison tool also provides a downloadable file that shows the level of identity across all the genomes

3.6.1 Finding the Tool

1. At the top of any PATRIC page, find the Services tab and click on it.

2. Click on Proteome Comparison.

3. This will open up the landing page (Fig. 6a) for where you can submit a Proteome Comparison job. This tool is a best bidirectional BLAST comparison of the annotated proteins from up to nine different genomes.

3.6.2 Setting Parameters and Selecting an Output Folder

1. To see what the advanced parameters are in the proteome comparison, click on the information icon, with is a blue "I." This opens a pop-up window that describes what can be adjusted.

2. The box to adjust the advanced parameters can be opened by clicking on the down arrow that follows Advanced Parameters (optional). Researchers can adjust the minimum percent coverage, the minimum percent identity, and the BLAST E-value.

3. Next the researcher must select an output folder where the proteome comparison job will be placed. To do this, click on the folder icon that follows the text box under the words Output Folder and click on preferred folder.

4. Provide a distinctive name for the proteome comparison in the text box underneath the words Output Name.

*3.6.3   Selecting the
Reference Genome*

1. The proteome comparison tools allows researchers to select genomes or a specific feature group that contains a set of proteins to serve as a reference that other genomes will be BLASTed against. To see and understand the available options, click on information icon next to the words "Reference Genome." This opens a pop-up window that describes the types of selections that can be made.

2. In this example, a private genome is selected. To do this, first click on the filter icon that is at the front of the text box directly under the words "Select a genome." This will open a box that allows a researcher to search across all of the public genomes available in PATRIC, or across the genomes that they have annotated and that are stored in their private workspace.

3. Click on the box in front of Public Genomes to deselect that box.

4. In the text box below Reference Genome, start typing some words that will identify the reference. Once the user starts typing in the text box, a list appeared below the box, providing the user with possible choices that match the text. Clicking on a name will auto-fill the name in the text box under Reference Genome.

*3.6.4   Selecting the
Comparison Genomes*

1. Locate the panel for selecting comparison genomes, or a set of proteins, that will be BLASTed against the selected reference.

2. Comparison genomes can be public or private. To select genomes that are publicly available, deselect the check box in front of Private Genomes.

3. Start typing a name into the text box. Once enough text has been entered to see the genome of interest, click on that name. This will auto-fill the text box with the selected name. If the choice is correct, click the "+" icon. The genome will then appear in the box below.

4. To finally select the genome, click on the "+" icon at the end of the text box that has the name of the selected genome. Clicking on the icon will move the genome to the Selected Genome table.

5. Repeat **step 3** to add as many genomes (up to 9) to compare to the reference genome you have selected.

6. Genomes that have been annotated by a different service, or a specific group of proteins, can also be used in the comparison. Researchers can upload a genome fasta file by clicking on the arrow or folder icon that follows the text box under the words AND/OR SELECT FASTA FILE, and then clicking on the plus icon to move the folder to the Select Genome Table.

7. The Proteome Comparison tool also allows researchers to compare genomes to a specific feature file that consists of a number of proteins by clicking on the arrow or folder icon that follows the text box under the words AND/OR SELECT FEATURE GROUP, and then clicking on the plus icon to move the folder to the Select Genome Table.

8. Once the nine genomes (or feature groups) are included, the Comparison Genome box will show all the members you have selected.

3.6.5 Submitting the Proteome Comparison Job

1. Click the Submit button at the bottom center of the page.

2. A message will appear above the submit button that confirms that the job has been submitted. This message is temporal and will disappear after several seconds.

3. Check the status of the annotation job by clicking on the Jobs indicator at the bottom left of the PATRIC page.

4. Clicking on Jobs opens the Jobs Status page, which shows the status of the proteome comparison job. The statuses of all the previous service jobs that have submitted to PATRIC are also available. You will be able to see when your job is complete.

3.6.6 Accessing the Proteome Comparison Job

1. To access the results of the submitted job, click on Workspace Home that is found at the top left of any PATRIC page. This will open up the workspace, where all folders are visible. Find the folder where the comparison job was placed and click on the folder icon that precedes the name.

2. This will open a page that shows all the comparisons available in that folder. Click on the icon in front of the job name. This opens up the landing page for that job that shows a diagram showing the sequence identity, a list of the names of the genomes in the job, and will also show a circular image that shows the relatedness. This will take a few seconds to load.

3. To see the entire image, find the download icon at the top of the page on the left and click on SVG image.

4. This will download the publication quality SVG image (Fig. 6b) that shows the percent identity across all the proteins in the comparison genomes compared to the reference genome.

5. To examine all the data that underlies the visualization, click on Genome Comparison Table.

6. This will open up a text file that can also be opened with excel (Fig. 6c). The document contains a lot of information, and users will be able to see all the genes in the comparison genomes that have the best BLAST hits to the reference genome. The first row will show the genome names in specific columns,

and the column heading in the second row shows the additional information. Data begins with the genome that was used as a reference and includes columns A–J. The data includes the following:

- accession number for the contig in the reference genome
- the order number of this gene in the genome
- size in amino acids
- PATRIC locus tag
- RefSeq locus tag
- gene name
- functional annotation
- start location for the gene on the contig
- end of the gene on the contig
- strand that the gene is located on

This is followed by information on the genomes used in the comparison. This data in columns K–T for row 2 (for the first comparison genome) includes:

- data on the type of BLAST hit (Column K, bi- or uni-directional, or missing)
- contig that the gene is located on
- the order number of this gene in the genome
- size in amino acids
- PATRIC locus tag
- RefSeq locus tag
- gene name
- functional description
- percent identity of the BLAST hit
- sequence coverage compared to the reference

This pattern is repeated for all comparison genomes in the same order.

References

1. Wattam AR et al (2013) PATRIC, the bacterial bioinformatics database and analysis resource. Nucleic Acids Res 42(Database issue): D581–D591. gkt1099

2. Aziz RK et al (2008) The RAST server: rapid annotations using subsystems technology. BMC Genomics 9(1):75

3. Brettin T et al (2015) RASTtk: a modular and extensible implementation of the RAST algorithm for building custom annotation pipelines and annotating batches of genomes. Sci Rep 5:8365

4. Branton D et al (2008) The potential and challenges of nanopore sequencing. Nat Biotechnol 26(10):1146–1153

5. Nikolenko SI, Korobeynikov AI, Alekseyev MA (2013) BayesHammer: Bayesian clustering for error correction in single-cell sequencing. BMC Genomics 14(1):1

6. Zerbino DR, Birney E (2008) Velvet: algorithms for de novo short read assembly using de Bruijn graphs. Genome Res 18(5):821–829

7. Peng Y et al (2010) IDBA–a practical iterative de Bruijn graph de novo assembler. In: Research in computational molecular biology. Springer, Berlin

8. Bankevich A et al (2012) SPAdes: a new genome assembly algorithm and its applications to single-cell sequencing. J Comput Biol 19(5):455–477

9. Li D et al (2015) MEGAHIT: an ultra-fast single-node solution for large and complex metagenomics assembly via succinct de Bruijn graph. Bioinformatics 31(10):1674–1676. btv033

10. Namiki T et al (2012) MetaVelvet: an extension of velvet assembler to de novo metagenome assembly from short sequence reads. Nucleic Acids Res 40(20):e155–e155

11. Clark SC et al (2013) ALE: a generic assembly likelihood evaluation framework for assessing the accuracy of genome and metagenome assemblies. Bioinformatics 29(4):435–443. bts723

12. Vicedomini R et al (2013) GAM-NGS: genomic assemblies merger for next generation sequencing. BMC Bioinformatics 14(7):1

13. Li H (2015) Minimap and miniasm: fast mapping and de novo assembly for noisy long sequences. Bioinformatics 32:2103–2110. arXiv preprint arXiv:1512.01801

14. Krzywinski M et al (2009) Circos: an information aesthetic for comparative genomics. Genome Res 19(9):1639–1645

15. Chen L et al (2005) VFDB: a reference database for bacterial virulence factors. Nucleic Acids Res 33(suppl 1):D325–D328

16. Chen L et al (2016) VFDB 2016: hierarchical and refined dataset for big data analysis-10 years on. Nucleic Acids Res 44(D1): D694–D697

17. Mao C et al (2015) Curation, integration and visualization of bacterial virulence factors in PATRIC. Bioinformatics 31(2):252–258

18. Xiang Z, Tian Y, He Y (2007) PHIDIAS: a pathogen-host interaction data integration and analysis system. Genome Biol 8(7):R150

19. Liu B, Pop M (2009) ARDB—antibiotic resistance genes database. Nucleic Acids Res 37 (suppl 1):D443–D447

20. McArthur AG et al (2013) The comprehensive antibiotic resistance database. Antimicrob Agents Chemother 57(7):3348–3357

21. Kanehisa M et al (2008) KEGG for linking genomes to life and the environment. Nucleic Acids Res 36(suppl 1):D480–D484

22. Kanehisa M et al (2004) The KEGG resource for deciphering the genome. Nucleic Acids Res 32(suppl 1):D277–D280

23. Davis JJ et al (2016) PATtyFams: protein families for the microbial genomes in the PATRIC database. Front Microbiol 7:118

24. Enright AJ, Van Dongen S, Ouzounis CA (2002) An efficient algorithm for large-scale detection of protein families. Nucleic Acids Res 30(7):1575–1584

25. van Dongen SM (2001) Graph clustering by flow simulation. University of Utrecht, Utrecht

26. Overbeek R et al (2014) The SEED and the rapid annotation of microbial genomes using subsystems technology (RAST). Nucleic Acids Res 42(D1):D206–D214

Chapter 5

Phylogenomics

José S. L. Patané, Joaquim Martins Jr., and João C. Setubal

Abstract

Phylogenomics aims at reconstructing the evolutionary histories of organisms taking into account whole genomes or large fractions of genomes. The abundance of genomic data for an enormous variety of organisms has enabled phylogenomic inference of many groups, and this has motivated the development of many computer programs implementing the associated methods. This chapter surveys phylogenetic concepts and methods aimed at both gene tree and species tree reconstruction while also addressing common pitfalls, providing references to relevant computer programs. A practical phylogenomic analysis example including bacterial genomes is presented at the end of the chapter.

Key words Phylogenomics, Phylogeny, Whole genome, Gene tree, Species tree, Phylogenetic networks

1 Introduction

The amount of available sequences in online data banks has been growing exponentially over the past decades (e.g., GenBank [1]). The growth rate became dramatic with the availability of the first next-generation sequencing (NGS) platform, starting around 2005. This allowed the inclusion of many more genes in phylogenetic studies than previously possible.

Phylogenomics [2, 3] aims at inferring detailed information about the evolutionary histories of organisms by using whole genomes rather than just a single gene or a few genes. The term was coined by Jonathan Eisen in the context of prediction of gene function [4, 5]. A "genome" in this context can be understood as its DNA sequence, or its gene content (generally the protein-coding genes only), or both. It would be difficult or impossible to understand the evolutionary history of an organism, even having available its whole genome sequence, in isolation. So it is always the case the phylogenomics is practiced for sets of genomes, justifying the inclusion of this chapter in this volume.

João C. Setubal et al. (eds.), *Comparative Genomics: Methods and Protocols*, Methods in Molecular Biology, vol. 1704, https://doi.org/10.1007/978-1-4939-7463-4_5, © Springer Science+Business Media LLC 2018

Our aim here is to give an overview of the theoretical aspects of the field, complemented by many references to computer programs that implement these theoretical concepts as well as a simple practical case study, given at the end. In order to explain phylogenomics methods we thought it necessary to provide a general overview of phylogenetic inference methods, which explains in part why this chapter is so long. Nevertheless we hope that this decision will have made this chapter more self-contained, and hence more useful, than it would have been otherwise.

2   Which Data to Use?

After the evolutionary range to be studied is known, the next important decision is about the data to be included. Even though the whole genome may be used for phylogenomics, there are many kinds of data that one can extract and use from whole genomes. In this section we describe the most commonly used data types.

2.1   Sequence Data

2.1.1   Whole Genomes

There are basically two ways in which whole genome nucleotide sequences can be compared: by computing whole genome distances between the genomes without relying on alignment between sequences (*alignment-free methods*) and by performing a multiple alignment with them (*alignment-based methods*). An example of alignment-free analysis is the phylogeny of 12 mammals using raw sequencing reads obtained by the "assembly and alignment-free" method, which is able to construct a phylogeny directly from unassembled genome sequence data, bypassing both genome assembly and alignment [6].

2.1.2   Local Collinear Blocks

An orthologous genomic block is a region that is present in all genomes being analyzed up to a user-defined (and software-dependent) similarity threshold. Local Collinear Blocks (LCBs) are the set of orthologous genomic blocks detected across genomes being compared, each LCB assumed to be internally free from genome rearrangements. The number of blocks that can be observed will vary depending on the evolutionary histories of the genomes being compared relative to each other; they can range from just a handful to several thousand (the latter is typical when organisms are evolutionary distant; these blocks also tend to be much smaller when compared to those of closely related organisms). ProgressiveMauve [7] is a whole genome multiple aligner that computes LCBs with the script stripSubsetLCBs. Sibelia [8] is another interesting option, as it can find synteny blocks repeated within genomes as well as blocks shared by multiple genomes.

2.1.3   Pan-Genome

We define *pan-genome* as the union of all gene sets in all genomes under study. Estimated pan-genomes provide information on two types of variation: genes that are maintained in all lineages (the *core genome*); and genes that are maintained in fewer lineages (or even in a single lineage), either due to losses in specific lineages (which are also informative; *see* "Indels" below), or due to gains by horizontal gene transfers (possibly contributing with local synapomorphies for unrelated clades in the tree, if those parallel gains occurred at the branch leading to each clade), constituting the *soft-core* genome. kSNP [9] (further discussed in Subheading 2.1.4) is an example of software determining the set of all variable positions across the pan-genome. The script get_homologues.pl (part of the Get_Homologues package [10]) with the option "-t 0" can also infer the pan-genome based on three alternative orthology assessment methods: bidirectional best hits using BLAST; OrthoMCL [11]; and COG triangles [12].

2.1.4   Core Genome

Using all single-copy genes present in all taxa (*core unicopy* genes) has become an important source of phylogenomic information as parsimoniously these were not gained by horizontal transmission, hence supposedly enriching the phylogenetic signal (assuming there was no homologous recombination within the gene). Another example of software that estimates orthologous groups from annotated genomes (besides get_homologues.pl with the option "-t" followed by the total number of taxa) is Parsnp within the Harvest suite [13].

Core-Coding Genes

Among core genes, some noncoding genes may induce bias in tree reconstruction (e.g., rRNA with similar convergent GC contents in unrelated hyperthermophilic Bacteria and Archaea [14]), therefore their use should in general be avoided. Data sets including only *core-coding* genes have become the standard, at least for prokaryotes; besides, they are amenable to translation into amino acids, which may be important for downstream analyses (for example, to reduce the effect of DNA saturation over distant divergences; Subheading 3.7.3).

Exons

Although there are pipelines for assembling the whole eukaryotic portion of a coding gene (e.g., from a transcriptome), sometimes it is easier to work directly with exons. An example is a study involving 3000 exons from a group of Australian skink lizards [15]. Exons are more informative for relatively divergent sequences, for they tend to be conserved across related eukaryote lineages.

Introns

Introns tend to be informative even for relatively shallow divergences compared to exons. A study including 280 loci was achieved based on a splice-site prediction method [16] in the plant genus *Heuchera* (Saxifragaceae), where it was shown that introns presented an overall fourfold increase in percent divergence as opposed to exons for the same dataset.

Other Regions

Ultra-conserved elements (UCEs) is a type of marker that has gained popularity within the past few years. They were first defined as segments of > 200 bp perfectly conserved between human and rodents [17]. Later they were redefined as conserved DNA sequences with ≥ 80% identity over ≥ 100 bp across taxa [18], but the thresholds can be different for other groups; an interesting example of their use is the inference of turtles as the sister group to archosaurs based on more than 1000 UCEs [19]. Besides vertebrates, they are also found in other eukaryotic groups, e.g. worms and yeast [20], insects [21], and plants [22]. Being extremely conserved across distantly related lineages, they are useful when comparing lineages spanning deep divergences; yet, their flanking regions harbor variation that increases with distance from the conserved core [18], validating their use at shallow evolutionary timescales as well [23]. Phyluce [24] includes a pipeline for assembly of UCEs and their phylogenomic analysis.

Caution When Using SNPs

All marker types shown above are based on sequence data, usually containing a few or many conserved positions. In order to reduce computational complexity, analyzing only variable sites may be an option. *Single nucleotide polymorphisms* (SNPs) are the smallest possible unit for phylogenetic analysis, being used in many phylogenomic studies. One issue about their use is known as *phylogenetic discovery bias* [25, 26], in which SNPs of interest are found by comparing a small panel of individuals; when genotyping new individuals based on the variable sites within that smaller panel, the latter will have larger branches in the complete tree (exactly because variation assessment was based on that panel) and furthermore they will tend to branch from a more derived node, impacting topological inference. Another issue has to do with *mapping bias* from reads of new genomes. A common strategy to call SNPs is to fix one of the genomes as the reference (usually the most complete), and then map all other reads/scaffolds/genomes to the reference. However, a level of 100% mapping (i.e., a totally collinear match between query and reference genomes) is unusual even for closely related lineages. This means that in most cases the SNPs detected will be a fraction of the total number of SNPs that exist in any given genome set, biasing branch lengths, which in extreme cases may bias tree inference. Finally, when using model-based methods, if the likelihood is not corrected for the fact that there are no invariant sites, *branch lengths will get overestimated*, and if the effect is relatively large it may impact tree inference as well [27]. This effect has been shown for morphological datasets (which always include variable characters only) [28].

When whole genomes are included, the first type of bias (phylogenetic discovery bias) is minimized; on the other hand, if markers were obtained by enrichment following variability assessment within a restricted taxon panel (e.g., as in target enrichment protocols), tree reconstruction may get biased. RealPHY [29] alleviates that kind of bias and also the second kind (mapping bias due to use of a single reference) by utilizing more references when calling SNPs, but the authors state that this mitigation works only for relatively close genomes (i.e., less than 5% divergence). Another way of minimizing the first and second biases is mapping against many (or all if computationally possible) genomes, instead of alignment with one or a few references. kSNP [9] implements an alignment-free algorithm that tests all genomes as references, allowing the program to find genome-wide SNPs even in non-core genomic regions; furthermore, it performs SNP detection based on k-mer comparisons across all taxa, minimizing the bias related to direct mapping of reads. However, kSNP considers variation only in the central site within each k-mer, so if there is variation in neighboring sites the k-mer will not map to that region, underestimating overall variability.

Likelihood-based programs such as RAxML [30] and IQTree [31] are able to employ evolutionary models correcting for the third type of bias (overestimation of branch lengths), by including "ASC" directives in the command line (for "ascertainment bias correction" of sites). MrBayes [32] is a Bayesian software with an even richer set of possible ASC corrections. Maximum parsimony (which counts the number of changes along a tree and then chooses the topology that minimizes the number of steps; Subheading 3.2.1) naturally uses only variable characters, not suffering from this type of bias, therefore being an alternative for SNP-based phylogeny estimation.

2.1.5 Taking Heterozigozity into Account

For studies including organisms with potential heterozygosity (i.e., diploid/polyploid) it is also important to estimate whether base call variations represent sequencing biases (wrong base calls, low quality scores, strand bias, read depth too low or too high, etc.) or real SNPs, and in the case of the latter whether the data support the hypothesis of heterozygosity for that site or not [33]. We will assume that in case of heterozygosity, the alleles have been parsed correctly (an important step, e.g., for some multi-species coalescent algorithms). Correctly identifying each haplotype is utterly important for shallow divergences (i.e., phylogenies including only closely related lineages), whereas it may not be as important for deeper divergences.

2.2 Other Types of Data

The following data types are not based on raw sequence information, but they can be very helpful for phylogenomic inference. Many of them are associated with *rare genomic changes* [34], being less prone to homoplasies and therefore more informative than DNA sequence analysis.

2.2.1 *Genome
Rearrangements*

Large-scale karyotypic evolution evolves at a slower pace compared to nucleotide evolution, providing rare, yet informative, footprints of common ancestries (e.g., inversions, transpositions, inverted transpositions). For example, variation in mitochondrial gene order showed that crustaceans and insects are closely related [35], in agreement with inclusive sequence-based studies carried much later (e.g., [36]). Also, an analysis based on inverted repeats of divergent chloroplast genomes including land plants and green algae recovered a phylogeny congruent with prior studies [37]; and an analysis of 15 Metazoan genomes reconstructed a tree that matched perfectly other results [38].

Most implementations use the *breakpoint distance* between genomes as the criterion for phylogenetic inference (where a breakpoint is when two genes present in both genomes are contiguous in one of the genomes, but not contiguous in the other either in direct or reverse order), not considering explicitly rearrangement types. GRAPPA [39] and its derivatives base their calculations on successive estimates of breakpoint median of three genomes, reconstructing a genome at their internal node by minimizing the breakpoint distance between the latter and each leaf's gene order. DCM-GRAPPA [40] scales to analyses of thousands of genomes by employing a variation of a *Disk-Covering Method* (DCM) that divides a set of taxa into overlapping subsets (the "disks"), constructing trees on the subsets using the same phylogenetic method on each, and then merges the subtrees into a final tree [40]. COGNAC further improves tree estimation by using an even more refined DCM, showing high accuracy and fast execution times [41]. UniMoG [42] implements many models that take into account different types of rearrangement using pairwise genomic distances (including models that allow for intra-species chromosome rearrangements, such as fusions, fissions, circularizations, and decircularizations), from which a tree can be estimated using distance methods (*see* Subheading 3.2.2). MLGO (Maximum Likelihood for Gene-Order Analysis [43]) performs binary encoding on gene-order data, also supporting a fairly general model of genomic evolution (rearrangements plus duplications, insertions, and losses of genomic regions). The encoding is done by transforming gene adjacencies (i.e., any two genes appearing next to each other in direct or inverse order) occurring at least once in any of the genomes into a unique character position in the sequence, and the presence or absence of any of these adjacencies in a given genome is recoded as 1 (presence) or 0 (absence), making maximum likelihood estimates possible by using a 2-state Markov model (*see* Subheading 3.4); also, because of such recoding, MLGO can deploy branch support by bootstrapping (*see* Subheading 3.2.2).

2.2.2 *Presence/Absence Data*

Indels

Deletions are a valuable source of phylogenetic information. Deletions occurring in the same region in different genomes, and having the same or similar sizes, may indicate phylogenetic relatedness. For example, different lineages of the bacteria *Mycobacterium tuberculosis* are characterized by the loss of specific segments from their common ancestor [44]. Nevertheless, a study of metazoan relationships [45] showed that even though indels bear reasonable phylogenetic signal (supporting the Ecdysozoa hypothesis as other analyses including molecular markers suggest) they are also recurrent targets of homoplasies. SeqState [46] has a complex coding algorithm that infers such different states per genomic region, or a binary coding can also be used for absence/presence, and then such a model can be analyzed by model-free or model-based phylogenetic methods. Such analyses are less biased if used with complete gene/genome information to avoid false positives (i.e., inference of a gap due to an incomplete sequenced genome, when the gap is not actually there), and furthermore ascertainment bias corrections must be employed (this being true for all presence/absence data described below).

Gene Content

Presence/absence and duplication of genes compose useful phylogenomic datasets, especially in the case of prokaryotes, where gains (by horizontal gene transfer), losses (due to deletions), and duplication of genomic regions are pervasive even between closely related lineages. States can be encoded as 0 in the case of gene absence, 1 in case of presence, and higher values in the case of other paralogs within the same genome. Alternatively, presence of one or more copies can be recoded as 1 if the user does not want to include information about duplications. The program Get_Homologues [10] exports such character matrices when full search of homologous families is chosen. Subsequently, such a matrix can be analyzed phylogenetically by maximum parsimony or by *n*-state Markovian models (Subheading 3.4) within a probabilistic framework. An analysis of anopheline mosquitoes [47] based on presence/absence of genes (but discarding duplications) had general agreement with phylogenies based on gene sequence. A more involved example is a distance-based tree reconstruction suggesting that eukaryotes arose from within both the Bacteria and the Archaea by an analysis involving comparison of conflicting support values [48]; the latter authors also used a modified distance that minimizes the effect of genomes of similar sizes attracting each other (which if not corrected can induce a biased topology).

Presence/Absence of Other Molecular Markers

Markers such as amplified fragment length polymorphism (AFLPs) [49] based on the action of restriction endonucleases along the whole genome and therefore relatively cheap to be produced can be a complementary source of phylogenomic signal.

Similarity (or dissimilarity) scores among all samples is generated based on presence/absence of DNA fragments of different sizes, being the input for distance-based phylogenetic methods (*see* Subheading 3.2.2). In a study of species in the rosid genus *Rosa*, which has a complicated and reticulate evolutionary history with many of the branches being poorly supported, AFLPs provided a tree resembling independent estimates based on morphology and molecular data [50]. Its scope is at shallower divergences, because such markers are prone to homoplasy.

Mobile Elements

Short and long interspersed nuclear elements (SINEs and LINEs) can get integrated into different regions of the genome. SINEs are retroposons that lack the ability for self-amplification, and therefore tend to "stay put" because their integration is apparently random and irreversible. They were successfully used to reconstruct relationships among Pacific salmonids [51]. An example of LINEs for phylogenetics (which have the ability for self-amplification) was in refining recent rodent relationships [52].

2.2.3 Repetitive Loci

All bacterial genomes contain batches of repetitive DNA along their genomes, where the number of repeat units per locus may define individual strains. Using numeric profiles compared by a categorical similarity coefficient, which were then subjected to a distance-based algorithm, lineages within the *Mycobacterium tuberculosis* complex could be divided into its constituent lineages with reasonable accuracy when compared to sequence-based phylogenies [53]. Such a method is meaningful only for closely related lineages due to the highly homoplastic nature of loci composed of repetitive segments (such as microsatellites in eukaryotes).

2.2.4 Morphology

Even though morphological characters cannot be readily assessed from genomic data, we mention their use as many studies incorporate them along sequence data, such as inferring placental phylogeny [54]. They constitute valuable phylogenetic information alone [28], especially for eukaryotes, as is the case of a large study of avian evolution based on morphology [55], whereby 2954 characters were employed across 150 taxa of major groups. However, the association of morphological characters to their underlying genomic source is not direct, due to one-to-many (pleiotropy), many-to-one (polygenic inheritance), and interaction (epistatic) effects; furthermore, they are affected by the environment, which may introduce further noise in the analysis.

2.3 Analyzing It All Together

Can different types of data be analyzed together to bring more power to phylogenomic inference? At least two of the main methods for summary analysis of multiple sets of data (supermatrix and supertrees; *see* Subheading 4) can be naturally extended to include mixed data types. A study on the evolution of species of the bacteria *Rickettsia* compared phylogenomic analyses using four complementary sources of genetic information: primary sequence, gene content, indels, and gene order [56], with results indicating similar relationships across datasets even though a few nodes were conflicting. A study based on different supertrees (morphological, molecular, and both combined [57]), obtained from previously published trees, agreed on suprafamilial taxa and orders of eutherian mammals (but showing conflicting interordinal clades). Another study focused on the same group of organisms included three different data types altogether (DNA, indels, morphology) in a concatenated phylogenomic analysis, also recovering important nodes though being an unresolved tree at its deeper levels, divided into Afrotheria, Xenarthra, Euarchontoglires, and Laurasiatheria [54].

3   Estimating Gene Trees

3.1 Multiple Alignment

Except for phylogenies based on alignment-free genomic distances or SNPs from reads/contigs, tree inference methods are based on a multiple sequence alignment (MSA) of genes or genomic regions across the taxa studied. Some multiple alignment methods also directly output an estimated phylogeny, bypassing the need of a subsequent phylogenetic analysis (e.g. POY [58]).

In general, MSA is performed by a *progressive alignment* algorithm, first generating a reference tree (which can be based on fast but approximate phylogenetic methods such as neighbor-joining; Subheading 3.2.2), and then pairwise alignments are performed following a post-order tree traversal, growing progressively until the root using (in general) a dynamic programming algorithm for the pairwise alignments. In the end, aligned site columns are obtained, with the expectation that they correspond to orthologous sites. Many programs refined this idea, using successive steps of re-estimation of the tree after the last alignment step for a given number of cycles, until a threshold is hit, or until a score stabilizes. Below we describe two commonly used algorithms for MSA estimation.

Muscle [59] is a relatively fast and widely used program that calculates pairwise distances by counting frequencies of k-mers and performing a progressive alignment using log-expectation scores, then refines the obtained neighbor-joining tree using a more involved distance measure (using a Markov model) that is used for MSA refinement in successive cycles. Tree refining is terminated if the set of internal nodes for which the branching order has changed has not decreased in size. Subsequently, the alignment is divided into two by deleting a tree edge, with MSAs being estimated for each partition, which facilitates local alignments, and then these alignment profiles are re-aligned against each other. If the sum-of-pairs (SP) score increases (see below), the MSA is once again divided into two and this refinement step is repeated. For calculating the SP, each column in an alignment is scored by summing the alignment scores of all pairs of symbols in that column; the score of the entire alignment is then summed over all column scores, computed as the sum of substitution matrix scores for each aligned pair of residues plus gap penalties.

Mafft [60] is another fast and relatively accurate software, having three general types of algorithms: progressive methods; iterative refinement methods using the WSP score (a weighted version of the SP score); and iterative refinement methods using the WSP summed with the consistency score for the alignment (which evaluates the consistency between a multiple alignment and pairwise alignments). The initial pairwise distances are based on shared 6-mers, and the tree is computed using a modified UPGMA method (see below for further explanation on the UPGMA algorithm). The simple progressive methods are the fastest, being able to analyze thousands of sequences in a reasonable time, while the second type of refinement method can be used for more difficult alignments (though limiting their use to at most hundreds of sequences).

There are alignment packages that drive existing MSA programs (e.g., Mafft), such as Guidance [61], PASTA (*Practical Alignment using SATe and Transitivity* [62]), and UPP (*Ultra-large alignments using Phylogeny-aware Profiles* [63]). PASTA is the fastest alternative for MSA of thousands of sequences, provided these are not too fragmented. It employs a divide-and-conquer strategy that is a variation of the DCM method mentioned above (Subheading 2.2.1), in which after a greedy progressive alignment, the tree is divided into disks (not necessarily subtrees) with fewer taxa that are aligned on each, and then these are merged together by transitivity, with further refinement cycles of tree inference and alignment [62]. UPP, which is also very fast and practical for thousands of sequences, first estimates a fast alignment and tree using PASTA, including only sequences with a minimum length threshold ("backbone alignment") to minimize error propagation in further steps; then, MSA hidden Markov models (HMMs) are estimated for the whole tree using the HMMER package [64], and then a different HMM is also estimated for each tree sector successively, until each sector reaches a minimum number of sequences (e.g., 10). The last step calculates a bit score of the alignment of a query sequence and each of those HMMs, and then the former is aligned with the MSA/HMM that has the top alignment score; this last step is repeated for all query sequences, until the whole set is multiply aligned [63]. PASTA may not be as accurate as UPP when sequences are too fragmented (a common situation when thousands of sequences are analyzed) or evolutionary rates are too high. The tree obtained in the last iteration of either PASTA or

UPP can be considered the best gene tree, bypassing the need for subsequent phylogenetic inference.

Guidance is aimed at finding MSA sites robust to alignment perturbations, while at the same time discarding sites that have too much ambiguity when aligned across different neighbor-joining guide trees (each tree obtained by bootstrapping the original MSA, e.g., ≥ 100 pseudoreplicates). This is interesting if the user wishes to be more conservative regarding the final result of a MSA, as many (possibly inaccurate) sites can be discarded. Guidance does not scale as well as PASTA or UPP in terms of handling thousands of sequences.

It is worth noting that, even with the conservative nature of Guidance, and the accuracy of PASTA and UPP, aligners may not perform well on some genes or on some regions of a gene, because of faster evolutionary rates at some sites or because there are exceedingly divergent species within the dataset. Therefore, local re-alignment of specific blocks should be tried manually in case they appear misaligned, using one of the above-mentioned programs. A fast and feature-rich program for such manual curation of alignments is Aliview [65].

3.2 Phylogenetic Methods

Some algorithms infer a single tree (such as UPGMA and Neighbor-Joining; see below), whereas others implement searches across the space of possible topologies. We begin this brief overview on phylogenetic methods by the latter, starting with maximum parsimony (MP), a method that does not assume explicit evolutionary models (although these can be employed under generalized parsimony; see below). Afterwards, we show ways to infer the best topology within the set of possible trees, which is the most demanding step for methods implementing tree search. Finally, we introduce Markov models, which are used by distance, likelihood, and Bayesian methods, while also describing such methods.

3.2.1 Maximum Parsimony

Maximum parsimony (MP) searches the tree(s) with lowest overall number of character changes across all characters (e.g., sites in an alignment). When changes are allowed to happen among unordered states (e.g., DNA, where each base can change to any other), this can be accomplished by the Fitch algorithm [77], which performs a post-order traversal of the tree while keeping track of the set of optimum states for internal nodes in the process, until the root is reached. This set is determined by testing for intersection first; if the latter is empty, then a set is built from the union of previously recorded states, and the number of overall steps for that character is incremented. The Wagner algorithm [66] is used to count changes for ordered multistate characters (e.g., size of a bone), being related to the Fitch algorithm: if state intervals overlap, then the set at a node is their union, but if the intersection is empty, then the set will include all values from smallest to largest.

Other important types of MP exist, and we cite a few of them here. *Camin-Sokal parsimony* [67] avoids reversals, being applicable to cases where a derived state (e.g., a deletion segment in a gene) would not spontaneously revert. *Dollo parsimony* [68, 69], on the other hand, permits reversals, but avoids parallel (or convergent) gains. Platt et al. [70] obtained a strongly supported phylogeny based on Dollo parsimony for almost 800,000 insertions of genome-wide short interspersed elements (SINEs) in specific genomic regions in the bat genus *Myotis* that was consistent with a tree obtained with other markers. *Transversion parsimony* (aimed at DNA analyses) counts only changes that result in transversions (i.e., purines ⇌ pyrimidines), a useful method if there is indication that transitions have occurred frequently and therefore homoplasies for this type of site substitution may be pervasive.

A generalized parsimony algorithm [71] can be used which addresses all types mentioned above by using different matrices of costs between states. Based on such a matrix, the minimum number of tree steps is obtained using the *Sankoff algorithm* [72], a dynamic programming algorithm that works for both unordered and ordered state changes. For analyses with a large number of taxa, maximum parsimony using TNT [73] is perhaps the best choice, implementing all parsimony variants described above while also being very fast.

3.2.2   Distance Methods

Distance methods first calculate pairwise distances (e.g., raw base differences, or percent, or percent corrected according to a *model of evolution*; see below), and then a tree is obtained such that the distance between any two taxa in the tree (patristic distance) conforms best with their pairwise distance. Among distance methods, Unweighted Pair Group Method with Arithmetic Mean (UPGMA) and neighbor-joining (NJ) are commonly used clustering algorithms that generate a single tree, contrarily to algorithms that search through tree space. UPGMA builds an ultrametric tree and hence assumes equal rates of evolution among all branches, a rare situation in real datasets. A fast implementation is found in the fastcluster package [74], with available interfaces for python and R. NJ relaxes this assumption by letting sister branches have different lengths (branch lengths are generally measured as amounts of expected substitutions/site for model-based phylogenetic methods, as opposed to MP, which calculates the raw number of substitutions at each branch). Fastphylo [75] is a fast implementation of NJ; PhyD* [76] also provides fast implementations of NJ including variants appropriate for species tree inference when taxa may be absent differentially across a set of genes (such as when genes were not sampled for all taxa, typical of phylogenomic analyses; *see* Subheading 4.5).

Other algorithms search the space of possible bifurcating trees for the "best" topology (where "best" depends on the specificities of the algorithm); in the case of distance methods, two such search algorithms are Minimum Evolution (ME) and Least-Squares (LS). Both infer, for each tree tested, the branch lengths by minimizing the error between pairwise and patristic distances using some least-squares function, but they differ in how to score each such tree: ME seeks the topology with minimum sum of branch lengths, whereas LS looks for the tree that minimizes the overall least-squares error between pairwise/patristic distances. A fast and accurate variation of ME can be found in the software FastME [77]. LS estimation of gene trees can be found in the program FITCH from the Phylip package [78].

3.2.3 Maximum Likelihood

Maximum likelihood (ML) methods are based on probability: by using a pre-specified model of evolution, they seek the tree that maximizes the overall probability of observing the sites in the current MSA alignment (or characters in a morphology matrix, among other possibilities), while at the same time estimating the model's best parameter values and branch lengths. Likelihood is not the same thing as probability though; actually, it can be considered its logical inverse: probability fixes a parameter value and estimates possible outcomes of data (e.g., given a transition/transversion rate, how many different sites can be generated and in which frequency?), whereas likelihood estimates parameter values given a fixed dataset (e.g., given a set of sites in an alignment, test for different values of transition/transversion rate). If we consider T = tree, m = model parameters, b = branch lengths, the general equation of the likelihood for a tree in a MSA (i.e. data) is:

$$L(T) = P(data|T, m, b), \qquad (1)$$

and then the tree with maximum likelihood (among all possibilities) is chosen. The likelihood is calculated independently for each site. The calculation involves the probability of each of the four nucleotides at each of the internal nodes changing to the nucleotide at the next node (or staying the same) until a leaf is found. Given a model of evolution represented by a matrix of rates Q, branch lengths (considered as a function of the rate matrix Q and time t, in substitutions per site) are optimized concomitantly based on Eq. 7 (*see* Subheading 3.4). After likelihoods are estimated under each site, these can be multiplied, but to avoid rounding errors due to multiplication of successive values between 0 and 1, the log-likelihood for each site is obtained and then these are added across the MSA. Fast ML implementations can be found in IQTree [79], RAxML [30], FastTree [80], PhyML [81], among others.

Bayesian inference (BI) is not an optimization criterion like LS, ME, MP, or ML. Instead, it finds an ensemble distribution of parameters based on the posterior probability of trees, model, and branch lengths, given the data according to the equation:

$$P(T, m, b|\text{data}) = \frac{P(\text{data}|T, m, b) \cdot P(T, m, b)}{P(\text{data})}, \qquad (2)$$

which is the Bayes theorem applied to general phylogenetics. The denominator can be further extended by:

$$P(T, m, b|\text{data}) = \frac{P(\text{data}|T, m, b) \cdot P(T, m, b)}{\sum P(\text{data}|T, m, b) \cdot P(T, m, b)}, \qquad (3)$$

It can be seen that it uses the likelihood function as well, while also depending on priors for the tree, model parameters, and branch lengths. Priors are discussed below. Actual estimation of parameters is done using the Markov Chain Monte Carlo (MCMC) algorithm based on [82] and later modified by Hastings [83]. The Metropolis-Hastings algorithm uses Markov chains as the connection mechanism between the actual state of the chain, and new states (where state means topology, branch lengths, and model parameters), which are obtained by proposals of new values according to perturbation algorithms (continuous in the case of parameters such as transition/transversion rates, discrete in the case of topology). During an MCMC run, trees are visited and then the above formula is used to calculate their probability. Because acceptance of a new state is based on the ratio of probabilities of this new proposed state relative to the old one, the denominator of Eq. 2 (or Eq. 3) cancels out.

In this way, different topologies are visited proportionally to their probabilities throughout the run, and eventually the likelihood and/or posterior probability of parameters reach a stationary region, in which the chain is said to have converged. In the end of the run, a distribution of values for all parameters (transition/transversion ratio, branch lengths, topologies, etc.) is obtained. The *burnin* (set of MCMC generations in which convergence has not been reached yet) must be discarded as its set is composed of low probability states. Ideally, at least two chains should be run concomitantly to avoid getting stuck in a local optimum. MrBayes allows the use of *heated chains*, which help the regular (*cold*) chain cross regions of low probability in the multi-dimensional space, hopefully escaping local optima, what is known as MCMCMC (Metropolis-coupled MCMC). The run is summarized by 95% highest posterior densities for continuous parameters, and a consensus tree (or a 95% credible set of trees) of all the trees whose states were accepted during the MCMC (except burnin). Good software options include MrBayes, BEAST [84], and Phycas [85].

3.2.5 What Is the Best Phylogenetic Method?

Distance methods that do not perform tree search tend to output reasonable trees in a fraction of the time that tree-search methods operate. Nevertheless, comparisons between sequences are averaged across the whole length of the alignment between them, so specific differences between two sequences are not assessed; character-based methods (such as MP, ML, and BI) have a finer resolution, assessing phylogenetic information on each character separately. However, distance methods are extremely useful for whole genomic phylogenomic analyses, and also for generating reasonable topologies that are used to initiate tree search for other algorithms.

Many studies compare MP and some probabilistic methods such as ML or BI. One of the most important drawbacks in MP is that it does not correct for multiple substitutions inciding in the same site, which tends to underestimate the total amount of change through time for distant divergences, impacting branch lengths and possibly tree shape. Felsenstein [86] showed that MP is also particularly prone to the effect of incorrectly approximating unrelated large branches (long branch attraction; Subheading 3.7.3). Contrarily, another study [87] found that when there is variation in the rate of evolution of lineages differently across sites (heterotachy; *see* Subheading 3.4.4), simple ML models tend to be outperformed by MP; nevertheless, at least three studies [88–90] contested those results, concluding that only a small region of the parameter space of arrangements of characters, branch lengths, and long branch position had been considered, and that for such an unbiased parameter space ML tends to be more accurate than MP. Nevertheless, ML can be inconsistent if the model used for its estimation is oversimplistic (e.g., [91]). As an example, ML accuracy is not guaranteed when indels are present and treated as missing data, even given arbitrarily long sequences [92]. BI, on the other hand, can also be inconsistent if reasonable prior distributions are not chosen for some parameters [93, 94].

The bottom line is that if the model is known, or not too different from the actual process of evolution that generated the data at hand, probabilistic methods tend to perform better than MP; but if the model applied to the data is oversimplistic, then ML and BI may become inconsistent as well, with lower accuracy than MP in at least a few cases. Running at least one probabilistic-based method (ME, ML, BI) altogether with MP is always recommended in order to test for differences in gene tree (or concatenated data) reconstruction.

3.3 Tree Search

Finding the best gene topology using optimality-based distance methods, MP, or ML, among all $2n - 5$ possible strictly bifurcating trees for n taxa ($2n - 3$ if rooted), is super-exponential in time. An exact shortcut exists, the *branch-and-bound method* [95], which first obtains a non-random tree with all taxa, estimates its optimality score (e.g., number of steps if MP), then restarts from scratch adding taxa to the tree, backtracking when a worse score is found with less taxa (i.e., adding more taxa will not improve the score). If a tree including all taxa is found with better score than the initial tree, it becomes the new upper limit; the search stops when successive trials fail to find a better tree. Nevertheless, this method is only feasible for up to ~ 20 taxa, above which the computational cost gets prohibitive. Heuristic searches were developed to improve tree search, yet these are not guaranteed to find a global optimum. Most common algorithms build a starting tree (either a random topology, or a topology in which taxa are added given some criterion such as lowest increase of number of steps, or a greedy tree that is closer to the true tree than a random tree, e.g. NJ), and then a different topology obtained by a specific type of *branch-swapping* is proposed. The score of this modified tree is calculated, being rejected if it is worse, or accepted if it is equal or better. Such tree proposals are done until all neighbors (i.e., all topologies with a distance of one such "atomic" move) are visited, or until a predefined number of cycles is reached; when the search is completed, the tree (or set of trees) with best score is reported.

An *NNI* (nearest neighbor interchange) rearrangement swaps subtrees on opposite sides of an internal edge. An *SPR* (subtree pruning and regrafting) rearrangement prunes a subtree and reattaches it to another edge without changing the former's local rooting. A *TBR* (tree bisection and reconnection) move reconnects a detached subtree in all possible ways. It can be seen from the above description that NNI $\subseteq$ SPR $\subseteq$ TBR. NNI will be more computationally efficient though less thorough, whilst TBR will search across tree space more thoroughly with less probability of getting stuck in local optima, though incurring in more computational burden. Most phylogenomic software implement NNI, SPR or some variation of it (e.g., RAxML implements the lazy-SPR move which performs a constrained SPR search, being actually a series of NNI moves up to a certain degree of edges away from the branch being considered). TNT is an example of software implementing TBR.

The types of branch swapping mentioned above are *hill-climbing* algorithms, always accepting better solutions during tree search. However, they do not cross "valleys" with transiently worse scores, and therefore may get stuck in local optima (or *islands*). To move between islands, further algorithms were developed, many of them also being relatively fast (sometimes even faster than global branch-swapping, such as sectorial and DCM searches). The *ratchet* [96] is based on perturbing trees whose score has stabilized after branch-swapping. It consists in re-weighting the characters in the dataset and then performing a new round of branch-swapping moves, until a topology stabilizes again. By doing this, the chances of escaping local optima increase. The original characters weights are then re-implemented, and the tree search restarts from there. It is implemented in TNT.

Genetic algorithms adapt evolutionary concepts to the optimization strategy, considering trees as individuals within a population, which can suffer mutations (branch-swapping) and recombination (exchange of the same subtree with different resolutions between trees) across many generations. After convergence the most adapted individuals (trees with best scores) are reported; examples include GARLI [97], MetaPIGA [98], and the *tree-fusing* algorithm [99] in TNT.

Simulated annealing methods accept suboptimal trees during branch-swapping with a certain probability, also helping in crossing valleys in tree space. *Tree-drifting* [99] is an example, consisting in accepting suboptimal rearrangements with a probability that depends on the tree-score difference between the new and the previous tree, being available in TNT. Another variation is implemented in MetaPIGA (using ML).

Divide-and-conquer algorithms reduce the dimension of the solution space by restricting a given problem to subsets of smaller problems. *Sectorial search* [99], and *disk-covering methods* (DCMs) and their variations (such as REC-I-DCM3; [100]) calculate scores for subsets of the original tree (a branch-swapped or starting tree) using the same base method (e.g., MP) by branch-swapping (or ratchet, etc.), which is less time consuming and more prone to find a better local solution than performing branch-swapping globally, and then the best resolution for each subset is returned. Sectorial searches optimizes non-overlapping subtrees, and then the best resolution is returned altogether with its original attachment position to the larger tree, to which subsequent TBR rounds may be applied; it is available in TNT. Contrarily, Rec-I-DCM3 chooses disjoint but overlapping subsets of the tree, further combining them using a supertree consensus method, and then a final round of refinement is performed to resolve any polytomies due to the latter step. It can be used in conjunction with PAUP* [101], GARLI, or RAxML available under the CIPRES Science Gateway portal (http://www.phylo.org).

TNT allows specific combinations of standard branch-swapping (NNI, SPR, TBR) with ratchet, tree-fusing, tree-drifting, and sectorial searches altogether, in different orders, and with a settable number of cycles, possibly being the fastest solution for computing gene trees under MP.

3.4 Models of Evolution

Probabilistic methods (such as ML and BI) depend on the use of molecular models of evolution for phylogenetic inference, which can be used with distance-based methods as well. The idea is to estimate quantitatively the rates of state change by employing continuous-time Markov models, in which the chance of a base

3.4.1 Markov Models

(or amino acid, or discrete characters, etc.) changing to another along a branch is described by an n-by-n matrix, where n is the alphabet size of the states composing the character set (four in the case of DNA, 20 for amino acids, etc.).

3.4.2 DNA Models

Considering the four DNA bases in alphabetical order (A, C, G, T) in the matrix below, the instantaneous rate matrix between any two states can be modeled by a non-stationary general Markov model (up to a substitutional rescaling parameter μ):

$$Q_{\text{GMMns}} = \mu \begin{bmatrix} - & a & b & c \\ g & - & d & e \\ h & j & - & f \\ i & k & l & - \end{bmatrix}. \tag{4}$$

This matrix has 11 free parameters, because one degree of freedom (d.f.) is lost as one of the rates is commonly fixed to 1.0 (or the average is set to 1.0). Such a model is *homogeneous* (the same throughout the tree), *non-stationary* (a unique vector of base frequencies may not be identifiable), and *non-reversible* (probability of evolutionary change may depend on directionality, so $A \leftrightarrow C$ may be different from $C \leftrightarrow A$). This was called the UNREST model (for "unrestricted"; [102]). Under the constraint of stationarity, the general model now becomes:

$$Q_{\text{GMMs}} = \mu \begin{bmatrix} - & \pi_c r_{ac} & \pi_g r_{ag} & \pi_t r_{at} \\ \pi_a r_{ca} & - & \pi_g r_{cg} & \pi_t r_{ct} \\ \pi_a r_{ga} & \pi_c r_{gc} & - & \pi_t r_{gt} \\ \pi_a r_{ta} & \pi_c r_{tc} & \pi_g r_{tg} & - \end{bmatrix}, \tag{5}$$

where each element q_{ij} of Q represents the instantaneous rate of change from a nucleotide to another. Decomposing q_{ij} into its elements, π_i are the stationary frequencies (e.g., empirically obtained from the data), and r_{ij} are 'exchangeability' rates of nucleotide substitutions. Each q_{ii} (diagonal elements) is such that each row sums to 0.0. A further assumption, on top of stationarity, is *time-reversibility*; it is generally assumed for mathematical tractability, in which $\pi_i q_{ij} = \pi_j q_{ji}$ (also called *detailed balance* property). It can be seen that the above formula is true if $r_{ij} = r_{ji}$, leading to the widely known general time reversible model (GTR; [103]) with 8 free parameters:

$$Q_{\mathrm{GTR}} = \mu \begin{bmatrix} - & \pi_c a & \pi_g b & \pi_t c \\ \pi_a a & - & \pi_g d & \pi_t e \\ \pi_a b & \pi_c d & - & \pi_t f \\ \pi_a c & \pi_c e & \pi_g f & - \end{bmatrix}. \tag{6}$$

Due to its better mathematical tractability and smaller parameter set (aiding at computations), most phylogenetic software implement GTR or some restriction of it (see below). To get the total amount of change after a time Δt (which is the branch length), the formula is:

$$P(t) = e^{Qt}, \tag{7}$$

which can be calculated by matrix diagonalization. Branch lengths are in number of substitutions, and therefore the product Qt is not identifiable (rates and times cannot be decomposed without extra information). The instantaneous substitution rate is then rescaled to expected number of substitutions per site (a relative unit), by equating $\mu = -1/\Sigma q_{ii}$. Values for each parameter can be estimated from the data by some kind of optimization, or obtained empirically (which is commonly used for base frequencies, aiding in computations). Typical reversible models of evolution (hence submodels of GTR) are JC69 [104], where all state changes have the same probability, K2P [105], where transitions (ti) have a different probability in relation to transversions (tv), HKY [106], where both π_i's are different and $ti \neq tv$, and of course GTR itself. These are commonly used models, but they represent only a few among the possible 406 reversible models (203 considering equal π_i's, 203 considering different π_i's). We will discuss how to choose among models further ahead.

3.4.3 Spatial
Heterogeneity of Rates

Due to differential selective constraints across DNA regions, such as regions under purifying selection, others closer to neutral evolution, and a few of them under positive selection, models not accounting for such spatial heterogeneities may lead to spurious phylogenetic reconstruction [107]. A possibility is using a two-rate model in which a proportion p of the sites is restricted to be invariable and $1 - p$ sites are allowed to change. Rate variation across sites can also be modeled by a discretized gamma distribution [107], in which a pre-specified number of rate classes is defined (usually four, due to computational constraints, but can be more), and then for each site the same Markov model is weighted across these classes. The latter is a simple example of a *mixture model*, in which there is an ensemble probability of each site belonging to all rate classes, instead of each being attributed to one class specifically. It is also possible to employ both a gamma distribution and a proportion of invariant sites in the same Markov model: GTR+G, HKY+I, and JC+I+G are a few examples of the models just discussed. Such models can be found in most probabilistic-based software.

Another possibility is the use of more complex mixture models, which employ two or more different matrices (each also having different distributions across sites if desired), in many cases fitting better the data. An example is [108] which showed that the use of two concomitant gamma distributions can lead to more improved phylogenies. Another example is the use of CAT profile mixture models [109], which allow the use of different stationary frequencies (of amino acids, originally) leading to an ensemble model with *n* profile matrices across sites (where each site has some probability of pertaining to any of the rate classes), again leading to better topological accuracy. CAT was later extended by models composed of *mixture of matrices* (e.g., [110]), allowing different empirical models to be considered simultaneously throughout the alignment, each of them also permitting inclusion of gamma rate categories. IQTree, among other packages, offers a wide range of possibilities of profile and matrix mixtures (either separated or jointly).

Hidden Markov models (HMMs) account for local correlations among sites, leading to better model fit in many cases (e.g., [111–113]). PhyML_multi [113] was shown to detect correct gene trees in the presence of recombination (generated by simulation), performing better than mixture models; its speed was also reasonable (considering that HMMs tend to be expensive algorithms), taking less than 4 min to estimate gene trees with 40 taxa on a single processor [113].

Site-partitioning models represent another reasonable way to account for spatial heterogeneity of rates. Each site is attributed to a single pre-specified rate class beforehand, based on previous biological knowledge (such as codon position, intron vs. exon, etc.), therefore constituting a type of *fixed-effects* models (contrarily to mixture models). They will be further discussed in Subheading 3.6.

3.4.4 Temporal Heterogeneity of Rates

A site under selection in a lineage may cease to be so upon entering a different niche; or it may be the other way around. In this context, models that do not permit variability of rates among branches across sites can induce systematic bias on tree reconstruction (e.g., [87, 114]). A *heterotachy mixture model* implemented in IQTree is a relatively fast procedure that allows different sites in a gene to have a separate set of branch lengths and model parameters, therefore being a kind of site-rate mixture model; the number of classes is user-defined a priori. The authors claim that extensive simulations obtained almost 100% accuracy for heterotachously evolved sequences (http://www.iqtree.org/doc/Heterotachy-Models/). Another possibility is to use *non-homogeneous models*, such as nhPhyML (http://pbil.univ-lyon1.fr/software/nhphyml/), which allows a separate GC-content for each branch of the phylogeny [115].

3.4.5 RNA Models

RNAs typically depend on their tertiary structure to perform their biological function, which in turn depends on secondary structure. The latter can be divided into regions with internal pairings (stems) and single-stranded regions (loops). A general 16-by-16 RNA model captures the dependencies between the substitutions at the paired stem sites, including all possible nucleotide pairings (e.g., [116–119]). Nevertheless, the dimensionality of such a model can be reduced by considering that most pairings are unstable (hence their frequency is negligible) except for the canonical ones, which are either AU, UA, CG, GC pairings, plus two other less stable non-canonical states, GU and UG, observable at lower frequencies. The latter leads to a six-dimensional matrix [119, 120]. Other models have 7 states, extending the six-dimensional model with a mismatch state encompassing all remaining states [119, 121, 122]. MrBayes, for example, implements the 16-state *doublet* model that assumes that the probability of a one-step double change is zero, therefore any double changes must go through an intermediate step (possibly transiently less fit within the evolving population). PHASE (https://github.com/james-monkeyshines/rna-phase-3) is another example, implementing 6, 7, and 16-state models, allowing for double changes within an infinitesimal time interval [119]; furthermore, the latter implements statistical state-space projection allowing comparison of likelihoods between DNA models, 7-state and 16-state RNA models (model selection is more complicated when the best model has to be chosen among different dimensions because likelihoods are not comparable; see below). An analysis encompassing 287 RNA families indicated that the choice of the appropriate dimensional model can have a substantial effect on tree estimation, with the greatest differences being between DNA and RNA models, but also with variation within the different RNA models. Furthermore, 281 out of 287 had RNA models selected in preference to 4-state DNA models, with 7-state models fitting better conserved families with shorter stems, and 16-state models best fitted for more divergent families with longer stems [123].

3.4.6 Protein Models

Under probabilistic models, a full 20-dimensional protein matrix is too expensive computationally, so reductions are necessary for the amino acid alphabet. Dayhoff et al. [124] introduced an empirical model based on *point accepted mutations* (PAM), which are a function of the estimated number of mutations per 100 amino acids (based on 1572 observed mutations in trees from 71 families of closely related proteins), and with the constraint that each alignment had at least 85% identity. Different PAM matrices have increasing values (e.g., PAM100, PAM120, etc.), with larger numbers indicating larger evolutionary distances. Alternatively, BLOSUM matrices (BLOcks SUbstitution Matrix; [125]) calculate substitutions in conserved motifs of related sequences, with associated indices (e.g., BLOSUM62, the default matrix for protein BLAST) defined by inclusion of pairwise identities of no more than $X\%$ (so for BLOSUM62, 62%), using local alignments, each being derived from observed alignments instead of extrapolated as in PAM matrices. The JTT model [126] continued the general idea of Dayhoff and colleagues creating an empirical matrix, but using a broader database, followed by other matrices (e.g., WAG and LG [127, 128]), including others focused at organelle types (e.g., mtMAM for mammals' mitochondria; [129]) or at specific organisms (e.g., FLU for influenza virus; [130]). Further refinements incorporated *protein mixture models* with either gamma rate heterogeneity or with distribution-free site rate bins [131]; the latter two matrix models were shown to outperform standard models, providing significant gains of log-likelihood units for different data sets. All such models can be found in ML software such as PhyML, IQTree, and RAxML, and in Bayesian software such as MrBayes and PhyloBayes (the latter also employing mixture models), among others.

Similarly to RNA stem models, protein models can explore higher-order structure. Le et al. [110] tested the fit of supervised and unsupervised mixture models encompassing exposed/buried AA sites (EX2), exposed/intermediate/buried AA sites (EX3), and extended/helix/other sites (EHO), indicating that mixture models using this kind of information improved likelihoods while also impacting tree estimation, in comparison to mixture models not considering exposure and/or secondary structure characteristics. IQTree implements these models along with other types of mixture models.

3.4.7 Codon Models

Different triplets may code for the same amino acid due to the degeneracy of genetic codes, with *synonymous* nucleotide changes maintaining the same amino acid, whereas *nonsynonymous* changes alter the amino acid. Codon models leverage both mutational tendencies among nucleotides and selective pressure on amino acid substitutions. The whole set of triplets leads to 64 codons, but for many models three stop codons are not entered into the calculations, so 61-dimensional matrices are used. Initial models allowed a single nucleotide change per infinitesimal time. The MG94 model [132] contended two rates (between synonymous codons, and between nonsynonymous codons), and equilibrium frequencies of target nucleotides. Goldman and Yang [133] presented a more complex model by including a parameter associated with transitions, and employing a normalized distance between amino acids based on several physico-chemical properties (GY94); furthermore, they used codon equilibrium frequencies instead of nucleotide frequencies (contrarily to MG94). Later on, this model was simplified (YN98; [134]) becoming completely parametric (or *mechanistic*), including a transversion/transversion rate ratio, and a parameter ω representing the nonsynonymous to synonymous rate ratio (dN/dS, becoming one of the most popular codon models due to its usefulness at estimating selection). Other models allow multiple substitutions combining parametric and empirical parameter values. WG04 [135] considers substitutions of two or three consecutive nucleotides as one possible evolutionary event, showing better fit than models not correcting for multiple substitutions. Another example is the ECM model [136], which has five different versions in which transition and transversion rates can be incorporated; a subset of 200 alignments from the Pandit database (http://www.ebi.ac.uk/research/goldman/software/pandit) indicated that the model with separate transition and transversion parameters had the best results, outperforming previous mechanistic and empirical models in phylogenetic reconstruction. Codon-PhyML [137] is a fast program for phylogenetic inference aimed at codon models, also having a large amount of models implemented. IQTree further allows complex codon mixture models, which in principle may lead to better fit models in at least some cases.

3.4.8 General Discrete-State Model

When using DNA data, it may be that transitions get saturated faster than transversions (Subheading 3.7.3), e.g. due to chemical similarities between pyrimidines (C and T), and between purines (A and G); in such cases, it may be more informative to consider only transversions by recoding purines as R and pyrimidines as Y, and then apply a *2-state Markov model*. Such binary state models are meaningful for morphological characters (e.g., presence/absence of wings), restriction site data such as AFLP (having a DNA band, or not), gene content, and indels. A natural extension is the use of *multi-ordered states* (nucleotide and amino acid data being subtypes), such as bone lengths within three or more size categories, or overlapping indel sizes with two or more categories (if indel length across taxa varies). Lewis [28] named this general model *Mk* (Markov k-states). A more appropriate version considers datasets in which constant characters are absent (such as SNPs), as stated before (Subheading 2.1.4), which Lewis named *Mkv* (v for "variable"). Variation across sites (e.g., gamma discretized rates) can also be incorporated (Subheading 3.4.3). Caution must be taken if frequencies of states are to be considered as parameters in the Q-matrix: differently than nucleotides (where an "A" is always an adenine across all characters), "0's" and "1's" are just codings that are reused across characters, not necessarily being comparable (can absence of a wing be summed with absence of beak in another character, to give an ensemble frequency of zeros across both characters?); incorporating state frequencies may be more justifiable for presence/absence data when it can be assumed (though only as an approximation) that the same process is operating across characters, as in restriction site and indel datasets. Examples of software where *Mkv* models can be used are IQTree, which considers variable characters only, and MrBayes, which includes different versions depending on the matrix: only variable sites (e.g., SNPs, morphology); parsimony-informative sites (a subset of the variable characters, aimed at MP analysis); and variable plus constant characters for one of the states only (e.g., restriction sites including a band visible in all taxa). A recent study [138] showed that Bayesian analyses using *Mk* models outperform MP under conditions that are commonly encountered in paleontological studies, even when assuming a wide range of scenarios including missing data and rate heterogeneity.

3.5 Model Choice

While it is true that an overly simplistic model may bias phylogenetic reconstruction by failing to take into account important evolutionary parameters affecting a dataset (e.g., transition/transversion ratios, missing in JC and F81 models), choosing an overly complex model may also be problematic because with too many parameters variances may get too large, compromising precision; moreover, there may not be enough information for estimating too many parameters in a dataset (e.g., G-T substitutions tend to be rare in individual gene multiple alignments). Therefore, it is not surprising that alternative models can change the results of phylogenetic analysis by affecting model parameter estimates (e.g., genetic distances and branch lengths; [139, 140]), branch support measures [140], and tree inference [86, 141, 142], so justified ways to perform model selection are warranted.

We start our discussion with likelihood-based indices, then move to Bayesian-based criteria. First of all, to avoid lengthy calculations, most likelihood-based model choice procedures allow estimation of model fit in a fixed tree, speeding up computations. This is based on the fact that model parameter values are not severely impacted by a topology obtained by a greedy algorithm [143, 144]. Hierarchical likelihood-ratio tests (hLRT) calculate chi-squared *P*-values to test between *nested* models, in terms of one being a restriction of the other (e.g., JC is a nested model within F81 as both are equal except for the latter allowing different base frequencies), and whenever a significant model is found, it is chosen as the new null hypothesis, but it is restricted to nesting schemes; moreover, it also depends on the starting point and the path through the hierarchy of models (should we start from the simpler model, or from the more complex?). The remaining procedures do not depend on nested models, therefore being able to test larger sets of models. The AIC is an asymptotically unbiased estimator of the expected relative Kullback-Leibler information distance [145], measuring the amount of information lost when we use an inferred model to approximate the (theoretically) real one, with smaller values indicating relatively better fit. Its equation is:

$$\text{AIC} = -2l + 2k, \tag{8}$$

where l is the log-likelihood of the model under the fixed tree, with the k parameters fixed at their ML estimates. AICc [146] is an AIC correction for parameters obtained from relatively small samples:

$$\text{AICc} = \text{AIC} + \frac{2k(k+1)}{(n-k-1)}, \tag{9}$$

where n is the number of samples (discussed below). BIC (Bayesian information criterion; [147]) is an approximation to the log marginal likelihood of a model, so taking the difference between the BICs of two models can be a reasonable approximation to the natural log of the Bayes factor between them [148]; even though BIC was developed having that Bayesian commonality in mind, it should not be confused with indices aimed at model choice under Bayesian inference, described further ahead. Its formula is:

$$\text{BIC} = -2l + k \cdot \log(n). \tag{10}$$

DT is another reasonable likelihood-based model choice procedure, based on a decision theory framework [149], where the best model is the one minimizing a function of relative branch-length error based on squared Euclidean distances. jModelTest 2 [150] implements all four criteria above; alternatively, the software can also employ *model averaging*, in which branch support values are calculated as the amount of different models supporting a specific tree [151].

What constitutes an appropriate quantity for n in the equations above is still debatable; usually n is considered the number of sites in the alignment, but it could also be number of sites times number of taxa, number of site patterns, etc. A recent study [152] found that only for a small percentage of models under simulation the use of different versions of n support another model, and therefore $n =$ *number of sites* should be satisfactory.

Two different simulation studies [144, 153] showed that BIC and DT have comparable performance while also outperforming other criteria; another study [152] also indicates that BIC finds the correct simulated model more often than other procedures, but only by a small margin. Collectively, these suggest that BIC is a reasonable and fast model choice criterion.

Another promising approach is *cross-validation* [154], in which each model can be tested using training sets (used to estimate parameters) and testing sets (used to assign likelihood values), and then the model showing less discrepancy between likelihoods of the training and testing sets is to be preferred. As an example, it showed that the CAT model had a better statistical fit than WAG in reconstructing the position of nematodes and platyhelminths within metazoans [155]. Cross-validation is available in

PhyloBayes, but it may be relatively slower for testing models in many gene trees.

Those likelihood-based criteria can only compare Markov models with the same number of dimensions (e.g., all 4-by-4 reversible models). What about comparisons among models of DNA (4-dimensional), amino acid (20-dimensional), and codon (61-dimensional), to test for the best model across dimensions? ModelOMatic [156] was developed as a means to leverage comparison across trans-dimensional datasets. It works by employing adapter functions, projecting aggregated models onto the originally observed sequence data. It performed relatively fast with alignments from the Pandit database, and showed that depending on the empirical dataset used, models with different dimensions can be preferred [156].

Under BI, *Bayes factors* (BFs) are typically used to measure model fit between two different models, by computing the ratio of the marginalized likelihoods between them [148]. Alternatively, BFs can be calculated individually for different models, and then the simplest model having the largest ΔBF is chosen. Originally, the marginalized likelihood (obtained by integrating over likelihood values in the posterior distribution) was estimated by a harmonic mean estimator which was found to be an inconsistent estimator, leading to strong overestimation of the marginal likelihood [157]). A modified BI version of AIC (AICM) performs better but still is, to a lesser degree, relatively unreliable [158]. However, more accurate ways of calculating a model's marginalized likelihood are still challenging for large datasets, such as *thermodynamic integration/ path sampling* [157], and the *stepping-stone* method [159], both performing samplings along paths in the space of the posterior and the prior distributions (or between the posterior and a reference distribution, in the case of *generalized stepping-stone* [159]), possibly increasing the number of MCMC runs by more than tenfold per estimate. All latter approaches are found in BEAST; *reversible-jump MCMC* [160], which tests among models with different dimensions during a single MCMC run, also induces a large computational burden on large numbers of gene trees or concatenated datasets (available in MrBayes). All considered, likelihood-based criteria (e.g., BIC and DT) are currently much faster than Bayesian alternatives, being also relatively accurate, and scaling better regarding large phylogenomic analyses.

3.6   Partitioning

The fact that different genomic regions (or sites within a gene) can have different rates of evolution must be taken into consideration for phylogenetics analysis, otherwise topology and/or branch length estimates can get biased (e.g., [161, 162]); the use of mixed models, explained above, is one way to implement it. Partitioning is another strategy, whereby sites are allocated to data partitions a priori. Such a division can be based on genes, on codon positions, on both, and even on other combinations (e.g., introns vs. exons, stems vs. loops, etc.), in most cases leading to better data fit. In general, a *proportional model* among partitions is assumed, in which branch lengths across partitions are kept proportional, up to individual rate multipliers, to avoid overparametrization. Nevertheless, individual partitions a priori may have lower fit compared to a model aggregating partitions into fewer classes. In this sense, PartitionFinder [163] estimates the relative fit of different combinations of partitions, the number of which can become explosive in phylogenomic datasets, reducing the complexity of the data; after the best partitioning scheme is chosen, the substitution model for each partition is done by model selection (e.g., BIC), significantly outperforming ad hoc selection of partitioning schemes on a range of published data sets [163]. Further combining partitioning scheme and mixture models (e.g., two GTR models for two genes, each model having a mixture model of site patterns) can be done in IQTree; ensemble analysis including partitions with different types of data can be done under many ML (e.g., PhyML, IQTree, RAxML) and BI-based software (e.g., MrBayes, PhyloBayes, BayesPhylogenies).

3.7 Controlling for Biases When Inferring Gene Trees

Gene trees are prone to both sampling errors (due to low amounts of data) and systematic errors (leading to incorrect inference even if amount of data is satisfactory). We will discuss both here; most issues also relate to reconstruction based on supermatrix methods (*see* Subheading 4.4), where we also address causes of gene tree variability among loci when estimating a tree using the latter method, but many of these biases can also impact supertrees and species tree methods. We start by noting some important sources of bias that may occur prior to the multiple alignment (issues with the alignment itself were discussed in Subheading 3.1).

3.7.1 Possible Sources of Bias Prior to a Multiple Alignment

When assembling genomes or contigs (either using a reference or de novo assembly), care must be taken to avoid *chimeric mapping*. This may occur in regions of low complexity, e.g. in genes embracing repetitive regions (e.g., virulence genes in some bacteria), or if there are paralogous genes that are relatively similar (e.g., globins in many vertebrates; IS elements in both prokaryotes and eukaryotes). Low complexity regions, and genes within, should be discarded previously to any phylogenetic analysis. Especially in the case of complete or near complete genomes (such as many prokaryotes), one tool that can identify regions of low complexity is Mummer [164], using its Nucmer script.

Annotation consistency is a desirable feature when comparing genomes through their predicted genes. Using the same annotation pipeline for all genomes is a way of achieving this consistency. However, not always this is possible, especially when using public annotations. In such cases, the resultant missing data across many genes may induce artifactual relationships, and auxiliary genomic information (such as indels and gene presence/absence) must be considered with caution in these cases.

When incorporating genes from online databases (an important source in many phylogenomic studies), it is important to check if the *taxonomy has changed*: different names may mean the same species (inflating the number of taxa being analyzed); or the opposite may have happened: some subspecies may have been unraveled as different (possibly paraphyletic) species (perhaps biasing relationship assessment if one of the sequences is chosen randomly). In case of many copies of the same gene for a taxonomic unit in the database, one can include the largest (or randomly among equally largest), or generate a consensus of partially overlapping sequences under that taxonomic unit to maximize size (among other possibilities); SCaFoS [165] was developed for such situations. Nevertheless, for analyses under the Multi-Species Coalescent paradigm (MSC; *see* Subheading 4.6), more than one sequence per gene of the same taxonomic unit should in general be included.

3.7.2   Sampling Errors

After a multiple alignment is obtained, and assuming its potential biases were minimized, biases due to lack of adequate sampling may still compromise gene tree reconstruction. Genes with small sizes (considering its DNA or AA length, depending on the data type chosen) may bias proper resolution due to an associated relatively larger variance. Too much *missing data* in a gene (if distributed quite randomly) can also incur in sampling error, especially if a gene is relatively small [166], while for genes ≥ 1000 bp, up to 80% of missing data across taxa under different scenarios is tolerable [166]. *Datasets with a few number of taxa*, when there is the possibility of including more, are another possible source of bias, because adding more taxa can help in breaking effects of long-branch attraction (see below) even if added OTUs also contain reasonable amounts of missing data, as observed from simulated data [166, 167].

3.7.3   Systematic Errors

We first mention typical biases affecting individual alignments or concatenated datasets, and then we discuss methods to detect and (if possible) overcome such biases; some of these have already been mentioned above, and are commented *en passant*. Such kinds of bias, if present, may not be minimized by the inclusion of more data, and in fact may lead to highly supported, but incorrect, clades. Furthermore, systematic errors (that lead to incorrect gene tree reconstructions) are not to be confused with legitimate sources of gene tree discordance, or gene-tree/species-tree discordance. The following list is representative of systematic errors, though not exhaustive.

Saturation is the effect of multiple substitutions impacting the same site in a multiple alignment, making the number of actual differences in a site between two taxa more than what is observable (which is always at most one, when nucleotides are different between two sequences). This kind of bias was one of the main reasons for the development of probabilistic methods (which incorporate models that correct for the extra substitutions). When saturation is extreme, the amount of substitutions is underestimated, leading to shorter branch lengths (especially at deeper divergences), which can lead to biased topologies in many cases [168].

Missing data, besides potentially generating sampling error, can also generate systematic errors when their distribution is not random [169], as is the case with datasets incorporating genes from the literature, e.g. when original studies focused on a subset of the taxa but other laboratories have not sequenced the same region for related lineages. Furthermore, under both ML and Bayesian frameworks, among-site rate variation can interact with ambiguous data to produce misleading estimates of topology and branch lengths [170].

An improper *evolutionary model* (Markov model) can also impact phylogenetic reconstruction, especially if an overly simplified model is employed, underestimating branch lengths [151]; this also includes properly adjusting for *variability in rates across sites* [107], with the rationale also extending to *proper partitioning* [163].

Compositional heterogeneity may also impact reconstruction because similar but unrelated nucleotide stretches can get closer due to their similarity even though they are not closest relatives, as is the case with thermophylic prokaryotes which have high GC content mostly due to their higher stability in hot environments [171].

Assuming a dataset follows a *homogeneous model* across lineages when in fact it is incorrect (*heterotachy being a subcase*) may also fail to capture correct relationships [87].

Selection in some cases can induce convergent tracts in distant lineages (convergent selection), or contrarily, suggest that closely related taxa are distant incorrectly (divergent selection). For example, an analysis of *rbcL* sequences (encoding the photosynthetic Rubisco enzyme, of crucial importance due to its role in photorespiratory carbon oxidation) from over 3000 species representing all lineages of green plants plus some phototrophs detected positive selection in many lineages of land plants [172].

Specific *priors* under BI can also lead to unrealistically large branches [173] and overconfident branch posterior probabilities [174].

Big genome artifacts relate to analyses based on gene content, in which lineages who lost (or gained) many genes in parallel may be highly supported as sister groups [48].

Rogue taxa are taxa with unstable placement in trees across datasets, or across data resamplings (e.g., bootstrap), which besides misguiding their own correct position in the tree, may also reduce overall support for branches across the tree [175].

Long-branch attraction (LBA) is one outcome expected by many of the above cited artifacts, related to the algorithm behavior of most phylogenetic models in different scenarios, where unrelated long branches attract each other due to shared homoplasies (e.g., due to symplesiomorphies, saturation, missing data, wrong model, heterotachy, etc.) [176].

All four *phylogenetic methods* described previously can also induce biases in different circumstances, as commented in Subheading 3.2.5.

Saturation is a pervasive problem in datasets including relatively distant divergences, even if the data as a whole is homogeneous in all other senses; hence, we approach ways of detecting it in more depth. Detection of saturation can be done by checking a distance plot, and alternatively by estimating the slope and comparing it with a transformed dataset supposedly less affected by multiple substitutions. Plotting p-distances in the *y*-axis (uncorrected distances) against patristic distances (edge distance in the tree connecting the same two taxa) obtained under the best-fit model can be done in PATRISTIC [177]. Here, the patristic distances in the *x*-axis are intended to be a proxy for the time between divergences, and it is expected that under a non-saturated dataset the slope should be linear; however for saturated datasets the p-distance will be underestimated, and if a curve leading to a plateau is observed, it is a sign of saturation. The next step could be data transforming/subsetting (see below), and then saturation in this new dataset can be compared to the original by checking the slope: if the slope is kept relatively the same or increases, then the new dataset is relatively better at counteracting saturation; and if the slope decreases sensibly, then the data transforming/subsetting did not work as expected. Another possible way of estimating saturation levels is using Xia's index [178], which is a function of the entropy of a site, based on the idea that the more saturated the dataset, the closer the average entropy across sites will be to the maximum entropy value, and then an empirically-derived critical value of significance is obtained; if the average alignment entropy is not significantly smaller, the interpretation is that the sequences have experienced severe substitution saturation [178]. DAMBE [179] obtains two critical values, one for a symmetrical tree, and another for an extremely asymmetrical tree, and ideally the value for the data should be significantly lower than both.

Once detected, there are many procedures that can be considered to minimize saturation, as well as minimizing other biases in gene trees. A few of them, along with their pros and cons, are depicted:

1. Discarding fast-evolving sites, e.g. using OV-method or TIGER [180, 181]. However, [182] depict cases in which both share systematic biases: against (1) characters with more symmetric distributions of states; (2) characters with greater observed character-state space; and (3) large clades in the context of character conflict. Downweighting such sites under an MP framework is also a feasible alternative.

2. Discarding 3rd codon positions, which tend to saturate faster than 1st and 2nd positions. A study employing phylogenetic reconstruction of vertebrate rhodopsin sequences [183] showed that by removing 3rd codon positions spurious reconstructions can be corrected. Nonetheless, third codon positions may also be highly informative even at deep divergences, bearing greater number of parsimony-informative characters compared to 1st and 2nd positions, as observed in a study of evolution of seed plants [184]. Alternatively, instead of discarding, downweighting 3rd positions under an MP framework can be useful (*see*, for example, [185], which studied cyt-b evolution in deer mice).

3. Recoding as amino acids if applicable, or even further reductions based on clustering by biochemical characteristics, such as Dayhoff recoding (as was done in [186], in analyzing the origin of eukaryotes, a dataset where strong levels of saturation are expected), available in PhyloBayes.

4. Recoding in a lower-dimensional state space, such as RY-coding for 3rd codon positions, in which purines are recoded as "R" and pyrimidines as "Y" to alleviate the excess of transitions (e.g., ReCoDer: http://web.pdx.edu/~stul/Software.html). Such a recoding was done in an avian phylogenomic study [187], which helped to identify potentially flawed clades. Other reductional recodings are also possible: SeqVis [188] displays the nucleotide composition of a set of sequences within a multiple alignment in a tetrahedron; the more points gather together, the more similar they are in composition, and the more they are spread apart from one another, the larger the variation. Tetrahedron plots can be obtained for the whole alignment or for each of the three codon positions separately. If reasonable spreading is detected in any of the latter, SeqVis can depict all 2-state and 3-state recodings in lower dimensional plots, possibly alleviating compositional heterogeneity without the use of heterogeneous models, which are much more costly to run.

5. Use of models that accommodate both site and lineage rate changes, such as mixture and/or heterotachy models. P4, PhyML, IQTree, PhyloBayes, BayesPhylogenies, and PHASE are some of the programs including such models. Some of these

algorithms retrieved phylogenies conforming better with morphology-driven taxonomy (based on putatively reliable evolutionary characters) in a mitogenomic study of beetles [189].

6. Automatically discarding sites including too many gaps, for example using TrimAl [190]. Non-random distribution of indels can induce artifactual gene tree relationships in some conditions [170].

7. Detecting rogue taxa and automatically excluding them in RogueNaRok [191] or RAxML, and then recalculating boot-strapped data without their presence. Removal of rogue taxa was shown to improve resolution in bee flies [192], on collec-tions of bootstrap trees from 26 real-world multiple sequence alignments [193], and in examples from the literature and from large biological data sets [194].

8. Increasing taxonomic sampling may help in breaking up long branches by revealing synapomorphies (as reviewed by Heath et al. [195]).

9. Trying different phylogenetic methods for gene tree estima-tion, at least a non-parametric (MP) and one parametric (e.g., ML or BI) if possible.

3.8 Inferring Clade Support

It is important to assess the amount of statistical support that clades in an estimated tree have. Below we describe the main measures used, further discussing their pros and cons.

3.8.1 Bootstrap

The most common procedure is the bootstrap [196], in which sites of the character matrix (e.g., derived from a MSA, or morphologi-cal) are resampled with replacement until the original number of sites is reached. Such resampling is done a large number of times (usually 1000), and for each such pseudoreplicate a tree is esti-mated, always based on the same phylogenetic method. In the end, a *majority-rule consensus tree* (MRC), which includes only the splits found in a majority of the input trees (therefore possibly inducing some polytomies) is generated. An extension of this algo-rithm, aimed at generating a more resolved tree (in terms of bifur-cations), keeps including less supported splits as long as they are compatible with splits already present in the tree, being called *extended majority-rule consensus* (eMRC) or *greedy consensus*; it is the most common variation found in many phylogenetic software. Many studies assume a threshold of 70% bootstrap proportion to consider a split reliable under bootstrapping (discussed below). Alternatively, supported clades in the consensus tree can be attrib-uted to bipartitions on the best tree (obtained previously by the same method). The *rapid bootstraping* method in RAxML (not to be confused with the ultra-fast bootstrap approximation of IQTree;

see below) is a modification that pre-computes prunings of all subtrees, then tests reinsertions of these but only within a fixed radius of neighboring branches (a type of *lazy* subtree pruning and regrafting), speeding up computations.

3.8.2 Ultra-Fast Bootstrap (UFBoot)

Though with a similar name, UFBoot [197] is more different than the algorithms above. It performs resampling of estimated log-likelihoods, and then it focuses only on relatively well-supported candidate trees using NNI moves. It can be up to $3.1\times$ (nucleotide) to $10.2\times$ (amino acid) faster than RAxML's rapid bootstrap, on average.

3.8.3 Jackknife

This measure involves resampling without reposition dropping a fixed percentage of characters on every turn, to test for sensitivity of character inclusion [196]. The latter suggests dropping 50% of the characters of a matrix, but only because then jackknife and bootstrap would have the same coefficient of variation, being more comparable with each other [196, 198]. Contrarily, Farris et al. [199] suggest deleting $1/e$ characters based on probabilities of support of a clade vs. a conflicting one. An advantage of the jackknife is its speed, as it uses less characters than bootstrap variations in its calculations. Even though it has not been used as much as other measures previously, it has been useful in some species tree studies (e.g., [200]), one of its main uses being in testing repeatability of different methods according to different subsampling schemes (*see* Subheading 4.8.3).

3.8.4 Posterior Probability

Under a Bayesian MCMC phylogenetic analysis, there are different ways to summarize clade support. One way is to calculate an eMRC topology containing clades occurring in at least x% of samples (e.g., 50%, 95%, 99%). Another way is to compute the MAP (maximum a posteriori tree) by means of a *maximum clade credibility tree* (MCC), which is the phylogeny among the samples having the largest product of clade probabilities (each clade of every MCMC tree being counted across all samples). A *median tree* can also be obtained by defining a metric on a high-dimensional tree space, such as Robinson–Foulds distances or variants (see below), and then estimating the tree that minimizes the distance to all MCMC trees, as in MulRF [201].

3.8.5 Local Support Measures

Another set of local indices measure the conflict between different bipartitions within the same quartet of subtrees, instead of simply quantifying the most frequent split. Different local support measures exist, based on some function of the likelihood (or probability) of the inferred resolution having the four observed subtrees adjacent to it, compared to the other two possible unrooted binary resolutions of the same four subtrees. In general, when the probabilities of alternative resolutions are being calculated, optimizations are done only locally (in the specific branch being tested plus the four adjacent ones), saving computations therefore allowing faster clade support estimates. The *aLRT* support measure (approximate likelihood ratio test; [202]) is based on the ratio of the likelihood of the best ML resolution vs. the second best using a chi-squared test with asymptotic distribution under a $50\% \chi_0^2 : 50\% \chi_1^2$ mixture, with resulting *P*-values that can be converted into support values ranging from 0.125 to 1. The *SH-aLRT* [81] is a non-parametric estimate of the latter, implementing a test akin to the Shimodaira-Hasegawa algorithm [203] (see below), by summing site log likelihoods over the alignment across pseudoreplicates (resampling sites with replacement); branch support is then the proportion of replicates for which the likelihood of the ML tree is significantly superior than the second best. *aBayes* [204] is a Bayesian extension of aLRT, in which a flat prior is used for the three possible rearrangements around an edge.

An extension to the above rationale would be to consider, within a set of trees, all observable splits that contradict an internal branch (instead of focusing only on the three possible ways that connect four subtrees locally), for example across bootstrapped trees. After applying Shannon's entropy formula, [205] derived:

$$\text{ICA} = 1 + \sum p_i \times \log_n(p_i), \qquad (11)$$

in which *n* is the number of resolutions being considered: two if only the two most frequent resolutions are considered, being called the *IC index* (Internode Certainty); or including all resolutions found in the tree set, in that case being called *ICA* (Internode Certainty All). p_i is the relative frequency of the *i*th bipartition across all resolutions within the set of trees; in practice (for computational reasons), only bipartitions appearing $\geq 5\%$ are considered [205]. A value of 1.0 in a consensus tree indicates absence of conflict (therefore the data strongly supports that split in the consensus), a value of 0.0 represents lack of support for any resolution, and negative values are incorporated in case the most supported split is not within the consensus tree (which may happen, e.g. if branch support values are being drawn in the MP/ML/MAP tree instead of the majority-rule consensus tree). These values can be summed up across the tree, leading respectively to *TC* (Tree Certainty) and *TCA* (Tree Certainty All) scores, where trees having higher scores denote less branch conflict overall. Values can also be compared across trees, in which case a normalized score for each tree is given by dividing TC (or TCA) by $n - 3$ (the total number of internal branches for the *n* taxa present in an unrooted binary tree). Due to their nature, those indices are also useful for assessing split conflict across gene trees in a phylogenomic context (*see* Subheading 4.4). A further extension [206] allows its use in a collection of partial gene trees (i.e., when the whole set of taxa is not present across all gene trees), a common scenario in phylogenomic datasets. All four indices are available in RAxML.

3.8.6 Decay and Double-Decay Indices

Developed under the parsimony framework, the *Bremer support* (or decay index; [207]) for a clade is the number of extra steps required to lose that same clade that is present in the set of most parsimonious trees. Therefore, it measures how resilient a hypothesis of relationship is under successively worse trees (i.e., trees with more steps). The larger the number of steps until a clade collapses, the more credible it can be considered. *Double decay analysis* [208] is the determination of the decay indices of all n-taxon statements/partitions common to the set of most-parsimonious trees, providing a comprehensive summary of the ensemble set of Bremer indices for all fully (i.e., clade with all of its taxa) and partially (i.e., subsets of taxa of a clade) supported relationships in the form of a reduced consensus support tree. RadCon [209] is a software that calculates both Bremer and double-decay indices. Decay and double-decay indices were used to assess relationships of crown Cetacea using concatenated morphological, paleontological, and genomic data [210].

3.8.7 Discussion

Many studies have investigated the properties of the standard bootstrap approach for phylogenetics (summarized in Felsenstein, 2004; and references therein), showing that it has many limitations. As an example, using simulations and a laboratory-generated virus phylogeny, [211] showed that bootstrap values are in general conservative, with values $\geq 70\%$ corresponding to a $\geq 95\%$ probability that the clade is real, but only under specific (and possibly unrealistic) circumstances (equal rates of change, symmetric phylogenies, and internodal change of $\leq 20\%$ of the characters); when these are not met, bootstrap values of 50% or more may be overestimates of accuracy [211]. Speed was also a limiting factor of the original bootstrap algorithm due to the many topology estimates that must be performed (one per each pseudoreplicate), which led to the development of the fast (RAxML) and ultrafast (IQTree) approximations discussed above.

Posterior probabilities were initially thought as a more direct measure of clade probability and therefore more appropriate than bootstrap, but then it was noted that it could also be inconsistent mostly due to some biased prior choices. Important issues were high support for non-existent branches (e.g., [93]), and branch lengths being unrealistic large [94]. Some solutions to the former was inclusion of polytomy priors [174], as in Phycas, acknowledging the possibility that some branches could be zero (therefore non-existent); and solutions to the issue of large branches involved the development of priors for separate internal and external branches, or also decreasing the mean of the exponential prior of all branches by an order of magnitude (as in MrBayes). Nevertheless, convergence of chains and speed are still an issue in cases of many genes and/or taxa.

Local support measures weigh over alternative splits within an internal branch, contrasting to consensus techniques which report the most frequent split only, at the same time being fast to calculate and having reasonable accuracy [204, 205]. A study using simulations and performance in a Metazoan phylogeny by Anisimova et al. [204] showed that the standard bootstrap was excessively conservative and much slower than aLRT-like methods. Rapid bootstrap (of RAxML) had better correlation with probability of a clade being true when compared to the standard bootstrap (but worse than aLRT-like local support measures), but still relatively slow. SH-aLRT was reasonably accurate (though aLRT and aBayes presented highest statistical power) while also more robust than other local support measures when key assumptions were not met, being the recommended index by the authors. Regarding IC, ICA, TC, and TCA, an example of their versatility is a phylogenomic study of 23 yeast lineages including 1070 genes, which showed that clade support (in terms of percentage of gene trees containing the bipartition) for the placements of *Saccharomyces bayanus* and *Zygosaccharomyces rouxii* were 52% and 62% respectively, but their IC/ICA were respectively 0.05/0.14, and 0.59/0.47, evincing that the *S. bayanus* grouping is much more disputed across the gene trees [205]. Furthermore, TC/TCA scores allow ordering of all the gene trees, which can be useful for subsequent selection of compatible trees. As an example, after ranking 1070 genes from the 23 yeast species according to their TC value (obtained from each gene's bootstrap trees), concatenation analysis of the 131 genes with the highest TC placed the lineage embracing *Candida glabrata* in a position not supported by the complete set of genes, though agreeing with the presence of several distinct rare genomic changes [212]. IC and ICA scores can also be used to test for resolution of different splits regarding a subset (or all) of the characters (regarded states are binary; RY-coding can be used for DNA data; *see* Subheading 3.7.3), such as rare genomic changes, indels, sites with radical amino acid changes, and so forth [205]: in the same yeast dataset just mentioned, a set of 20,289 sites containing single radical substitutions was shown to support splits that were incongruent with the tree supported by the whole set of characters [205]. This character-based version of ICA can be particularly important to identify conflict among characters in a supermatrix analysis, as it tends to be less impacted by a specific type of statistical bias (large sample effect) than other support measures (see further discussion in Subheading 4.4).

UFBoot correlates better with the true probability of a clade, as well as behaving better under some model violations [197] when compared to SH-aLRT, at least in simulations; furthermore, it was shown to have a median speedup gain in the range [3.1–10.2] (under real DNA and amino acid data, respectively) compared with RAxML rapid bootstrapping.

The double-decay index provides a better comprehension of complex phylogenetic hypotheses than other indices, as it focuses on the decay indices of all n-taxon statements/partitions common to the most-parsimonious tree, being visualized by, e.g., reduced consensus support trees; it highlights weaknesses of phylogenetic hypotheses rather than its strengths, without depending on a priori exclusion of poorly known taxa from phylogenetic analyses [208].

3.9 Tree Distances

It is important to test for tree differences among gene trees, between gene trees and a species tree, or among different phylogenomic methods, to name a few examples. A commonly used measure is the *unweighted Robinson-Foulds distance* (RF-distance; [213]), also called symmetric difference, or partition metric. It measures the number of internal branches that generate different splits between two topologies (Fig. 1). A normalized distance score can be obtained upon dividing RF-distance by the sum of all bipartitions observed across the two trees, or by dividing by the maximum possible number of split differences between two fully resolved trees with the same number of taxa (which is always $2n - 6$);

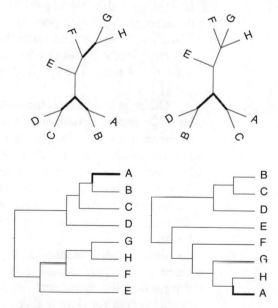

Fig. 1 *Top:* Different internal branches between the two trees are highlighted; their RF-distance is 5. *Bottom:* RF-distances may get too large even when general structure is similar, depending on taxon rearrangement; as an example, when position of taxon A is changed, maximal distance between the two trees is achieved because no splits are shared

the former normalization returns a distance of 1.0 (maximal distance) between a fully resolved tree vs. a bush tree, and also 1.0 for two completely dissimilar bifurcating trees (therefore relatively conservative), whilst the latter normalization returns a distance of 0.5 between a fully resolved tree and a bush tree (more liberal). RF-distance (either normalized or not) is widely used in the literature, even though it may attribute large distances between trees having similar structures in some cases (Fig. 1). An unrelated, but also strictly topological measure, is the *path-length* distance [214], based on the ensemble difference of the number of branches separating pairs of tips in two different trees.

Other measures include branch lengths, such as the *weighted RF-distance* and the *branch score distances*. The general idea is to sum absolute values of differences in branch lengths (if weighted-RF), or to take the square root of the sum of squared differences (if branch score), across all branches (internal and external) present on either tree or both (a length of 0.0 is attributed to a branch absent in one of the trees), with more similar trees having smaller values. The *geodesic distance* [215] is based on the generation of a tree space that assumes each of the possible $2n - 3$ topologies is defined by an $\mathbb{R}^+$ *orthant* (i.e., the general n-dimensional Euclidean analogue of a quadrant in 2D-space). Each axis delimiting an orthant represents the length of a specific branch; the dimensionality of each orthant depends on the set of branches being considered (if it is only the internal branches, then each orthant has $n - 3$ dimensions), and each possible tree can be represented by a vector in such a tree space. Then, the shortest path between two trees that lies completely inside the space is calculated. Its computation is polynomial-time [216], but can be approximated in linear time [217].

Other types of tree distances are based on a reduced set of leaves in common that they induce. *Quartets-based distance* [218] measures the amount of quartets different between two trees. The *triplets distance* [219] follows the same rationale, but in terms of induced three-taxon trees dissimilar between rooted trees. The *MAST distance* (maximum agreement subtrees [220]) is based on the size of the maximum shared subtree identical in two trees, being converted into a distance by subtracting it from the total size of the tree.

Kuhner and Yamato [221], using simulations (and including more distance measures), found that for trees involving recent divergences distances incorporating length information performed best, whereas for deeper divergences topology-only metrics had a better performance. Gori et al. [222] simulated different "cluster trees" (i.e., a tree common to more than one locus) within a species tree, showing that branch-score and geodesic distances (both taking branch lengths into account) performed better than RF-distances at identifying gene trees corresponding to loci of common evolutionary history (which were then submitted to clustering procedures to test for the optimal number of such clusters [222]).

A different set of distances is based on the minimum number of topological rearrangements that transform a tree into another. The minimum number of NNI, SPR, and TBR moves (Subheading 3.3) between two trees can also be employed as distance measures. All those rearrangements are NP-hard, but even though there are heuristic solutions to compute them, they are not as commonly used for large studies being expensive to calculate when trees are too dissimilar [221].

Suggestions of software implementing many such metrics are treedist (within package phangorn in R), treescape (also in R), and a set of scripts in python by Kuhner and Yamato [221].

3.10 Assessing Significance of Non-optimal Trees

Assessing statistical significance of trees is warranted if one wishes to report reasonable trees besides the best tree, or to compare different trees a priori. Instead of focusing on the amount of support for each internal branch as discussed above, the aim is to test how likely is a topology (or a set of topologies) as a whole under the given optimality criterion (e.g., parsimony). The general idea is to test for significance of differences of score between trees (i.e., sitewise or overall scores), and then if such a difference is significant, the suboptimal tree is considered significantly worse than the tree with better score. It is important to consider whether the trees being compared were chosen a priori (e.g., testing for alternative sister-group relationships that may have been raised in the literature) or a posteriori (e.g., testing for suboptimal trees against the best tree found), as some tests are appropriate for the former, others for the latter framework.

In terms of MP, the *Templeton test* [223] aims at testing two trees chosen a priori. It assesses the magnitude of difference (in number of steps) for each character in each of the two trees, replaces absolute values of differences by their ranks, and then re-applies the signs. The sum of the less numerous sign is used for a two-tailed Wilcoxon signed rank test. The *KH-test* (Kishino-Hasegawa test; [224]) can also be used under parsimony; it uses a t-test to compare the difference in steps between two trees chosen a priori.

Under ML, sitewise differences in log-likelihoods are computed, and then significance of the sum of differences (δ) can be assessed either by a t-test approximation or by resampling procedures. In most implementations, the ML-version of KH-test can use both versions. Regular resampling (i.e., bootstrapping and then re-estimating all model parameters and branch lengths) can be employed when it is reasonable to assume non-normality of the data, but it can be costly computationally. A workaround is bootstrapping over δ, as it is in general reasonable to assume that parameter values are stable around non-optimal trees [143, 144]. This was termed the RELL (resampling estimated log-likelihood; [224]) bootstrap, which speeds computations by a large amount as nothing needs to be estimated. Susko [225] showed that the KH-test is conservative and provides a corrected version. Another study [226] presented a KH-test that adjusts for alignment uncertainty, which can be implemented currently only by scripting.

The *SH-test* (Shimodaira-Hasegawa test; [203]) can be used to compare multiple trees chosen either a priori or a posteriori (commonly used with RELL bootstrapping as well). The null hypothesis is that the set of specified trees can explain the data equally well, and the alternative hypothesis is that one or more trees are better approximations of the data. It computes normalized values of δ that account for the contribution of the maximum likelihood tree to the null distribution, therefore avoiding the bias of a posteriori tree selection. A problem with the SH-test is that a set of reasonable a priori or a posteriori trees must be provided (such as trees obtained using other phylogenetic methods, based on other datasets, and/or by also considering second-best ML trees under the same dataset). If implausible trees are included, they will tend to increase the mean log-likelihood differences, therefore making the test too conservative [227]. A workaround in such cases is using a *weighted SH-test* [203]. Another possibility to reduce such bias is the use of the *AU-test* (approximately unbiased test; [228]), that calculates the null distribution and *p*-values based on multi-scale bootstraping, in which pseudoreplicates are of different sizes, being the most recommended test of significance for topologies considered in a set of reasonable trees (either a priori or a posteriori trees).

The *SOWH-test* (Swofford–Olsen–Waddell–Hillis test; [229]) uses the parametric bootstrap technique (which simulates an alignment with pre-specified choices of parameters under a chosen tree) to simulate datasets under the null hypothesis (e.g., a tree with a locally polytomic region of interest; [225]) using the same model selected for the original dataset, and for each pseudoreplicate the log-likelihood of the null and ML trees are estimated (therefore it uses full optimization instead of RELL); the significance of the original difference (by comparing to the distribution of values throughout the datasets) is then assessed. Nevertheless, the SOWH-test can be very dependent on the correct specification of the evolutionary model, and it also appears to be affected by heterogeneity in branch lengths [227, 229, 230].

Another way to assess the credible set of a posteriori topologies is using Bayesian inference, already mentioned above. At the end of an MCMC run in MrBayes, for example, an output file reporting the confidence set including all trees which summed frequencies are within the $1 - \alpha$ threshold (such as 95%) can be obtained. However, if many taxa are included, or if the run has not converged properly, the credible set may be biased, and it may also not include some desired a priori trees.

Like all significance tests, the above tests are meaningful only if the dataset is fixed; it is legitimate to compare the best and the second best ML topologies (e.g., using AU-test) using a core-coding dataset, or to test for a priori tree based on a previous study under that same dataset (e.g., using KH-test), but if the dataset is changed, *p*-values become non-comparable. In that sense, it is important to provide reasonable arguments for the dataset to be used for assessing significance of trees (e.g., if it is limited to the set of morphological characters, or a reduced set of the genes studied). The above tests can be used for species trees (under concatenation) as well.

An example of software that estimates significance of trees is CONSEL [231]. IQTree has fast implementations of all the tests above (except for SOWH) which are adequate for very large datasets (such as supermatrices). The SOWHAT package [232] automates the process of performing SOWH tests considering different variables such as number of replicates, ML software (GARLI or RAxML currently), possibility of including gaps in the simulations, choosing different models, and use of polytomic trees as null vs. fully resolved trees.

4   Estimating the Species Tree

We start by reviewing the main evolutionary forces that can lead to gene trees that are *actually* different from their containing species trees, and different among themselves (therefore disregarding systematic biases discussed previously). More in-depth reviews on these processes can be found in sources such as [233–236]. Subsequently, we discuss three general ways to gather information from gene trees to estimate a species tree: supermatrix (also called concatenation, or total evidence), supertrees (including consensus methods), and species tree methods (including summary methods and others). We discuss each of them, subsequently showing in which cases their use is reasonable.

4.1   Incomplete Lineage Sorting (ILS)

When two populations start to diverge, different alleles inherited from the ancestral population may get reduced to a single allelic variant through time (e.g., by genetic drift); this is complete lineage sorting (referring to the single allele that was "sorted" by each population), and results in populations (either terminal or internal to the phylogeny) that are reciprocally monophyletic regarding that allele. Contrarily, if more than one allele survives between internodes, this is called *incomplete lineage sorting* (ILS). In such a scenario, if the allele fixed in a population is not the closest relative to the allele fixed in the other diverging population, the outcome is

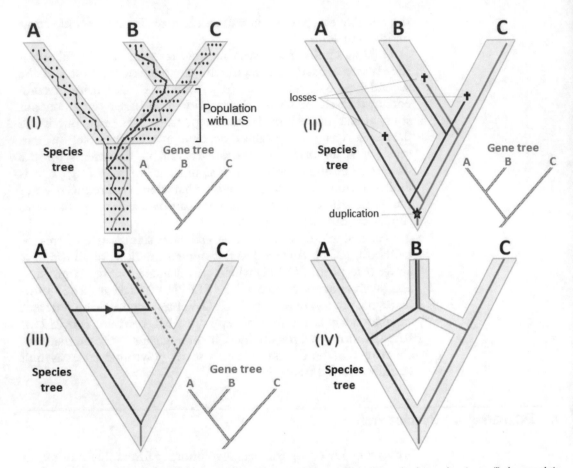

Fig. 2 Processes that may induce gene trees that are different than the actual species tree. (I) *Incomplete Lineage Sorting* (ILS): each quadrilateral is a population/species, with dots representing individuals within a same generation. Colored lines indicate different alleles (i.e., bearing different mutations) that eventually were fixed differentially across populations due to genetic drift; looking backwards in time (as in a coalescent framework), ILS can be treated as failure of allele lineages from diverging populations in coalescing at the level of the immediate ancestral population. (II) *Duplication and Loss* (DL): a locus may generate a duplicate somewhere in the genome, and then both may be inherited or just a single copy is maintained in each lineage. (III) *Horizontal Gene Transfer* (HGT): a donor DNA segment (from taxon A) is transmitted and incorporated into the host's genome (taxon B); see text for different types of HGT. In both prokaryotes and eukaryotes, closely related taxa tend to exchange more material, but transfers can also occur between distantly related taxa (in this case, more frequently between prokaryote lineages). (IV) *Hybridization/Introgression*: in extreme cases of lateral transfer, or upon mixing of related species, different regions of the genome will bear two distinct evolutionary histories; in general, it happens between closely related species/populations (prokaryotes and eukaryotes), many examples occurring in plants and animals [238, 239]

deep coalescence, whereby coalescence of those alleles is previous to the immediate ancestral population, inducing an incorrect species tree (Fig. 2, case I). ILS (even without deep coalescences) is one natural outcome of the *multispecies coalescent* model (MSC), which is itself an extension of coalescent theory that provides the link between phylogenetic models and the underlying population genetics [237]. When considered within a phylogenetic perspective, MSC provides a theoretical framework for estimating species trees based on individual (or ensemble) analysis of gene trees, while also accounting for possible deep coalescences due to ILS. Incorporating ILS as a natural possibility of the MSC translates to assuming it is a pervasive force, a reasonable assumption given the stochastic nature of lineage sorting when species diverge from each other. Most implementations assume linkage equilibrium among loci, and with each locus being free from recombination internally. The model has been applied more commonly to eukaryotes, where cross-overs during meiosis reduce levels of linkage between loci across time even for closely related lineages, matching to some extent the assumption of free recombination between loci. In practice, to infer a species tree assuming the MSC model, the following formula is applied:

$$P(S|X) \propto P(S) \cdot P(G|S) \cdot P(X|G), \qquad (12)$$

where X is the data, S is a species tree being proposed, and G is a compatible gene tree within S (in terms of absolute or relative divergence times) with model parameters according to an evolutionary model. Estimating the best tree (or actually the set of credible species trees) regarded the formula above is generally done under a Bayesian framework, after marginalizing over the species trees sampled from the joint posterior density.

4.2 Duplication and Loss (DL)

It is an important source of gene/species tree conflict when some of the sampled genes are homologous, but paralogous instead of orthologous. Even when there is no loss of paralogs, the sampling of lineages that are not true orthologs will make them appear more closely related to each other than they are in the actual topology (*undetected paralogy*; Fig. 2, case II). Many cases of past duplications and losses have been inferred in plants, insects and ray-finned fishes, among other eukaryotic lineages. Those are also common processes in prokaryotes.

4.3 Horizontal Gene Transfer (HGT)

Here we restrict the term HGT to instances where allelic variants from an outer population/species get incorporated by the recipient population's gene pool, which is the definition mostly used in phylogenomic studies (whereas the general definition also embraces the possibility of incorporation of new genes). This is similar to the concept of *gene flow*, a definition more commonly found in eukaryote studies. Different ways of incorporating new allelic variation include *homologous recombination*, such as during meiosis in eukaryotes, in that case being reciprocal; when non-reciprocal (i.e., the transfer is unidirectional), it is called *gene conversion*, such as following conjugation in bacteria, as well as in eukaryotes by paralogous gene conversion (Fig. 2, case III). Even when unidirectional regarding the individuals participating in the event, the net effect may be interchanges between two or more populations through time. In case homologous recombination occurs within a locus, it will lead to different phylogenetic stories depending on which segment the analysis is based on [240] (Fig. 2, case III). Homologous recombination is pervasive in Bacteria even among more distant lineages, whereas in eukaryotes it tends to be restricted to genetically similar populations (due to meiosis restrictions). *Non-homologous recombination* can also aggregate novel regions within a gene (e.g., fragments of insertion elements due to transposition). *Hybridization* is a massive mixture of genomic components from two genomes, such as in salamanders [241] (Fig. 2, case IV). Alternatively, *introgression* may also happen when there are successive backcrosses with a parental genome after acquiring variation by hybridization (Fig. 2, case IV), such as in *Campylobacter* proteobacteria [242], salamanders [243], and in many plant lineages.

4.4 Supermatrix Analysis

This is a method based on concatenating all genomic regions into a single matrix including all taxa present in at least one of the datasets (Fig. 3). Also, different types of characters can be aggregated into a

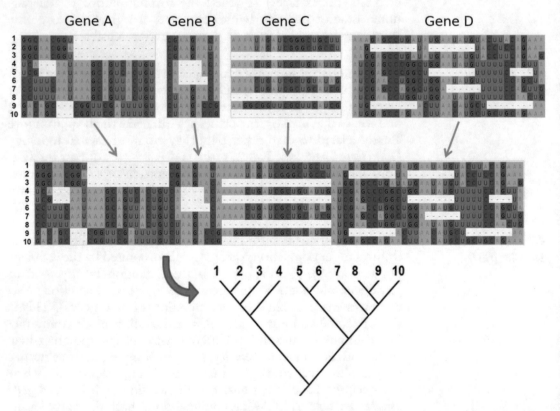

Fig. 3 A schematic view of supermatrix generation. Taxa are represented by numbers (1–10). Missing data entries are represented by "-"

supermatrix, such as morphology, restriction site data, etc. [210], with the possibility of using morphological/binary evolutionary Markov models for the appropriate partitions (such as Lewis' Mk/Mkv models) alongside DNA, codon, and amino acid models (e.g., IQTree). Such a concatenated dataset is then subjected to phylogenomic inference using the desired phylogenetic method (distance, MP, ML, or BI).

Many programs able to analyze single gene tree are able to perform supermatrix analyses up to a few genes, but some programs scale better when thousands of genes are included (e.g., TNT, IQTree, RAxML, ExaML, FastTree). Goloboff and colleagues [244] published a concatenated analysis of 73,060 taxa, including major eukaryotic lineages (under MP, using TNT), being the largest de novo supermatrix analysis thus far and reconstructing most groups as known previously. TNT is probably the fastest supermatrix software, employing advanced tree searches and mixing different algorithms [73] based on the maximum parsimony criterion.

Supermatrices are particularly appropriate when genes follow the same tree without strong levels of recombination among loci, as is the case with organelles such as mitochondrial and chloroplasts, and for prokaryotes within short evolutionary distances. Important drawbacks of concatenated analyses are: (1) it hinders variation among gene trees by assuming implicitly that all of them conform to a single species tree; (2) if sampling was heterogeneous across species there may be too much missing data, which can affect topological reconstruction; (3) *large data sampling effects* inflate credibility in some clades; (4) *spurious hidden support* can lead to support for non-existent clades; and (5) in case of moderate to severe levels of ILS, supermatrix can become statistically inconsistent. The latter three issues are further discussed now.

One important characteristic of some support measures in the context of supermatrices, such as bootstrap and posterior probabilities, is that they can be plagued by large data sampling effects, similarly to the pattern of overconfidence of p-values in large statistical analyses [245]. An example is given in Fig. 4 regarding the ((A,B),(C,D)) split in a quartet tree, where a set of four sites is repeated in powers of ten, generating datasets from 4×10^0 (4 sites) up to 4×10^5 (400,000 sites). In each unit of four sites, the split (A,B) is supported by two sites (first and second), but negated by the other two (which support the other two possible splits). Common sense suggests even though (A,B) would be relatively better supported across bootstrapped datasets, support would still be present for the remaining splits; instead, that is not what happens: support for (A,B) is already 100% under either MP or ML with only 400 sites in total! A similar simulation was presented in [246], where units of 100 sites contained 53 of them favoring a tree bipartition (say phylogeny A) vs. 47 sites supporting

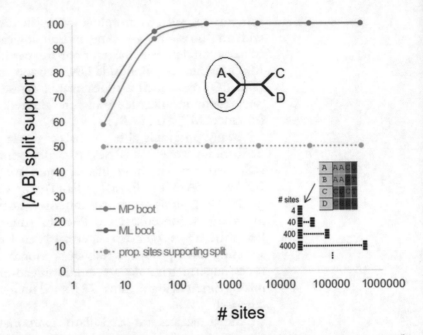

Fig. 4 The same "alignment unit" of four sites repeated in powers of 4×10^n ($0 \leq n \leq 5$), with support for the (A,B) partition being analyzed by either MP bootstrap (in MEGA) or ML (UFBoot in IQTree). Two sites favor (A,B) in each unit, but the other two contradict it. The curves of this contrived example show that support indices (here, bootstrap) can get easily inflated in cases where there is not a *definitive* support for that bipartition across gene trees. *Gray*: a naive character support measure, that nevertheless acknowledges the relative contribution of different sites, would suggest 50% support, precluding inflated branch support when more data is gathered; a similar idea is employed with the character-based versions of IC and ICA indices [205, 206] (*see* Subheading 3.8.5)

another. When this character set was expanded (but again proportion of sites supporting each phylogeny remained the same), bootstrap for phylogeny A increased to ~97% with only 1000 bp in total (530 sites vs. 470 sites). Therefore, even in the presence of a reasonable proportion of contrasting characters, the hypotheses with slightly more sites supporting it across genes may lead to inflated support, possibly being the main reason why so many concatenation studies reach supporting values close to 100% for all bipartitions, even in cases where contrasting clades are estimated using different methods [247]. Such a bias suggests the use of indices that take into account the proportion of sites supporting contrasting patterns in each gene tree, or in the whole supermatrix, such as the character-based versions of IC and ICA indices (mentioned above).

This is not to be confounded with phylogenetic hidden support, which can reveal consistent signal across concatenated genes in cases where most sites within a gene *do not support* the intended bipartition, but a few sites are consistent with it; when such a hidden signal is summed across genes the overall support may become high [248]. Nevertheless, non-linear association of sites favoring contradicting bipartitions in large alignments may induce *biased hidden support* as well.

Notwithstanding, even when such biases are minimized, spurious species tree reconstruction can still be obtained by supermatrices if ILS levels are moderate to severe in at least part of the tree [249]. This is because regions with specific combinations of short branch lengths and/or large past population sizes (which increase the probability of ILS) may induce the evolution of gene trees that do not match the species tree topology [250]. In fact, the bias can get quite severe for specific combinations of those factors, to a point where the most probable gene tree is different from the species tree, making supermatrices statistically inconsistent under such scenarios. This is called the *anomaly zone* of species tree reconstruction, and the respective high probability (but incorrect) gene tree is called *anomalous gene tree* [250]. For this reason, methods that explicitly acknowledge ILS, or others that are proven to be consistent in its presence, may be preferable to supermatrices in those circumstances [251]. This will be further discussed in Subheading 4.6.

4.5 Supertree Methods

Instead of forcing all gene trees to comply to a single tree, supertree methods infer the best topology for each gene (using the same phylogenetic method for each), and then a topological consensus is obtained. Such methods are able to make consensus trees even if the number of leaves among gene trees differs but overlaps to some extent, for example when a gene has not been sequenced for some taxa (Fig. 5). Input trees obtained from different types of data (molecular, morphological, paleontological, etc.) can be analyzed separately and then combined within such a framework. The rationale is that each dataset can "speak for itself," while also minimizing biases related to missing data (though indels within a gene and associated gene tree biases may still be present). Also, for datasets overlapping only partially, gene trees involve less taxa and much smaller individual alignment lengths when compared to the whole supermatrix, decreasing computational cost if gene trees are estimated de novo (at least for simpler/faster methods such as MRP; see below), and especially when parallel processing is available. The sparser the concatenated alignment, the larger the speed gain.

The first practical (and widely used) supertree method was based on the MRP method (*Matrix Representation with Parsimony*), proposed in the same year by Baum [252] and Ragan [253]. It consists in treating nodes of each input tree as characters, ordering them consecutively starting from the first tree and moving up until the last node in the last gene tree (Fig. 5), whereby taxa to one side of each node in an unrooted gene tree are encoded as "0",

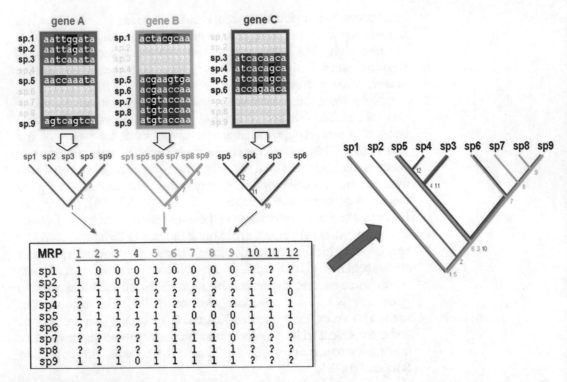

Fig. 5 From gene trees to a supertree. The algorithm used for this example was MRP (matrix reconstruction using parsimony; see text for details)

"1" if on the other side, and taxa not present in that gene tree are encoded as '?'. After that, this matrix of 0s and 1s is submitted to tree search (e.g., by parsimony), generating a supertree at the end. An example using rooted gene trees is shown in Fig. 5. MRP is an example of the *indirect* approach of achieving a supertree, by generating an intermediate matrix that is analyzed afterwards. Other algorithms use a *direct* approach, in which a consensus is obtained directly from input trees (for example, the extended consensus majority when employed for supertree reconstruction).

Individual gene trees can be estimated de novo, or they can be obtained from gene trees published in different studies. The latter procedure is not recommended, because different input trees may be the result of different phylogenetic methods, they can propagate possible systematic errors that may have been overlooked by some of the original studies, and because they can bear a large amount of structural correlation if different studies inferred phylogenies including the same gene. Therefore it is *highly* recommended that each character dataset has its tree re-estimated when inferring a supertree.

The original MRP method works reasonably well for phylogenomic reconstruction in many studies [254–256], especially a boosted version based on TNT heuristics and Superfine (the latter itself a supertree heuristic [257, 258]). However, MRP (and variations of it) can lead to undesired behavior, which subsequent algorithms were able to overcome. Below we present common past criticisms, together with associated reasonable and relatively fast solutions for the use of supertrees in phylogenomic analyses:

1. Lack of branch support. Methods that allow for resampling of source trees have been developed (analogously to bootstrap for standard characters), as in CLANN [259].

2. Non-existent clades. PhySIC_IST [260] is an algorithm that includes only relationships present in input trees, or induced by them, providing supertrees of placental mammals and animals that agreed with previous results.

3. Inability to include duplications (therefore duplicated taxa). MulRF [201] is a software that infers relatively accurate supertrees by minimizing multi-labeled RF-distances to source trees, processing almost 7000 gene trees from 36 mammalian species under 2 h using only two processors [201], while having accuracy comparable to PHYLDOG (an accurate species tree method acknowledging duplication-and-loss processes; Subheading 4.6).

4. Lack of branch lengths. ERaBLE (Evolutionary Rates and Branch Length Estimation) is an example of a method capable of estimating supertree branch lengths, based on distance estimates for individual genes either directly or from previously calculated gene trees [261].

5. Lack of an objective function. FastRFS [262] is based on a dynamic programming method that finds an exact solution to a constrained version of the minimum RF-distance between the inferred supertree and its input trees, substantially improving on accuracy regarding competing methods on a large collection of biological and simulated data; it is also very fast, finishing in a few minutes an analysis involving 2228 species [262].

Presently, even though better algorithms have been developed, supertree methods still do not resolve conflict among the source trees with respect to explicit evolutionary events. Nevertheless, many species tree methods can be considered special types of supertrees in which specific evolutionary events are acknowledged, such as ILS and HGT. That is why many researchers perceive species tree methods as the natural evolution of supertrees and therefore prefer the former [263], hence polarizing the debate of phylogenomic accuracy between supermatrix and species tree methods [251, 263]. Nevertheless, this is not a universal point of view especially given the accuracy of some supertree methods, even of older and naive methods such as MRP [264], as in a study reconstructing accepted avian clades embracing 2/3 of all species [265]. The reasonable performance of supertrees at phylo-genomic reconstruction is reminiscent of the behavior (and also similar points of view) of maximum parsimony for single gene tree (or supermatrix) analyses, as previously discussed.

4.6 Species Tree Methods

A step beyond supertrees is the use of methods that take into consideration specific evolutionary processes that may be responsible for differences in gene topologies, and then estimate the species tree which would most likely have generated such gene trees, under different scenarios (Fig. 2).

Considering analyses including estimated orthologous genes only (and assuming undetected paralogies are minimized in that case), ILS is generally considered the main process responsible for gene/species tree discordance in eukaryotes, as free recombination between genomic regions during meiosis may induce independent gene trees among loci. Therefore, many proposed species tree algorithms aim at testing first for phylogenetic reconstruction under ILS, either by proving it mathematically or by showing robustness of the algorithm under different levels of ILS. Some methods co-estimate gene trees and their containing species tree altogether assuming specific evolutionary processes.

The iGTP software [266] minimizes the number of steps for reconciliation among gene trees assuming ILS (but also other processes; see below), by counting the number of deep coalescences across gene trees and minimizing it under MP. The *Infer_ST_MD-C_UR* module within Phylonet [267] also performs a similar task. Parametric examples incorporating ILS include *BEAST [84, 268] and BEST [269], both Bayesian methods. Nevertheless, those programs are restricted to a relatively low number of species due to the computational cost of inferring too many parameters explicitly while also accounting for gene tree uncertainty. BPP is a promising alternative under MSC that speeds up the process of co-estimating gene/species trees; it implements efficient SPR and node-slider move proposals, while simultaneously altering the gene trees at multiple genetic loci to automatically avoid conflicts with the newly proposed species tree, being computationally more efficient than the fully parametric algorithms mentioned above, and statistically more efficient than summary methods (the latter are discussed below).

Other species tree methods based on MSC+ILS were developed to make parametric species tree estimation even faster (though with reasonable accuracy) by estimating gene tree uncertainty beforehand, by skipping gene tree estimation altogether, and/or by focusing on smaller subsets of data for which a consensus is obtained afterwards; these are called *summary methods*. Examples include GLASS [270], STAR [271], STEAC [272], STEM [273], BUCKy [274, 275], MP-EST [276], ASTRAL [249, 277], ASTRID [278], BBCA [279], SNAPP [280], and SVDQuartets [281, 282]. These and other software were derived assuming ILS is prevalent, or some contrived scenarios of ILS+HGT, either mathematically or by simulations.

Assuming ILS may have impacted evolution, distances between all pairs of terminal taxa can be obtained for all gene trees separately, and then these can get compared (and a species tree estimated) either by calculating average ranks of coalescence times (STAR), average coalescence times (STEAC), or the minimum number of nodes until coalescence happens (GLASS). Then, those distances can be input into a distance-based phylogenetic method such as NJ. A simulation study suggested that STAR outperforms STEAC and GLASS when substitution rates among lineages are highly variable [271]; also, two real genomic data analyzed by STAR and STEAC (eight *Saccharomyces* yeast species, and 54 mammals) led to species trees consistent with previous results [271].

BUCKy works by inferring concordance factors (CFs), which are estimates of the proportion of genes having a specific clade, working on distributions for each gene tree estimated previously (e.g., using MrBayes), therefore integrating over gene tree estimation errors. Two types of consensus trees can be obtained subsequently: *concordance trees*, based on the greedy consensus of CFs of clades including all full splits across genes (which can generate biased clade support for a species tree if ILS or HGT are impacting the dataset, and also if there are rogue taxa which will tend to lower average support across all splits); and *population trees*, based on an adapted version of the R*-consensus (which is originally based on rooted triplets; [283]) of CFs of unrooted quartets. The latter was shown to be consistent under the MSC+ILS as the distribution of unrooted quartets identifies the underlying unrooted species tree topology [284]. This algorithm variation is sometimes called *BUCKy-pop*.

MP-EST and ASTRAL (versions I and II) use pseudo-likelihood maximization (which are consensus likelihood estimates that ignore correlations among different gene trees bearing taxon overlaps, reducing computing time), the former using rooted tripled trees, the latter using unrooted quartets. ASTRID is based on internode distances resembling the distance-based algorithms above, where a matrix of average leaf-to-leaf topological distances is obtained, and then a tree is generated using FastME [285], a modified and faster implementation of the minimum-evolution algorithm.

BBCA randomly partitions the loci into bins having the same approximate size (which can be chosen by the user), runs *BEAST (a completely parametric species tree method, as mentioned above) on each such bin to co-estimate gene trees and species tree for the bin, and then runs MP-EST on those estimated gene trees; it follows the same rationale as BUCKy in terms of leveraging gene tree uncertainty, making it possible to use *BEAST on datasets containing hundreds of loci.

SNAPP and SVDQuartets are species tree methods aimed at unlinked SNP data, and they make computations faster because they bypass the necessity of computing gene trees. The general idea justifying their use is that ideally genic regions (used to estimate gene trees) should be recombination-free to guarantee statistical consistency under the MSC, but then each chosen recombination-free region can become arbitrarily short if many recombination events took place through the history of the lineages considered (the so-called *recombination ratchet*; [286]), possibly leading to high gene tree estimation error; therefore, methods that could estimate a species tree directly from widely spaced SNPs in the genome, skipping gene tree estimation altogether, could minimize the impact of the recombination ratchet, while also being faster. SNAPP is aimed at biallelic markers (also accepting AFLP data as input), being a Bayesian algorithm based on a population genetic model of finite-sites model of mutation, therefore estimating altogether mutation rate, generation time, and effective population size. SVDQuartets is a probabilistic species tree method based on algebraic statistics and singular value decomposition applied to site patterns that are evaluated across quartet trees. A score for each split is calculated for each given quartet, the split with best score is selected, and then a consensus tree (currently, in PAUP*) is built from these validated quartets; nevertheless, its derivation currently assumes a strict clock rate [281, 282].

Regarding inferences acknowledging duplication-and-loss, non-parametric algorithms include GTP (gene tree parsimony analysis), which minimizes the number of steps for reconciliation among gene trees (under either ILS, simple duplications, or DL frameworks) using maximum parsimony, such as in the iGTP software [266]. Dynadup [287] also aims at minimizing duplications or duplication and losses, being polynomial in the number of gene trees and taxa. Other algorithms are parametric, such as PHYL-DOG, that can analyze thousands of gene families in dozens of genomes simultaneously, using an ML algorithm incorporating a duplication-loss model [288].

We defer our discussion of species tree methods taking into account HGT to Subheading 5, when we mention them in conjunction with network methods.

4.7 What is the Best Phylogenomic Method?

Any comparison between supermatrices, supertrees, and species tree methods is necessarily contrived, because details varying even within a single method may matter a lot. So for example, if supermatrix is chosen, one must take into account which phylogenetic method was used, and whether partitioning has been undertaken or not; if supertree, which phylogenetic method was used for inference of gene trees, and which consensus method was chosen; and if species tree, whether it was a de facto species tree or a summary method, and if the latter, how individual trees were obtained (phylogenetic method and whether gene tree uncertainty was considered, e.g., bootstrapped or from a Bayesian analysis), and which consensus method was used to merge the gene trees.

Supermatrices, at least methodologically, can be considered as an extension of single gene analyses, as concatenation assumes all gene trees implicitly follow the species tree; the only drawback is that the analysis will take much longer with many genes, and potential systematic biases may get multiplied. Some pre-analytical issues can be more prominent though, such as the natural tendency of supermatrix of including much higher levels of missing data due to imbalance of genes sequenced across taxa. Supermatrices can be more justified in the case of shallow divergences within prokaryotes, as genes are linked in a single circular genome, minimizing differences in ILS effects across genes; linkage disequilibrium may take some time to induce independent gene trees within the species tree (e.g., within deeper divergences such as among bacterial families or higher divisions). A study based on 24 unicopy core-coding genes of almost 3000 complete bacterial and archaeal genomes [289] found that a partitioned supermatrix had better clade support than a species tree method (the latter using BUCKy) when compared to its respective 16S rRNA tree (a commonly used marker to infer phylogenetic relationships). Therefore, even in such an extreme case in which it is reasonable to assume linkage equilibrium among genomic segments (due to many putative recombination events along the tree time span) and gene trees could tell different stories suggesting species tree would be more appropriate, the ensemble signal contained within the supermatrix is still strong, at least when distant prokaryote lineages are compared; but comparisons were done against the 16S tree, which is not necessarily a universal benchmark for "all-true" relationships [290].

Species trees are theoretically sound methods for inference as they can incorporate important factors impacting the evolution of gene trees. Some of them (e.g., ASTRAL-2) can have good accuracy even when reasonable amounts of ILS and HGT are incorporated in simulations [291], as the software is theoretically consistent under bounded amounts of HGT. Nevertheless, comparisons between supermatrices and species tree methods have shown that depending on the exact conditions, supermatrices can have comparable accuracy. A study by Davidson et al. [291] showed that (unpartitioned) supermatrix can be highly accurate under highly heterogeneous model conditions, even when low amounts of ILS and HGT were simulated; but with larger amounts of ILS and HGT, supermatrix had a worse behavior [291]. Another study showed that under a range of simulation conditions of ILS, both methods reached statistically indistinguishable accuracy [292]. The problem is that most of the time it is not obvious to know whether ILS or HGT have an important impact on a dataset or not, so supermatrix may still be an effective method for inferring species trees.

Supertree analyses were also employed for relationships of distant lineages across the tree of life (including lineages from Archaea, Bacteria, and Eukarya) using MRP based on a set of core of genes that support similar species phylogeny (therefore supposedly maximizing vertical signal), obtaining relevant phylogenomic relationships [293]. Therefore, they can be a valid alternative for studies including distant lineages of prokaryotes. For eukaryotes, examples of their usefulness at estimating species trees were given in Subheading 4.5. Furthermore, use of a supertree is a mandatory step within species tree summary methods, by making a consensus of the quartets (or rooted triplets in the case of MP-EST). One such example is weighted quartets maxCut (wQMC), a highly accurate algorithm even in the presence of substantial amounts of ILS and HGT under simulations [291]; therefore, the development and use of supertrees continues to be important at estimating species trees. One good option in this sense is MulRF, which minimizes the RF-distance to multi-copy gene trees, therefore being useful for cases in which gene trees are different than species trees by either ILS, HGT, and DL.

4.8 Exploring and Filtering Data

Below, we describe some useful approaches aimed at exploring the behavior and filtering of data, under different scenarios.

4.8.1 Data Reduction

We have already discussed some possibilities of site exclusion to minimize gene tree artefacts; those are also useful hints for phylogenomics. Now we continue that discussion by extending the rationale to phylogenomic datasets. Removal of specific genes may be important if these have large evolutionary rates, which could induce biases such as LBA. One way of doing it is by using DistR [294]. Another interesting option is keeping only genes containing parsimony-informative sites [295]. Maintaining only genes that comply to a test of composition homogeneity may also be warranted, as it is not guaranteed that heterogeneous models (mixture, heterotachous, and non-homogeneous models) will correct it [189]. Phylo-MCOA [296] detects genes with different phylogenetic signal in a projected space, where genes deviant from the average pattern can be detected. Caution must be taken here, because removing contrastant genes may increase bias if the most common gene tree is an anomalous gene tree; hence, this procedure is more applicable for shallow prokaryote comparisons and/or organellar evolution, as in these cases ILS is not deemed relevant (due to linkage disequilibrium between loci). In cases where ILS is suspected to have operated, BUCKy is also a reasonable alternative for data reduction, as it builds a *primary concordance tree* (i.e., the R*-consensus tree of quartets including splits with largest CFs); because such a tree is consistent even under ILS, then the gene trees with supported splits (e.g., obtained by bootstrap or posterior probability) that were not included in the primary concordance tree can be eliminated without substantial risk of incurring in anomalous gene trees (and supposing other types of errors are not influencing gene tree estimates sensibly). Aliscore (https://www.zfmk.de/en/research/research-centres-and-groups/aliscore) can identify genic regions showing random similarity within multiple alignments, cutting those regions out. MARE (Meyer, Karen Meusemann & Bernhard Misof, April 2011, https://www.zfmk.de/en/research/research-centres-and-groups/mare) aims at decreasing the amount of missing data, by reducing a supermatrix to an incomplete edge-weighted bipartite graph, representing a subset of taxa and genes.

4.8.2 Binning Data Under Supertree or Species Tree Analyses

As a way of counter-weighting a possible (and important) source of bias in supertree and species tree methods, which is the possible lack of sufficient data within each genomic region analyzed separately, data binning methods were developed. The idea is to join genomic regions with similar phylogenetic signals into *supergenes*, perform tree search on each such supergene using a supermatrix approach (including supergene partitioning by locus), and then proceed to species tree (or supertree) inference based on these supergene trees. Based on that idea, [297] developed *unweighted statistical binning*. It involves first estimating individual gene trees and associated support values, then the respective genes are combined into a single bin if they do not present highly supported but conflicting branches; in case of gene trees that can fit equally into different supergene bins, attribution is done by minimizing size differences among bins. It was shown that the original method was statistically inconsistent under MSC. A *weighted* version of statistical binning was further developed to better address the fact that a supergene tree should be weighted according to the number of loci it embraces, which corrected for the above inconsistency [298]. Nevertheless, using biological and simulated datasets (under the MSC plus GTR model) both algorithms had similar accuracy under MP-EST and ASTRAL [298], being superior to the unbinned version except in cases of very high level of ILS, low average bootstrap support for the gene trees, and a few species altogether [298]. The "binning" pipeline (available at https://github.com/smirarab/binning) implements both versions of the algorithm. A possible caveat with both procedures is that in cases of closely related organisms lacking sufficient phylogenetic signal to evince putative conflicting clade resolutions, or if long-branch attraction (or other biases) affecting data with more distantly related taxa lead to gene trees incorrectly grouped in the same bin, biased hidden support may lead to wrong supergene tree reconstructions, possibly affecting species tree estimation (even though such issues should be less pronounced under the weighted version). For closely related species in particular, it may be that attributing genes to bins becomes sufficiently random due to lack of gene tree signal, possibly compromising its general superiority at species tree reconstruction in comparison to unbinned analysis. BUCKy's secondary concordance trees (and tertiary, etc.), obtained by applying the R*-consensus of quartets a second time to those clades that were not added to the primary concordance tree, are another way of binning genes with similar evolutionary histories (but different than the ones included in the primary tree), even though such bins can be prone to the same artifacts just mentioned.

4.8.3 Testing Subsamples of Data

A different direction regarding data combinability is whether different subsamples of genes (or gene trees) lead to the same topology, or some clades specifically, being a test of phylogenetic stability under different types of analyses. The Random Addition Concatenation Analysis (RADICAL) [299] does this under a supermatrix framework, by sequentially concatenating randomly chosen gene partitions, starting with a single-gene partition and ending with the entire genomic data set; for each subsample size, different replicates are performed. The authors found congruent signal among core and shell gene sets in general in a cyanobacterial dataset, with phylogenetic disagreements being restricted to a few specific genes [299].

Beyond comparing stability of phylogenetic methods (e.g., supermatrix vs. species tree; parsimony vs. likelihood) or datasets, Edwards [300] also suggests phylogenomic subsampling to assess the effect of evolutionary rate on phylogenomic inference (in which genes can be added sequentially in order of rate, for example), and in assessing the effect of missing data. He proposes subsampling both loci (testing for different combinalities of gene trees) and sites within loci (accounting for gene tree error) to minimize both types of biases. Using this methodology, he found a "flip-flop" effect (Fig. 6) of supported clades in a mammal dataset under a supermatrix approach, finding "strong support for a clade on the one hand, and an alternative, incompatible clade on the other, even within replicates of the same matrix size, and even more regularly across matrices of different sizes," but that under MSC (MP-EST) the support increased more monotonically [300]. If such a different pattern between supermatrix vs. species tree (or any other type of comparison) is shown to be mirrored in other datasets, then this would suggest that the latter is more robust to data choice/filtering; this can be an important piece of information, because at least a few partitions suspected of bias (e.g., having too much missing

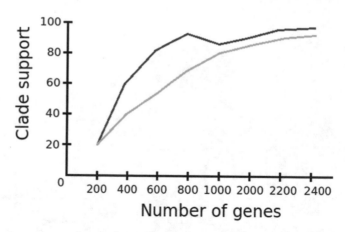

Fig. 6 Phylogenetic data subsampling, used to compare internal consistency of phylogenomic methods (e.g., supermatrix vs. species tree methods) or phylogenetic frameworks (e.g., parsimony vs. likelihood, under the same desired phylogenomic method) in rescuing a priori clade relationships given the data. A method that lacks repeatability (regarding support of a specific resolution) across data subsamplings becomes suspicious in its results, at least regarding that resolution. Each point in the y-axis represents average support across N subsampled pseudoreplicates for the same number of genes. Red line: method without monotonic increase for the desired clade association, or "flip–flop" effect, in which support for the desired relationship falls below 95% (on average) when 1000 genes are used, but with increasing number the support rises again. Green line: monotonic method, support values suggest internal consistency (though not necessarily statistical consistency) if more genes keep being added

data, or heterogeneity in base composition across taxa, or LBA artifacts) could be dismissed without impacting substantially robustness of inference; contrarily, if such a test is not performed, an important source of bias (conjunctural support) may be overlooked, possibly leading to highly supported but non-existent branches. Obviously, a monotonic pattern may also be a sign of an inconsistent estimator, but in any case a "flip-flopped" pattern keeps being more suspicious (Fig. 6). Regarding the distribution of gene trees, Simmons and colleagues [301] recommend using plots of pairwise congruence among gene trees regularly to assess extent and distribution of gene tree incongruence. Similarly to subsampling genes directly, this methodology helps in determining primary causes of incongruence between supermatrix and coalescent-based results, to reconcile conflicting phylogenetic results based on different phylogenomic methods, and to identify genes that may have been impacted by reconstruction artifacts.

4.8.4 Testing Only Relationships of Interest

It is often the case that we are more interested in specific clade relationships as opposed to the topology as a whole. In order to focus on genomic markers (or other marker types) necessarily

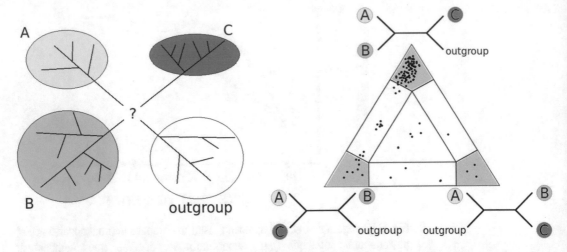

Fig. 7 The likelihood mapping test [302]. Gray: regions with high relative probability for a specific quartet; quartets falling outside those regions are considered uninformative. Some gene trees (or particular sets of taxa in a supermatrix) may map into a different high probability area in the simplex, which may be due to some kind of bias, or to real evolutionary forces operating (e.g., recombination, selection, etc.); in the example above, most support is for [A, B], though a few gene trees (or some taxa within the supermatrix) support the other two resolutions

present only in lineages of interest, different tests were proposed, of which a few are discussed below.

Assuming in advance which lineages are monophyletic (e.g., from previously known hypotheses, and/or by finding which lineages received high support in different preliminary phylogenomic analysis using different methods), one may select genomic markers for which at least one taxon from each desired lineage is present, and therefore an analysis based on this restricted dataset would be maximally informative for the specific question being asked. One such test, *likelihood mapping* [302], is focused at quartets of trees (Fig. 7). Contrived search of quartets is performed within a larger taxon set being analyzed (either gene-wise or within a distribution of trees based on the concatenated dataset), in which every proposed quartet must contain at least one taxon from each of four pre-defined lineages whose evolutionary relationship is to be tested (A, B, C, and outgroup), serving as proxies of support for the respective subtrees they represent. Posterior probability for each quartet is given by $p_i = \frac{L_i}{L_1 + L_2 + L_3}$, where L_i are the individual maximum likelihood tree estimates. Each value is then mapped onto an equilateral triangle (also called a two-dimensional *simplex* by the authors). Some gene trees (or particular sets of taxa) may map to some other probability region, due to some kind of bias or to real evolutionary forces (e.g., recombination, selection, etc.).

A paper testing different hypotheses of relationships of the primarily wingless insects [303] employed this test to unravel arthropod relationships within Protura, Collembola, and Diplura (vs. other lineages) using a supermatrix method, finding that inter-ordinal phylogenetic relationships are still inconclusive. Furthermore, after removing all genes that covered all three entognathous groups (which they called a *maximally indecisive data set*), they still found spurious support for some clade associations, which they attributed to systematic bias of *uneven distribution of missing data* (a reasonable hypothesis after other factors were ruled out during their analyses).

Concomitant tests including five taxa (or subtrees) or more would make the analysis harder to interpret in 2-D; with five sub-trees, a 15-vertex simplex is needed, not easily visualized even in 3-D. Yet, nothing precludes such hypotheses to be analyzed individually. In a study of the largest freshwater fish radiation, the Otophysi [304], the complexity of tree space was reduced to the 15 possible topological constraints (representing five main radiations), ten of them being supported by preliminary analysis of the whole dataset (using supermatrix and species tree methods). Subsequently, they established the ranking of alternative trees and their probabilities (akin to AU test) using constrained ML searches to optimize site likelihood scores for each gene alignment, a process they called *gene genealogy interrogation*. They found that the vast majority of gene genealogies supported a single tree topology grounded on morphology, not previously obtained by molecular studies.

5 Reticulated Trees and Phylogenetic Networks

In many occasions, it may not be possible to obtain a single bifurcating phylogenetic tree that best fits a dataset, but still different resolutions get high support due to stochastic/systematic errors, legitimate gene/allele tree incongruence (particularly hybridization and recombination). Furthermore, no strictly bifurcating (nor multifurcating) tree can represent graphically instances in which ancestors and derived taxa co-exist, such as when virus or bacteria demographic expansions occur abruptly (in many cases leading to epidemic bursts). In such cases, phylogenetic networks better represent evolutionary relationships. Phylogenetic networks are defined as a set of nodes (leafs and internal nodes) connected by vertices, and allowing cycles.

Implicit networks indicate non-treelike relationships without considering any model of evolution or specific force; instead, they focus on graphically representing regions where the data appears to be non-treelike whatever the reason, evincing ambiguous and/or incompatible signals, therefore working as a summary statistics. They are useful tools for preliminary data analyses, in showing whether

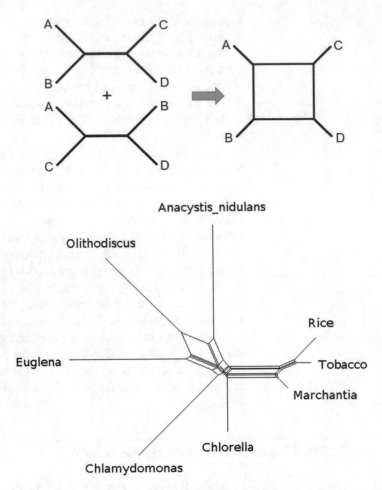

Fig. 8 On top, the general idea behind networks: two different trees place taxon A either close to B or to C, but never to D. This incompatibility induces a pair of "bands of parallel edges," generating a parallelogram, in which A is represented as neighbor to both B and C, but with a larger path to D. The bottom figure is an implicit phylogenetic network based on the Neighbor-Net algorithm [306], a type of split network, based on the example datafile algae.nex from the SplitsTree4 distribution

(and if so, where) there is substantial signal for "non-treelikeness" in a data graph or not, and if not a bifurcating (or multifurcating) tree may indeed be more appropriate. The program SplitsTree4 [305] has many options regarding split networks (which are implicit networks derived from character incompatibilities) and other types. The software also provides a test to determine whether a tree or network fits better the data. Consensus algorithms are also embraced: the consensus network is aimed at gene trees having the full set of taxa, while supernetworks are aimed at consensus across gene trees bearing missing taxa. Bands of parallel edges are drawn whenever there is an incompatible set of splits between trees (Fig. 8).

On the other hand, explicit phylogenetic networks (or evolutionary phylogenetic networks) aim at modeling reticulate evolutionary events (such as sexual recombination in which each parent contributes half of the nuclear complement, meiotic recombination, recombination due to HGT such as in viruses and Bacteria, and hybrid speciation). Because such events flow through time from root to tips, they are directed acyclic graphs (DAGs); hence, they have no directed cycles (as opposed to trees, which have no cycles at all, not even undirected). Internal nodes in explicit networks denote ancestral taxa, and nodes having more than two parents are an inference of reticulate events. The HGT-consensus method in T-rex [307], along with the interactive method within the same package, offers the possibility of finding an optimal scenario of HGT in which many gene trees are within a species tree, with support given by the number of gene trees compatible with inferred reticulations. For explicit networks, it has been shown that when it is used in datasets that are non-reticulate, but are in fact noisy (due to systematic errors), the method may produce false inferences of reticulation [305, 308]. Some explicit phylogenetic networks aim at finding the best network given large sets of gene trees while incorporating specific processes related to real discordance among gene trees, being discussed below.

Phylonet [267] and SNaQ [309] contain algorithms to find the best explicit network (given a fixed number of hybridization events) taking into account both ILS and/or HGT. Both are pseudo-likelihood methods, speeding up the analysis by orders of magnitude while being proven to be robust to ILS [267, 309]. Phylonet is based on the use of likelihood or either pseudo-likelihood as applied to rooted triples, and based on it infer either species trees or networks, under either parsimony (by minimizing deep coalescences it is possible to account for ILS), likelihood, or Bayesian strategies. When searching for hybridizations, estimates inheritance probabilities (the vertical part of the signal, in percentage). Under Bayesian analysis incorporating ILS + HGT, it is able to estimate the number of hybridizations and their locations in the tree by reversible jump Markov Chain Monte Carlo (rjMCMC). Tests done by the authors point towards its accuracy in simulations and in detecting known introgression events from previous studies [267]. It scales to up to 30 taxa if parsimony or pseudo-likelihood methods are used, less for other methods.

SNaQ is a package developed within the Julia programming language, inside which there is the PhyloNetworks module, which infers explicit networks. It uses unrooted quartets estimated by other methods (e.g., BUCKy, ASTRAL) which are proven to be robust against ILS (see above), explicitly estimating reticulations by inferring a γ parameter that relates to the amount of genetic information coming horizontally from a donor in the same tree, whilst $1 - \gamma$ is the percent of vertical signal. It has been deemed robust by its authors [309] and more scalable than Phylonet in terms of increase in number of taxa, but a recent paper comparing Phylonet and SNaQ [310] indicated instead that both have comparable regarding run times.

ClonalFrame [311] uses a Bayesian MCMC algorithm to search for the best phylogenomic tree based on genomic regions (e.g., genes or LCBs) and taking into account gene conversion, a typical HGT outcome of bacterial conjugation. It reports the inferred clonal tree among the organisms, together with parameters ρ/θ (ratio of the relative rates on recombination in relation to mutation), r/m, and average segment import size δ per branch. ClonalOrigin [312] goes one step further and detects origin of putative "donor branches" within the phylogeny being analyzed; the authors found broad regions of elevated levels of recombination when analyzing a set of 13 whole genomes from the *Bacillus cereus* group. Networks can be obtained by the trees generated from either software (e.g., by SplitsTree), one example being a consensus network inferred from 6000 phylograms produced by ClonalFrame analyses of 45 *Vibrio fischeri* taxa using concatenation of four loci [313].

6   Concluding Remarks

It is possible that some divergences are not resolvable, either because the signal of very ancient branches has been mostly erased due to accumulation of many homoplasies in the branches leading to their extant taxa (where the ancestral state of characters cannot be estimated reliably anymore), or because there has been rapid speciation events in some lineages (for example, due to radiations), whereby identifiable synapomorphies may indeed be absent in the ancestral branch. In any case, it is important to search for possible sources of error and biases, circumventing them where possible, but even if not possible a rich discussion of such inconsistencies may clarify further studies down the line. Comparing different data subsets and taxonomic inclusion (because more is not always better as seen above) or different phylogenetic/phylogenomic methods is always warranted. There is probably a larger debate over the latter (parsimony vs. probabilistic, supermatrix vs. species tree methods), and as discussed above, there appear to be no clear winners under all circumstances so far, not the least because all of them are subject to potential sources of bias. It is interesting to try parsimony (a - non-parametric method) and at least one probabilistic method for gene tree (or supermatrix) estimation (e.g., likelihood), and it is not a bad idea to try concatenation as well as a consensus technique, at least for eukaryotes (e.g., species tree method). Also, beware some branch support measures because statistical inconsistency can also lead to increasingly strong support as more data is added. Lastly, networks and supernetworks can be employed if local resolutions remain unresolved even after using different approaches, or if there is enough signal for non-treelike evolutionary processes locally.

An interesting example of all of the above is the evolution of Neoaves (all avian lineages except the ones derived from relatively ancient nodes such as ostriches, tinamous, fowls and ducks), in a review study done by Suh [314]. He reanalyzed different sets of molecular markers (e.g., UCEs, introns, retroposons) and also compared the levels of conflicting resolutions among previous phylogenomic studies, some of the analyses having been done under a supermatrix approach, others using species trees. He observed that the amount of reticulation obtained by networks calculated for each data set was *on par* with networks based on simulated sets of gene trees on a completely unresolved tree (or alternatively based on simulated MSAs on this unresolved tree, whose gene trees were subsequently estimated). Furthermore, he tested for the effect of taxon inclusion by using a single taxon representative of each of the nine well-resolved major lineages (instead of the 48 or more taxa used in previous studies/analyses), and yet the amount of conflict observable in the resulting network remained similar, therefore also rejecting such an bias. Noise in data has also been ruled out: different sets of markers, and particularly an analysis including only retroposons (a marker type within the set of "rare genomic changes" markers, as defined previously), still led to large amounts of reticulation at the base of Neoaves; and it did not matter what phylogenomic method was used as well. Therefore, a radiation becomes a reasonable hypothesis in this case, raising the possibility that it can also be likely for other clades in the tree of life. We researchers are always wishing for fully resolved trees, but it may be that depending on the case, this may not be possible. Finally, that study also highlights the issue of having excessive confidence in bootstrap or posterior probabilities as reliable indices for clade support: the above author mentions that two previous phylogenomic studies on avian evolution had shown very high support for contrasting clades! As mentioned before, instead of such discrepant results regarding naive indices associated to some splits being the exception, they are probably the rule in phylogenomic studies.

To sum up, there is no single phylogenomic appraisal that is robust across the whole set of possible biases, at least among the ones developed so far. So it is always a good idea to explore the data at hand.

7 Practice

In this section we present a brief case study demonstrating some of the theoretical concepts we have discussed above. The following hands-on phylogenomics analysis example uses bacterial genomes,

Table 1
The ten genomes (plus plasmids) used in the practice session

Accession	Species name	Strain name	Short name
NC_007086.1	*Xanthomonas campestris* pv. *campestres*	8004	campestris_8004
NZ_CP009037.1 (chr); NZ_CP009035.1 (plasmid pXAW19); NZ_CP009036.1 (plasmid	*X. citri* subsp. *citri*	AW15	citri_AW15
NC_016010.1	*X. axonopodis* pv. *citrumelo*	F1	citrumelo_F1
NC_007508.1 (chr); NC_007507.1 (plasmid pXCV183); NC_007505.1 (plasmid pXCV19); NC_007504.1 (plasmid pXCV2); NC_007506.1 (plasmid pXCV38)	*X. campestris* pv. *euvesicatorica*	85-10	euvesicatoria_85_10
NC_022541.1 (chr); NC_022539.1 (plasmid pla); NC_022540.1 (plasmid plb); NC_022542.1 (plasmid plc)	*X. fuscans* subsp. *fuscans*	4834-R	fucans_4834R
NZ_CM002264.1 (chr); NZ_CM002265.1 (plasmid unnamed 1); NZ_CM002266.1 (plasmid unnamed 2)	*X. axonopodis* pv. *glycines*	CFBP 7119	glycines_CFBP7119
NZ_CP012947.1	*X. oryzae* pv. *oryzae*	PXO83	oryzae_PX083
NZ_CP017271.1	*X. campestris* pv. *raphani*	756C	raphani_756C
NC_013722.1 (chr); NC_017557.1 (plasmid 1); NC_017556.1 (plasmid 2); NC_017555.1 (plasmid 3)	*X. albilineans*	GPE PC73	albilineans_GPE_PC73
NC_004556.1 (chr); NC_004554.1 (plasmid pXFPD1.3)	*Xylella fastidiosa*	Temecula 1	Xf_temecula1

GenBank accessions are depicted

but many of the analyses presented are also applicable to eukaryotes. Because the dataset is based on closely related genomes, we employ a supermatrix method (*see* Subheading 4.4). For eukaryotes, supertree or species tree methods should be tried as well.

The dataset consists of species of the bacterial genus *Xanthomonas*, all of them plant pathogens, infecting plants such as citrus (oranges, lemons, grapefruits, etc.) and soybean. Ten species with complete genomes (nine *Xanthomonas* plus an outgroup, *Xylella fastidiosa temecula*) were gathered from GenBank (Table 1), making the analyses feasible within 1 or 2 days of computing time.

7.1 Gathering the Data Matrices

7.1.1 Retrieving Homologous Families

In this step, we will infer all gene families shared between all genomes in the input dataset. First, it is important to prepare the input files to avoid any incompatibility with the steps downstream, because afterwards it gets much more complicated to make header corrections. It is highly recommended to rename input files to intuitive names, avoiding spaces and less common characters (alphanumeric and underline are always safe).

Now we move on to inferring the homologous families. There are many programs that could be used to perform this step. We chose Get_Homologues [315] because it is a wrapper of common algorithms for homologous inference, such as Bi-Directional Best Hits and OrthoMCL. As input, Get_Homologues accepts Gen-Bank files (.gbk) or amino acid (aa) sequence fasta files (one per input genome) and nucleotide (nuc) sequence fasta files (optional; needed if inference is to be based on DNA rather than aa). Either gbk files or aa/nuc files should be in the same single input folder. In addition, aa and nuc files must have the same file name but extensions ".faa" and ".fna", respectively. Detailed information can be found at github repository (https://github.com/eead-csic-com pbio/get_homologues/releases). For the purpose of this tutorial we chose inference using DNA, for which both protein multifasta and nucleotide multifasta files (.faa/.fna) are needed. These files can be downloaded directly from NCBI's RefSeq genome database or extracted from GenBank files (.gbk) using in-house scripts. Prepare.faa/.fna headers of each sequence like this:

>SeqID|[species_name] ATCGATCGAATTG...

where SeqID can include the GI of the gene product, its description, and other useful information (fields can be separated by "|"). The basic command line to launch search for homologues is:

```
$ get_homologues.pl −d <input_folder> −M −n <n_threads> −r
<ref_genome> −S <min_%_Identity> −C <min_%_Coverage> −t 0
```

where "−M" is the flag for the clustering algorithm OrthoMCL, and "-r" indicates the name of each gene file output based on the reference genome chosen. With "-t 0", each gene file will contain all inferred homologues for that gene, containing any clusters which include at least one sequence per genome; other values of "-t < n > " will report all clusters containing sequences from at least *n* taxa. CDSs are searched, but alternatively the user can use the option "-a" in which user-selected sequence features such as rRNA or tRNA are searched instead of CDSs, and in that case sequences are compared by BlastN instead of BlastP. Also, one could choose between other two algorithms, BDBH (Bi-Directional Best Hit) or COG (COGtriangles). More details about them can be found in the software manual. With the command line above, Get_Homologues will run all-vs.-all BlastP searches followed by a clustering step employing

OrthoMCL [316]. This is done for either protein-based or DNA search, the only difference is that for the latter a mapping between Protein - > DNA file is done in the end. A total of 8272 homologous families were found (there may have small fluctuations from run to run because the search is stochastic).

7.1.2 Filtering Orthologous Families

Once the homologous searching is done, we can filter only the inferred orthologous gene families, so all families containing paralogs (both inparalogs or outparalogs) are discarded for this step. To accomplish this task, we run an auxiliary script in Get_Homologues called compare_clusters.pl, with the following parameters:

```
$ compare_clusters.pl -d ;<input_folder> -t <n_input_genomes> -o
<output_folder> -n
```

This command will export *unicopy* orthologous gene families (i.e., families having one copy per genome, for all taxa) of nuc fasta files to the desired output folder; for amino acid fasta files, remove the option "-n". A total of 1226 unicopy core-coding genes was found after our run was completed.

7.1.3 Multiple Alignment of Orthologous Families

For each orthologous family exported, we will perform a multiple alignment. In this tutorial, we are going to use Guidance [317], which performs the sequence alignment followed by a validation step based on guide trees obtained by bootstrap, checking the quality of the produced alignment and removing (according to a pre-configured threshold) the low confidence sites (or an entire sequence if it is cast as an outlier), if desired. In general, hundreds to thousands of families will have to be aligned, so a script that runs tasks in parallel is recommended (or by using the linux—xargs directive). If we choose to use alignment by codons, export sequences in the same order as in the input, and using Mafft as the base aligner, the basic command line to run Guidance is:

```
$ guidance.pl --seqFile <fasta_file> --seqType codon --outOrder
    as_input --proc_num <n_threads> --dataset <outfile_prefix>
    --bootstraps <n_bootstraps> --msaProgram mafft
```

More options and details can be found at http://guidance.tau.ac.il/ver2/overview.php. Manual curation of each alignment should be done (e.g., in Aliview; [65]) even if it takes some time to be completed, because misaligned regions can induce wrong assessments of topology, branch lengths, selection and recombination levels, and divergence dating.

7.1.4 Building the Supermatrix

Now, we concatenate all individual alignments into a single alignment. Here, we use FasconCAT (https://www.zfmk.de/en/research/research-centres-and-groups/fasconcat), a Perl script capable of generating output files in most common formats required for phylogenetic tree building programs. A window with options is displayed once the program is run, in which the user can choose some format options, as well as if all or part of the genes will be concatenated (we will include all of them). It is important that the fasta header of each taxon across alignment files is identical, otherwise the concatenation process will fail.

7.1.5 Generating the Matrix of Gene Presence/Absence

In addition, it is possible to compute the presence/absence profile of homologous gene families in the form of a numeric matrix, where "0" represents absence of a gene, "1" presence of a single copy, and larger values are inferred duplications. For this matrix to include all homologous families encountered (even those including only a single sequence for a single genome), it is important that the previous Get_Homologues run included the option "-t 0". In order to generate a multistate numerical matrix, compare_clusters.pl must be re-run as follows:

```
$ compare_clusters.pl —d <input_folder> —m —o <output_folder>
```

7.1.6 Generating the Matrix of Indels

The explicit use of indels was shown to be phylogenetically informative for both prokaryotes [318] and eukaryotes [319]. Under maximum parsimony, indels can be treated as a 5th character (e.g., TNT, PAUP), but in this way sequential gaps in a same taxon will be treated as multiple indel events, potentially distorting topological inference. SeqState [46] detects sequential gaps in the same taxon transforming it in a single state character ("1"). Other taxa having this same indel, with equal length, will also be considered "1"; in other taxa having indels overlapping it but with a different length, states will have higher values ("2", or if there is yet another indel variant "3", and so forth). A taxon with absence of indels in the ensemble gap region has "0" for that character. To generate the indel matrix, choose *File > Open* and open the concatenated core-coding alignment file in fasta format. Next, choose *indelCoder > modified complex coding* (suggested by the authors as the more meaningful gap coding scheme). It is recommended that the concatenated matrix be script-edited to include user-defined nucleotide flag marks at the beginning and end of each gene alignment. This is to avoid wrongly assuming a single indel state in cases where a taxon has an indel that crosses from the end of a gene to the start of the next contiguous one in the concatenated matrix. One possible flag is adding 20 As ("AAAAA..."), or any other mononucleotide string, at the beginning and end of every gene alignment, across all sequences present in that alignment. Then concatenation can be done in the usual way (e.g., by FasconCAT), and it is this alternative matrix that shall be input into SeqState to have indel states inferred. After that, this alternative concatenation matrix can be discarded. The output is a nexus file from which the numeric matrix can be extracted with little bioinformatic effort.

7.2 Phylogenomic Inference

In the following steps a mixed-data based phylogeny (combining all three types of data) is inferred and compared to the separate trees. We will base the analyses in IQTree [79], a command line program with many options regarding data types, evolutionary models, partitioning, model testing, tree search, branch support, and mixed data analysis. Its multithreaded version (iqtree-omp) will be used here.

7.2.1 Unicopy Core-Coding Phylogeny

We will first suggest a priori data blocks to the program (e.g., three data blocks: 1st, 2nd, and 3rd codon positions). Amalgamation of the data blocks is subsequently tested by BIC, and if two or more of them have better BIC score when joined, these will form a subset (= partition), and then Markov models are tested for each subset. We use the PartitionFinder algorithm [163] as implemented in IQTree for this purpose. We use the three data blocks relative to different codon positions to facilitate calculations; with the three partitions, all permutations lead to five possible partitioning schemes: unpartitioned dataset, 3 codon-based partition, and then another three combinations of two partitions vs. the remaining. If gene data blocks are input (or codon positions within each gene block) the computation would take an exceedingly amount of time (recall we obtained 1226 unicopy orthologous genes, think permutations of these). A modified nexus file (.nex) containing the description of the data blocks must be generated. Its content follows:

#NEXUS
begin sets;
    CHARSET Codon_p1 = alignment_file.phy: 1-1227495\3;
    CHARSET Codon_p2 = alignment_file.phy: 2-1227495\3;
    CHARSET Codon_p3 = alignment_file.phy: 3-1227495\3;
end;

The command line to run the above-mentioned partitioning test (plus tree search with bootstraps) is:

```
$ iqtree-omp -spp <partition_file.nex> -nt <n_threads> -bb
<n_fast_bootstrap> -m TESTNEWMERGE
```

The option "-spp" means that rates among partitions are calculated assuming that relative proportions of branch lengths in each partition are fixed (as well as the topology), up to a constant of proportionality among partitions, and then these constants are optimized altogether with tree search. "-m TESTNEWMERGE" means choosing the best partitioning scheme altogether with models for each, for a total of 22 base models (spanning from JC to GTR) considered with or without G (discretized gamma rate

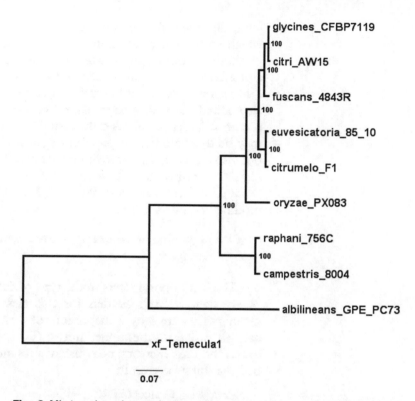

Fig. 9 ML tree based on unicopy core-coding sequences. Bootstrap support values based on 1000 ultrafast bootstrap replicates are indicated

categories), I (proportion of invariable sites), Rn (FreeRate model, in which the same model is tested with *n* different rates, from 2 to 10 being default if *n* is not specified). Alternatively, ASC (ascertainment correction) is also included during model testing if the alignment does not include constant sites, such as SNPs and morphology. With the option "-bb", an amount of 1000 fast bootstraps [197] is reasonable. Our result in terms of best partitioning scheme and best model for each subset was:

Codon_p1: GTR + R3
Codon_p2: GTR + R3
Codon_p3: GTR + R2,

meaning the best BIC score was for the partitioning scheme where the three positions are kept separated, all of them having a mix of 2–3 different rates optimized within the base GTR model. Figure 9 shows the estimated core-coding tree.

7.2.2 Presence/Abscence of Genes

When deciding for the use of presence/absence of genes in the pangenome of all the taxa involved (= all genes present at least in one taxon), one could use all the homologous gene alignments. However, there would be problems when considering paralogous copies of a taxon across gene alignments: if a taxon has two copies in gene alignment A, the same taxon in alignment B would align to which of the copies in A? In such cases, supertree or specie tree methods are more appropriate for sequence data. For supermatrix, a numeric matrix of precence/absence is workable, even though it throws away sequence information across taxa. Furthermore, we also edited the matrix to transform entries ≥ 2 to "1" to stick to precence/absence entries only, avoiding duplications, as the latter may be due to different processes (gains by HGT, losses by deletion); in any case, the choice is up to the user. After obtaining such a matrix, any phylogenetic method could be employed (e.g., parsimony), but here we stick to ML in IQTree. We run it with a slightly modified command line:

```
$ iqtree-omp -s <alignment file> -st BIN -m TESTNEW -nt <n_threads>
-bb <n_fast_bootstrap>
```

The "-st" option refers to the type of data, which in the case of binary data is BIN. Models for this class are JC2 and GTR2, meaning they are 2-by-2 adaptations of their original 4-by-4 matrices. All variations mentioned above (G, I, Rn) and also ASC are tested (because there are no constant sites including only "0"s). We had the following result:

Pres_Abs_Genes: GTR2 + FO,

where FO means optimized state frequencies of 0s and 1s (instead of being fixed or empirical). A total of 8272 characters were found (this should match the number of homologous families found previously). Figure 10 shows the estimated tree of gene presence/absence.

7.2.3 Indels

In this case, different indel lengths overlapping in the same genomic region translate into different character states. The command line is:

```
$ iqtree -omp -s <alignment file> -st MORPH -m TEST-
NEW -nt <n_threads> -bb <n_fast_bootstrap>
```

The difference between "BIN" and "MORPH" is that the latter is aimed at numeric matrices with states >1. Here is the result:

Indels: ORDERED+FQ+ASC+R2

It means that the best model includes the assumption of ordered states (compared to instantaneous rate changes between any two states), so any change is possible only between adjacent state values. "FQ" means state frequencies are all equal. A total of 2319 characters were found. Figure 11 shows the estimated ML tree based on indel coding.

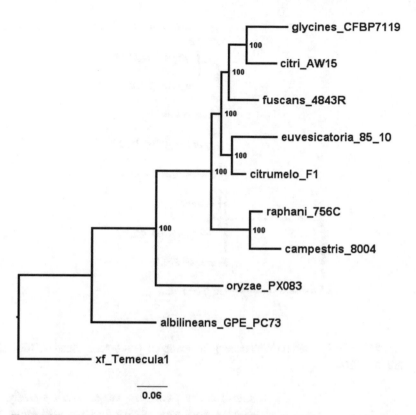

Fig. 10 ML tree based on presence/absence of genes. Bootstrap support values based on 1000 ultrafast bootstrap replicates are indicated

7.2.4 Concatenation of All Three Data Sets

We further proceed to an ensemble analysis, involving the three sets of data described above, each being considered a different partition. We subdivide the core-coding dataset into the three codon positions, for a final partitioning scheme with five partitions, and implement the proportional model of rate multipliers across them. Below, we show the nexus partition file:

```
#NEXUS
begin sets;
    CHARSET Codon_p1 = alignment_file.phy: 1-1227495\3;
    CHARSET Codon_p2 = alignment_file.phy: 2-1227495\3;
    CHARSET Codon_p3 = alignment_file.phy: 3-1227495\3;
    CHARSET Pres_Abs_Genes = gene_pres_abs.phy: 1-8272;
    CHARSET Indels = indels_file.phy: 1-2319;
    CHARPARTITION Multidata = GTR+R3:Codon_p1,
GTR+R3:Codon_p2, GTR+R2:Codon_p3,
    GTR2+FO:Pres_Abs_Genes,    ORDERED+FQ+ASC+R2:
Indels ;
end;
```

Notice above that the command "charpartition" has been included, it specifies the intended model for each partition as

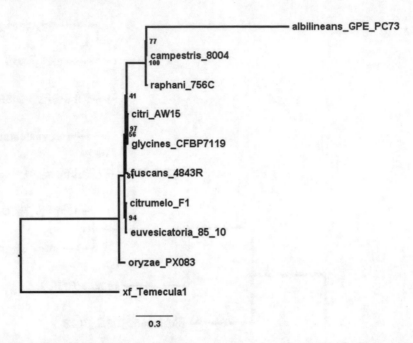

Fig. 11 ML tree based on indel coding. Bootstrap support values based on 1000 ultrafast bootstrap replicates are indicated

obtained in previous runs. Alternatively, the best partitioning scheme and models for each could be estimated concomitantly with tree search like we did for core-coding, because the likelihood of each model/partitioning scheme may change when the ensemble data is considered (therefore changing BIC). However, we assume for simplicity that any changes in parameter estimates do not impact partitioning, models, or tree search significantly. Because the models were already defined in the.nex file, the "-m" directive is dropped:

```
$ iqtree-omp -spp partition_file.nex -bb 1000 -nt <n_threads>
```

Figure 12 shows the estimated ML tree based on concatenation of the three types of data (whole set of core-coding, pres./abs. of genes, indels).

It can be seen that core-coding and gene presence/absence trees are very similar, except for the position of *oryzae_PX083*, which is closer to the root in the pres./abs tree. We also get to see that the mixed data tree (Fig. 12) is identical in topology and very close in branch lengths to the core-coding tree; this is not surprising since most of the signal comes from the latter due to its much larger size, and furthermore the whole tree represents a relatively shallow evolutionary window. However, the behavior can be different in other situations (e.g., for some deeper divergences it may be that base substitutions saturate faster than indels

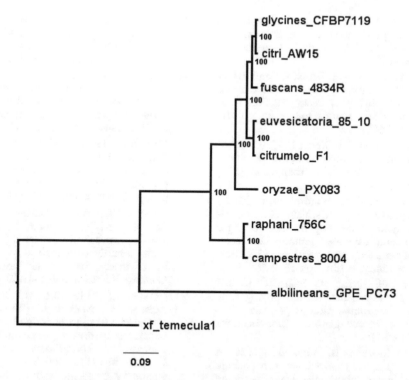

Fig. 12 ML tree based on core-coding + pres./abs. genes + indels. Bootstrap support values based on 1000 ultrafast bootstrap replicates are indicated

or gene gains/losses, and in that case focusing on non-saturated data such as indels could be more meaningful, even if core-coding matrix length is much larger).

Contrarily, the indel tree is highly discordant compared to the mixed data tree, and with *albilineans_GPE_PC73* exhibiting a long branch. This species is possibly the most ancient among *Xanthomonas* lineages [320], so its position in the indel tree is highly suspicious, as well as other (supposedly) wrong taxonomic placements. One possible explanation for this loss of indel-based phylogenetic signal is that gene losses and gains have been occurring too frequently, hampering phylogenomic assessment based in this datatype alone.

References

1. Benson DA, Cavanaugh M, Clark K, Karsch-Mizrachi I, Lipman DJ, Ostell J, Sayers EW (2013) Genbank. Nucleic Acids Res 41(D1): D36–D42

2. O'Brien SJ, Menotti-Raymond M, Murphy WJ, Nash WG, Wienberg J, Stanyon R, Copeland NG, Jenkins NA, Womack JE, Graves JAM (1999) The promise of comparative genomics in mammals. Science 286 (5439):458–481

3. Delsuc F, Brinkmann H, Philippe H (2005) Phylogenomics and the reconstruction of the tree of life. Nat Rev Genet 6(5):361–375

4. Eisen JA, Kaiser D, Myers RM (1997) Gastrogenomic delights: a movable feast. Nat Med 3 (10):1076

5. Eisen JA (1998) Phylogenomics: improving functional predictions for uncharacterized genes by evolutionary analysis. Genome Res 8(3):163–167

6. Fan H, Ives AR, Surget-Groba Y, Cannon CH (2015) An assembly and alignment-free method of phylogeny reconstruction from next-generation sequencing data. BMC Genomics 16(1):522

7. Darling AE, Mau Bob, Perna NT (2010) pro-gressiveMauve: multiple genome alignment with gene gain, loss and rearrangement. PloS One 5(6):e11147

8. Minkin I, Patel A, Kolmogorov M, Vyahhi N, Pham S (2013) Sibelia: a scalable and comprehensive synteny block generation tool for closely related microbial genomes. In: International workshop on algorithms in bioinformatics. Springer, Berlin, pp 215–229

9. Gardner SN, Slezak T, Hall BG (2015) kSNP3.0: SNP detection and phylogenetic analysis of genomes without genome alignment or reference genome. Bioinformatics 31:2877–2878

10. Contreras-Moreira B, Vinuesa P (2013) Get_homologues, a versatile software package for scalable and robust microbial pangenome analysis. Appl Environ Microbiol 79 (24):7696–7701

11. Li L, Stoeckert CJ, Roos DS (2003) Orthomcl: identification of ortholog groups for eukaryotic genomes. Genome Res 13 (9):2178–2189

12. Kristensen DM, Kannan L, Coleman MK, Wolf YI, Sorokin A, Koonin EV, Mushegian A (2010) A low-polynomial algorithm for assembling clusters of orthologous groups from intergenomic symmetric best matches. Bioinformatics 26(12):1481–1487

13. Treangen TJ, Ondov BD, Koren S, Phillippy AM (2014) The harvest suite for rapid core-genome alignment and visualization of thousands of intraspecific microbial genomes. Genome Biol 15(11):524

14. Galtier N, Tourasse N, Gouy M (1999) A nonhyperthermophilic common ancestor to extant life forms. Science 283 (5399):220–221

15. Bragg JG, Potter S, Bi K, Moritz C (2015) Exon capture phylogenomics: efficacy across scales of divergence. Mol Ecol Resour

16. Folk RA, Mandel JR, Freudenstein JV (2015) A protocol for targeted enrichment of intron-containing sequence markers for recent radiations: a phylogenomic example from heuchera (saxifragaceae). Appl Plant Sci 3(8):1500039

17. Bejerano G, Pheasant M, Makunin I, Stephen S, Kent WJ, Mattick JS, Haussler D (2004) Ultraconserved elements in the human genome. Science 304(5675):1321–1325

18. Faircloth BC, McCormack JE, Crawford NG, Harvey MG, Brumfield RT, Glenn TC (2012) Ultraconserved elements anchor thousands of genetic markers spanning multiple evolutionary timescales. Syst Biol 61:717–726

19. Crawford NG, Faircloth BC, McCormack JE, Brumfield RT, Winker K, Glenn TC (2012) More than 1000 ultraconserved elements provide evidence that turtles are the sister group of archosaurs. Biol Lett 8(5):783–786

20. Siepel A, Bejerano G, Pedersen JS, Hinrichs AS, Hou M, Rosenbloom K, Clawson H, Spieth J, Hillier LW, Richards S et al (2005) Evolutionarily conserved elements in vertebrate, insect, worm, and yeast genomes. Genome Res 15(8):1034–1050

21. Glazov EA, Pheasant M, McGraw EA, Bejerano G, Mattick JS (2005) Ultraconserved elements in insect genomes: a highly conserved intronic sequence implicated in the control of homothorax mrna splicing. Genome Res 15(6):800–808

22. Zheng W-X, Zhang C-T (2008) Ultraconserved elements between the genomes of the plants arabidopsis thaliana and rice. J Biomol Struct Dyn 26(1):1–8

23. Smith BT, Harvey MG, Faircloth BC, Glenn TC, Brumfield RT (2013) Target capture and massively parallel sequencing of ultraconserved elements (uces) for comparative studies at shallow evolutionary time scales. Syst Biol 63:83–95

24. Faircloth BC (2015) PHYLUCE is a software package for the analysis of conserved genomic loci. Bioinformatics 32:786–788

25. Pearson T, Busch JD, Ravel J, Read TD, Rhoton SD, U'ren JM, Simonson TS, Kachur SM, Leadem RR, Cardon ML et al (2004) Phylogenetic discovery bias in bacillus anthracis using single-nucleotide polymorphisms from whole-genome sequencing. Proc Natl Acad Sci USA 101(37):13536–13541

26. Pearson T, Okinaka RT, Foster JT, Keim P (2009) Phylogenetic understanding of clonal populations in an era of whole genome sequencing. Infect Genet Evol 9 (5):1010–1019

27. Leaché AD, Banbury BL, Felsenstein J, Nieto-Montes de Oca A, Stamatakis A (2015) Short tree, long tree, right tree, wrong tree: new acquisition bias corrections for inferring snp phylogenies. Syst Biol 64:1032–1047

28. Lewis PO (2001) A likelihood approach to estimating phylogeny from discrete morphological character data. Syst Biol 50 (6):913–925

29. Bertels F, Silander OK, Pachkov M, Rainey PB, van Nimwegen E (2014) Automated reconstruction of whole-genome phylogenies from short-sequence reads. Mol Biol Evol 31 (5):1077–1088

30. Stamatakis A (2014) Raxml version 8: a tool for phylogenetic analysis and post-analysis of large phylogenies. Bioinformatics 30 (9):1312–1313

31. Nguyen L-T, Schmidt HA, von Haeseler A, Minh BQ (2015) Iq-tree: a fast and effective stochastic algorithm for estimating maximum-likelihood phylogenies. Mol Biol Evol 32(1):268–274

32. Ronquist F, Teslenko M, Van Der Mark P, Ayres DL, Darling A, Höhna S, Larget B, Liu L, Suchard MA, Huelsenbeck JP (2012) Mrbayes 3.2: efficient Bayesian phylogenetic inference and model choice across a large model space. Syst Biol 61(3):539–542

33. Nielsen R, Paul JS, Albrechtsen A, Song YS (2011) Genotype and snp calling from next-generation sequencing data. Nat Rev Genet 12(6):443–451

34. Rokas A, Holland PWH (2000) Rare genomic changes as a tool for phylogenetics. Trends Ecol Evol 15(11):454–459

35. Boore JL, Lavrov DV, Brown WM (1998) Gene translocation links insects and crustaceans. Nature 392(6677):667

36. Regier JC, Shultz JW, Zwick A, Hussey A, Ball B, Wetzer R, Martin JW, Cunningham CW (2010) Arthropod relationships revealed by phylogenomic analysis of nuclear protein-coding sequences. Nature 463 (7284):1079–1083

37. Yue F, Cui L, Moret BME, Tang J et al (2008) Gene rearrangement analysis and ancestral order inference from chloroplast genomes with inverted repeat. BMC Genomics 9(1): S25

38. Hu F, Lin Y, Tang J (2014) Mlgo: phylogeny reconstruction and ancestral inference from gene-order data. BMC Bioinf 15(1):354

39. Moret BME, Wyman S, Bader DA, Warnow T, Yan M (2001) A new implementation and detailed study of breakpoint analysis. In: Pacific symposium on biocomputing, vol 6, pp 583–594

40. Tang J, Moret BME (2003) Scaling up accurate phylogenetic reconstruction from gene-order data. Bioinformatics 19(suppl 1): i305–i312

41. Kang S, Tang J, Schaeffer SW, Bader DA (2011) Rec-DCM-Eigen: reconstructing a less parsimonious but more accurate tree in shorter time. PloS One 6(8):e22483

42. Hilker R, Sickinger C, Pedersen CNS, Stoye J (2012) Unimog—a unifying framework for genomic distance calculation and sorting based on DCJ. Bioinformatics 28 (19):2509–2511

43. Hu F, Lin Y, Tang J (2014) MLGO: phylogeny reconstruction and ancestral inference from gene-order data. BMC Bioinf 15(354)

44. Mostowy S, Behr MA (2005) The origin and evolution of mycobacterium tuberculosis. Clin Chest Med 26(2):207–216

45. Belinky F, Cohen O, Huchon D (2010) Large-scale parsimony analysis of metazoan indels in protein-coding genes. Mol Biol Evol 27(2):441–451

46. Müller K (2005) Seqstate. Appl Bioinf 4 (1):65–69

47. Rosenfeld JA, Oppenheim S, DeSalle R (2017) A whole genome gene content phylogenetic analysis of anopheline mosquitoes. Mol Phylogenet Evol 107:266–269

48. Lake JA, Rivera MC (2004) Deriving the genomic tree of life in the presence of horizontal gene transfer: conditioned reconstruction. Mol Biol Evol 21(4):681–690

49. Vos P, Hogers R, Bleeker M, Reijans M, Van de Lee T, Hornes M, Friters A, Pot J, Paleman J, Kuiper M et al (1995) Aflp: a new technique for dna fingerprinting. Nucleic Acids Res 23(21):4407–4414

50. Koopman WJM, Wissemann V, De Cock K, Van Huylenbroeck J, De Riek J, Sabatino GJH, Visser D, Vosman B, Ritz CM, Maes B et al (2008) Aflp markers as a tool to reconstruct complex relationships: a case study in rosa (rosaceae). Am J Bot 95(3):353–366

51. Murata S, Takasaki N, Saitoh M, Okada N (1993) Determination of the phylogenetic relationships among pacific salmonids by using short interspersed elements (sines) as temporal landmarks of evolution. Proc Natl Acad Sci 90(15):6995–6999

52. Verneau O, Catzeflis F, Furano AV (1998) Determining and dating recent rodent speciation events by using l1 (line-1) retrotransposons. Proc Natl Acad Sci 95 (19):11284–11289

53. Gibson A, Brown T, Baker L, Drobniewski F (2005) Can 15-locus mycobacterial interspersed repetitive unit-variable-number tandem repeat analysis provide insight into the evolution of mycobacterium tuberculosis? Appl Environ Microbiol 71(12):8207–8213

54. Asher RJ (2007) A web-database of mammalian morphology and a reanalysis of placental phylogeny. BMC Evol Biol 7(1):108

55. Livezey BC, Zusi RL (2007) Higher-order phylogeny of modern birds (theropoda, aves: Neornithes) based on comparative anatomy. ii. analysis and discussion. Zool J Linnean Soc 149(1):1–95

56. Murray GGR, Weinert LA, Rhule EL, Welch JJ (2016) The phylogeny of rickettsia using different evolutionary signatures: how tree-like is bacterial evolution? Syst Biol 65 (2):265–279

57. Liu F-GR, Miyamoto MM, Freire NP, Ong PQ, Tennant MR, Young TS, Gugel KF (2001) Molecular and morphological supertrees for Eutherian (placental) mammals. Science 291(5509):1786–1789

58. Wheeler WC, Lucaroni N, Hong L, Crowley LM, Varón A (2015) Poy version 5: phylogenetic analysis using dynamic homologies under multiple optimality criteria. Cladistics 31(2):189–196

59. Edgar RC (2004) Muscle: multiple sequence alignment with high accuracy and high throughput. Nucleic Acids Res 32 (5):1792–1797

60. Katoh K, Standley DM (2013) Mafft multiple sequence alignment software version 7: improvements in performance and usability. Mol Biol Evol 30(4):772–780

61. Sela I, Ashkenazy H, Katoh K Pupko T (2015) Guidance2: accurate detection of unreliable alignment regions accounting for the uncertainty of multiple parameters. Nucleic Acids Res 43(W1):W7–W14

62. Mirarab S, Nguyen N, Guo S, Wang L-S, Kim J, Warnow T (2015) Pasta: ultra-large multiple sequence alignment for nucleotide and amino-acid sequences. J Comput Biol 22(5):377–386

63. Nguyen N-PD, Mirarab S, Kumar K, Warnow T (2015) Ultra-large alignments using phylogeny-aware profiles. Genome Biol 16 (1):124

64. Eddy SR (2011) Accelerated profile HMM searches. PLoS Comput Biol 7(10):e1002195

65. Larsson A (2014) Aliview: a fast and lightweight alignment viewer and editor for large datasets. Bioinformatics 30(22):3276–3278

66. Farris JS (1970) Methods for computing Wagner trees. Syst Biol 19(1):83–92

67. Camin JH, Sokal RR (1965) A method for deducing branching sequences in phylogeny. Evolution 311–326

68. Le Quesne WJ (1974) The uniquely evolved character concept and its cladistic application. Syst Biol 23(4):513–517

69. Farris JS (1977) Phylogenetic analysis under Dollo's law. Syst Biol 26(1):77–88

70. Platt RN, Zhang Y, Witherspoon DJ, Xing J, Suh A, Keith MS, Jorde LB, Stevens RD, Ray DA (2015) Targeted capture of phylogenetically informative ves sine insertions in genus Myotis. Genome Biol Evol 7(6):1664–1675

71. Swofford DA, Olsen GJ (1990) Phylogeny reconstruction. In: Hillis DM, Moritz C (eds) Molecular systematics. Sinauer Associates, Sunderland, MA, pp 411–501

72. Sankoff D, Rousseau P (1975) Locating the vertices of a steiner tree in an arbitrary space. Math Program 9:240–246

73. Goloboff PA, Farris JS, Nixon KC (2008) Tnt, a free program for phylogenetic analysis. Cladistics 24(5):774–786

74. Müllner D (2011) fastcluster: Fast hierarchical clustering routines for R and Python

75. Khan MA, Elias I, Sjölund E, Nylander K, Guimera RV, Schobesberger E, Schmitzberger P, Lagergren J, Arvestad L (2013) Fastphylo: fast tools for phylogenetics. BMC Bioinf 14(1):334

76. Criscuolo A, Gascuel O (2008) Fast NJ-like algorithms to deal with incomplete distance matrices. BMC Bioinf 9(1):166

77. Lefort V, Desper R, Gascuel P(2015) Fastme 2.0: a comprehensive, accurate, and fast distance-based phylogeny inference program. Mol Biol Evol 32(10):2798–2800

78. Felsenstein J (2016) {PHYLIP}: phylogenetic inference package, version 3.5 c

79. Nguyen L-T, Schmidt HA, von Haeseler A, Minh BQ (2015) Iq-tree: a fast and effective stochastic algorithm for estimating maximum-likelihood phylogenies. Mol Biol Evol 32(1):268–274

80. Price MN, Dehal PS, Arkin AP (2010) Fasttree 2–approximately maximum-likelihood trees for large alignments. PloS One 5(3): e9490

81. Guindon S, Dufayard J-F, Lefort V, Anisimova M, Hordijk W, Gascuel O (2010) New algorithms and methods to estimate maximum-likelihood phylogenies: assessing the performance of phyml 3.0. Syst Biol 59 (3):307–321

82. Metropolis N, Rosenbluth AW, Rosenbluth MN, Teller AH, Teller E (1953) Equation of state calculations by fast computing machines. J Chem Phys 21(6):1087–1092

83. Hastings WE (1970) Monte carlo sampling methods using Markov chains and their applications. Biometrika 57(1):97–109

84. Drummond AJ, Suchard MA, Xie D, Rambaut A (2012) Bayesian phylogenetics with beauti and the beast 1.7. Mol Biol Evol 29 (8):1969–1973

85. Lewis PO, Holder MT, Swofford DL (2015) Phycas: software for Bayesian phylogenetic analysis. Syst Biol 64(3):525–531

86. Felsenstein J (1978) Cases in which parsimony or compatibility methods will be positively misleading. Syst Zool 401–410

87. Kolaczkowski B, Thornton JW (2004) Performance of maximum parsimony and likelihood phylogenetics when evolution is heterogeneous. Nature 431(7011):980–984

88. Philippe H, Zhou Y, Brinkmann H, Rodrigue N, Delsuc F (2005) Heterotachy and long-branch attraction in phylogenetics. BMC Evol Biol 5(1):50

89. Gadagkar SR, Kumar S (2005) Maximum likelihood outperforms maximum parsimony even when evolutionary rates are heterotachous. Mol Biol Evol 22(11):2139–2141

90. Spencer M, Susko E, Roger AJ (2005) Likelihood, parsimony, and heterogeneous evolution. Mol Biol Evol 22(5):1161–1164

91. Ripplinger J, Sullivan J (2008) Does choice in model selection affect maximum likelihood analysis? Syst Biol 57(1):76–85

92. Warnow T (2012) Standard maximum likelihood analyses of alignments with gaps can be statistically inconsistent. PLOS Curr Tree Life 4:RRN1308

93. Simmons MP, Pickett KM, Miya M (2004) How meaningful are Bayesian support values? Mol Biol Evol 21(1):188–199

94. Rannala B, Zhu T, Yang Z (2012) Tail paradox, partial identifiability, and influential priors in Bayesian branch length inference. Mol Biol Evol 29(1):325–335

95. Hendy MD, Penny D (1982) Branch and bound algorithms to determine minimal evolutionary trees. Math Biosci 59(2):277–290

96. Nixon KC (1999) The parsimony ratchet, a new method for rapid parsimony analysis. Cladistics 15(4):407–414

97. Bazinet AL, Zwickl DJ, Cummings MP (2014) A gateway for phylogenetic analysis powered by grid computing featuring garli 2.0. Syst Biol 63(5):812–818

98. Helaers R, Milinkovitch MC (2010) Metapiga v2. 0: maximum likelihood large phylogeny estimation using the metapopulation genetic algorithm and other stochastic heuristics. BMC Bioinf 11(1):379

99. Goloboff PA (1999) Analyzing large data sets in reasonable times: solutions for composite optima. Cladistics 15(4):415–428

100. Roshan UW, Warnow T, Moret BME, Williams TL (2004) Rec-i-dcm3: a fast algorithmic technique for reconstructing phylogenetic trees. In: Proceedings of 2004 I.E. computational systems bioinformatics conference, 2004. CSB 2004. IEEE, New York, pp 98–109

101. Swofford DL (2003) Paup*. phylogenetic analysis using parsimony (* and other methods). version 4.

102. Yang Z (1994) Estimating the pattern of nucleotide substitution. J Mol Evol 39 (1):105–111

103. Tavaré S (1986) Some probabilistic and statistical problems in the analysis of dna sequences. Lect Math Life Sci 17:57–86

104. Jukes TH, Cantor CR (1969) Evolution of protein molecules. Mamm Protein Metab 3 (21):132

105. Kimura M (1980) A simple method for estimating evolutionary rates of base substitutions through comparative studies of nucleotide sequences. J Mol Evol 16 (2):111–120

106. Hasegawa M, Kishino H, Yano T-A (1985) Dating of the human-ape splitting by a molecular clock of mitochondrial dna. J Mol Evol 22(2):160–174

107. Yang Z (1996) Among-site rate variation and its impact on phylogenetic analyses. Trends Ecol Evol 11(9):367–372

108. Mayrose I, Friedman N, Pupko T (2005) A gamma mixture model better accounts for among site rate heterogeneity. Bioinformatics 21(suppl 2):ii151–ii158

109. Lartillot N, Philippe H (2004) A Bayesian mixture model for across-site heterogeneities in the amino-acid replacement process. Mol Biol Evol 21(6):1095–1109

110. Le SQ, Lartillot N, Gascuel O (2008) Phylogenetic mixture models for proteins. Philos Trans R Soc B 363(1512):3965–3976

111. Felsenstein J, Churchill GA (1996) A hidden Markov model approach to variation among sites in rate of evolution. Mol Biol Evol 13 (1):93–104

112. McGuire G, Wright F, Prentice MJ (2000) A Bayesian model for detecting past recombination events in dna multiple alignments. J Comput Biol 7(1–2):159–170

113. Boussau B, Guéguen L, Gouy M (2009) A mixture model and a hidden Markov model to simultaneously detect recombination breakpoints and reconstruct phylogenies. Evol Bioinf 5:67

114. Lopez P, Casane D, Philippe H (2002) Heterotachy, an important process of protein evolution. Mol Biol Evol 19(1):1–7

115. Galtier N, Gouy M (1998) Inferring pattern and process: maximum-likelihood implementation of a nonhomogeneous model of dna sequence evolution for phylogenetic analysis. Mol Biol Evol 15(7):871–879

116. Schöniger M, Von Haeseler A (1994) A stochastic model for the evolution of autocorrelated dna sequences. Mol Phylogenet Evol 3 (3):240–247

117. Muse SV (1995) Evolutionary analyses of dna sequences subject to constraints of secondary structure. Genetics 139(3):1429–1439

118. Rzhetsky A (1995) Estimating substitution rates in ribosomal RNA genes. Genetics 141 (2):771–783

119. Savill NJ, Hoyle DC, Higgs PG (2001) Rna sequence evolution with secondary structure constraints: comparison of substitution rate models using maximum-likelihood methods. Genetics 157(1):399–411

120. Renée E, Tillier M (1994) Maximum likelihood with multiparameter models of substitution. J Mol Evol 39(4):409–417

121. Higgs PG (2000) RNA secondary structure: physical and computational aspects. Q Rev Biophys 33(3):199–253

122. Tillier ERM, Collins RA (1998) High apparent rate of simultaneous compensatory basepair substitutions in ribosomal rna. Genetics 148(4):1993–2002

123. Allen JE, Whelan S (2014) Assessing the state of substitution models describing noncoding RNA evolution. Genome Biol Evol 6 (1):65–75

124. Dayhoff MO, Schwartz RM, Orcutt BC (1978) 22 a model of evolutionary change in proteins. In: Atlas of protein sequence and structure, vol 5. National Biomedical Research Foundation, Silver Spring, MD, pp 345–352

125. Henikoff S, Henikoff JG (1992) Amino acid substitution matrices from protein blocks. Proc Natl Acad Sci 89(22):10915–10919

126. Jones DT, Taylor WR, Thornton JM (1992) The rapid generation of mutation data matrices from protein sequences. Comput. Appl. Biosci. 8(3):275–282

127. Whelan S, Goldman N (2001) A general empirical model of protein evolution derived from multiple protein families using a maximum-likelihood approach. Mol Biol Evol 18(5):691–699

128. Le SQ, Gascuel O (2008) An improved general amino acid replacement matrix. Mol Biol Evol 25(7):1307–1320

129. Yang Z, Nielsen R, Hasegawa M (1998) Models of amino acid substitution and applications to mitochondrial protein evolution. Mol Biol Evol 15(12):1600–1611

130. Dang CC, Le QS, Gascuel O, Le VS (2010) Flu, an amino acid substitution model for influenza proteins. BMC Evol Biol 10(1):99

131. Le SQ, Dang CC, Gascuel O (2012) Modeling protein evolution with several amino acid replacement matrices depending on site rates. Mol Biol Evol 29:2921–2936

132. Muse SV, Gaut BS (1994) A likelihood approach for comparing synonymous and nonsynonymous nucleotide substitution rates, with application to the chloroplast genome. Mol Biol Evol 11(5):715–724

133. Goldman N, Yang Z (1994) A codon-based model of nucleotide substitution for protein-coding dna sequences. Mol Biol Evol 11 (5):725–736

134. Yang Z, Nielsen R (1998) Synonymous and nonsynonymous rate variation in nuclear genes of mammals. J Mol Evol 46 (4):409–418

135. Whelan S, Goldman N (2004) Estimating the frequency of events that cause multiple-nucleotide changes. Genetics 167 (4):2027–2043

136. Kosiol C, Holmes I, Goldman N (2007) An empirical codon model for protein sequence evolution. Mol Biol Evol 24(7):1464–1479

137. Gil M, Zanetti MS, Zoller S, Anisimova M (2013) CodonPhyML: fast maximum likelihood phylogeny estimation under codon substitution models. Mol Biol Evol, page mst034

138. Wright AM, Hillis DM (2014) Bayesian analysis using a simple likelihood model outperforms parsimony for estimation of phylogeny from discrete morphological data. PLoS One 9(10):e109210

139. Ho SYW, Jermiin LS (2004) Tracing the decay of the historical signal in biological sequence data. Syst Biol 53(4):623–637

140. Lemmon AR, Moriarty EC (2004) The importance of proper model assumption in Bayesian phylogenetics. Syst Biol 53 (2):265–277

141. Sullivan J, Swofford DL (1997) Are guinea pigs rodents? The importance of adequate models in molecular phylogenetics. J Mamm Evol 4(2):77–86

142. Sullivan J, Joyce P (2005) Model selection in phylogenetics. Annu Rev Ecol Evol Syst 36:445–466

143. Posada D, Crandall KA (2001) Selecting the best-fit model of nucleotide substitution. Syst Biol 50(4):580–601

144. Abdo Z, Minin VN, Joyce P, Sullivan J (2005) Accounting for uncertainty in the tree topology has little effect on the decision-theoretic approach to model selection in phylogeny estimation. Mol Biol Evol 22(3):691–703

145. Kullback S, Leibler RA (1951) On information and sufficiency. Ann Math Stat 22 (1):79–86

146. Anderson DR, Burnham KP (2002) Avoiding pitfalls when using information-theoretic methods. J Wildl Manag 66:912–918

147. Schwarz G et al (1978) Estimating the dimension of a model. Ann Stat 6(2):461–464

148. Kass RE, Raftery AE (1995) Bayes factors. J Am Stat Assoc 90(430):773–795

149. Minin V, Abdo Z, Joyce P, Sullivan J (2003) Performance-based selection of likelihood models for phylogeny estimation. Syst Biol 52(5):674–683

150. Darriba D, Taboada GL, Doallo R, Posada D (2012) jModelTest 2: more models, new heuristics and parallel computing. Nature methods 9(8):772–772

151. Posada D, Buckley TR (2004) Model selection and model averaging in phylogenetics: advantages of Akaike information criterion and Bayesian approaches over likelihood ratio tests. Syst Biol 53(5):793–808

152. Hoff M, Orf S, Riehm B, Darriba D, Stamatakis A (2016) Does the choice of nucleotide substitution models matter topologically? BMC Bioinf 17(1):143

153. Luo A, Qiao H, Zhang Y, Shi W, Ho SYW, Xu W, Zhang A, Zhu C (2010) Performance of criteria for selecting evolutionary models in phylogenetics: a comprehensive study based on simulated datasets. BMC Evol Biol 10 (1):242

154. Duchêne S, Duchêne DA, Di Giallonardo F, Eden J-S, Geoghegan JL, Holt KE, Ho SYW, Holmes EC (2016) Cross-validation to select Bayesian hierarchical models in phylogenetics. BMC Evol Biol 16(1):115

155. Lartillot N, Brinkmann H, Philippe H (2007) Suppression of long-branch attraction artefacts in the animal phylogeny using a site-

heterogeneous model. BMC Evol Biol 7(1): S4

156. Whelan S, Allen JE, Blackburne BP, Talavera D (2015) Modelomatic: fast and automated model selection between RY, nucleotide, amino acid, and codon substitution models. Syst Biol 64(1):42–55

157. Lartillot N, Philippe H (2006) Computing bayes factors using thermodynamic integration. Syst Biol 55(2):195–207

158. Baele G, Lemey P, Bedford T, Rambaut A, Suchard MA, Alekseyenko AV (2012) Improving the accuracy of demographic and molecular clock model comparison while accommodating phylogenetic uncertainty. Mol Biol Evol 29(9):2157–2167

159. Fan Y, Wu R, Chen M-H, Kuo L, Lewis PO (2011) Choosing among partition models in Bayesian phylogenetics. Mol Biol Evol 28 (1):523–532

160. Huelsenbeck JP, Larget B, Alfaro ME (2004) Bayesian phylogenetic model selection using reversible jump Markov chain monte carlo. Mol Biol Evol 21(6):1123–1133

161. Brandley MC, Schmitz A, Reeder TW (2005) Partitioned Bayesian analyses, partition choice, and the phylogenetic relationships of scincid lizards. Syst Biol 54(3):373–390

162. Li C, Lu G, Orti G (2008) Optimal data partitioning and a test case for ray-finned fishes (actinopterygii) based on ten nuclear loci. Syst Biol 57(4):519–539

163. Lanfear R, Calcott B, Ho SYW, Guindon S (2012) Partitionfinder: combined selection of partitioning schemes and substitution models for phylogenetic analyses. Mol Biol Evol 29 (6):1695–1701

164. Kurtz S, Phillippy A, Delcher AL, Smoot M, Shumway M, Antonescu C, Salzberg SL (2004) Versatile and open software for comparing large genomes. Genome Biol 5(2):R12

165. Roure B, Rodriguez-Ezpeleta N, Philippe H (2007) SCaFoS: a tool for selection, concatenation and fusion of sequences for phylogenomics. BMC Evol Biol 7(1):S2

166. Wiens JJ (2003) Missing data, incomplete taxa, and phylogenetic accuracy. Syst Biol 52 (4):528–538

167. Wiens JJ (2006) Missing data and the design of phylogenetic analyses. J Biomed Inform 39 (1):34–42

168. Jeffroy O, Brinkmann H, Delsuc F, Philippe H (2006) Phylogenomics: the beginning of incongruence? Trends Genet 22(4):225–231

169. Simmons MP (2012) Misleading results of likelihood-based phylogenetic analyses in the

presence of missing data. Cladistics 28 (2):208–222

170. Lemmon AR, Brown JM, Stanger-Hall K, Lemmon EM (2009) The effect of ambiguous data on phylogenetic estimates obtained by maximum likelihood and Bayesian inference. Syst Biol 58(1):130–145

171. Foster PG (2004) Modeling compositional heterogeneity. Syst Biol 53(3):485–495

172. Kapralov MV, Filatov DA (2007) Widespread positive selection in the photosynthetic rubisco enzyme. BMC Evol Biol 7(1):73

173. Yang Z, Rannala B (2005) Branch-length prior influences Bayesian posterior probability of phylogeny. Syst Biol 54(3):455–470

174. Lewis PO, Holder MT, Holsinger KE (2005) Polytomies and Bayesian phylogenetic inference. Syst Biol 54(2):241–253

175. Aberer AJ, Stamatakis A (2011) A simple and accurate method for rogue taxon identification. In: 2011 I.E. international conference on bioinformatics and biomedicine (BIBM). IEEE, New York, pp 118–122

176. Bergsten J (2005) A review of long-branch attraction. Cladistics 21(2):163–193

177. Fourment M, Gibbs MJ (2006) Patristic: a program for calculating patristic distances and graphically comparing the components of genetic change. BMC Evol Biol 6(1):1

178. Xia X, Xie Z, Salemi M, Chen L, Wang Y (2003) An index of substitution saturation and its application. Mol Phylogenet Evol 26(1):1–7

179. Xia X, Xie Z (2001) DAMBE: software package for data analysis in molecular biology and evolution. J Hered 92(4):371–373

180. Goremykin VV, Nikiforova SV, Bininda-Emonds ORP (2010) Automated removal of noisy data in phylogenomic analyses. J Mol Evol 71(5-6):319–331

181. Cummins CA, McInerney JO (2011) A method for inferring the rate of evolution of homologous characters that can potentially improve phylogenetic inference, resolve deep divergence and correct systematic biases. Syst Biol 60(6):833–844

182. Simmons MP, Gatesy J (2016) Biases of tree-independent-character-subsampling methods. Mol Phylogenet Evol 100:424–443

183. Chang BSW, Campbell DL (2000) Bias in phylogenetic reconstruction of vertebrate rhodopsin sequences. Mol Biol Evol 17(8):1220–1231

184. Simmons MP, Zhang L-B, Webb CT, Reeves A (2006) How can third codon positions outperform first and second codon positions

in phylogenetic inference? an empirical example from the seed plants. Syst Biol 55(2):245–258

185. Bradley RD, Durish ND, Rogers DS, Miller JR, Engstrom MD, Kilpatrick CW (2007) Toward a molecular phylogeny for Peromyscus: evidence from mitochondrial cytochrome-b sequences. J Mammal 88(5):1146–1159

186. Cox CJ, Foster PG, Hirt RP, Harris SR, and Embley TM (2008) The archaebacterial origin of eukaryotes. Proc Natl Acad Sci 105(51):20356–20361

187. Benoit Nabholz, Axel Künstner, Rui Wang, Erich D Jarvis, and Hans Ellegren (2011) Dynamic evolution of base composition: causes and consequences in avian phylogenomics. Mol Biol Evol 28(8):2197–2210

188. Jermiin LS, Ho JWK, Lau KW, Jayaswal V (2009) SeqVis: a tool for detecting compositional heterogeneity among aligned nucleotide sequences. Bioinf DNA Seq Anal 65–91

189. Sheffield NC, Song H, Cameron SL, Whiting MF (2009) Nonstationary evolution and compositional heterogeneity in beetle mitochondrial phylogenomics. Syst Biol 58(4):381–394

190. Capella-Gutiérrez S, Silla-Martínez JM, Gabaldón T (2009) trimAl: a tool for automated alignment trimming in large-scale phylogenetic analyses. Bioinformatics 25(15):1972–1973

191. Aberer AJ, Krompaß D, Stamatakis A (2011) RogueNaRok: an efficient and exact algorithm for rogue taxon identification. Heidelberg Institute for Theoretical Studies: Exelixis-RRDR-2011-10

192. Trautwein MD, Wiegmann BM, Yeates DK (2011) Overcoming the effects of rogue taxa: evolutionary relationships of the bee flies. PLOS Currents Tree of Life

193. Aberer AJ, Krompass D, Stamatakis A (2013) Pruning rogue taxa improves phylogenetic accuracy: an efficient algorithm and webservice. Syst Biol 62(1):162–166

194. Pattengale N, Aberer A, Swenson K, Stamatakis A, Moret B (2011) Uncovering hidden phylogenetic consensus in large data sets. IEEE/ACM Trans Comput Biol Bioinf 8(4):902–911

195. Heath TA, Hedtke SM, Hillis DM (2008) Taxon sampling and the accuracy of phylogenetic analyses. J Syst Evol 46(3):239–257

196. Felsenstein J (1985) Confidence limits on phylogenies: an approach using the bootstrap. Evolution 39:783–791

197. Minh BQ, Nguyen MAT, von Haeseler A (2013) Ultrafast approximation for phylogenetic bootstrap. Mol Biol Evol 30:1188–1195

198. Felsenstein J, Felenstein J (2004) Inferring phylogenies, vol 2. Sinauer Associates, Sunderland

199. Farris JS, Albert VA, Källersjö M, Lipscomb D, Kluge AG (1996) Parsimony jackknifing outperforms neighbor-joining. Cladistics 12(2):99–124

200. Yang Y, Smith SA (2014) Orthology inference in nonmodel organisms using transcriptomes and low-coverage genomes: improving accuracy and matrix occupancy for phylogenomics. Mol Biol Evol 31(11):3081–3092

201. Chaudhary R, Fernández-Baca D, Burleigh JG (2014) Mulrf: a software package for phylogenetic analysis using multi-copy gene trees. Bioinformatics 31:432–433

202. Anisimova M, Gascuel O (2006) Approximate likelihood-ratio test for branches: A fast, accurate, and powerful alternative. Syst Biol 55(4):539–552

203. Shimodaira H, Hasegawa M (1999) Multiple comparisons of log-likelihoods with applications to phylogenetic inference. Mol Biol Evol 16:1114–1116

204. Anisimova M, Gil M, Dufayard J-F, Dessimoz C, Gascuel O (2011) Survey of branch support methods demonstrates accuracy, power, and robustness of fast likelihood-based approximation schemes. Syst Biol 60:681–699

205. Salichos L, Stamatakis A, Rokas A (2014) Novel information theory-based measures for quantifying incongruence among phylogenetic trees. Mol Biol Evol 31:1261–1271

206. Kobert K, Salichos L, Rokas A, Stamatakis A (2016) Computing the internode certainty and related measures from partial gene trees. Mol Biol Evol 33:1606–1617

207. Bremer K et al. (1994) Branch support and tree stability. Cladistics 10(3):295–304

208. Wilkinson M, Thorley JL, Upchurch P (2000) A chain is no stronger than its weakest link: double decay analysis of phylogenetic hypotheses. Syst Biol 49(4):754–776

209. Thorley JL, Page RDM (2000) RadCon: phylogenetic tree comparison and consensus. Bioinformatics 16(5):486–487

210. Geisler JH, McGowen MR, Yang G, Gatesy J (2011) A supermatrix analysis of genomic, morphological, and paleontological data from crown cetacea. BMC Evol Biol 11(1):112

211. Hillis DM, Bull JJ (1993) An empirical test of bootstrapping as a method for assessing confidence in phylogenetic analysis. Syst Biol 42(2):182–192

212. Scannell DR, Byrne KP, Gordon JL, Wong S, Wolfe KH (2006) Multiple rounds of speciation associated with reciprocal gene loss in polyploid yeasts. Nature 440(7082):341–345

213. Robinson DF, Foulds LR (1981) Comparison of phylogenetic trees. Math Biosci 53 (1-2):131–147

214. Williams WT, Clifford HT (1971) On the comparison of two classifications of the same set of elements. Taxon 519–522

215. Billera LJ, Holmes SP, Vogtmann K (2001) Geometry of the space of phylogenetic trees. Adv Appl Math 27(4):733–767

216. Owen M, Provan JS (2011) A fast algorithm for computing geodesic distances in tree space. IEEE/ACM Trans Comput Biol Bioinf 8(1):2–13

217. Amenta N, Godwin M, Postarnakevich N, John KS (2007) Approximating geodesic tree distance. Information Processing Letters 103(2):61–65

218. Estabrook GF, McMorris FR, Meacham CA (1985) Comparison of undirected phylogenetic trees based on subtrees of four evolutionary units. Syst Biol 34(2):193–200

219. Critchlow DE, Pearl DK, Qian C (1996) The triples distance for rooted bifurcating phylogenetic trees. Syst Biol 45(3):323–334

220. Gordon AD (1983) On the assessment and comparison of classifications. University of St. Andrews. Department of Statistics

221. Kuhner MK, Yamato J (2015) Practical performance of tree comparison metrics. Syst Biol 64(2):205–214

222. Gori K, Suchan T, Alvarez N, Goldman N, Dessimoz C (2016) Clustering genes of common evolutionary history. Mol Biol Evol 33:1590–1605

223. Templeton AR (1983) Phylogenetic inference from restriction endonuclease cleavage site maps with particular reference to the evolution of humans and the apes. Evolution 37:221–244

224. Kishino H, Hasegawa M (1989) Evaluation of the maximum likelihood estimate of the evolutionary tree topologies from dna sequence data, and the branching order in hominoidea. J Mol Evol 29(2):170–179

225. Susko E (2014) Tests for two trees using likelihood methods. Mol Biol Evol 31:1029–1039

226. Karin EL, Susko E, Pupko T (2014) Alignment errors strongly impact likelihood-based

tests for comparing topologies. Mol Biol Evol 31(11):3057–3067

227. Buckley TR (2002) Model misspecification and probabilistic tests of topology: evidence from empirical data sets. Syst Biol 51 (3):509–523

228. Shimodaira H (2002) An approximately unbiased test of phylogenetic tree selection. Syst Biol 51(3):492–508

229. Goldman N, Anderson JP, Rodrigo AG (2000) Likelihood-based tests of topologies in phylogenetics. Syst Biol 49(4):652–670

230. Strimmer K, Rambaut A (2002) Inferring confidence sets of possibly misspecified gene trees. Proc R Soc Lond B Biol Sci 269 (1487):137–142

231. Shimodaira H, Hasegawa M (2001) Consel: for assessing the confidence of phylogenetic tree selection. Bioinformatics 17 (12):1246–1247

232. Church SH, Ryan JF, Dunn CW (2015) Automation and evaluation of the SOWH test with SOWHAT. Syst Biol 64 (6):1048–1058

233. Madison WP (1997) Gene trees in species trees. Syst Biol 46(3):523–536

234. Nakhleh L (2013) Computational approaches to species phylogeny inference and gene tree reconciliation. Trends Ecol Evol 28 (12):719–728

235. Szöllősi GJ, Tannier E, Daubin V, Boussau B (2014) The inference of gene trees with species trees. Syst Biol 64:e42–e62

236. Degnan JH, Rosenberg NA (2009) Gene tree discordance, phylogenetic inference and the multispecies coalescent. Trends Ecol Evol 24 (6):332–340

237. Rannala B, Yang Z (2003) Bayes estimation of species divergence times and ancestral population sizes using DNA sequences from multiple loci. Genetics 164(4):1645–1656

238. Arnold ML (1997) Natural hybridization and evolution. Oxford University Press, Oxford

239. Mallet J (2007) Hybrid speciation. Nature 446(7133):279

240. Lewis-Rogers N, Crandall KA, Posada D (2004) Evolutionary analyses of genetic recombination. Dyn Genet 408:49–78

241. Riley SPD, Shaffer HB, Voss SR, Fitzpatrick BM (2003) Hybridization between a rare, native tiger salamander (ambystoma californiense) and its introduced congener. Ecol. Appl.13(5):1263–1275

242. Sheppard SK, Didelot X, Jolley KA, Darling AE, Pascoe B, Meric G, Kelly DJ, Cody A, Colles FM, Strachan NJC et al (2013) Progressive genome-wide introgression in agricultural campylobacter coli. Mol Ecol 22 (4):1051–1064

243. Storfer A, Mech SG, Reudink MW, Ziemba RE, Warren J, Collins JP, Wood RM (2004) Evidence for introgression in the endangered sonora tiger salamander, ambystoma tigrinum stebbinsi (lowe). Copeia 2004(4):783–796

244. Goloboff PA, Catalano SA, Mirande JM, Szumik CA, Arias JS, Källersjö M, Farris JS (2009) Phylogenetic analysis of 73 060 taxa corroborates major eukaryotic groups. Cladistics 25(3):211–230

245. Sullivan GM, Feinn R (2012) Using effect size—or why the p value is not enough. J Grad Med Educ 4(3):279–282

246. Rokas A, Carroll SB (2006) Bushes in the tree of life. PLoS Biol 4(11):e352

247. Phillips MJ, Delsuc F, Penny D (2004) Genome-scale phylogeny and the detection of systematic biases. Mol Biol Evol 21 (7):1455–1458

248. Gatesy J, O'Grady P, Baker RH (1999) Corroboration among data sets in simultaneous analysis: hidden support for phylogenetic relationships among higher level artiodactyl taxa. Cladistics 15(3):271–313

249. Mirarab S, Reaz R, Bayzid MS, Zimmermann T, Swenson MS, Warnow T (2014) Astral: genome-scale coalescent-based species tree estimation. Bioinformatics 30(17):i541–i548

250. Degnan JH, Rosenberg NA (2006) Discordance of species trees with their most likely gene trees. PLoS Genet 2(5):e68

251. Warnow T (2011) Concatenation analyses in the presence of incomplete lineage sorting. PLoS Currents 7

252. Baum BR (1992) Combining trees as a way of combining data sets for phylogenetic inference, and the desirability of combining gene trees. Taxon 3–10

253. Ragan MA (1992) Phylogenetic inference based on matrix representation of trees. Mol Phylogenet Evol 1(1):53–58

254. Beck RMD, Bininda-Emonds ORP, Cardillo M, Liu F-GR, Purvis A (2006) A higher-level mrp supertree of placental mammals. BMC Evol Biol 6(1):93

255. Kupczok A, Schmidt HA, von Haeseler A (2010) Accuracy of phylogeny reconstruction methods combining overlapping gene data sets. Algorithms Mol Biol 5(1):37

256. Swenson MS, Suri R, Linder CR, Warnow T (2011) An experimental study of quartets maxcut and other supertree methods. Algorithms Mol. Biol. 6(1):7

257. Swenson MS, Suri R, Linder CR, Warnow T (2012) Superfine: fast and accurate supertree estimation. Syst Biol 61(2):214–227

258. Nguyen N, Mirarab S, Warnow T (2012) MRL and SuperFine+ MRL: new supertree methods. Algorithms for Molecular Biology 7 (1):3

259. Creevey CJ, McInerney JO (2005) Clann: investigating phylogenetic information through supertree analyses. Bioinformatics 21(3):390–392

260. Scornavacca C, Berry V, Lefort V, Douzery EJP, Ranwez V (2008) Physic_ist: cleaning source trees to infer more informative supertrees. BMC Bioinf 9(1):413

261. Binet M, Gascuel O, Scornavacca C, Douzery EJP, Pardi F (2016) Fast and accurate branch lengths estimation for phylogenomic trees. BMC Bioinf 17(1):23

262. Vachaspati P, Warnow T (2016) FastRFs: fast and accurate Robinson-Foulds supertrees using constrained exact optimization. Bioinformatics 33:631–639

263. Edwards SV, Xi Z, Janke A, Faircloth BC, McCormack JE, Glenn TC, Zhong B, Wu S, Lemmon EM, Lemmon AR et al (2016) Implementing and testing the multispecies coalescent model: a valuable paradigm for phylogenomics. Mol Phylogenet Evol 94:447–462

264. Bayzid SM, Warnow T (2012) Estimating optimal species trees from incomplete gene trees under deep coalescence. J Comput Biol 19(6):591–605

265. Davis KE, Page RD (2014) Reweaving the tapestry: a supertree of birds. PLoS Curr 6. https://doi.org/10.1371/currents.tol.c1af68dda7c999ed9f1e4b2d2df7a08e

266. Chaudhary R, Bansal MS, Wehe A, Fernández-Baca D, Eulenstein O (2010) iGTP: a software package for large-scale gene tree parsimony analysis. BMC Bioinf 11(1):574

267. Yu Y, Dong J, Liu KJ, Nakhleh L (2014) Maximum likelihood inference of reticulate evolutionary histories. Proc Natl Acad Sci 111(46):16448–16453

268. Bouckaert R, Heled J, Kühnert D, Vaughan T, Wu C-H, Xie D, Suchard MA, Rambaut A, Drummond AJ (2014) Beast 2: a software platform for Bayesian evolutionary analysis. PLoS Comput Biol 10(4):e1003537

269. Edwards SV, Liu L, Pearl DK (2007) High-resolution species trees without concatenation. Proc Natl Acad Sci 104(14):5936–5941

270. Mossel E, Roch S (2010) Incomplete lineage sorting: consistent phylogeny estimation from multiple loci. IEEE/ACM Trans Comput Biol Bioinf 7(1):166–171

271. Liu L, Yu L, Pearl DK, Edwards SV (2009) Estimating species phylogenies using coalescence times among sequences. Syst Biol 58 (5):468–477

272. Liu L, Yu L, Kubatko L, Pearl DK, Edwards SV (2009) Coalescent methods for estimating phylogenetic trees. Mol Phylogenet Evol 53 (1):320–328

273. Kubatko LS, Carstens BC, Knowles LL (2009) Stem: species tree estimation using maximum likelihood for gene trees under coalescence. Bioinformatics 25(7):971–973

274. Ané C, Larget B, Baum DA, Smith SD, Rokas A (2007) Bayesian estimation of concordance among gene trees. Mol Biol Evol 24 (2):412–426

275. Larget BR, Kotha SK, Dewey CN, Ané C (2010) Bucky: gene tree/species tree reconciliation with Bayesian concordance analysis. Bioinformatics 26(22):2910–2911

276. Liu L, Yu L, Edwards SV (2010) A maximum pseudo-likelihood approach for estimating species trees under the coalescent model. BMC Evol Biol 10(1):302

277. Mirarab S, Warnow T (2015) ASTRAL-II: coalescent-based species tree estimation with many hundreds of taxa and thousands of genes. Bioinformatics 31(12):i44–i52

278. Vachaspati P, Warnow T (2015) Astrid: accurate species trees from internode distances. BMC Genomics 16(10):S3

279. Zimmermann T, Mirarab S, Warnow T (2014) Bbca: improving the scalability of* beast using random binning. BMC Genomics 15(6):S11

280. Bryant D, Bouckaert R, Felsenstein J, Rosenberg NA, RoyChoudhury A (2012) Inferring species trees directly from biallelic genetic markers: bypassing gene trees in a full coalescent analysis. Mol Biol Evol 29 (8):1917–1932

281. Chifman J, Kubatko L (2014) Quartet inference from SNP data under the coalescent model. Bioinformatics 30(23):3317–3324

282. Chifman J, Kubatko L (2015) Identifiability of the unrooted species tree topology under the coalescent model with time-reversible substitution processes, site-specific rate variation, and invariable sites. J Theor Biol 374:35–47

283. Degnan JH, DeGiorgio M, Bryant D, Rosenberg NA (2009) Properties of consensus methods for inferring species trees from gene trees. Syst Biol 58(1):35–54

284. Allman ES, Degnan JH, Rhodes JA (2011) Identifying the rooted species tree from the distribution of unrooted gene trees under the coalescent. Journal of mathematical biology 62(6):833–862

285. Lefort V, Desper R, Gascuel O (2015) FastME 2.0: a comprehensive, accurate and fast distance-based phylogeny inference program. Mol Biol Evol 32(10):2798–2800

286. Springer MS, Gatesy J (2016) The gene tree delusion. Mol Phylogenet Evol 94:1–33

287. Bayzid MS, Mirarab S, Warnow TJ (2013) Inferring optimal species trees under gene duplication and loss. In: Pacific symposium on biocomputing, vol 18, pp 250–261

288. Boussau B, Szöllősi GJ, Duret L, Gouy M, Tannier E, Daubin V (2013) Genome-scale coestimation of species and gene trees. Genome Res 23(2):323–330

289. Lang JM, Darling AE, Eisen JA (2013) Phylogeny of bacterial and archaeal genomes using conserved genes: supertrees and supermatrices. PloS One 8(4):e62510

290. Pride DT, Meinersmann RJ, Wassenaar TM, Blaser MJ (2003) Evolutionary implications of microbial genome tetranucleotide frequency biases. Genome Res 13(2):145–158

291. Davidson R, Vachaspati P, Mirarab S, Warnow T (2015) Phylogenomic species tree estimation in the presence of incomplete lineage sorting and horizontal gene transfer. BMC Genomics 16(10):S1

292. Tonini J, Moore A, Stern D, Shcheglovitova M, Ortí G (2015) Concatenation and species tree methods exhibit statistically indistinguishable accuracy under a range of simulated conditions. PLOS Curr Tree Life

293. Daubin V, Gouy M, Perriere G (2002) A phylogenomic approach to bacterial phylogeny: evidence of a core of genes sharing a common history. Genome Res 12(7):1080–1090

294. Bevan RB, Lang BF, Bryant D (2005) Calculating the evolutionary rates of different genes: a fast, accurate estimator with applications to maximum likelihood phylogenetic analysis. Syst Biol 54(6):900–915

295. Manthey JD, Campillo LC, Burns KJ, Moyle RG (2016) Comparison of target-capture and restriction-site associated dna sequencing for phylogenomics: a test in cardinalid tanagers (aves, genus: Piranga). Syst Biol 65:640–650

296. de Vienne DM, Ollier S, Aguileta G (2012) Phylo-MCOA: a fast and efficient method to detect outlier genes and species in phylogenomics using multiple co-inertia analysis. Mol Biol Evol 29(6):1587–1598

297. Mirarab S, Bayzid MS, Boussau B, Warnow T (2014) Statistical binning improves species tree estimation in the presence of gene tree incongruence. Science 346:1250463

298. Bayzid MS, Mirarab S, Boussau B, Warnow T (2015) Weighted statistical binning: enabling statistically consistent genome-scale phylogenetic analyses. PLoS One 10(6):e0129183

299. Narechania A, Baker RH, Sit R, Kolokotronis S-O, DeSalle R, Planet PJ (2012) Random addition concatenation analysis: a novel approach to the exploration of phylogenomic signal reveals strong agreement between core and shell genomic partitions in the cyanobacteria. Genome Biol Evol 4(1):30–43

300. Edwards SV (2016) Phylogenomic subsampling: a brief review. Zool Scr 45(S1):63–74

301. Simmons MP, Sloan DB, Gatesy J (2016) The effects of subsampling gene trees on coalescent methods applied to ancient divergences. Mol Phylogenet Evol 97:76–89

302. Strimmer K, Von Haeseler A (1997) Likelihood-mapping: a simple method to visualize phylogenetic content of a sequence alignment. Proc Natl Acad Sci 94(13):6815–6819

303. Dell'Ampio E, Meusemann K, Szucsich NU, Peters RS, Meyer B, Borner J, Petersen M, Aberer AJ, Stamatakis A, Walzl MG et al (2014) Decisive data sets in phylogenomics: lessons from studies on the phylogenetic relationships of primarily wingless insects. Mol Biol Evol 31(1):239–249

304. Arcila D, Ortí G, Vari R, Armbruster JW, Stiassny MLJ, Ko KD, Sabaj MH, Lundberg J, Revell LJ, Betancur-R R (2017) Genome-wide interrogation advances resolution of recalcitrant groups in the tree of life. Nat Ecol Evol 1:0020

305. Huson DH, Bryant D (2006) Application of phylogenetic networks in evolutionary studies. Mol Biol Evol 23(2):254–267

306. Bryant D, Moulton V (2004) Neighbor-net: an agglomerative method for the construction of phylogenetic networks. Mol Biol Evol 21(2):255–265

307. Boc A, Makarenkov V et al (2012) T-rex: a web server for inferring, validating and visualizing phylogenetic trees and networks. Nucleic Acids Res 40(W1):W573–W579

308. Legendre P, Makarenkov V (2002) Reconstruction of biogeographic and evolutionary networks using reticulograms. Syst Biol 51(2):199–216

309. Solís-Lemus C, Ané C (2016) Inferring phylogenetic networks with maximum

pseudolikelihood under incomplete lineage sorting. PLoS Genet 12(3):e1005896

310. Hejase HA, Liu KJ (2016) A scalability study of phylogenetic network inference methods using empirical datasets and simulations involving a single reticulation. BMC Bioinf 17(1):422

311. Didelot X, Falush D (2007) Inference of bacterial microevolution using multilocus sequence data. Genetics 175(3):1251–1266

312. Didelot X, Lawson D, Darling A, Falush D (2010) Inference of homologous recombination in bacteria using whole-genome sequences. Genetics 186(4):1435–1449

313. Wollenberg MS, Ruby EG (2012) Phylogeny and fitness of Vibrio fischeri from the light organs of euprymna scolopes in two Oahu, Hawaii populations. ISME J 6(2):352–362

314. Suh A (2016) The phylogenomic forest of bird trees contains a hard polytomy at the root of neoaves. Zool Scr 45(S1):50–62

315. Contreras-Moreira   B,   Vinuesa P. Get_homologues, a versatile software package for scalable and robust microbial pan-genome analysis. Appl Environ Microbiol 79 (24):7696–7701 (2013)

316. Li L, Stoeckert CJ, Roos DS (2003) Orthomcl: identification of ortholog groups for eukaryotic genomes. Genome Res 13 (9):2178–2189

317. Penn O, Privman E, Landan G, Graur D, Pupko T (2010) An alignment confidence score capturing robustness to guide tree uncertainty. Mol Biol Evol 27(8):1759–1767

318. Gupta RS (1998) Protein phylogenies and signature sequences: a reappraisal of evolutionary relationships among archaebacteria, eubacteria, and eukaryotes. Microbiol Mol Biol Rev 62(4):1435–1491

319. Ajawatanawong P, Baldauf SL (2013) Evolution of protein indels in plants, animals and fungi. BMC Evol Biol 13(1):1

320. Rodriguez-R LM, Grajales A, Arrieta-Ortiz ML, Salazar C, Restrepo S, Bernal A (2012) Genomes-based phylogeny of the genus Xanthomonas. BMC Microbiol 12(1):1

Chapter 6

Comparative Genome Annotation

Stefanie König, Lars Romoth, and Mario Stanke

Abstract

Newly sequenced genomes are being added to the tree of life at an unprecedented fast pace. Increasingly, such new genomes are phylogenetically close to previously sequenced and annotated genomes. In other cases, whole clades of closely related species or strains ought to be annotated simultaneously. Often, in subsequent studies *differences* between the closely related species or strains are in the focus of research when the shared gene structures prevail. We here review methods for comparative structural genome annotation. The reviewed methods include classical approaches such as the alignment of protein sequences or protein profiles against the genome and comparative gene prediction methods that exploit a genome alignment to annotate a target genome. Newer approaches such as the simultaneous annotation of multiple genomes are also reviewed. We discuss how the methods depend on the phylogenetic placement of genomes, give advice on the choice of methods, and examine the consistency between gene structure annotations in an example. Further, we provide practical advice on genome annotation in general.

Key words Gene prediction, Multi-genome alignment, Clade annotation, Annotation consistency, Annotation mapping

1 Introduction

In this chapter we will mainly discuss methods for *structural* eukaryotic genome annotation of protein-coding genes, here *genome annotation* for short, and will briefly mention some practical considerations for *functional* genome annotation in Subheading 7. Genome annotation in general encompasses the identification of the location and the structure of all genes, including the untranslated regions (UTRs) and multiple transcripts or protein isoforms for an alternatively spliced gene. However, some of the methods discussed, in particular methods that exploit homology through protein sequence similarity, may predict the coding sequence of genes only, and do that only for a subset of genes with close enough homology to existing annotated species. We will therefore also discuss non-comparative, RNA-Seq based methods in Subheading 2. Genes that are neither expressed in the RNA-Seq samples nor show sufficient similarity to previously

João C. Setubal et al. (eds.), *Comparative Genomics: Methods and Protocols*, Methods in Molecular Biology, vol. 1704, https://doi.org/10.1007/978-1-4939-7463-4_6, © Springer Science+Business Media LLC 2018

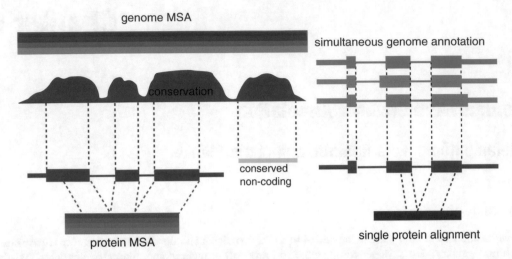

genome MSA

simultaneous genome annotation

conservation

conserved
non-coding

protein MSA

single protein alignment

Fig. 1 Overview of approaches for comparative gene prediction. Spliced alignments of proteins (bottom right) or protein families (multiple sequence alignment (MSA) on bottom left) provide evidence for splicing and translation and are discussed in Subheading 3. Note that in above sketch parts of the protein(s) and the coding regions remain unaligned, as typical in a setting with only remote homology. A multiple alignment of genomes can either be used to predict genes in a single target genome, mostly through exploiting conservation information (top left, *see* Subheading 4) or to predict genes in several aligned genomes exploiting also conservation of intron positions (top right, *see* Subheading 5)

annotated homologs need to be predicted with ab initio or de novo methods that use a statistical model of genes only. As the species- or clade-specific statistical models of ab initio gene predictors are also used by many homology-based methods, we briefly discuss parameter estimation in Subheading 6. Figure 1 gives an overview of types of approaches for comparative gene prediction and states in which Subheadings the actual methods and programs will be discussed. We will here only report on eukaryotic genome annotation methods. However, also in the structural genome annotation of bacterial strains "many inconsistencies in annotated gene structures" have been reported [1]. These "inconsistencies may indicate errors in the annotated gene structures" [1], thus, comparative approaches may improve prokaryotic gene prediction, too.

Accurate genome annotation is important because further downstream analysis may fail or itself deliver a low quality when the structural annotation has low quality. An example of downstream analysis is the study of protein family evolution, such as the orthologous groups stored in OrthoDB [2] or as displayed in the EnsemblCompara GeneTrees [3]. Another example—one where the number of failed experiments is directly related to errors in the annotation—is a large-scale RNA interference (RNAi) screen to study the function of genes via their knockdown using double-stranded RNA constructed from the predicted transcripts [4]. An example of downstream applications from structural bioinformatics is coevolutionary analysis to predict contacts between residues, e.g. in a protein complex. This requires phylogenetically deep alignments of orthologous proteins [5]. Another ongoing development is the batch sequencing and assembly of closely related genomes, for example subsets of the i5k initiative to sequence 5000 arthropod genomes, the Genome 10K project to sequence and annotate 10,000 vertebrate genomes and the Bird 10K project to sequence about 10,500 bird genomes and to study the links between genotypes and phenotype [6]. For such clade sequencing or annotation projects the challenge is the accurate and efficient annotation of large numbers of genomes of species that are closely enough related to exploit homology through genome alignments. In some cases different strains from the same species are sequenced, such as in ongoing projects to sequence and de novo assemble 20 new mouse strains and species. We here explicitly do not refer to resequencing projects that are followed only by variation-calling on a reference genome. In clade sequencing projects, often one or a few species or genomes are already relatively well annotated and for many of the (other) species RNA-Seq data is available. In Subheading 5 methods for multi-genome annotation will be presented.

Some of the below described methods assume that repeat families have been identified, e.g. using RepeatModeler [7], and that the occurrences of repeats have been masked in the genome. Softmasking (lower case masking) is preferable for some programs such as AUGUSTUS (option `--softmasking=on`) and the genome aligner CACTUS [8], so they have the option to consider repeat regions.

2 Noncomparative Approaches

In this section we briefly summarize annotation approaches that consider a single target genome only and that do not make use of homology information. Such noncomparative approaches constitute a general alternative to comparative approaches as they do not depend on the phylogenetic proximity of the species to other sequenced species. Further, these methods can in principle be complemented or combined with the comparative methods described below.

Nearly always, current genome sequencing projects are accompanied by RNA-Seq transcriptome sequencing. We briefly describe here the three major types of approaches for RNA-Seq based gene finding. All approaches require the spliced alignment of transcript sequences—either single reads or assemblies thereof—to a genome of the same or closely related species. Suitable tools for the spliced alignment of RNA-Seq reads are, for example, STAR [9], GSNAP [10], and TopHat2 [11].

1. Reference-genome assisted transcriptome assemblers like StringTie [12], Cufflinks [13] and MITIE [14] construct from the read alignments a set of transcripts for each locus but do not directly predict whether they encode a protein. This can be done in an additional step, e.g. using TransDecoder (Brian Haas, http://transdecoder.github.io).

2. Transcripts and transcript fragments can first be assembled de novo, i.e. without using the genome as a reference, e.g. using Oases [15] or Trinity [16] and then be aligned against the genome to infer the likely gene structures.

3. Several gene prediction programs can integrate evidence from RNA-Seq alignments (raw or assembled) such as AUGUSTUS [17], Fgenesh++ [18], and MGENE [19]. These programs specifically search for protein-coding genes and can provide the option to consider additional evidence such as from homology simultaneously.

In 2013, results of the RNA-Seq Genome Annotation Assessment Project (RGASP) were published [20], independently assessing results of 14 transcriptome reconstruction and gene prediction methods. The submissions included examples of the three types of approaches above, on human, *Drosophila melanogaster* and *Caenorhabditis elegans* and were submitted by the tool authors themselves in 2010. RGASP was open to submissions from the field of de novo transcript reconstruction and methods that infer transcript structures from read alignments to the genome; six of the participating tools predicted coding sequences in the transcripts (e.g. AUGUSTUS [17], MGENE [19, 21], Transomics [22]), the others, e.g. Cufflinks [13], did not. On *D. melanogaster*, the best performing tools for protein-coding gene prediction were AUGUSTUS (48.53%/44.03%), Transomics (46.95%/33.54%), and MGENE (43.99%/44.02%), all of the third type. These numbers refer to sensitivity and precision (often called "specificity" in publications about gene finding) on the gene level. For example, for 48.53% of the genes in the FlyBase reference gene set, AUGUSTUS predicted at least one of its protein isoforms exactly, i.e. without any errors. A more stringent evaluation criterion is the percentage of the reference protein isoforms that were predicted correctly, including all reference alternative transcripts. Here, the maximum achieved value was only about 24% on *Drosophila* and about 20% on human (achieved by AUGUSTUS and exonerate [23], respectively). In his comment, Korf calls the RGASP results "a little depressing" because of the disappointingly low accuracy [24] and concludes that the methods that contain a model of gene structure (AUGUSTUS, MGENE, Transomics) perform better because they know what genes are supposed to look like.

The application of single molecule real time sequencing [25], that allows sequencing of whole or near-whole transcripts, is on the rise (e.g., [26]). Improvements in annotation quality are to be expected from such improvements of sequencing technology, of alignment programs and of transcriptome reconstruction tools. However, still many open challenges in the utilization of this data remain and in any case, genes with insufficient expression in the RNA-Seq samples need to be identified with other approaches. Further, when independently annotating orthologous alternatively spliced genes in multiple even closely related species based on RNA-Seq, one is likely to obtain differing sets of transcripts, even for many genes that are sufficiently expressed. This can merely be expected from the random nature of RNA-Seq, that is due to the fact that it constitutes a sample and due to expression differences between species, differences between individuals of the same species and possibly differing conditions, tissues or even sequencing methods. Further, the total number of transcripts in a genome annotation is currently influenced by the amount of data and manual annotation efforts, if any. For example, the average number of transcripts per gene in the GENCODE annotation is 4.0 in human, 2.3 in mouse, and of the Ensembl annotation 1.3 in rat, 1.06 in chicken, and 1.04 in cat. When performing detailed comparative genomics studies on gene structure differences between genomes, artifactual differences create problems and can be addressed by comparative prediction methods as presented in Subheading 5 and by methods exploiting protein sequence similarity as presented in the next Subheading.

3 Protein Homology

In this Subheading we describe approaches that use a database of gene sequences, usually protein sequences but sometimes transcript sequences, to predict genes in a target genome, based on the assumption that sequence similarity of a region to a known gene very often implies that the region encodes for a homolog of the protein.

The core algorithm of protein spliced alignment methods uses as input either a single protein sequence (e.g., GenomeThreader [27], exonerate [23], Spaln [28], ProSplign [29], GeneSeqer [30]) or a representation of a protein family obtained from a multiple alignment of proteins (GeneWise [31], AUGUSTUS-PPX [32]). Using a whole and diverse protein family as input has the advantage that additional information about conserved domains can be used. The conservation of intron positions is not exploited by above methods. However, recently, Keilwagen et al. [33] presented the method GeMoMa that uses a single source gene sequence and splits it into its exons (in the source genome).

GeMoMa then TBLASTNs it against the target genome and assembles a gene structure from the matches with dynamic programming. The authors show that their approach is better than the variant of GeMoMa in which the source protein is not split by its introns and argue that "exploiting intron position conservation improves homology-based gene prediction" [33].

As can be expected, the accuracy of homology-based gene finding decreases with the distance of the input proteins from the target protein, whose structure is sought. The decrease is faster for methods that rely mostly on the alignment (exonerate, Genome-Threader) than for methods that use statistical models on gene structures, such as ab initio gene finders [28, 32]. In Fig. 2 we compare several homology-based gene finders and vary the input genes. As accuracy measure we here use the harmonic mean (F1 score) of the exon-level sensitivity (=recall) and specificity (=precision). In particular, exonerate and the newer Genome-Threader, that is based on enhanced suffix arrays and was about 77 times faster in our experiments than exonerate, lose accuracy when the query species have increasing distance to the target genome of *D. melanogaster* (dmel). Both spliced aligners were run with default settings. However, as exonerate had by default a very low specificity, we imposed minimum thresholds on the score (400) and the percent identity (70% for *Drosophilas* and 60% for the house fly) for transcripts predicted by exonerate. These thresholds were chosen to achieve a high exon F1 score. With increasing distance to *D. melanogaster*, it is mainly the sensitivity that decreases rapidly. For example, the nucleotide sensitivity of GenomeThreader is only 20% when mapping the housefly proteins to the genome of the fruit fly *D. melanogaster*. Remarkably, both spliced alignment programs perform worse when given the proteins from four more distant species in addition to *D. ananassae* (experiment dana + · · · + dgri), showing that multiple sources can interfere unfavorably and that choosing a target-specific subset of a given protein set improves the accuracy. Even though AUGUSTUS, when using the predictions of GenomeThreader as hints (blue curve in Fig. 2), is much more accurate than the spliced aligner itself, the accuracy gain over a simple ab initio prediction (dashed line) is low in remote homology settings.

For the example from Fig. 2 with *D. melanogaster* as hypothetical target genome we compared (1) the genetic distance implied by the phylogenetic tree constructed from genomic alignments to (2) the percent identity of protein sequence alignments of closest homologs. Genomic alignments with substantial aligned portions of the genomes are only available for genomes at a closer distance. We here only aligned the genomes from the *Drosophila* clade using the CACTUS aligner [8] and did not include the genome of the house fly. The furthest genomes of *D. virilis* (dvir) and *D. grimshawi* (dgri) are already separated from the genome of *D. melanogaster*

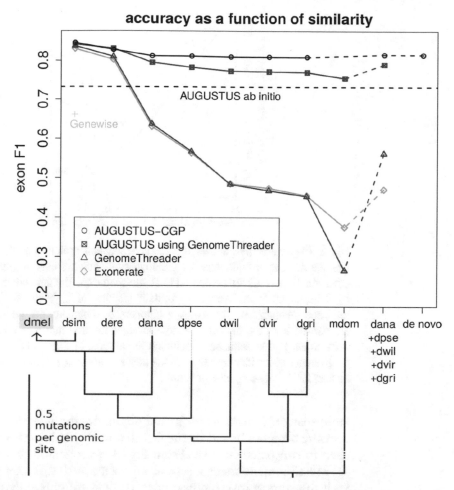

Fig. 2 Whole genome exon accuracy of homology based gene finding methods are shown on the target genome of *D. melanogaster* (dmel highlighted in yellow). Source protein sets from nine reference annotations were used as informants (sorted by phylogenetic distance to dmel on the horizontal axis). The closest seven source species are also from the *Drosophila* clade (dsim to dgri). The house fly *Musca domestica* (mdom) was used as a close outgroup. The second from right data points refer to the use of five source protein sets together (dana to dgri). AUGUSTUS-CGP (black curve at the top) refers to a method that additionally uses an alignment of 12 *Drosophila* genomes and is described below in Subheading 5. For the rightmost data point (de novo) only this genome alignment was used

by a little more than one average mutation per genomic site. In order to provide a reference point when transferring these results to other clades we compared for each genome these two distance measures in Fig. 3. The genetic distance on the horizontal axis is—in the theory of the phylogenetic model and under the molecular clock hypothesis—proportional to time, while the protein identity decreases nonlinear with divergence time as multiple mutations of the same amino acid do not decrease the identity more than a single mutation. When the distance between genomes becomes so

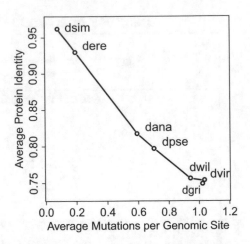

Fig. 3 The scatter plot shows the relation between protein identity and the average number of mutations per genomic site when proteins or genomes of other fruit fly species are compared to *D. melanogaster*. The dots are connected by lines, in order of decreasing protein identity, to highlight an assumed functional relationship. The average numbers of mutations per genomic site are derived from the distances in the phylogenetic tree that was constructed from ortholog gene sequences including the introns. The protein identities are the averages of the identity values of the best `exonerate` hit for each protein against the *D. melanogaster* genome

large that only small portions are alignable, the genetic distance measure becomes biased by the fact that unalignable parts were not used to construct the tree. From Fig. 3 we conclude that protein spliced alignment methods have an accuracy that is competitive with the comparative method AUGUSTUS-PPX roughly only below a distance of about 20% on the genome level or above 93% protein identity. If the source and target species are less closely related than that, the protein spliced alignment methods can still provide a good specificity: The worst nucleotide-level specificity is achieved for both spliced aligners in the experiment where all proteins of the five species are input (dana + ⋯ + dgri), yet, it is still high with about 97% for GenomeThreader and about 96% for `exonerate`. However, the rapid loss of sensitivity means that a near-comprehensive whole-genome annotation can only be achieved if also other methods are used, like RNA-Seq and gene-finders described in the next two sections.

Another disadvantage of this simple approach is its susceptibility to errors such as the split gene error, which are not properly captured in above exon-level evaluation. If a protein is unalignable in some regions, a combined approach such as AUGUSTUS using GenomeThreader may predict two or more genes in the genomic range of a single protein. For example, with such an approach members of the dynein heavy chain (DHC) protein family, with more than 4000 amino acids and up to a hundred exons in mammals, will typically be split up in many predicted genes in a test setting with only remote homology. Therefore, the PPX extension to AUGUSTUS was developed [32]. Here, the usually two-dimensional dynamic programming table of the Viterbi algorithm is replaced by a three-dimensional dynamic programming algorithm so that the partial alignment of a profile of a protein-family to the genome and the search for a gene structure are done simultaneously: AUGUSTUS-PPX searches for gene-structures encoding proteins that match the query protein-family well. Thereby, a protein-family is represented by a sequence of block profiles parametrizing conserved, gapless regions of the protein multiple sequence alignment (MSA). In addition, minimum and maximum length constraints may be given for the number of amino acids between blocks, derived from the observed insertions in the given family. Inserted sequences between conserved blocks are not modeled and the structure in the corresponding genomic region is predicted with statistical and other external evidence only. With this extension, 62.5% of the DHC members in the human genome were predicted with high accuracy in a test on informant proteins with at most 60% identity to the targets. This was a significant improvement, e.g. GENEWISE finds in this demanding setting few gene structures highly accurately (6.3% highly accurate genes) [32].

Spliced aligners often require very long running times but are easy to use and flexible. They are commonly used in genome annotation pipelines such as the Ensembl genebuild pipeline (exonerate and GeneWise) or the NCBI Eukaryotic Genome Annotation Pipeline (ProSplign). However, they have a conceptual disadvantage over genome alignments, as the *query genome* is not used. Figure 4 gives an example, why genome alignments—if possible—have an advantage over protein alignments. Genome alignment programs can use the sequence context around an exon to correctly align the exon boundaries. In this example, the initial exon has a coding part with only four amino acids, which is nearly impossible to find using the query protein sequence only. The

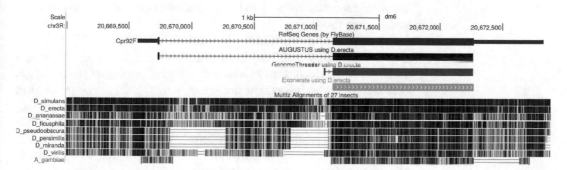

Fig. 4 An example gene of *D. melanogaster* that highlights the limits of protein spliced alignments: very short exons

genome of the source genome of *D. erecta* can however be very well aligned also in the UTR and intron surrounding this short coding sequence. As a gedankenexperiment, consider what would happen in Fig. 2 if the curves were continued on the left side and the phylogenetic distance between source and target even further decreased. In the ideal limiting case of identical source and target and an error-free and complete source annotation, the accuracy of a method based on mapping annotations along genome alignments could approach 100%. However, the accuracy of spliced aligners is limited on genes with very short protein-coding exons. In realistic settings, however, homology-based methods have to solve more difficult problems, in which the source annotation has errors, is missing transcripts and with differences in both sequence and structure.

4   Annotating a Single Target Genome Using Genome Alignments

4.1   Comparative Gene Prediction

Another homology-based approach is *single species comparative gene prediction*, which makes use of the genome sequences of closely related species rather than protein sequences and, thus, does not rely on the availability and correctness of known genes. Methods that only use raw genomes or an alignment thereof are in literature also known as de novo methods. It is good practice, however, to combine de novo methods with methods like RNA-Seq, as they provide complementary information.

Early comparative gene prediction methods such as TWIN-SCAN [34] and SLAM [35] were designed for two input genomes only (e.g., of human and mouse). As they predict genes in both genomes at the same time, they conceptually belong to the methods of the next section, but are not discussed in any further detail here, because they are rather early proofs-of-concepts and do not seem to be applied in current projects. In general they are not suitable as stand-alone tools for whole-genome annotation, as gene finding is limited to pairs of homologous sequences. TWIN-SCAN was actually used in further genome projects, e.g. for *Drosophila pseudoobscura* [36] in conjunction with other gene prediction tools.

Programs like N-SCAN [37] and CONTRAST [38] are better fitted for whole-genome annotation, albeit for a single target genome only. Both require a genome alignment between the target and two or more informant genomes, which inform the prediction in the target, e.g. through sequence conservation. In particular, CONTRAST achieved remarkable results for human (92% sensitivity and 72% specificity on exon level), when using 11 informants (mostly from the mammalian clade), and was celebrated by Brent as "breakthrough" in a review from 2008 on gene finding [39]. Despite these substantial progresses in de novo gene finding, the restriction of the gene model to a single target genome increases the general difficulty of comparative approaches to distinguish between protein-coding and conserved non-coding regions (*see* Fig. 1), as the information is lost, how well a conserved gene structure in the target also fits into a biologically meaningful gene structure in the informant genomes.

For accurate and consistent annotation of large numbers of species within a clade, programs like N-Scan and CONTRAST are less suited. In the typical clade annotation setting, transcriptome data such as RNA-Seq is available for the majority of species, while for a few species (e.g., for model organisms) trusted annotations exist. The challenge is to find practicable solutions to annotate all genomes given the combined evidence, that scale well with an increasing number of genomes in the clade. Both N-SCAN and CONTRAST can only annotate a single target genome at a time and require a target-specific training. In order to annotate several genomes within a clade, not only the prediction step, but also the training step has to be repeated for each genome. The training is computationally very expensive and can represent technical challenges for third party users. In fact, it appears that both tools are barely—if at all—used in any recent annotation projects. N-SCAN, indeed, has been used in a honey bee genome project [40], however with only two other bee species (*Apis florea* and *Bombus terrestris*) as informants.

4.2 Annotation Mapping

A special case of comparative gene prediction is the "mapping" of the sequence coordinates of exons from a source genome to a target genome via a pairwise alignment of the genomes. This is particularly useful for closely related genomes, where one can expect that many gene structures have exactly corresponding structures or structures that are very similar. The tool TRANSMAP (`pslMap` in the UCSC Genome Browser code) transitively maps the coordinates of a transcript sequence R of the source genome S to the target genome T using the alignment of S with T. In close homology settings the alignment of R with T thereby usually implies an approximate gene structure, in which small indels typically correspond to deletions and insertions of codons. When the indels are larger or some part of the query R is unmapped, the corrections that would be required to modify the alignment into a valid gene structure of T are not always trivial and are therefore best solved by a gene finder. This has been done with AUGUSTUS, whereby simultaneously native transcript evidence from genome T can be used to fill in gaps in the gene structure as implied by the transMap alignment [17]. Figure 5 shows such an example.

In practice, the pairwise alignment can be induced by a multiple alignment of many genomes, for example, when a single source annotation, e.g. from a reference genome, is mapped in turn to many new strains of the same species. The gene predictor AUGUSTUS-

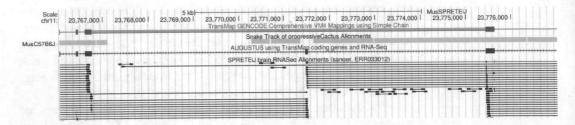

Fig. 5 Example of a transcript that is mapped from the reference mouse strain (C57B6J) as source to the wild mouse species *Mus spretus* (target). The exon in the middle of the displayed region is missed by the TRANSMAP alignment as the genome alignment (blue rectangles in the "Snake Track") misses this particular region. AUGUSTUS using TRANSMAP and RNA-Seq alignments (displayed at the bottom) fills in the missing exon but otherwise reproduces the exon suggested by TRANSMAP

CGP described in Subheading 5.1 provides an other approach for annotation mapping. It is especially useful when many genomes are the target of annotation mapping, and—in contrast to the one described here—can also find new genes.

5   Multi-Genome Annotation

Besides the protein sequence itself, the exon–intron structure of a gene can be fairly conserved through wide branches of the tree of life. For example, Csuros et al. report that introns have mostly been lost since the intron-dense most recent common ancestor of all Metazoans [41], which suggests that many of the introns occur multiple times when many genomes are compared. In particular for above-mentioned clade annotation challenges, it is natural to consider methods that simultaneously try to find the structure of orthologous genes in multiple genomes. This way, theoretically, the information which gene structures or exons are biologically possible, plausible or even supported by experimental evidence can be shared and complemented across genomes. Also, one can expect to have fewer inconsistencies between the annotations of closely related species. However, considering multiple gene structures at the same time poses algorithmic challenges, and exact and efficient solutions to the corresponding formal optimization problem—such as dynamic programming algorithms for single genomes—may not exist.

5.1   Simultaneous Gene Prediction in Multiple Genomes

Recently, two methods for the simultaneous prediction of genes in multiple genomes have been proposed. The first method is called gene-structure-aware multiple protein sequence alignment (GSA-MPSA) and was presented by Gotoh et al. [42]. As the name suggests, it is derived from a tool for multiple alignments of proteins. The locations of the introns in the protein sequences are used for scoring the multiple alignment, which is iteratively improved. For example "lonesome" introns that are not shared in other proteins are considered candidates for false positives. When a protein does not yet contain a satisfactory homologous structure, its genomic region is aligned to the profile of the protein family, incentivizing matching intron positions. In their tests, Gotoh et al. very often obtained a new set of protein sequences that are in better agreement with each other. This method, however, merely corrects inconsistencies in an initial annotation for individual protein families. It is unlikely to find exons that were originally missed in all species and is not a whole-genome annotation method.

The second method is AUGUSTUS-CGP, a comparative gene prediction version of AUGUSTUS that we recently developed [43, 44]. AUGUSTUS-CGP predicts genes simultaneously in multiple aligned genomes. It can be used both de novo using only the raw genomes and, if available, with further evidence, e.g. from RNA-Seq and existing annotations. The evidence is species-specific and can be provided for all or a subset of the genomes. With the multiple genome alignment, evidence is transferred between the species and evolutionary evidence is exploited, such as sequence conservation and selective pressure. A phylogenetic model of exon evolution rewards gene structures that are in agreement across the genomes and, thus, increases consistency among the gene sets, while at the same time allowing for true structural differences, such as the loss or gain of an exon or entire gene, which can be observed in more distantly related species. The parameters for ab initio model components only have to be trained for one species in place of the clade or, alternatively, can be reused from single-genome AUGUSTUS. The underlying optimization problem is NP-hard (manuscript in prep.), however, an approximate algorithm based on dual decomposition is presented in [43], that scales well with an increasing number of input genomes and still yields good approximative solutions.

Figure 2 shows the results of AUGUSTUS-CGP when an alignment of 12 *Drosophila* genomes is input, as well as the reference annotation of one or a few source genomes. This simulates a setting in which a few reference genomes in a clade are already annotated and others (here *D. melanogaster*) have no annotation or direct evidence. The black line in Fig. 2 shows that annotation evidence coming from close relatives of *D. melanogaster* increases the accuracy beyond what is possible with de novo predictions. Annotations of species that are further away than *D. erecta* virtually have no effect on the accuracy. However, whereas the accuracy of protein-homology based approaches rapidly decreases with distance as they entirely depend on the alignability of the proteins, the de novo model in AUGUSTUS-CGP is still effective, yielding accuracy values well beyond the ab initio prediction.

The multi-genome annotation method can be applied to any alignment—we have used the current AUGUSTUS with both

MULTIZ and PROGRESSIVE CACTUS alignments. CACTUS is not refer-ence based, i.e. it does not make the improper assumption that everything that is alignable, must also align to a reference genome. It uses efficient indexed data structures (.hal format) and algo-rithms that scale well, which is important for the ultimate goal of creating a single alignment of 10,000 vertebrate genomes [45]. The .hal-formatted alignments can conveniently be used to create a comparative assembly hub—an index structure that allows users to browse the locally hosted aligned genomes of their clade on the UCSC browser [46].

5.2 Cross-Species Consistency of Gene Sets

Inconsistent gene structure annotation within clades makes com-parative analysis very hard, in particular, when the aim of the study is to investigate the biological differences between species. For example, Hiller et al. link phenotypic traits, such as the ability of mammals to synthesize vitamin C, that were independently lost in several mammalian subclades, to genotypic changes, such as exon deletions or splice site mutations [47]. In this approach, which Hiller et al. term "forward genomics," they try to identify causal changes among the very large number of changes between gen-omes. Differences that are a result of inconsistency in annotation and annotation errors result in a loss of statistical power for approaches like the above or could be mistaken for real biological differences and therefore lead to false interpretations. For consis-tency, an important accuracy criterion is the *specificity of the pre-dicted differences*, the fraction of predicted structural differences between genes from different genomes, that are actually true. This specificity of predicted differences can actually be low, even if the overall average accuracy of the compared gene sets is high, if the compared genomes are closely related and therefore the overall number of differences is small. Comparative gene finding has the potential to produce more accurate and consistent gene structure annotations than non-comparative approaches that only consider a single genome at a time, as it can exploit homology relations within a clade.

To provide an example, we investigated the consistency between *D. melanogaster* and *D. simulans* coding (parts of) exons (CDS), once obtained by comparative gene finding and once obtained by single-species gene finding with AUGUSTUS and com-pare it with the consistency of annotated exons from FlyBase. In the comparative approach, a genome alignment of 12 *Drosophila* spe-cies is used to simultaneously annotate all 12 genomes. A *D. mel.* exon is considered consistent with *D. sim.*, if both its boundaries are aligned to a *D. sim.* exon in the same open reading frame (ORF), and vice versa. Observe that an exon can be consistent with more than one exon in another species (e.g., paralogous exons after gene duplication). Thus, the number of *D. mel.* exons consistent with

Table 1
Consistency of *D. simulans* exons with *D. melanogaster* exons obtained from single-species prediction, comparative predictions and from FlyBase

	Exons in *D. simulans*	
	Total	% consistent with *D. mel.*
Single-species	54,859	81.3%
Comparative	55,849	89.2%
FlyBase	56,627	89.4%

The *D. sim.* exons from single-species gene finding show a higher inconsistency with the *D. mel.* prediction than the ones from comparative gene finding that have a value very close to the consistency of the FlyBase exons

D. sim. may slightly differ from the number of *D. sim.* exons consistent with *D. mel.*

It is reasonable to assume that the FlyBase annotation for *D. mel.* has a more complete status than the annotation for *D. sim.* (e.g., we observe that the *D. mel.* annotation has 61,746 annotated coding exons—almost 10% more, than the *D. sim.* annotation). To avoid counting a *D. mel.* exon as inconsistent, that for example is exclusive to an alternative splice form that has not yet been annotated in *D. sim.*, we only look at the other direction, i.e. how consistent the *D. sim.* annotation is with *D. mel.*.

In the case of single-species gene finding 81. 3% of the predicted *D. simulans* exons are consistent with the *D. melanogaster* prediction, whereas in the case of comparative gene finding, 89.2% of the exons are consistent, very close to the 89.4% consistent exons of the *D. simulans* FlyBase annotation (*see* Table 1).

The exon accuracy (F1 score) of single-species predictions is below 80% for both flies (for the ab initio exon accuracy in *D. melanogaster*, see dashed line in Fig. 2). This implies that single-species predictions are more consistent than we would expect under the assumption that prediction errors are made independently in *D. melanogaster* and *D. simulans*. The reason, why errors are correlated, is due to the fact that ab initio models that are based on statistical properties of coding and non-coding sequences and therefore prone to making the same errors in similar sequences. Thus, even noncomparative single-genome methods have some tendency towards consistency, albeit it is lower than what can be achieved with comparative methods.

Furthermore, we took a closer look at inconsistencies that are related to gene prediction errors. For this purpose, we identified false positive (FP) and false negative (FN) exons in the *D. melanogaster* prediction, that are inconsistent (or likely inconsistent) with the *D. simulans* prediction. A *D. mel.* exon is considered to be inconsistent with *D. sim.*, if it is not consistent with any exon in *D. sim.*, but both its boundaries align to *D. sim.* (on the same

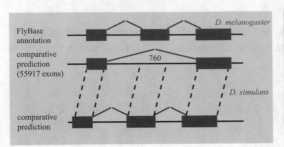 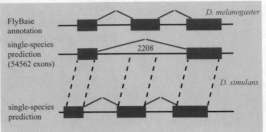

Fig. 6 False negative exons in the *D. melanogaster* prediction that are inconsistent with the *D. simulans* prediction. The single-species prediction has 2208 inconsistent FN exons, whereas the comparative prediction only has 760, thus, reducing the number of inconsistent FN exons by 65%

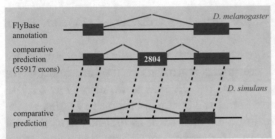 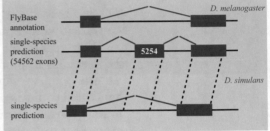

Fig. 7 False positive exons in the *D. melanogaster* prediction that are likely inconsistent with the *D. simulans* prediction. The single-species prediction has 5254 likely inconsistent and FP exons, whereas, the comparative prediction only has 2804

chromosome or scaffold), and vice versa. Note that there is a third class of exons that are not aligned to the other species. These exons are assumed to be exclusive to a species and, therefore, neither consistent nor inconsistent with the other species.

Figure 6 shows the number of FN *D. mel.* exons inconsistent with *D. sim.* in comparative gene finding (left) and in single-species gene finding (right). With approximately the same total number of exons, the single-species prediction contains 2208 inconsistent FN exons, whereas the comparative prediction only contains 760 inconsistent FN exons, thus, reducing the number of inconsistent FN exons by 65%.

Likewise Fig. 7 shows the number of inconsistent FP exons in *D. melanogaster*. Observe that, above inconsistency of FN exons is somewhat stronger, because the ORF and exon boundary signals (e.g. splice sites, start or stop codon) are present in both species. In the case of the FP exons, the aligned sequence in *D. simulans* does not necessarily represent a valid exon. Therefore, the term *likely inconsistent* is preferred to take account of the possibility for species-specific exons that are nevertheless aligned. In single-species prediction the number of likely inconsistent FP exons

(5254) is considerably larger than in comparative gene finding (2804), which again leads to a reduction of likely inconsistent FP exons by 46%.

FP and FN exons may also lead to more consequential inconsistencies, e.g. an FP exon may split a gene and an FN exon may join two genes in one species. This can, for example, result in different numbers of genes that are assigned to a gene family within the clade.

Also in applications following annotation, inconsistencies may cause problems. From the above, we have learned that FN and FP exons are correlated in close species. While phylogenetic tree reconstruction methods are robust against FN exons, FP exons could lead to wrong estimates in branch lengths and even incorrect topologies, when they are correlated in a subclade of the species.

In the above-mentioned work of Hiller, which attempts to tie genotypic differences to the loss of phenotypes, inconsistent gene structure annotation increases the overall number of genes with differences. In the unfavorable case, a unique genotype cannot be determined, as there are several candidates that could be related to the phenotype.

The same applies in opposite direction, when specifically looking at differences in gene structures of closely related species or strains with the purpose of linking them to biological differences. Gene knockdown experiments, that are carried out for both versions of the genes with the expectation of observing an altered function, will fail, if the differences are merely a result of inconsistent annotations.

6 Parameter Training

Parameters of ab initio gene finders may need to be estimated for the given target species because applying the parameters from a distance species can yield a low accuracy. The necessity to train a gene finder depends on the phylogenetic proximity to other well-annotated species or to a species with pre-trained parameters. As an example to give orientation, the exon accuracy as measured by the F1 score of ab initio AUGUSTUS on a holdout set of zebrafish genes is 75.3%, 69.6%, and 65.0%, respectively, when the parameters were trained on zebrafish itself, chicken, and human, respectively. For closely related species, such as mammals, for example, a separate training is not necessary. Also, parameters of splice pattern models of some spliced aligners such as spaln2 [28] may be adjusted to the target genome to achieve optimal performance.

Ab initio models of biological signals are required for those genes that are weakly or not at all represented in any RNA-Seq library, that have insufficient similarity to any known protein and lack other evidence [48]. In addition, ab initio components are used to identify the protein translation of a transcript with otherwise known exon–intron structure or to identify the structure of the non-conserved parts of a gene with partial homology information. Further, ab initio components can help to choose correct splicing structures in the common case that other evidence is ambiguous. The parameters of signal models such as the translation initiation site, the splice sites, the branch-point signal, polyadenylation site and promoters are estimated by training a gene-finder for a target genome. This is often done in a supervised fashion, but sometimes also unsupervised [49, 50].

The possibilities for the training depend on the availability of transcriptome data or a training set of gene structures and of the phylogenetic proximity to previously annotated genomes. One method is the prediction of the structure of a subset of universal eukaryotic proteins via the BUSCO pipeline [51]. Homolog proteins highly similar to a gene in the target genome can also serve as a source to build initial genes with Scipio [52]. Alternatively or additionally, if EST or RNA-Seq data is available, the PASA pipeline [53] and MAKER2 [54] produce training gene structures. If only the genome is available, one can still train the gene finder GeneMark-ES, whose training procedure iterates prediction and training on a predicted subset for increasingly complex models [55].

WebAugustus [56] is a web server implementation of the fully automatic autoAug pipeline of the AUGUSTUS distribution. Among others, it trains AUGUSTUS from sequence input alone (protein or transcript sequences, employing PASA or Scipio) and may also be used to predict genes genome-wide.

When RNA-Seq is available, the RNA-Seq based genome annotation pipeline BRAKER1 [50] can be used to obtain parameters for AUGUSTUS and GENEMARK. In BRAKER1 GENEMARK-ET [49] automatically trains the ab initio gene finder GeneMark from RNA-Seq [49]. A subset of the genes filtered using the RNA-Seq evidence is then used for parameter estimation of AUGUSTUS and for RNA-Seq based gene predictions. With the parameters trained automatically through the BRAKER1 pipeline, the ab initio performance of AUGUSTUS is on *A. thaliana* and on *C. elegans* not significantly worse than when AUGUSTUS is trained in a supervised fashion [50].

7   Related Tasks: Visualization, Quality Control, Noncoding Genes, Functional Annotation and Submission

7.1   *Visualization*

Tools are being developed for the challenging task of visualizing and comparing the assemblies and annotations of multiple aligned genomes. The UCSC browser offers "assembly hubs," which constitute a convenient method to browse assemblies on the web server instance in Santa Cruz (http://genome.ucsc.edu) or Bielefeld (http://genome-euro.ucsc.edu), while the data is stored on a local web server in an indexed format [57]. A recent extension "comparative assembly hubs" allows users to browse aligned genomes, where a single reference genome is selected at a time and assemblies of the other genomes are displayed alongside it as well as annotation tracks of other genomes that are mapped to the chosen reference genome via the genome alignment [46]. Another visualization tool suitable for comparative genome annotation is GBrowse_syn which is able to display up to three genomes and corresponding annotation tracks simultaneously, as well as to visualize aligned region pairs by trapezoids connecting these genome regions from different genomes [58].

7.2 Noncoding Genes

There are different classes of noncoding RNA (ncRNA) belonging to non-protein coding genes (e.g., lincRNAs, snRNAs, snoRNAs, tRNAs, and microRNAs) often with an important or even essential function [59, 60]. Just as protein-coding genes, non-protein coding genes can be spliced. The splice sites exhibit standard canonical splice site patterns and alternative splicing occurs [61]. However, ab initio detection by statistical methods is difficult due to the lack of some strong statistical signals that can be found in protein-coding genes. RNA-Seq and cDNA based methods appear to be widespread within recent research. Thereby, reconstructed transcripts that may be protein-coding, e.g. because some candidate reading frame exhibits a non-neutral ratio of synonymous to non-synonymous substitutions, are filtered out (PHYLOCSF [62]) [63].

Comparative prediction of noncoding genes was performed as early as 2001, in the case of two bacterial genomes [64]. However, this approach used a pair-HMM. Besides lacking an intron model, it is therefore restricted to two genomes. We suspect that future methods of multi-genome prediction of noncoding genes could be successful in particular in large clades of closely relates species, where enough sequence variation occurs to detect conservation of structures.

7.3 Quality Control

One way to assess the completeness of the assembly and its annotation is to check how many protein families, that have one or only a few members in most other eukaryotes, are represented in it. The benchmarking set of universal single-copy orthologs (BUSCO) of OrthoDB contains such proteins [2]. Waterhouse et al. use the protein-profile-extension of AUGUSTUS-PPX to predict members of these families in the genome and compute the percentage of orthologous groups with near full alignment to the genes predicted by AUGUSTUS-PPX, a proxy for the completeness of the assembly [51]. Similarly, the completeness of any other genome annotation can be estimated. This approach has the obvious caveat that, if homology has previously been used for the genome annotation, this is likely to be a biased evaluation. We recommend the usage of visualization tools such as JBrowse [65] or the UCSC browser to identify possible systematic issues with the annotation and to iterate the prediction accordingly.

7.4 Functional Annotation for a GenBank Submission

In the context of a submission of the genome annotation to GenBank, "functional annotation" refers to choosing a name for each protein sequence, such as "cytochrome b," for example. This can be done automatically through a homology search in a database of proteins or protein families and in the easiest case by copying the name of the best hit if its E-value is below a cutoff. Pirovano et al. have recently given some recommendation for databases, tools and for the cutoff [66]. Functional names can also be omitted, in which case the name "hypothetical protein" is typically chosen. The annotation is expected by NCBIs `tbl2asn` program to be in a particular tabular format. However, since the spring of 2016 the NCBI also allows the submission of genome annotations in the more common GFF3 format (Terrence Murphy, personal communication). Pirovano et al. recommend to submit the genome assembly to GenBank first and to wait for their acceptance before annotating the genome, as the possible presence of foreign DNA may require a change of the assembly and therefore a reannotation [66].

8 Discussion

The tree of life is increasingly densely populated with sequenced genomes and with clade sequencing projects such as Bird 10K and Genome 10K but also with medium projects such as the roughly 50 switchgrass strains, that are sequenced at the Joint Genome Institute, or with small projects such as that of three bee species from the genus *Apis*. At the same time, the requirements on the precision of genome annotation methods increase, when close relatives are compared and phenotypic or functional differences are related to gene structure differences. Annotation pipelines can produce inconsistent annotations, in which a gene structure in one genome is predicted different from the structure of the ortholog in another genome, although that difference is not warranted by the evidence and not true. This is in particular a problem when each genome is annotated independently, e.g. based on native RNA-Seq only. Homology-based methods that use a database of source protein sequences, e.g. including those of a closely related reference species, introduce a comparative element to annotation. However, the accuracy is limited by the mere fact that only the query proteins are used and not also the source genome sequence outside the coding parts of exons. Pairwise genome alignments allow the mapping of annotation from one aligned genome to another.

However, when the number of genomes is 10,000, for example, the choice of genome pairs to consider may either be prohibitive or may itself introduce a bias against the discovery of structures specific to subclades. The construction of multi-genome alignments, that align base pairs that actually are homologous with high sensitivity and specificity, is itself a hard challenge due to rearrangements, duplications and in particular when the number of genomes gets large. They, however, form the basis for comparative single- and multi-genome annotation methods which can exploit evidence from the multiple comparison such as conservation and negative selection and which have been shown to achieve a high accuracy [38, 44]. Many challenges in comparative genome annotation remain, among them, a further increase in accuracy, in particular when the homology is only remote or medium, the comparative prediction of alternatively spliced genes and the development of scalable, automatized clade annotation tools, similar to automatic single genome annotation pipelines.

Acknowledgement

The research was supported by the German National Academic Foundation (to S.K.) and the German Research Foundation (DFG RTG 1870).

References

1. Salzberg SL, Angiuoli SV, Dunning Hotopp JC, Tettelin H (2011) Improving pan-genome annotation using whole genome multiple alignment. BMC Bioinf 12(1):272

2. Waterhouse RM, Tegenfeldt F, Li J, Zdobnov EM, Kriventseva EV (2012) OrthoDB: a hierarchical catalog of animal, fungal and bacterial orthologs. Nucleic Acids Res 41:D358–D365

3. Vilella AJ, Severin J, Ureta-Vidal A, Heng L, Durbin R, Birney E (2009) EnsemblCompara GeneTrees: complete, duplication-aware phylogenetic trees in vertebrates. Genome Res 19 (2):327–335

4. Schmitt-Engel C, Schultheis D, Schwirz J, Ströhlein N, Troelenberg N, Majumdar U, Grossmann D, Richter T, Tech M, Dönitz J, Gerischer L, Theis M, Schild I, Trauner J, Koniszewski NDB, Küster E, Kittelmann S, Hu Y, Lehmann S, Siemanowski J, Ulrich J, Panfilio KA, Schröder R, Morgenstern B, Stanke M, Buchholz F, Frasch M, Roth S, Wimmer EA, Schoppmeier M, Klingler M, Bucher G (2015) The iBeetle large-scale RNAi screen reveals gene functions for insect development and physiology. Nat Commun 6:7822

5. Avila-Herrera A, Pollard KS (2015) Coevolutionary analyses require phylogenetically deep alignments and better null models to accurately detect inter-protein contacts within and between species. BMC Bioinf 16(1):1–18

6. Zhang G (2015) Genomics: bird sequencing project takes off. Nature 522(7554):34–34

7. Smit AFA, Hublcy R (2008–2015) RepeatModeler Open-1.0. http://www.repeatmasker.org

8. Paten B, Earl D, Nguyen N, Diekhans M, Zerbino D, Haussler D (2011) Cactus: algorithms for genome multiple sequence alignment. Genome Res 21(9):1512–1528

9. Dobin A, Davis CA, Schlesinger F, Drenkow J, Zaleski C, Jha S, Batut P, Chaisson M, Gingeras TR (2013) STAR: ultrafast universal RNA-seq aligner. Bioinformatics 29(1):15–21

10. Wu TD, Nacu S (2010) Fast and snp-tolerant detection of complex variants and splicing in short reads. Bioinformatics 26:873–881

11. Daehwan K, Pertea G, Trapnell C, Pimentel H, Kelley R, Salzberg SL (2013) TopHat2: accurate alignment of transcriptomes in the presence of insertions, deletions and gene fusions. Genome Biol 14:R36

12. Pertea M, Pertea GM, Antonescu CM, Chang TC, Mendell JT, Salzberg SL (2015) StringTie enables improved reconstruction of a transcriptome from RNA-seq reads. Nat Biotech 33:290–295. StringTie transcript assembler. http://ccb.jhu.edu/software/stringtie. Accessed 28 Oct 2014

13. Trapnell C, Williams BA, Pertea G, Mortazavi A, Kwan G, van Baren MJ, Salzberg SL, Wold BJ, Pachter L (2010) Transcript assembly and quantification by RNA-Seq reveals unannotated transcripts and isoform switching during cell differentiation. Nat Biotechnol 28:511–515

14. Behr J, Kahles A, Zhong Y, Sreedharan VT, Drewe P, Rätsch G (2013) MITIE: simultaneous RNA-Seq-based transcript identification and quantification in multiple samples. Bioinformatics 29(20):2529–2538

15. Schulz MH, Zerbino DR, Vingron M, Birney E (2012) Oases: robust de novo RNA-seq assembly across the dynamic range of expression levels. Bioinformatics 28(8):1086–1092

16. Haas BJ, Papanicolaou A, Yassour M, Grabherr M, Blood PD, Bowden J, Brian Couger M, Eccles D, Li B, Lieber M, et al (2013) De novo transcript sequence reconstruction from RNA-seq using the Trinity platform for reference generation and analysis. Nat Protoc 8(8):1494–1512

17. Stanke M, Diekhans M, Baertsch R, Haussler D (2008) Using native and syntenically mapped cDNA alignments to improve de novo gene finding. Bioinformatics 24(5):637–644

18. Solovyev V, Kosarev P, Seledsov I, Vorobyev D (2006) Automatic annotation of eukaryotic genes, pseudogenes and promoters. Genome Biol 7(Suppl 1):S10

19. Behr J, Bohnert R, Zeller G, Schweikert G, Hartmann L, Rätsch G (2010) Next generation genome annotation with mGene.ngs. BMC Bioinf 11(S10):O8

20. Steijger T, Abril JF, Engstrom PG, Kokocinski F, Akerman M, Alioto T, Ambrosini G, Antonarakis SE, Behr J, Bohnert R, et al (2013) Assessment of transcript reconstruction methods for RNA-seq. Nat Methods 10(12):1177–1184

21. Schweikert G, Zien A, Zeller G, Behr J, Dietrich C, Ong GS, Philips P, De Bona F, Hartmann L, Bohlen A, et al (2009) mGene: accurate SVM-based gene findng with an application to nematode genomes. Genome Res 19:2133–2143

22. Seledtsov I, Molodtsov V, Kosarev P, Solovyev V (2014) Transomics transcript assembly pipeline. http://www.softberry.com. Accessed 28 Oct 2014

23. Slater GSC, Birney E (2005) Automated generation of heuristics for biological sequence comparison. BMC Bioinf 6(1):31

24. Korf I (2013) Genomics: the state of the art in RNA-seq analysis. Nat Methods 10(12):1165–1166

25. Levene MJ, Korlach J, Turner SW, Foquet M, Craighead HG, Webb WW (2003) Zero-mode waveguides for single-molecule analysis at high concentrations. Science 299:682–686

26. Martin JA, Johnson NV, Gross SM, Schnable J, Meng X, Wang M, Coleman-Derr D, Lindquist E, Wei C-L, Kaeppler S, Chen F, Wang Z (2014) A near complete snapshot of the zea mays seedling transcriptome revealed from ultra-deep sequencing. Sci Rep 4:4519

27. Gremme G (2013) Computational Gene Structure Prediction. PhD thesis, Universität Hamburg

28. Iwata H, Gotoh O (2012) Benchmarking spliced alignment programs including Spaln2, an extended version of Spaln that incorporates additional species-specific features. Nucleic Acids Res 40(20):e161

29. ProSplign (2014). http://www.ncbi.nlm.nih.gov/sutils/static/prosplign/prosplign.html. Accessed 17 Oct 2014

30. Usuka J, Brendel V (2000) Gene structure prediction by spliced alignment of genomic DNA with protein sequences: increased accuracy by differential splice site scoring. J Mol Biol 297(5):1075–1085

31. Birney E, Clamp M, Durbin R (2004) GeneWise and Genomewise. Genome Res 14:988–995

32. Keller O, Kollmar M, Stanke M, Waack S (2011) A novel hybrid gene prediction method employing protein multiple sequence alignments. Bioinformatics 27(6):757–763

33. Keilwagen J, Wenk M, Erickson JL, Schattat MH, Grau J, Hartung F (2016) Using intron position conservation for homology-based gene prediction. Nucleic Acids Res 44(9):e89

34. Korf I, Flicek P, Duan D, Brent MR (2001) Integrating genomic homology into gene structure prediction. Bioinformatics 1 Suppl. 1:S1–S9

35. Alexandersson M, Cawley S, Pachter L (2003) SLAM: cross-species gene finding and alignment with a generalized pair hidden Markov model. Genome Res 13:496–502

36. Richards S, Liu Y, Bettencourt BR, Hradecky P, Letovsky S, Nielsen R, Thornton K, Hubisz MJ, Chen R, Meisel RP, et al (2005) Comparative genome sequencing of drosophila pseudoobscura: chromosomal, gene, and cis-element evolution. Genome Res 15(1):1–18

37. Gross SS, Brent MR (2005) Using multiple alignments to improve gene prediction. In: Proceedings of RECOMB 2005

38. Gross S, Do C, Sirota M, Batzoglou S (2007) CONTRAST: a discriminative, phylogeny-free approach to multiple informant de novo gene prediction. Genome Biol 8(12):R269

39. Brent MR (2008) Steady progress and recent breakthroughs in the accuracy of automated genome annotation. Nat Rev Genet 9:62–73

40. Elsik C, Worley K, Bennett A, Beye M, Camara F, Childers C, de Graaf D, Debyser G, Deng J, Devreese B, et al (2014) Finding the missing honey bee genes: lessons learned from a genome upgrade. BMC Genomics 15(1):86

41. Csuros M, Rogozin IB, Koonin EV (2011) A detailed history of intron-rich eukaryotic ancestors inferred from a global survey of 100 complete genomes. PLoS Comput Biol 7 (9):e1002150

42. Gotoh O, Morita M, Nelson DR (2014) Assessment and refinement of eukaryotic gene structure prediction with gene-structure-aware multiple protein sequence alignment. BMC Bioinf 15(1):189

43. König S, Romoth LW, Gerischer L, Stanke M (2016) Simultaneous gene finding in multiple genomes. Bioinformatics 32:3388–3395

44. König S, Romoth L, Gerischer L, Stanke M (2015) Simultaneous gene finding in multiple genomes. PeerJ PrePrints 3:e1296v1

45. Hickey G, Paten B, Earl D, Zerbino D, Haussler D (2013). HAL: a hierarchical format for storing and analyzing multiple genome alignments. Bioinformatics 29(10):1341–1342

46. Nguyen N, Hickey G, Raney BJ, Armstrong J, Clawson H, Zweig A, Karolchik D, Kent WJ, Haussler D, Paten B (2014) Comparative assembly hubs: web-accessible browsers for comparative genomics. Bioinformatics 30:3293–3301

47. Hiller M, Schaar BT, Indjeian VB, Kingsley DM, Hagey LR, Bejerano G (2012) A "forward genomics" approach links genotype to phenotype using independent phenotypic losses among related species. Cell Rep 2 (4):817–823

48. Goodswen SJ, Kennedy PJ, Ellis JT (2012) Evaluating high-throughput ab initio gene finders to discover proteins encoded in eukaryotic pathogen genomes missed by laboratory techniques. PloS One 7(11):e50609

49. Lomsadze A, Burns PD, Borodovsky M (2014) Integration of mapped RNA-Seq reads into automatic training of eukaryotic gene finding algorithm. Nucleic Acids Res 42(15):e119

50. Hoff KJ, Lange S, Lomsadze A, Borodovsky M, Stanke M (2015) BRAKER1: unsupervised RNA-Seq-based genome annotation with GeneMark-ET and AUGUSTUS. Bioinformatics 32(5):767–769

51. Simão FA, Waterhouse RM, Ioannidis P, Kriventseva EV, Zdobnov EM (2015) Busco: assessing genome assembly and annotation completeness with single-copy orthologs. Bioinformatics 31(19):3210–3212

52. Keller O, Odronitz F, Stanke M, Kollmar M, Waack S (2008) Scipio: using protein sequences to determine the precise exon/intron structures of genes and their orthologs in closely related species. BMC Bioinf 9(1):278

53. Haas B, Salzberg S, Zhu W, Pertea M, Allen J, Orvis J, White O, Buell CR, Wortman J (2008) Automated eukaryotic gene structure annotation using EVidenceModeler and the program to assemble spliced alignments. Genome Biol 9 (1):R7

54. Holt C, Yandell M (2011) MAKER2: an annotation pipeline and genome-database management tool for second-generation genome projects. BMC Bioinf 12:491

55. Lomsadze A, Ter-Hovhannisyan V, Chernoff YO, Borodovsky M (2005) Gene identification in novel eukaryotic genomes by self-training algorithm. Nucleic Acids Res 33 (20):6494–6506

56. Hoff KJ, Stanke M (2013) WebAUGUSTUS – a web service for training AUGUSTUS and predicting genes in eukaryotes. Nucleic Acids Res 41:W123–W1238

57. Raney BJ, Dreszer TR, Barber GP, Clawson H, Fujita PA, Wang T, Nguyen N, Paten B, Zweig AS, Karolchik D, Kent WJ (2013) Track data hubs enable visualization of user-defined genome-wide annotations on the UCSC Genome Browser. Bioinformatics 30 (7):1003–1005

58. McKay SJ, Vergara IA, Stajich JE (2010) Using the generic synteny browser (gbrowse_syn). Curr Protoc Bioinformatics UNIT 9.12

59. Mercer TR, Dinger ME, Mattick JS (2009) Long non-coding RNAs: insights into functions. Nat Rev Genet 10(3):155–159

60. Mattick JS, Makunin IV (2006) Non-coding RNA. Hum Mol Genet 15(Suppl 1):R17–R29

61. Derrien T, Johnson R, Bussotti G, Tanzer A, Djebali S, Tilgner H, Guernec G, Martin D, Merkel A, Knowles DG, et al (2012) The GENCODE v7 catalog of human long non-coding RNAs: analysis of their gene structure, evolution, and expression. Genome Res 22 (9):1775–1789

62. Lin MF, Jungreis I, Kellis M (2011) PhyloCSF: a comparative genomics method to distinguish protein coding and non-coding regions. Bioinformatics 27(13):i275–i282

63. Ulitsky I, Bartel DP (2013) lincRNAs: genomics, evolution, and mechanisms. Cell 154 (1):26–46

64. Rivas E, Eddy SR (2001) Noncoding RNA gene detection using comparative sequence analysis. BMC Bioinformatics 2(1):1

65. Skinner ME, Uzilov AV, Stein LD, Mungall CJ, Holmes IH (2009) JBrowse: a next-generation genome browser. Genome Res 19:1630–1638

66. Pirovano W, Boetzer M, Derks MF, Smit S (2015) NCBI-compliant genome submissions: tips and tricks to save time and money. Brief Bioinform 18(2):179–182

Chapter 7

A Practical Guide for Comparative Genomics of Mobile Genetic Elements in Prokaryotic Genomes

Danillo Oliveira Alvarenga, Leandro M. Moreira, Mick Chandler, and Alessandro M. Varani

Abstract

Mobile genetic elements (MGEs) are an important feature of prokaryote genomes but are seldom well annotated and, consequently, are often underestimated. MGEs include transposons (Tn), insertion sequences (ISs), prophages, genomic islands (GEIs), integrons, and integrative and conjugative elements (ICEs). They are intimately involved in genome evolution and promote phenomena such as genomic expansion and rearrangement, emergence of virulence and pathogenicity, and symbiosis. In spite of the annotation bottleneck, there are so far at least 75 different programs and databases dedicated to prokaryotic MGE analysis and annotation, and this number is rapidly growing. Here, we present a practical guide to explore, compare, and visualize prokaryote MGEs using a combination of available software and databases tailored to small scale genome analyses. This protocol can be coupled with expert MGE annotation and exploited for evolutionary and comparative genomic analyses.

Key words Transposons, Insertion sequences, Prophages, Clustered regularly interspaced short palindromic repeats, Genomic islands, Integrons, Integrative conjugative elements, Evolution, Genomics

1 Introduction

Most genome annotation pipelines developed to date are dedicated to the prediction and characterization of coding regions and their putative products, signal peptides, pseudogenes, and noncoding RNAs. Surprisingly, annotation of ubiquitous genomic features such as Mobile Genetic Elements (MGEs) is generally not fully addressed and/or is neglected in most of these pipelines, and thus MGEs are seldom well characterized and annotated. Consequently, they are generally underestimated, impacting the quality of the annotation and potentially affecting downstream genome analyses.

Transposons (Tn), Insertion Sequences (ISs), Prophages, Clustered Regularly-Interspaced Short Palindromic Repeats (CRISPRs), Genomic Islands (GEIs), Integrons and Integrative

João C. Setubal et al. (eds.), *Comparative Genomics: Methods and Protocols*, Methods in Molecular Biology, vol. 1704, https://doi.org/10.1007/978-1-4939-7463-4_7, © Springer Science+Business Media LLC 2018

and Conjugative Elements (ICEs) are the most common MGEs found in prokaryote genomes and their properties and behavior are important in lateral gene transfer events (LGT). These elements are known to promote genomic expansion and rearrangements, and the emergence of virulence, pathogenicity, and symbiosis. Over the last 15 years, several reviews have focused on the impact of LGT mediated by MGEs [1–13]. It is now generally recognized that MGEs are central to bacterial and archaeal genome evolution.

To begin an analysis of the MGE content of a given genome, it is first necessary to identify and annotate ordinary genome features such as coding sequences (CDSs), rRNAs, and tRNAs. There are several useful genome annotation pipelines that use a combination of distinct methods based on computer predictions for CDS detection and product assignment. Putative gene product attribution for each identified CDS is generally based on sequence similarity obtained by using BLAST [14] and Hidden Markov Model [15] searches against trusted databases such as RefSeq [16], Interpro [17], Pfam [18], and TIGRFAMs [19]. However, few sequencing projects include manual curation and validation, mostly relying on the annotation results of automatic computer predictions. Indeed, this generally results in quite variable annotation qualities [20], impacting downstream analyses.

For MGE detection and annotation it is essential to use a variety of approaches including additional specialized pipelines and software which are normally not implemented in a regular annotation pipeline. Most MGE de novo-detection software are not integrated into the most popular genome annotation pipelines, such as Prokka [21], the NCBI Prokaryotic Genome Annotation Pipeline (PGAP), the Rapid Annotation using Subsystem Technology (RAST) [22, 23], or the Integrated Microbial Genomes System/Expert Review (IMG/ER) [24]. The absence of MGE predictions is therefore an important example of the deficiencies in expert genome annotation. The resulting incomplete annotation files are regularly deposited in public databases and used by the scientific community for detailed evolutionary and comparative genomic analyses. Identification, annotation, and classification of each MGE type are becoming central in the prokaryote genomics field. A correct MGE annotation will ultimately lead to new insights into how prokaryotes are genetically tailored to their lifestyles [25].

A considerable number of software and databases have been developed for MGE detection and analysis in the last decades. This makes it tiresome and time consuming to evaluate the programs that are most suited for a given work-flow. Some MGE software and databases provide very precise and curated information, together with gold standard methods and protocols for annotation. These include the ISfinder Database [26] and ISsaga2 [25], for IS analysis and annotation, respectively, while other databases such as ICEberg [27], INTEGRALL [28], and PHAST [29] for ICEs, integrons and prophages, respectively, provide valuable information concerning other MGEs. Conversely, there are a number of predictors that provide de novo methods for MGE detection, giving the user the opportunity to investigate the detailed role of MGE in novel complete and draft genomes.

Tables 1 and 2 provide a list of software and databases published and currently available for MGE research and some of their features. There are several software and/or databases for each MGE, and therefore there is no single solution to deal with all MGE types at once. This makes it difficult to choose the most reliable and appropriate software and databases. In view of the number of possibilities available (as shown in Table 1), a novice in this research area will probably spend a considerable time switching between programs and deciding which should be included in their projects and methodologies. Figure 1 illustrates the canonical mechanisms of known lateral gene transfer events (transduction, conjugation, and transformation) in a prokaryotic cell, and the databases and software for detection and analysis of each MGE type used by this protocol. It is worth mentioning that it is not unusual to find chimeras between different MGE types (Fig. 1, dashed boxes), making it difficult to distinguish their boundaries. These concepts are discussed in this protocol.

To provide an easier introduction to this subject, we will present a standard MGE bioinformatics work-flow for prediction and annotation using established methods and tools and provide tips for MGE investigation and analysis. This chapter will show how to run de novo MGE predictors, how to extract and interpret results, and how to visualize these results in circular or linear genome maps by using public bioinformatics software. Overall, the results of the analyses generated by this protocol can be exploited for expert annotation and comparative genomics analysis with genome browsers and annotation tools, such as Gview [96] and Artemis [97].

2 Materials

For de novo MGE prediction and comparative genomics analysis, a modern computer containing a 64-bit processor, with at least 4 GB of RAM, a 500 GB hard drive, and broadband Internet access are usually enough for meeting the minimum requirements of most software. Additionally, as presented in Table 1, a Unix-like operating system (OS) is required by the majority of the available MGE analysis software.

In these examples, we use Ubuntu 16.04, a free and open source Linux distribution that can be downloaded from https://www.ubuntu.com. In most hardware, the 64-bit version of Ubuntu can be installed either as your sole OS, alongside a preexisting OS (such as Microsoft Windows or Apple OS X) or in a virtual machine

Table 1
Features from available software and databases for prokaryotic MGEs. Operating system was assumed as including both Linux and Apple Mac OS X when none was mentioned in documentation. When no license was specified, the software was assumed to be proprietary unless source code is available

Tool	Use	Availability	License	OS	References
A: Software and databases for transposon (insertion sequence) analysis					
ESSENTIALS	Transposons insertion analysis	Web server, Perl/R scripts	AGPL 3	Linux, Mac, Windows (browser-based)	[30]
ISbrowser	Insertion sequences visualization	Web server	Proprietary	Linux, Mac, Windows (browser-based)	[31]
IScan	Insertion sequences identification	Perl/C package	GPL 2	Linux	[32]
ISCR elements	Insertion sequences common region (ISCR) database	Web database	Proprietary	Linux, Mac, Windows (browser-based)	[7]
ISfinder	Insertion sequences database	Web server	Proprietary	Linux, Mac, Windows (browser-based)	[26]
ISMapper	Transposase insertion sites identification	Python package	Modified BSD	Linux, Mac	[33]
ISQuest	Insertion sequences identification	C/C++ package	GPL 3	Linux, Windows	[34]
ISsaga	Insertion sequences identification and annotation	Web server	Proprietary	Linux, Mac, Windows (browser-based)	[25]
OASIS	Insertion sequences identification and annotation	Python scripts	Unspecified (source available)	Linux, Mac	[35]
PRAP	Transposons identification	Perl scripts	GPL 3	Linux, Mac	[36]
Recon	Transposons identification and classification	C/Perl package	GPL 2	Linux	[37]
Red	Transposons detection	C++ package	Public domain	Linux, Mac	[38]
RepeatFinder	Transposons detection	C++/Perl package	Artistic	Linux, Mac	[39]
RepeatMasker	Transposons detection	C++/Perl package	OSL 2.1	Linux	[40]

(continued)

Table 1
(continued)

Tool	Use	Availability	License	OS	References
Repseek	Transposons detection	C package	LGPL 2	Linux, Mac	[41]
RISCI	Transposons identification	Perl scripts	Unspecified (source available)	Linux	[42]
TnpPred	Insertion sequences prediction	Web server	Proprietary	Linux, Mac, Windows (browser-based)	[43]
B: Software and databases for prophage and CRISPR analysis					
ACLAME	Prophages database	Web server	Unspecified (available for download)	Linux, Mac, Windows (browser-based)	[44]
Phage_Finder	Prophages identification	Perl scripts	GPL 2	Linux, Mac	[45]
PHAST	Prophages identification and annotation	Web server	Unspecified (available for download)	Linux, Mac, Windows (browser-based)	[29]
PhiSpy	Prophages prediction	Python/R/ C++ package	Unspecified (source available)	Linux, Mac	[46]
Prophage database	Prophages database	Web server	Proprietary	Linux, Mac, Windows (browser-based)	[47]
Prophinder	Prophages prediction	Web server	Proprietary	Linux, Mac, Windows (browser-based)	[48]
VirSorter	Prophages prediction	Perl/C package	GPL 2	Linux	[49]
CRASS	CRISPR assembly in metagenomic data	C++/Shell package	GPL 3	Linux, Mac	[50]
CRISPI	CRISPR database	Web server	Proprietary	Linux, Mac, Windows (browser-based)	[51]
CRISPRcompar	CRISPR comparison	Web server	Proprietary	Linux, Mac, Windows (browser-based)	[52]

(continued)

Table 1
(continued)

Tool	Use	Availability	License	OS	References
CRISPRdb	CRISPR database and prediction	Web server	Proprietary	Linux, Mac, Windows (browser-based)	[53]
CRISPResso	CRISPR analysis	Web server, Python/Java/C package	AGPL 3	Linux, Mac, Windows (browser-based)	[54]
CRISPRfinder	CRISPR prediction	Web server	Proprietary	Linux, Mac, Windows (browser-based)	[55]
CRISPRmap	CRISPR classification	Web server	Proprietary	Linux, Mac, Windows (browser-based)	[56]
CRISPR recognition tool	CRISPR prediction	Java package	Public domain	Linux, Mac, Windows	[57]
CRISPRstrand	CRISPR prediction	Web server	Proprietary	Linux, Mac, Windows (browser-based)	[58]
CRISPR target	CRISPR prediction and analysis	Web server	Proprietary	Linux, Mac, Windows (browser-based)	[59]
MINCED	CRISPR prediction	Java package	GPL 3	Linux, Mac, Windows	[60]
PILER-CR	CRISPR prediction	C package	Public domain	Linux, Mac	[61]
C: Software and databases for genomic and pathogenicity island analysis					
EGID	Genomic islands prediction	Perl/Java/C++ package	Custom (source available)	Linux	[62]
GIDetector	Genomic islands classification	Perl/Java package	GPL 2	Windows	[63]
GIHunter	Genomic islands prediction	Perl/Java/C++ package	Custom (source available)	Linux	[64]
GIPSY	Genomic islands prediction	Java package	GPL	Linux, Windows	[65]
GIST	Genomic islands prediction	Perl/Java/C++ package	Custom (source available)	Linux	[66]

(continued)

Table 1
(continued)

Tool	Use	Availability	License	OS	References
GIV	Genomic islands visualization	C++ package	Proprietary	Linux, Mac	[67]
IGPIT	Genomic islands prediction	Web server	Proprietary	Linux, Mac, Windows (browser-based)	[68]
Islander	Genomic islands identification and database	Perl scripts, web server	Unspecified (source available)	Linux, Mac; Linux, Mac, Windows (browser-based)	[69]
IslandHunter	Genomic islands prediction	Java package	Proprietary	Linux, Mac, Windows	[70]
IslandPath	Genomic islands prediction	Perl scripts	GPL 2	Linux	[71]
IslandPick	Genomic islands comparison and identification	Perl scripts	GPL 2	Linux	[72]
IslandViewer	Genomic islands identification and visualization	Perl scripts	GPL 2	Linux	[73]
Mobilome-FINDER	Genomic islands detection	Web server	Proprietary	Linux, Mac, Windows (browser-based)	[74]
MSGIP	Genomic islands prediction	Java package	Unspecified (source available)	Linux, Mac, Windows	[75]
OligoWords	Genomic islands identification	Python script	CC-BY	Linux, Mac	[76]
SeqWord genome browser	Genomic islands identification and visualization	Web server, python scripts	Unspecified (source available)	Linux, Mac, Windows (browser-based)	[77]
Colombo/ SIGI-HMM	Genomic islands prediction	Java package	Proprietary	Linux, Mac, Windows	[78]
tRNAcc	Genomic islands identification	C++/Perl package	Proprietary (source available)	Windows	[79]
Alien_Hunter	Pathogenicity islands prediction	Perl/Java package	GPL 2	Linux, Mac	[80]
PAIDB	Pathogenicity islands database	Web server	Proprietary	Linux, Mac, Windows (browser-based)	[81]
PIPS	Pathogenicity islands prediction	Perl scripts	GPL 3	Linux, Mac	[82]

(continued)

Table 1
(continued)

Tool	Use	Availability	License	OS	References
PredictBias	Genomic and pathogenicity islands prediction	Web server	Proprietary	Linux, Mac, Windows (browser-based)	[83]
D: Databases for integron and integrative conjugative elements (ICE)					
ACID	Integrons database	Web server	Proprietary	Linux, Mac, Windows (browser-based)	[84]
ICEberg	Integrative and conjugative elements database	Web server (available for download)	Proprietary	Linux, Mac, Windows (browser-based)	[27]
INTEGRALL	Integrons database	Web server	Proprietary	Linux, Mac, Windows (browser-based)	[28]

Table 2
Currently unavailable software for prokaryotic MGE analysis. Some of these programs might be obtained upon request from authors

Tool	Target MGE	Reference
Centroid	Genomic islands	[85]
GI-POP	Genomic islands	[86]
PAI-IDA	Genomic islands	[87]
SIGI	Genomic islands	[88]
DOASIS/NOASIS	Insertion sequences	[89]
ISA	Insertion sequences	[90]
Prophage finder	Prophages	[91]
Unamed script	Prophages	[3]
SSFinder	CRISPR	[92]
IRs search	Transposable elements	[93]
MUST	Transposable elements	[94]
Profile HMM search	Transposable elements	[93]
Repeats search	Transposable elements	[93]
Transposon express	Transposable elements	[95]

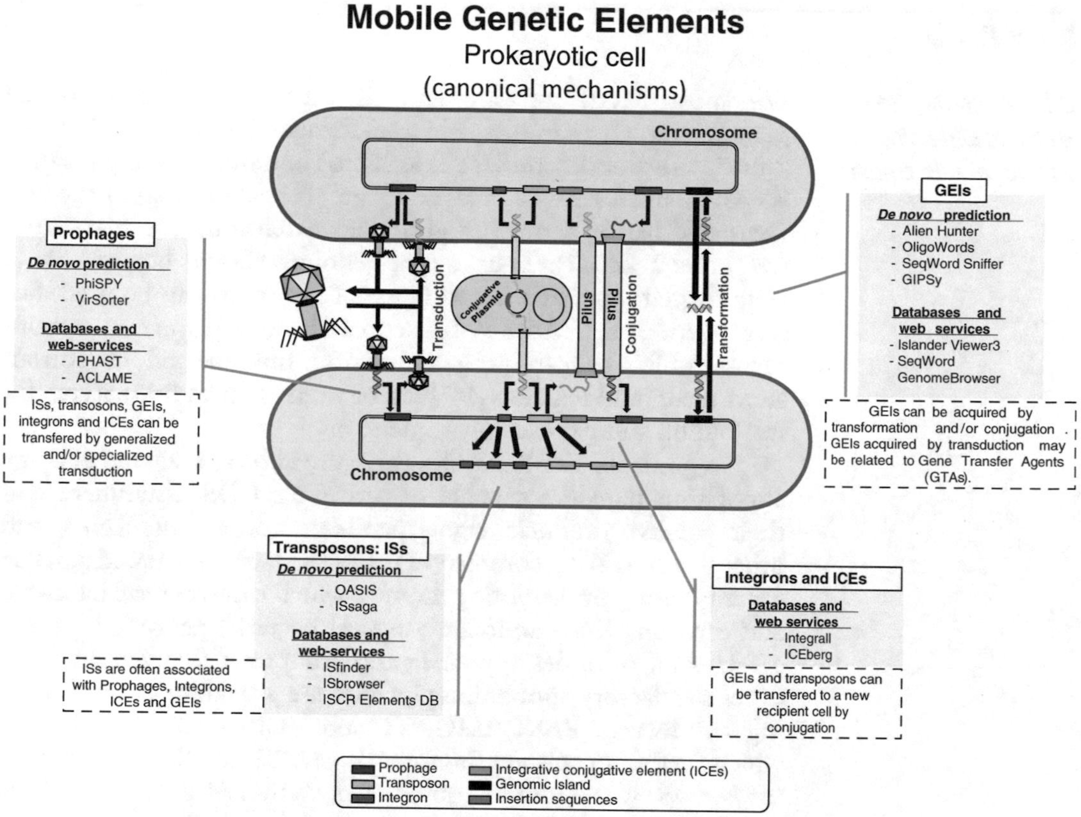

Fig. 1 Canonical lateral gene transfer mechanisms present in a prokaryotic cell and their respective software and databases for analyses included in this guide. The dashed box shows chimeras between different MGE types which may occur

following instructions from the Ubuntu community help wiki (https://help.ubuntu.com/community/installation). However, for better performance, it is best to avoid virtual machines and install Ubuntu directly on the computer instead. To follow this guide a basic knowledge in management and analysis of directories, files and genomic data in a command line interface is also necessary.

We used 21 genomes from different bacterial and archaeal classes bearing distinct MGE types and numbers as examples for the methods described in this protocol. Final results for the analyses of these genomes can be obtained from https://github.com/danillo-alvarenga/mogece/blob/master/Analyses.tar.gz. To download these results, open the GitHub webpage, click on the "Download ZIP" link located on the right of your screen, and save it to an appropriate directory. We advise visualizing these files in addition to reading this chapter for a better understanding of what results the following methods should produce.

3   Methods

3.1   Preparing Your Dataset: Obtaining Prokaryote Genomes

For most MGE software and databases, either unannotated genome sequences in the plain fasta format (".fasta", ".fas", ".fa", ".fna", ".fnt" and ".fnn" file extensions) or annotated sequences in the GenBank format (".gbk" and ".gb" file extensions) or the new GenBank flatfile format (".gbff" file extension) are mandatory (*see*Notes 1 and 2). Thus, target genomes should be available in both formats so that a broad range of programs can be used. For novel genomes, SPAdes [98] is currently among the best options for assembling prokaryotic genomes from Illumina and Ion Torrent short reads, and Platanus [99] can be used as an additional step for scaffolding and gap-closing sequences.

To generate GenBank files there are several available genome annotation pipelines capable of providing CDS assignment and their putative products, signal peptides, non-coding RNAs, and other features. We recommend Prokka [21], an automated pipeline for annotating prokaryotic genomes, which runs on local hardware and can completely annotate a typical bacterial genome in under 10–15 min on a desktop or laptop computer. Conversely, three other satisfactory annotation pipelines are available on the following web-servers: RAST, IMG/ER, and NCBI Pipeline PGAP (for which further details are found in the NCBI handbook chapter at https://www.ncbi.nlm.nih.gov/books/NBK174280). All these pipelines generate standard-compliant output files.

If the user is not interested in analyzing novel genomes or wants to compare them to available genomes, two useful sources of bacterial and/or archeal genomes are the NCBI ftp server and the Genomes OnLine Database (GOLD) [100]. Available genomes can be retrieved by visiting ftp://ftp.ncbi.nlm.nih.gov/genomes/ on a web browser and navigating to *genbank/* at the bottom of the page, or browsing the GOLD website at https://gold.jgi.doe.gov/. Both databases include updated files on virtually every prokaryotic genome publicly released thus far.

3.2   Preparing Your Computer for MGE Analysis: Installing Dependencies

While some MGE analysis software provides web servers with browser-based user interfaces or graphical user interfaces, most available programs are based on command-line interfaces and need to be installed on a local computer running a Linux-based OS before analysis can be carried out (*see*Note 3). In some cases this can be difficult even with bioinformatics experience. Out-of-the-box Ubuntu lacks a few software elements and libraries on which these programs depend. Nevertheless, several of these dependencies can be easily installed by typing a few commands in a terminal emulator, a program that allows users to interact with computer programs by a text-based interface.

Ubuntu's terminal emulator can be accessed by typing "terminal" in the dash (the first button from top on the left-sided launcher bar) or pressing the <ctrl>+<alt>+<T> key combination. Although there are alternative terminal implementations, all commands described in this chapter are assumed to be typed in the standard Ubuntu terminal emulator. Before starting the analyses, follow the procedures below using this terminal emulator to prepare the system for the software described in the subsequent sections (*see* **Notes 4** and **5**).

First, it is important to install essential software for building programs and make sure the system has all that is needed for compiling sources. For this purpose, issue the following command to the apt-get package manager (*see* **Note 6**): *sudo apt-get install build-essential*.

Navigation in the terminal is achieved by the command *cd* followed by a space and the directory name. Since it takes some time to familiarize oneself with this method, it is useful to install a shortcut for opening a directory in the terminal directly from the Ubuntu file manager also using the apt-get manager: *sudo apt-get install nautilus-open-terminal*.

Software written in the Java programming language is commonly distributed as .jar files. These files depend on a runtime environment that does not come pre-installed in Ubuntu systems. To run Java-based applications, install the Open Java Development Kit: *sudo apt-get install openjdk-7-jdk*.

R is an open-source computing language widely used for statistics on which some bioinformatics tools rely. Most R packages are included in the Comprehensive R Archive Network (CRAN), but the Ubuntu repositories include some of these packages, which can also be installed with the apt-get manager for an easier process. Install the basic R files and the randomForest package with the following command: *sudo apt-get install r-base r-cran-randomforest*.

Bioinformatics software written in the Python programming language may sometimes depend on Biopython, a library containing several bioinformatics tools, or TkInter, an interface to the GUI toolkit Tk. Both libraries can be easily installed with the apt-get manager: *sudo apt-get install python-biopython python-tk*.

A different approach to dependencies is implemented by Docker, which is able to install a program and all its dependencies and create containers for this software. For bioinformatics programs that use this distribution method, reboot the operating system after installing Docker and adding your username to the Docker group with the following command: *sudo apt-get install docker.io; sudo usermod -aG docker $USER*.

The NCBI BLAST suite is another popular dependency for bioinformatics programs. At present there are two BLAST versions in the Ubuntu repositories. Some programs rely on the legacy version while others depend on the current version (*see* **Note** 7). To avoid incompatibility issues, both versions can be installed concomitantly: *sudo apt-get install blast2 ncbi-blast+*.

3.3   Insertion Sequence Prediction

ISs are the smallest and simplest autonomous mobile genetic elements, ranging from 0.7 to 3.5 kbp, and generally include a transposase gene encoding the enzyme that catalyzes IS movement. They are classified into about 28 different families on the basis of the relatedness of transposases and overall genetic organization [13]. The ISfinder database (https://www-is.biotoul.fr/) is the reference center for IS analysis, providing a gold standard method and protocol for IS identification, name attribution, annotation, and classification [25]. We strongly recommend following the ISfinder annotation protocol, using a manual expert annotation of each predicted IS, with the ISsaga web-service. These instructions can be found on the ISsaga Manual in the "About" section of the ISsaga main webpage (http://issaga.biotoul.fr/ISsaga2/issaga_manual.pdf). Other available software, such as OASIS [35] and ISQuest [59], are dedicated to de novo predictions, providing valuable resources for IS discovery in a given genome. This guide focuses on ISsaga and OASIS, but can be exploited with ISQuest and other IS software and databases shown in Table 1-A (*see* **Note** 8).

3.3.1   IS Detection with the ISsaga2 Web-Service

1. Open the ISsaga2 webpage at http://issaga.biotoul.fr.

2. Log-in into the system, or create a new account.

3. On the "ISsaga public section", click on Start Annotation.

4. Fill-in the forms, and choose which type of genome file (".fasta" or ".gbk") is to be analyzed. Click on the "Send/Run" button, and wait for the results.

5. Follow the ISfinder/ISsaga gold standards for IS annotation, naming and validating each predicted IS, according to the ISsaga manual (optional).

6. On the "Annotation Report" webpage of your submitted genome, click on the pull-down menu "Annotation," and choose the "Extract Annotation" option.

7. Click on the "Excel annotation file" button, and download the ".xls" file to your genome folder.

8. Open the ".xls" file in your favorite spreadsheet program, convert it to the comma-separated values format (".csv") and save this new file in your genome folder.

9. If the ISfinder/ISsaga gold standards for IS annotation were followed to the end, extract the final annotation results in the "Annotation" tab, and choose "Extract Annotation" option. On the new webpage, click on the "GenBank annotation file", and use this new GenBank file to visualize the results in the GView or Artemis genome viewers (optional).

1. Download the OASIS source code from https://github.com/dgrtwo/OASIS.

2. Go to the Downloads folder in the file manager, right-click on the downloaded file and select "extract here."

3. Move the extracted folder to the directory where software and database files will be stored. In this and the following examples, we will use */home/bioinfo/software* as the default path for the installed software and */home/bioinfo/genomes* for genome files. Replace this path with your own directory paths whenever necessary (*see* **Note 9**).

4. Go to the folder where a *setup.py* file can be found, right-click on a blank space and select "open in terminal." In the opened terminal, install the software:

   python setup.py build; sudo python setup.py install

5. Find the data subdirectory inside the src directory and modify the *data.cfg* file to the following:

   [BLAST]
   BLAST_EXE=/usr/bin/blastall
   FORMAT_EXE=/usr/bin/formatdb

6. On these examples, we also use *TargetGenome* as proxy for the genome filename and *AnalysisDirectory* for the results directory, which should be replaced with the names of your file and directory. Open a terminal from your genome folder and run OASIS with the appropriate file and directory names:

   OASIS -g TargetGenome.gb -o OASISAnalysisDirectory

7. Repeat the previous step for each genome you wish to analyze.

8. OASIS will produce two files – a fasta file containing both nucleotide and amino acid sequences of each detected IS, and a General Feature Format file (".gff" extension) containing information about the predicted insertion sequences. Please note that, unlike ISsaga, OASIS does not classify ISs into families. The data obtained from OASIS must be parsed through ISfinder for this purpose (*see* **Note 10**).

3.4   Prophage and Clustered Regularly Interspaced Short Palindromic Repeat Prediction

Temperate or lysogenic phages generally integrate their genomes into the bacterial chromosome as prophages, which replicate passively with the host chromosome until conditions favor their reactivation. Integration occurs by site-specific recombination often into tRNA/tmRNA genes [46] (*see* **Note 11**). Prophages can encode virulence-related genes converting non-pathogenic bacteria into pathogens. It is well known that prophage identification in bacterial genomes is a difficult process [46]. Indeed, the longer and more complex the MGE the more difficult it is to correctly identify it. Prophages can also be confounded with Gene Transfer Agents (GTAs), which also resemble phages in a subtle way

[101]. GTAs are widespread in bacteria and may also be involved in virulence and adaptation [102].

CRISPRs are specific loci which provide acquired immunity against viruses and plasmids [103]. Therefore, in addition to the prophage prediction and analysis, CRISPR detection also provides valuable information concerning the history of phage infection of the analyzed genome (*see* **Note 12**). CRISPR analysis should use both de novo approaches, such as MinCED and CRISPRdb (http://crispr.u-psud.fr/crispr/), one of the most complete databases for CRISPR analysis.

3.4.1 Prophage Detection with PhiSpy 2.3

1. Download the PhiSpy source code from https://sourceforge.net/projects/phispy/, extract the package and move it to your software directory.

2. Go to the folder where a makefile can be found, open a terminal from the right-click menu, and compile the executable files:

   make

3. Make all Python scripts executable:

   chmod +x *.py */*.py

4. Add the directory to your global environment variables (*see* **Note 13**):

   echo 'export PATH=$PATH:'$(pwd) >> ~/.bashrc; source ~/.bashrc

5. Add the Python interpreter path to the main PhiSpy scripts:

   sed -i '1i#!/usr/bin/env python' phiSpy.py; sed -i '1i#!/usr/bin/env python' genbank_to_seed.py

6. Go to the directory where the target genomes are hosted:

   cd /home/bioinfo/genomes

7. Transform the target genome file from the GenBank file format to a SEED directory:

   genbank_to_seed.py TargetGenome.gb GenomeSEEDDirectory

8. Run PhiSpy on the newly-created SEED directory:

   phiSpy.py -i GenomeSEEDDirectory -o PhiSpyAnalysisDirectory

9. Repeat **steps 9** and **10** for the other target genomes.

10. After the analysis is finished, the output directory will host several files, including a subdirectory named "results" containing a file named *prophage.tbl*. This file contains the location of the predicted prophages.

3.4.2 Prophage Detection with VirSorter 1.0.3

1. Download VirSorter with Docker:

   docker.io pull discoenv/virsorter:v1.0.3

2. Download the VirSorter database from http://mirrors.iplantcollaborative.org/browse/iplant/home/shared/imicrobe/VirSorter/virsorter-data.tar.gz.

3. Extract the downloaded file and move the VirSorter database folder to your software directory.

4. Create a VirSorter analysis folder in your genomes folder and copy the fasta files for your target genomes there.

5. Open a terminal and run VirSorter from Docker (*see* **Note 14**):

   docker.io run -v /home/bioinfo/software/virsorter-data:/data -v/home/bioinfo/genomes/VirSorterAnalysisDirectory:/wdir -w/wdir --rm. discoenv/virsorter:v1.0.3 --db 2 --fna/wdir/TargetGenome.fasta

6. Claim ownership on the created files and change permissions:

   *sudo chown -R $USER: *; chmod -R 755 ***

7. Repeat **steps 5** and **6** for each target genome.

8. VirSorter main results will be output to a comma-separated table named VIRSorter_global_phage_signal.csv, containing possible viral and prophage sequences divided into categories according to the certainty of prediction. However, this table does not provide genomic coordinates for theses prophages. These coordinates can be found in the headers from fasta sequences written to the Predicted_viral_sequences directory.

3.4.3 CRISPR Detection with MinCED

1. Download the MinCED source code from https://github.com/ctSkennerton/minced.

2. Go to the Downloads folder in the file manager, right-click on the downloaded file and select "extract here."

3. Move the extracted folder to the directory where you wish to keep software and databases files.

4. Go to the folder where a makefile can be found, right-click on a blank space, and select "open in terminal." In the opened terminal, compile the executable files:

   make

5. Export the MinCED directory by issuing the following command:

   echo 'export PATH=$PATH:'$(pwd) >> ~/.bashrc; source ~/.bashrc

6. Still in the terminal, change to your genomes directory:

   cd /home/bioinfo/genomes

7. Run MinCED on your target genome:

   minced -gff TargetGenome.fasta MinCEDResults.gff

8. Repeat the previous step for each genome you wish to analyze.

9. By default, MinCED outputs a tab-separated values table to the terminal. However, by adding the *-gff* parameter to its command and pointing a filename for writing, MinCED will produce a ".gff" file containing information about the predicted CRISPRs.

**3.5   Genomic Island
Prediction**

GEIs are central to the dissemination and evolution of a broad spectrum of bacteria [8]. GEIs can be correlated with pathogenicity, virulence, fitness, symbiosis, and cell metabolism, depending on the gene composition of the given GEIs. Therefore, the better the CDS annotation, the better the GEI classification. There are several available GEI detection software packages. Genomic Island Prediction software (GIPSy) [65] is one of the most complete and user-friendly GEI detection software currently available, and it is capable of distinguishing pathogenicity islands, metabolic islands, resistance islands, and symbiotic islands. We recommend downloading and following the GIPSy annotation through their interface (http://www.bioinformatics.org/groups/?group_id=1180). The instructions below show how to use Alien_Hunter and SeqWord Gene Island Sniffer software for GEI prediction (*see* **Note 15**).

**3.5.1   GEI Prediction
with Alien_Hunter 1.7**

1. Download the Alien_Hunter source code from http://www.sanger.ac.uk/science/tools/alien-hunter, extract the package and move it to your software folder.

2. Go to the folder where an *alien_hunter* file can be found, right-click on a blank space, and select "open in terminal." In the opened terminal, add the directory to your global environment variables:

   echo 'export PATH=$PATH:'$(pwd) >> ~/.bashrc; source ~/.bashrc

3. Change to your genome directory in the terminal:

   cd /home/bioinfo/genomes

4. Run Alien_Hunter on your fasta-formatted genome:

   alien_hunter TargetGenome.fasta AlienHunterOutputFile

5. You may opt to view the resulting prediction file on the Artemis genome browser. To do so, follow the procedure for installing Artemis described in the first step of Subheading 3.4.2. To open the resulting prediction file on Artemis after analysis, add the *-a* parameter to the command illustrated in the **step 3**:

   alien_hunter TargetGenome.fasta AlienHunterOutputFile -a

6. Alien_Hunter will generate three result files: two feature tables and a plot file. Look for the ".sco" file, which indicates coordinates and scores for the predicted genomic islands.

**3.5.2   GEI Prediction
with OligoWords 1.2
and SeqWord Gene Island
Sniffer 1.0**

1. Download OligoWords and SeqWord Gene Island Sniffer from http://www.bi.up.ac.za/SeqWord/downloads/OligoWords_1.2.1_linux.zip and http://www.bi.up.ac.za/SeqWord/downloads/SWGIS_1.0.zip, respectively, extract the packages, and move them to your software folder.

2. Open a terminal in the directory where the OligoWords and the SeqWord Sniffer scripts can be found and add their paths to your environment variables:

echo 'export PATH=$PATH:'$(pwd) >> ~/.bashrc; source ~/.bashrc

3. Add the Python interpreter path to the main scripts in their corresponding directories:

    sed -i '1i#!/usr/bin/env python' OligoWords1.2.1.1.py
    sed -i '1i#!/usr/bin/env python' SeqWordSniffer.py

4. Change executable permissions for the scripts:

    chmod +x OligoWords1.2.1.1.py ; chmod +x */*
    chmod +x SeqWordSniffer.py; chmod +x */*

5. Find the *input* folder inside the extracted directories and copy target genomes in the fasta file format, renaming extensions from ".fasta" to ".fna."

6. Open a terminal in the scripts directories and run the main scripts:

    OligoWords1.2.1.1.py
    SeqWordSniffer.py

7. When prompted, type Y to analyze the genomes using the default parameters or follow the instructions for changing the settings according to your preferences.

8. For each genome, a ".out" file with the results will be written to the *output* folder inside the software directories.

9. SeqWord Gene Island Sniffer 1.0 generates a circular genomic map showing GEI location and nucleotide composition using different metrics. This map is useful to visualize the detected island, and must be compared with the GIPSy results for high-quality GEI annotation.

3.6 ICE and Integron Analysis and Prediction

ICEs are self-transmissible integrative elements found in both Gram-positive and Gram-negative bacteria encoding conjugation-related genes [27], whereas integrons show a diverse genetic organization, containing a number of combinations of gene cassettes, mostly related to antibiotic resistance and often associated with transposons and conjugative plasmids [28, 104, 105]. GEI prediction software, such as Alien_Hunter, may detect these anomalous regions; however, they are not capable of distinguishing GEIs, ICEs, and integrons. Therefore, in addition to the IS, prophage, and GEI predictions, a complete MGE analysis should include searches against the ICE and integron reference databases, such as ICEberg (http://db-mml.sjtu.edu.cn/ICEberg), and INTE-GRALL (http://integrall.bio.ua.pt).

3.7 Visualizing Prediction Results in Circular and Linear Genomic Maps

GView is a program for visualizing genomes. Although not developed specifically for MGE analyses, it can be used for viewing the results obtained in the previous steps in a broader genomic context, either for complete genomes or single contigs. It is also possible to visualize the previous results with the Artemis genome browser, which additionally allows users to perform manual curation of annotations, thus making it very useful for refining automated predictions (*see* **Note 16**). However, most MGE prediction software does not generate results in formats compatible with these programs. To integrate predictions with these viewers, we have developed Mobile Genetic Element Coordinates Extractor (MoGECE), which extracts mobile genetic element locations in prokaryotic genomes from outputs created by the MGE analysis software described in the previous section and generates files compatible with GView and Artemis. The following instructions show how to draw linear and circular genomic maps and visualize CDS annotations coupled with the MGE predictions.

3.7.1 Formatting Prediction Results with MoGECE 1.0.1

1. Download the MoGECE package from https://www.github.com/danillo-alvarenga/mogece/, extract it and move it to a folder in your software directory.

2. Enter a terminal from the MoGECE folder and add it to your environment:

   echo 'export PATH=$PATH:'$(pwd) >> ~/.bashrc; source ~/.bashrc

3. Go to the directories containing the relevant output files described in the previous subsections and run the program indicating the output file, the program in which this file was created, and which program visualization should be used. For Alien_Hunter, for example, issue the following command to the terminal in the outputs directory:

   MoGECE.py -f alienhunter.sco -l -a -g

4. MoGECE will output either a feature table for visualization in Artemis, a comma-separated values table for GView, or both according to the parameters you have chosen when running the program. The files produced will be named according to the program output in which they were based, e.g., an Alien_Hunter output file used as input for MoGECE with the *-a* and *-g* parameters will be processed and two files will be created: alienhunter.csv and alienhunter.ft.

3.7.2 Visualizing Results on Artemis 16.0.0

1. Download and extract the Artemis compressed file on your software folder from ftp://ftp.sanger.ac.uk/pub/resources/software/artemis/artemis.tar.gz, open the directory in the terminal, and enter the following command:

   echo 'export PATH=$PATH:'$(pwd) >> ~/.bashrc ; source ~/.bashrc

2. Start Artemis from a terminal by typing *art*.

3. In the "Options" menu, select the bacterial and plant plastid Genetic Code Table 11.

4. In the "File" menu, select "Open" and open the target genome in the GenBank file format.

5. In the genome annotation window, go to the "File" menu and click on "Read an Entry." Navigate to the directory containing the feature table created with MoGECE, change file types to "all files," and select the table (*see* **Note 17**).

3.7.3 Visualizing Results on GView 1.7

1. Download the Ubuntu/Debian GView package from https://www.gview.ca/wiki/GViewDownload/.

2. Double-click on the downloaded ".deb" file and install it from the Ubuntu Software Center.

3. Open GView by searching for its name in the dash.

4. In the "Open Files" window, go to the folder where your target genome is stored and select the ".gb" genome file as your sequence data. You may also indicate a previous GView Style Sheet in this window. Click on "Build Map" for visualizing the target genome.

5. GView can provide additional plots from ranges represented in comma-separated values. To create the necessary csv files from outputs produced by the software described in the previous steps, move the csv files created with MoGECE and the GView-StyleSheet.gss file included with it to the same directory where the GenBank-formatted file is stored and indicate both the genome file and the style sheet in the "Open Files" window (*see* **Notes 18** and **19**).

6. The circular and linear genomic maps can be exported to ".svg," ".png," and ".jpg" figures format.

3.8 How to Interpret the Results

Figures 2 and 3 show examples of analyses generated by this protocol. These circular genomic maps were produced by the GView software, and are used as a template for interpreting the results obtained. GView can generate a circular or linear genomic representation which can be zoomed-in or zoomed-out with point-and-click capabilities, showing CDS annotations. This is very useful to analyze each prediction, as described below. Linear and circular layouts can be interchanged in the "View" drop-down menu.

Figure 2 shows a global representation of all predicted MGEs together with CDS annotations of the *Escherichia coli* O26-H11 11368 genome. This genome is known to carry a large number of ISs and prophages and dozens of regions with potential anomalous nucleotide composition. Four examples of anomalous regions marked with dashed boxes were further explored. Figure 2-region A illustrates a typical laterally acquired island. This region was detected by both Alien_Hunter and SeqWord Sniffer, showing an anomaly in the GC content. In this example, the anomalous regions show lower GC content when compared to the genome average.

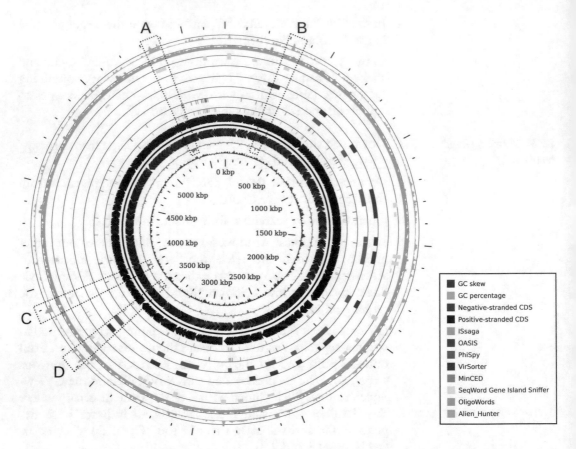

Fig. 2 Circular genomic representation of CDS and MGEs. GView circular representation of the *Escherichia coli* O26-H11 11368 genome illustrating from the inner to the outer circle in the following order: GC skew, GC content, CDS annotation, ISsaga, OASIS, PhiSpy, VirSorter, MinCED, SeqWord Gene Island Sniffer, OligoWords, and Alien_Hunter predictions. Dashed boxes A–D illustrate anomalous regions identified by different software

Depending on the analyzed genome, the laterally acquired island may show either higher or lower GC content when compared to the genome average. Abrupt changes in the GC content and GC skew are well-characterized landmarks of laterally acquired regions. However, this should not be taken as a rule, as GC characteristics are not unique parameters to identify laterally acquired islands. For instance, other cellular mechanisms such as intra-molecular recombination may generate similar patterns, and thus result in false positive predictions. Therefore, further manual inspection of the gene content in these regions is mandatory, and explained below. The CDS content of this region shows open reading frames (ORFs) encoding several hypothetical genes, IS transposases, chaperones, a lytic transglycosylase, and several genes from the type III secretion system, suggesting that it is a pathogenicity island. Figure 2-region B illustrates a typical GEI region, showing an integrase gene located on the border of the GEI. In addition, other ORFs, such as phage-

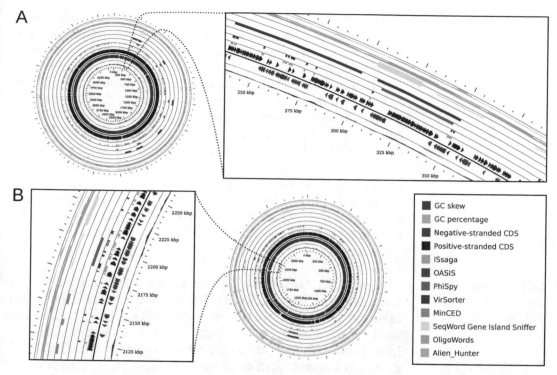

Fig. 3 Interpreting the circular maps results. Detailed Gview map (zoom-in) highlighting genomic regions with MGE predictions in bacterial and archaeal strains. (**a**) *Shigella flexneri* 2002017. (**b**) *Sulfolobus solfataricus* SULA

and flagellar-related genes, and several hypothetical ORFs were identified. Figure 2-region C illustrates a typical pathogenicity island detected by Alien_Hunter and SeqWord Sniffer, with atypical GC content and encoding ORFs related to a type III secretion system. Figure 2-region D and the other regions marked by PhiSpy and VirSorter are a typical prophage region, encoding integrases, holin, lysozyme and structural phages genes with homology to the lambda phage.

The left panel of Fig. 3a shows that *Shigella flexneri* carries a large number of ISs spread over its chromosome, together with some prophage regions and GEIs. The right panel of Fig. 3a shows a zoom-in of a specific region pointing that both ISsaga and OASIS generated similar IS predictions, indicating a consistent result. However, some differences were noted between PhiSpy and Vir-Sorter predictions: while PhiSpy detected only one prophage (blue bar), VirSorter detected two regions (pink bar). CDS analyses of the region detected only by VirSorter indicate a typical GEI, containing integrase, phage-related and IS transposase ORFs. The region detected by both PhiSpy and VirSorter was also marked by SeqWord Sniffer (yellow bar) and OligoWords (gray lines) predictions, which indicates a prophage region encoding several phage-related genes.

The right panel of Fig. 3 shows that *Sulfolobus solfataricus* carries large numbers of ISs and GEIs, and few prophages. The low number of prophages might be due to the presence of at least three CRISPR loci detected by MinCED (orange bars on the left panel). The CDS analysis of the surrounding genes of the CRISPR loci indicate the presence of Cas1 to 7 ORFs (CRISPR-associated genes), suggesting that this archaea may have had a long history of battle against phages. Indeed, a comparative analysis with the use of the CRISPRdb indicates that this genus carries several CRISPR loci. The other regions marked on the right panel follow the pattern shown in previous figure examples.

Overall, these results emphasize that multiple predictors and databases must be used for a proper MGE analysis (*see* **Note 20**), and that manual expert annotation is a mandatory second annotation step.

3.8.1 Chimeric MGEs

As mentioned above and illustrated in Figs. 2 and 3, it is relatively frequent to find chimeric MGEs. For instance, prophages and GEIs often carry ISs which are the product of different LGT events and must be considered separate entities with a distinct evolutionary history. Similarly, prophages are often integrated into GEIs, and these can undergo further IS invasion. Indeed, in certain cases, some GEIs may be generated by a number of different combinations and recombinations between prophages and IS.

Excluding plasmids, which exist as autonomously replicating extrachromosomal entities and are generally annotated separately, elements that are normally integrated into the chromosome but are self-transmissible by conjugation are classified as ICE. Interestingly, some GEIs are transferred by conjugation and carry genes with similarities to known plasmid transfer systems, indicating a common origin, whereas others can be transferred by packaging into phages [8]. ISCRs (Insertion Sequence with a Common Region) are related to ISs of the IS*91* family, but unlike IS*91* family members are generally associated with several antibiotic resistance genes [7]. In addition, an IS can insert within other ISs, resulting in structures like "russian dolls." A similar phenomenon, generated by a number of consecutive phage invasions, is also observed with prophages [2].

Thus, certain MGEs may include a combination of ISs, prophages, GEIs, integrons, and ICEs, generating chimeric structures by illegitimate and homologous recombination. The logic to be used in their analysis is often complex, especially since certain MGEs are fast evolving and can be interdigitated in a number of subtle ways. MGE annotation best practices must commence with a bottom-up approach: first detecting the simplest and smallest elements before passing to the more complex and bigger elements (e.g., ISs → prophages → GEIs/ICEs and integrons). This maximizes annotation efficiency, and largely avoids misinterpretation of these "intertwined" MGEs and the identification of false negatives and positives. This is an important concept which must be taken into account before starting MGE analysis of a prokaryote genome. A second concept is that all predictions must be validated by manual and expert annotation (*see* **Notes 21** and **22**).

3.8.2 Non-autonomous and Partial Elements

The occurrence of non-autonomous MGEs in Prokaryotic genomes is quite common. These mainly include: (a) MITEs (Miniature Inverted-Repeat Transposable Elements), composed of the inverted repeats of an IS or Tn and some short, interstitial, non-coding DNA, capable of impacting prokaryotic genome evolution by acting as substrates for genome rearrangements and by modifying gene expression by creating new promoters; (b) partial MGEs representing relics of prophages, ISs, and GEIs, mostly generated by genome decay or other recombination events.

In spite of their abundance, the predictors and software used in this guide are not able to detect MITEs, or to classify complete and partial MGEs. This level of MGE analysis requires manual and expert annotation of the predicted results, mainly based on BLAST analysis against the MGEs databases, such as ISfinder, PHAST, ACLAME, ICEberg and INTEGRAL, and literature search (*see* **Note 23**).

4   Notes

1. Some programs can recognize files only when they have certain extensions. If you are running into file recognition errors, try changing the extension. The GenBank flatfile format (.gbff) is virtually identical to the previous GenBank format (.gb or .gbk), but most prediction software only recognizes the ".gbk" or ".gb" file extensions. In such circumstances, the ".gbff" extension should be renamed ".gbk."

2. For bacteria with multiple chromosomes, it is better to analyze each chromosome separately instead of grouping them into a multi-fasta or multi-gb file. This is due to the different ways that programs deal with such files, which might result in errors when comparing their outputs.

3. Although some software has been developed for Linux distributions and OS X, they may work on other Unix-like systems such as BSD and Solaris as well. Likewise, some software that apparently targets bacteria exclusively may also work for archaeal genomes. Try including the software in your workflow before discarding it.

4. When using the command line, press <enter> after every command, type your password when required, and type *yes* or *y* whenever required. Make sure you have memorized the password you registered when installing Ubuntu, as it will

frequently be requested after commands requiring superuser authorization (the ones preceded by *sudo*).

5. Typing errors are the major source of errors when using the command line. Getting used to using auto-completion for filenames and programs by typing their first letters and then pressing <tab> prevents several mistakes.

6. If you are not using Ubuntu or another Debian-based Linux distribution as your operating system, the apt-get package manager may not be available. Alternatively, most Python packages may be installed using the *pip* or *easy_install* managers, and Perl packages are also available from *cpan*.

7. Some programs include a compiled version of the BLAST software that may run into library issues. If you encounter this issue, remove the embedded BLAST executable and create a symbolic link to your system's executable by starting a terminal on the executable directory and typing the following command:

   rm blastn; ln -s $(which blastn) blastn

8. The general IS annotation pipelines do not consider the ISCR (Insertion Sequence with Common Regions) elements. For that level of analysis and annotation it is necessary to follow the standards proposed by Toleman and collaborators [7] and to use the ISCR Database (http://medicine.cf.ac.uk/infect-immun/research/infection/antibacterial-agents/iscr-elements/). After drawing the Gview map, investigate the IS genomic context of the gene to identify possible ISCRs.

9. Avoid using spaces in file or directory names as some commands and programs (such as Alien_Hunter) may have trouble recognizing them. Suppress spaces or replace them with underlines.

10. New ISs should be submitted to ISfinder for attribution of a standard name and inclusion in the database.

11. Since many prophages are inserted near tRNA/tmRNA genes, results from tRNA predictor software compared by BLASTn with the complexity filter disabled against the given genome should be used to improve the detection of insertion sites and to define the prophage borders. This can be done with tRNAScan-SE [106] or Aragorn [107].

12. For prophage prediction refinement, further comparisons can be made by using the PHAST (http://phast.wishartlab.com) and ACLAME (http://aclame.ulb.ac.be/) databases.

13. After compiling a program and exporting its path to the global environment, it is necessary to reload bash, the default Ubuntu terminal interpreter, so that its location can be updated. If the exported program path is no longer accessible after closing a

terminal emulator window, reload bash by typing the command *source ~/.bashrc* in a terminal or by restarting your computer.

14. If you have trouble starting Docker, first make sure that the service is still running by typing *sudo service docker start* in the terminal.

15. For GEI prediction refinement, further comparisons can be made by using the SeqWord Genome Browser (http://www. bi.up.ac.za/SeqWord/mhhapplet.php) and IslandViewer3 (http://www.pathogenomics.sfu.ca/islandviewer).

16. Artemis is not particularly well suited for visualizing analyses from programs that generate coordinates for large sections of the genome (such as Alien_Hunter and OligoWords). GView is a better tool for such cases.

17. In Artemis, it is possible to visualize concurrently the results for different feature tables. To do so, first create a directory containing the feature tables alone and concatenate them into a single file by using the following command in the terminal:

*cat *.ft > all.ft*

18. If you are analyzing a draft genome, which is made up of a number of contigs, it is possible to visualize results for single contigs with GView if you analyze each contig separately and ignore the circular view.

19. Always compare the GView MGEs circular map results against the GIPSy predictions and the SeqWord Gene Island Sniffer circular map. If you followed the ISfinder/ISsaga gold standards for IS annotation, you can also compare these maps with the ISsaga circular map. For that go to the ISsaga webpage, and on the "Annotation" tab, click on the "ISbrowser preview."

20. Sometimes, the latest versions of some programs have not been thoroughly tested and present execution errors that the original versions described in the published papers do not. If you suspect you may be encountering such errors, look for previous versions.

21. Annotations regarding joined genes at the extremities of sequences may lead some programs to errors. Workarounds may include deleting such annotations or manually joining these genes (e.g., taking a part from the beginning of the genomic sequence to its end) and reannotating the genome.

22. Some programs rely on previous genome annotation for detecting MGE sequences. However, annotation is often not reliable for this purpose as it may overlook some elements. In addition, false positives are commonly produced by MGE analysis software. Always try generating a consensus from different software and refine the results by manual curation.

23. Last and most important: the results generated by this protocol are based on automated predictions. For high-quality results and downstream analysis, all predictions must be validated by manual, expert annotation through your preferred genome browser. Validated results can be exported to GView by editing the csv files generated by the MoGECE script. The final circular map can be exported as an svg figure for publication.

Acknowledgments

This work was supported by a project from the Coordenação de Aperfeiçoamento de Pessoal de Nível Superior (CAPES-BIGA, number 3385/2013). DOA was supported by a postdoctoral research fellowship from the São Paulo Research Foundation (FAPESP n° 2015/14600-5).

References

1. Canchaya C, Proux C, Fournous G et al (2003) Prophage genomics. Microbiol Mol Biol Rev 67:238–276

2. Canchaya C, Fournous G, Chibani-Chennoufi S et al (2003) Phage as agents of lateral gene transfer. Curr Opin Microbiol 6:417–424

3. Canchaya C, Fournous G, Brüssow H (2004) The impact of prophages on bacterial chromosomes. Mol Microbiol 53:9–18

4. Burrus V, Waldor MK (2004) Shaping bacterial genomes with integrative and conjugative elements. Res Microbiol 155:376–386

5. Frost LS, Leplae R, Summers AO et al (2005) Mobile genetic elements: the agents of open source evolution. Nature Rev Microbiol 3:722–732

6. Mazel D (2006) Integrons: agents of bacterial evolution. Nature Rev Microbiol 4:608–620

7. Toleman MA, Benett PM, Walsh TR (2006) ISCR elements: novel gene-capturing systems of the 21st century? Microbiol Mol Biol Rev 70:296–316

8. Juhas M, van der Meer JR, Gaillard M et al (2009) Genomic islands: tools of bacterial horizontal gene transfer and evolution. FEMS Microbiol Rev 33:376–393

9. Wozniak RA, Waldor MK (2010) Integrative and conjugative elements: mosaic mobile genetic elements enabling dynamic lateral gene flow. Nature Rev Microbiol 8:552–563

10. Varani AM, Monteiro-Vitorello CB, Nakaya HI et al (2013) The role of prophage in plant-pathogenic bacteria. Annu Rev Phytopathol 51:429–451

11. Fortier LC, Sekulovic O (2013) Importance of prophages to evolution and virulence of bacterial pathogens. Virulence 4:354–365

12. Siguier P, Gourbeyre E, Chandler M (2014) Bacterial insertion sequences: their genomic impact and diversity. FEMS Microbiol Rev 38:865–891

13. Siguier P, Gourbeyre E, Varani AM et al (2015) Everyman's guide to bacterial insertion sequences. In: Craig N, Chandler M, Gellert M et al (eds) Mobile DNA III. ASM Press, Washington

14. Camacho C, Coulouris G, Avagyan V et al (2009) BLAST+: architecture and applications. BMC Bioinformatics 10:421

15. Eddy SR (2011) Accelerated profile HMM searches. PLoS Comput Biol 7:e1002195

16. O'Leary NA, Wright MW, Brister JR et al (2016) Reference sequence (RefSeq) database at NCBI: current status, taxonomic expansion, and functional annotation. Nucleic Acids Res 44:D733–D745

17. Hunter S, Apweiler R, Attwood TK et al (2009) InterPro: the integrative protein signature database. Nucleic Acids Res 37:D211–D215

18. Punta M, Coggill PC, Eberhardt RY et al (2012) The Pfam protein families database. Nucleic Acids Res 40:D290–D301

19. Haft DH, Selengut JD, White O (2003) The TIGRFams database of protein families. Nucleic Acids Res 31:371–373

20. Lima T, Auchincloss AH, Coudert E et al (2009) HAMAP: a database of completely sequenced microbial proteome sets and manually curated microbial protein families in UniProtKB/Swiss-Prot. Nucleic Acids Res 37:D471–D478

21. Seemann T (2014) Prokka: rapid prokaryotic genome annotation. Bioinformatics 30:2068–2069

22. Aziz RK, Bartels D, Best AA et al (2008) The RAST server: rapid annotations using subsystems technology. BMC Genomics 9:75

23. Overbeek R, Olson R, Pusch GD et al (2014) The SEED and the rapid annotation of microbial genomes using subsystems technology (RAST). Nucleic Acids Res 42:D206–D214

24. Markowitz VM, Mavromatis K, Ivanova NN et al (2009) IMG ER: a system for microbial genome annotation expert review and curation. Bioinformatics 17:2271–2278

25. Varani AM, Siguier P, Gourbeyre E et al (2011) ISsaga is an ensemble of web-based methods for high throughput identification and semi-automatic annotation of insertion sequences in prokaryotic genomes. Genome Biol 12:R30

26. Siguier P, Perochon J, Lestrade L et al (2006) ISfinder: the reference centre for bacterial insertion sequences. Nucleic Acids Res 34: D32–D36

27. Bi D, Xu Z, Harrison EM et al (2012) ICEberg: a web-based resource for integrative and conjugative elements found in bacteria. Nucleic Acids Res 40:D621–D626

28. Moura A, Soares M, Pereira C et al (2009) INTEGRALL: a database and search engine for integrons, integrases and gene cassettes. Bioinformatics 25:1096–1098

29. Zhou Y, Liang Y, Lynch KH et al (2011) PHAST: a fast phage search tool. Nucleic Acids Res 39:W347–W352

30. Zomer A, Burghout P, Bootsma HJ et al (2012) ESSENTIALS: software for rapid analysis of high throughput transposon insertion sequencing data. PLoS One 7:e43012

31. Kichenaradja P, Siguier P, Pérochon J et al (2010) ISbrowser: an extension of ISfinder for visualizing insertion sequences in prokaryotic genomes. Nucleic Acids Res 38: D62–D68

32. Wagner A, Lewis C, Bichsel M (2007) A survey of bacterial insertion sequences using ISScan. Nucleic Acids Res 35:5284–5293

33. Hawkey J, Hamidian M, Wick RR et al (2015) ISMapper: identifying transposase insertion sites in bacterial genomes from short read sequence data. BMC Genomics 16:667

34. Biswas A, Gauthier DT, Ranjan D et al (2015) ISQuest: finding insertion sequences in prokaryotic sequence fragment data. Bioinformatics 31:3406–3412

35. Robinson DG, Lee MC, Marx CJ (2012) OASIS: an automated program for global investigation of bacterial and archaeal insertion sequences. Nucleic Acids Res 40:e174

36. Chen CL, Chang YJ, Hsueh CH (2013) PRAP: an ab initio software package for automated genome-wide analysis of DNA repeats for prokaryotes. Bioinformatics 21:2683–2689

37. Bao Z, Eddy SR (2002) Automated de novo identification of repeat sequence families in sequenced genomes. Genome Res 12:1269–1276

38. Girgis HZ (2015) Red: an intelligent, rapid, accurate tool for detecting repeats de-novo on the genomic scale. BMC Bioinformatics 16:227

39. Volfovsky N, Haas BJ, Salzberg SL (2001) A clustering method for repeat analysis in DNA sequences. Genome Biol 2: research0027.1–researc0027.11

40. Smit AFA, Hubley R, Green P (2015) RepeatMasker. http://www.repeatmasker.org. Accessed 24 Mar 2016

41. Achaz G, Boyer F, Rocha EPC et al (2007) Repseek, a tool to retrieve approximate repeats from large DNA sequences. Bioinformatics 23:119–121

42. Singh V, Mishra RK (2010) RISCI–repeat induced sequence changes identifier: a comprehensive, comparative genomics-based, in silico subtractive hybridization pipeline to identify repeat induced sequence changes in closely related genomes. BMC Bioinformatics 11:609

43. Riadi G, Medina-Moenne C, Holmes DS (2012) TnpPred: a web service for the robust prediction of prokaryotic transposases. Comp Funct Genomics 2012:678761

44. Leplae R, Lima-Mendez G, Toussaint A (2010) ACLAME: a classification of mobile genetic elements, update 2010. Nucleic Acids Res 38:D57–D61

45. Fouts DE (2006) Phage_Finder: automated identification and classification of prophage regions in complete bacterial genome sequences. Nucleic Acids Res 34:5839–5851

46. Akhter S, Aziz RK, Edwards RA (2012) PhiSpy: a novel algorithm for finding prophages in bacterial genomes that combines similarity- and composition-based strategies. Nucleic Acids Res 40:e126

47. Srividhya KV, Alaguraj V, Poornima G et al (2007) Identification of prophages in bacterial genomes by dinucleotide relative abundance difference. PLoS One 11:e1193

48. Lima-Mendez G, Van Helden J, Toussaint A et al (2008) Prophinder: a computational tool for prophage prediction in prokaryotic genomes. Bioinformatics 24:863–865

49. Roux S, Enault F, Hurwitz BL et al (2015) VirSorter: mining viral signal from microbial genomic data. PeerJ 3:e985

50. Skennerton CT, Imelfort M, Tyson GW (2013) Crass: identification and reconstruction of CRISPR from unassembled metagenomic data. Nucleic Acids Res 41:e105

51. Rousseau C, Gonnet M, Le Romancer M et al (2009) CRISPI: a CRISPR interactive database. Bioinformatics 25:3317–3318

52. Grissa I, Vergnaud G, Pourcel C (2008) CRISPRcompar: a website to compare clustered regularly interspaced short palindromic repeats. Nucleic Acids Res 36:W145–W148

53. Grissa I, Vergnaud G, Pourcel C (2007) The CRISPR database and tools to display CRISPRs and to generate dictionaries of spacers and repeats. BMC Bioinformatics 8:172

54. Pinello L, Canver MC, Hoban MD et al (2015) CRISPResso: sequencing analysis toolbox for CRISPR-Cas9 genome editing. bioRxiv. https://doi.org/10.1101/031203

55. Grissa I, Vergnaud G, Pourcel C (2007) CRISPRFinder: a web tool to identify clustered regularly interspaced short palindromic repeats. Nucleic Acids Res 35:W52–W57

56. Lange SJ, Alkhnbashi OS, Rose D et al (2013) CRISPRmap: an automated classification of repeat conservation in prokaryotic adaptive immune systems. Nucleic Acids Res 41:8034–8044

57. Bland C, Ramsey TL, Sabree F et al (2007) CRISPR recognition tool (CRT): a tool for automatic detection of clustered regularly interspaced palindromic repeats. BMC Bioinformatics 8:209

58. Alkhnbashi OS, Costa F, Shah SA et al (2014) CRISPRstrand: predicting repeat orientations to determine the crRNA-encoding strand at CRISPR loci. Bioinformatics 30:i489–i496

59. Biswas A, Gagnon JN, Brouns SJJ et al (2013) Bioinformatic prediction and analysis of crRNA targets. RNA Biol 10:817–827

60. Angly F, Skennerton C (2015) MinCED. https://github.com/ctSkennerton/minced. Accessed 24 Mar 2016

61. Edgar RC (2007) PILER-CR: fast and accurate identification of CRISPR repeats. BMC Bioinformatics 8:18

62. Che D, Hasan MS, Wang H et al (2011) EGID: an ensemble algorithm for improved genomic island detection in genomic sequences. Bioinformation 7:311–314

63. Che D, Hockenbury C, Marmelstein R et al (2010) Classification of genomic islands using decision trees and their ensemble algorithms. BMC Genomics 11:S1

64. Che D, Wang H, Fazekas J et al (2014) An accurate genomic island prediction method for sequenced bacterial and archaeal genomes. J Proteomics Bioinform 7:214–221

65. Soares SC, Geyik H, Ramos RTJ et al (2015) GIPSY: genomic island prediction software. J Biotechnol 232:2–11. https://doi.org/10.1016/j.jbiotec.2015.09.008

66. Hasan MS, Liu Q, Wang H et al (2012) GIST: genomic island suite of tools for predicting genomic islands in genomic sequences. Bioinformation 8:203–205

67. Che D, Wang H (2013) GIV: a tool for genomic islands visualization. Bioinformation 9:879–882

68. Jain R, Raminemi S, Parekh N (2011) IGIPT–integrated genomic island prediction tool. Bioinformation 7:307–310

69. Hudson CM, Lau BY, Williams KP (2015) Islander: a database of precisely mapped genomic islands in tRNA and tmRNA genes. Nucleic Acids Res 43:D48–D53

70. Baichoo S, Goodur H, Ramtohul V (2014) IslandHunter–a java-based GI detection software. PeerJ Preprints 2:e716v1

71. Hsiao W, Wan I, Jones SJ et al (2003) IslandPath: aiding detection of genomic islands in prokaryotes. Bioinformatics 19:418–420

72. Langille MGI, Hsiao WWL, Brinkman FSL (2008) Evaluation of genomic island predictors using a comparative genomics approach. BMC Bioinformatics 9:329

73. Langille MGI, Brinkman FSL (2009) IslandViewer: an integrated interface for computational indentification and visualization of genomic islands. Bioinformatics 25(5):25664–25665

74. Ou HY, He X, Harrison EM et al (2007) MobilomeFINDER: web-based tools for *in silico* and experimental discovery of bacterial genomic islands. Nucleic Acids Res 35:W97–W104

75. Brito DM, Maracaja-Coutinho V, Farias ST et al (2016) A novel method to predict genomic islands based on mean shift clustering algorithm. PLoS One 11:e0146352

76. Reva ON, Tümmler B (2005) Differentiation of regions with atypical oligonucleotide composition in bacterial genomes. BMC Bioinformatics 6:251

77. Ganesan H, Rakitianskaia AS, Davenport CF et al (2008) The SeqWord genome browser: an online tool for the identification and visualization of atypical regions of bacterial genomes through oligonucleotide usage. BMC Bioinformatics 9:333

78. Waack S, Keller O, Asper R et al (2006) Score-based prediction of genomic islands in prokaryotic genomes using hidden Markov models. BMC Bioinformatics 7:142

79. Ou HY, Chen LL, Lonnen J et al (2006) A novel strategy for the identification of genomic islands by comparative analysis of the contents and contexts of tRNA sites in closely related bacteria. Nucleic Acids Res 34:e3

80. Vernikos GS, Parkhill J (2006) Interpolated variable order motifs for identification of horizontally acquired DNA: revisiting the *Salmonella pathogenicity* islands. Bioinformatics 22:2196–2203

81. Yoon SH, Park YK, Lee S et al (2007) Towards pathogenomics: a web-based resource for pathogenicity islands. Nucleic Acids Res 35:D395–D400

82. Soares SC, Abreu VAC, Ramos RTJ et al (2012) PIPS: pathogenicity island prediction software. PLoS One 7:e30848

83. Pundhir S, Vijayvargiya H, Kumar A (2008) PredictBias: a server for the identification of genomic and pathogenicity islands in prokaryotes. In Silico Biol 8:0019

84. Joss MJ, Koenig JE, Labbate M et al (2009) ACID: annotation of cassette and integron data. BMC Bioinformatics 10:118

85. Rajan I, Aravamuthan S, Mande SS (2007) Identification of compositionally distinct regions in genomes using the centroid method. Bioinformatics 23:2672–2677

86. Lee CC, Chen YPP, Yao TJ (2013) GI-POP: a combinational annotation and genomic island prediction pipeline for ongoing microbial genome projects. Gene 518:114–123

87. Tu Q, Ding D (2003) Detecting pathogenicity islands and anomalous gene clusters by iterative discriminant analysis. FEMS Microbiol Lett 221:269–275

88. Merkl R (2004) SIGI: score-based identification of genomic islands. BMC Bioinformatics 5:22

89. Al-Nayyef H, Guyeux C, Bahi J (2014) A pipeline for insertion sequence detection and study for bacterial genome. Lect Notes Infor matics 235:85–99

90. Zhou F, Olman V, Xu Y (2008) Insertion sequences show diverse recent activities in cyanobacteria and Archaea. BMC Genomics 9:36

91. Bose M, Barber RD (2006) Prophage finder: a prophage loci prediction tool for prokaryotic genome sequences. In Silico Biol 6:0020

92. Upadhyay SK, Sharma S (2014) SSFinder: high throughput CRISPR-Cas target sites prediction tool. Biomed Res Int 2014:742482

93. Kamoun C, Payen T, Hua-Van A et al (2013) Improving prokaryotic transposable elements identification using a combination of de novo and profile HMM methods. BMC Genomics 14:700

94. Chen Y, Zhou F, Li G et al (2009) MUST: a system for identification of miniature inverted-repeat transposable elements and applications to *Anabaena variabilis* and *Haloquadratum walsbyi*. Gene 436:1–7

95. Herron PR, Hughes G, Chandra G (2004) Transposon express, a software application to report the identity of insertions obtained by comprehensive transposon mutagenesis of sequenced genomes: analysis of the preference for in vitro Tn5 transposition in to GC-rich DNA. Nucleic Acids Res 32:e113

96. Petkau A, Stuart-Edwards M, Stothard P et al (2010) Interactive microbial genome visualization with GView. Bioinformatics 26:3125–3126

97. Carver T, Harris SR, Berriman M et al (2012) Artemis: an integrated platform for visualization and analysis of high-throughput sequence-based experimental data. Bioinformatics 28:464–469

98. Bankevich A, Nurk S, Antipov D (2012) SPAdes: a new genome assembly algorithm and its applications to single-cell sequencing. J Comput Biol 19:455–477

99. Kajitani R, Toshimoto K, Noguchi H et al (2014) Efficient de novo assembly of highly heterozygous genomes from whole-genome shotgun short reads. Genome Res 24:1384–1395

100. Reddy TBK, Thomas AD, Stamatis D et al (2015) The genomes OnLine database (GOLD) v.5: a metadata management system based on a four level (meta)genome project classification. Nucleic Acids Res 43: D1099–D1106

101. Lang AS, Zhaxybayeva O, Beatty JT (2012) Gene transfer agents: phage-like elements of genetic exchange. Nat Rev Microbiol 10:472–482

102. Guy L, Nystedt B, Toft C et al (2013) A gene transfer agent and a dynamic repertoire of secretion systems hold the keys to the explosive radiation of the emerging pathogen *Bartonella*. PLoS Genet 9:e1003393

103. Horvath P, Barrangou R (2010) CRISPR/Cas, the immune system of bacteria and archaea. Science 327:167–170

104. Escudero JA, Loot C, Nivina A et al (2015) The integron: adaptation on demand. In: Craig N, Chandler M, Gellert M et al (eds) Mobile DNA III. ASM Press, Washington

105. Gillings M, Boucher Y, Labbate M et al (2008) The evolution of class 1 integrons and the rise of antibiotic resistance. J Bacteriol 190:5095–5100

106. Lowe TM, Eddy SR (1997) tRNAscan-SE: a program for improved detection of transfer RNA genes in genomic sequence. Nucleic Acids Res 25:955–964

107. Laslett D, Canback B (2004) ARAGORN, a program to detect rRNA genes and tmRNA genes in nucleotide equences. Nucleic Acids Res 32:11–16

Chapter 8

Comparative Metagenomics

Andrew Maltez Thomas, Felipe Prata Lima, Livia Maria Silva Moura, Aline Maria da Silva, Emmanuel Dias-Neto, and João C. Setubal

Abstract

Thanks in large part to newer, better, and cheaper DNA sequencing technologies, an enormous number of metagenomic sequence datasets have been and continue to be generated, covering a huge variety of environmental niches, including several different human body sites. Comparing these metagenomes and identifying their commonalities and differences is a challenging task, due not only to the large amounts of data, but also because there are several methodological considerations that need to be taken into account to ensure an appropriate and sound comparison between datasets. In this chapter, we describe current techniques aimed at comparing metagenomes generated by 16S ribosomal RNA and shotgun DNA sequencing, emphasizing methodological issues that arise in these comparative studies. We provide a detailed case study to illustrate some of these techniques using data from the Human Microbiome Project comparing the microbial communities from ten buccal mucosa samples with ten tongue dorsum samples in terms of alpha diversity, beta diversity, and their taxonomic and functional profiles.

Key words Microbiome, 16S rRNA, DNA shotgun, Comparative metagenomics, Metagenome

1 Introduction

The main biological topic of this chapter is the *microbiome*. Different and sometimes conflicting definitions of this term and the related terms *microbiota* and *metagenome* can be found in the literature. Following Whiteside et al. [1] we define **microbiota** as the set of microorganisms in a given environmental niche; **metagenome** as the genes and genomes of the microbiota, including plasmids; and **microbiome** as the set of genes and genomes of the microbiota, as well as the products of the microbiota and the host environment.

The study of microbiomes has gained considerable attention in the past few years [2–5] thanks in large part to newer, better, and cheaper DNA sequencing technologies [6], and to the technique of metagenomics [7]. Microbes are everywhere, but two contexts concentrate the bulk of research efforts: the human microbiome

João C. Setubal et al. (eds.), *Comparative Genomics: Methods and Protocols*, Methods in Molecular Biology, vol. 1704,
https://doi.org/10.1007/978-1-4939-7463-4_8, © Springer Science+Business Media LLC 2018

[3, 8] and environmental microbiomes [9, 10], resulting in an enormous number of metagenomic sequence datasets and covering an unprecedented variety of environmental niches, including several different human body sites.

In this chapter, we define comparative metagenomics as the problem of computationally comparing different metagenomes from different samples to learn about their commonalities and differences. There must, however, be a rationale for comparing a given sample set. Some usual reasons include time-series samples (the environment is "the same" and samples are collected at different time points; the ultimate goal is understanding the *dynamics* of a given microbiota), disease versus healthy states (e.g., cancer tumor versus normal tissue) [11, 12], different diets [13], or different geographical locations. A good review comparing the human microbiome in health and disease is Pflughoeft & Versalovic [14]; and also Lloyd-Price et al. [15].

Given a sample set, the two basic questions that can be posed about their metagenomes are: (1) How do they differ in terms of their taxonomic profile? This includes both presence/absence of taxa as well as differences in relative abundance; and (2) How do they differ in terms of their functional potential? In the sections that follow we will present an overview of various techniques that can be used to help answer these and related questions.

2   Metagenomic Data

The term metagenomics usually implies two kinds of sequencing data. One is 16S ribosomal RNA (rRNA) amplicon data (in the case of prokaryotes) or 18S rRNA amplicon data (in the case of eukaryotes). The other is genome shotgun DNA, in which the entire genome of organisms living in the niche to be studied is fragmented and sequenced. From now on, without loss of generality, we will refer to these two types as **16S** and **shotgun**. It should be noted that it is becoming more common to also sequence metatranscriptomic data (mRNA) [16] and metaproteomic data [17]. In this chapter we cover only metagenomic data.

Before we leave the topic of data, it is important to mention that *metadata* is an all-important aspect of microbiome studies. This includes all information about samples that is not molecular in nature. It may include geographic location, time and date when it was sampled, physical-chemical properties, individual characteristics of the sample donor, detailed disease aspects, and others [18]. Any microbiome project needs to pay special attention to metadata, without which it may be impossible to make biological sense of sequencing data, no matter how abundant.

3   Normalization

When conducting comparative metagenomic analyses researchers should keep in mind some factors that can significantly influence their results. For example, differences between sequence sampling depths (also known as library size) can affect both 16S and (to a lesser extent) shotgun derived data. For 16S-derived data, there are several normalization procedures aimed at decreasing this bias: total sum scaling (TSS), cumulative sum scaling (CSS), relative abundance and rarefaction, among others [19]. 16S copy number differs among bacteria and can also cause bias [20]. A number of methods and tools exist to deal with this bias; for example, CopyRighter [21], RDP classifier (new feature) [22], and the method of Kembel and colleagues [20]. A big caveat when dealing with shotgun metagenomic data, along with library size, is different genome sizes among prokaryotes. Tools such as MicrobeCensus [23] and GAAS [24] try to address this issue.

4   Comparative Analyses

Depending on the input data type (16S or shotgun), the number of samples (2, 3 or more groups with more than 1 sample/group), and other variables, there are a number of analyses that can be performed. When using public 16S data, researchers should be aware that data generated using different 16S primers, different variable regions, or different sequencing platforms [25] should not be compared, as differences in primer coverage rates, amplification biases, and sequencing error rates and patterns can interfere with these comparisons. For shotgun data, sequencing can produce nonuniform coverage (for example, less coverage of GC-rich regions), skewing representation of both genomes and genes [26]. Another caveat when dealing with comparative metagenomics is uneven coverage (or lack of representatives) of the natural phylogenetic diversity in reference databases [27]. Even in well-explored environments like the human gut, 43% of prokaryotic species abundance cannot be captured by current reference genome-based methods [28]. In other less studied environments such as soil and seawater, 90–98% of microbes have no sequenced genome at the species level [29].

4.1   Ecological Measures

In this section, we describe the comparative ecological measures *alpha diversity, beta diversity,* and *microbial interaction/association networks.* Such measures are typically evaluated in 16S-generated datasets, as data heterogeneity tends to have less impact.

Alpha diversity: It pertains to a single sample's microbial community, with regard to its richness, evenness, and diversity. *Richness* refers to the number of different species or units present in a community; *evenness* refers to variations in the abundance of species/units, and *diversity* takes into account both richness and evenness. Some diversity measures may give more weight to dominant members of the community, as is the case with the Simpson diversity index. The Shannon and Simpson diversity indexes are common ways to evaluate diversity within a given sample and have been implemented in tools such as *Qiime* [30], phyloseq [31], vegan [32], and DiversitySeq [33]. Once researchers have calculated these measures for each sample of their comparison groups, they can compare how these measures differ between them. For a more detailed description of the mathematical formulations, purposes, and properties of different diversity indices, we refer readers to Finotello et al. [33].

Beta diversity: It pertains to the variation in community structure among a set of sample units (*variation*) or change in community structure from one sampling unit to another along a spatial, temporal, or environmental gradient (*turnover*) [34]. Usually, researchers calculate distances between all pairs of samples based on how similar/dissimilar their microbial communities are, and then pairwise distance matrices are generated. For 16S-based analysis, this can be done using count data at a certain taxonomical level and distances such as Bray-Curtis or using phylogenetic trees and UniFrac [35] distances. For a more detailed review on distance calculations and beta diversity fundamentals, we point readers to the review by Tuomisto [36]. For shotgun data, nucleotide distances can be calculated between different samples using tools such as MASH [37]. Researchers can then compare intra-group variabilities as well as differences in inter-group variabilities [38]. These distance matrices can also be used to analyze associations with categorical or numerical metadata, as well as with distance matrices created using only metadata (not a taxon table).

Microbial association networks: Microbial association networks for each of the comparison groups can also be generated; network properties such as topology, density, and clustering coefficients, among others, can be computed and compared. These networks can be created at the Operational Taxonomic Unit (OTU) level (which is more sensitive to OTU clustering algorithms and sequencing depth) or at the genus level. Examples of tools to create such networks include SparCC [39], Molecular Ecological Network Analysis Pipeline (MENAP) [40], Sparse InversE Covariance estimation for Ecological Association Inference (SPIEC-EASI) [41], and Local Similarity Analysis (LSA) [42]. A nice review of network association analysis techniques is given by Layeghifard et al. [43].

4.2 Abundance

Differential Abundance: Differences in microbial community structure can be determined between samples and/or groups. The absolute abundance of a taxon or gene in a community cannot be fully retrieved from metagenomic shotgun/16S sequencing alone; however, relative abundances and copy numbers can capture comparative biological properties. Relative abundance may be sufficient to compare taxa or genes that vary by several orders of magnitude across communities, whereas copy number is more sensitive in detecting smaller ranges. This type of analysis can be conducted at different taxonomic levels, depending on the researcher's preference and/or the nature of the data. For example, some datasets may have a small percentage of sequences classified at the genus level, therefore needing a higher taxonomical level (such as phylum) in order to compare community structure, taking into account larger (and therefore representative) fractions of the data. Differential abundance analysis works best when researchers have more than one sample in each comparison group, as most statistical methods require more than one sample per group. Examples of tools that conduct such analysis include LEfSe [44], Metagenome-Seq [45], and MetaStats [46]. Instead of analyzing relative or normalized abundances for each taxon, researchers may choose to compute the ratio of all possible taxa. For example, one could simply compute the *Bacteroidetes/Firmicutes* ratio for all samples and compare it between groups.

Differential abundance analysis can also be conducted on KEGG modules and pathways [47], allowing the determination of differences in the abundance of microbial pathways [48]. Researchers can also compare samples in terms of the presence or absence of gene functions of interest. Examples of tools include HUMAnN [49], MG-RAST [50], MUSiCC [51], and FMAP [52]. A hypothesis-driven approach is to identify and quantify specific protein sequences using ShortBRED [53], aiming to investigate differences in protein abundance between comparison groups. For a more in-depth review on how to accurately and quantitatively compare metagenomes in terms of their taxonomic and functional profiles, we refer readers to Nayfach and Pollard [26].

Presence/Absence: Researchers seeking to reveal broader trends between communities can also analyze differences in microbial community membership. Such analysis has some technical caveats, which include differing sequencing/sampling depths of the comparison groups. One such caveat is attempting to correct zero values, which can fall into two categories: zeros that are a consequence of under-sampling (known as "rounded zeros") and zeros that truly represent the absence of taxa (known as "essential" or "structural" zeros). Paulson et al. [45] present a statistical method for dealing with these two kinds of zero values.

An alternative to this analysis is computing the core microbiome, which can be defined as the set of microbes present in at least a predetermined percentage of samples. This type of analysis is helpful when researchers want to know what microbes are essential and contribute to the stability of the community; different communities may have different key members. This analysis has been implemented in *Qiime* [30] and MetagenomeSeq [45], among others. Researchers should bear in mind that differences in composition between core microbiomes do not necessarily imply differences in their overall functional profiles [54].

High-level phenotypes: Depending on the source material of the metagenomic data, researchers may choose to analyze differences in phenotypes between samples. This is normally done using taxonomic information derived from the data in order to calculate proportions of phenotypes such as Gram-negative, Gram-positive, aerobic, anaerobic, and biofilm-forming bacteria. Researchers should proceed with caution when opting to run this type of analysis because not all microbial communities may be represented in taxonomy databases for which phenotypic data are available. Generally, well-explored environments tend to have greater representativeness of such microbe information. Example tools for this analysis are BugBase (https://bugbase.cs.umn.edu or https://github.com/danknights/bugbase) and TRAITAR for shotgun data [55].

Community types: Also known as *enterotypes*, community types stratify samples based on the relative abundances of their microbes at a certain taxonomic level. Generally, this analysis is run at the genus level. This analysis is helpful when researchers want to know whether there are underlying subgroups or gradients between their samples that are independent of the predetermined comparison groups. Underlying community types may be associated with several community characteristics, such as diversity, predominance of certain genera, and dysbiosis. R packages available for enterotyping analysis include Dirichlet Multinomial Models (DMM) [56] and Partitioning Around Medoids (PAM) [57].

Association with metadata: Researchers can also search for associations between microbes and numerical and categorical metadata associated with their samples. Because of the compositional nature of metagenomic datasets, certain precautions need to be taken due to spurious correlations. The tool MaAsLin (Multivariate Association with Linear Models) (https://bitbucket.org/biobakery/maaslin/) addresses this issue.

Feature subset selection: This analysis aims at discovering microbial taxa or genes that can accurately and reproducibly classify samples into two or more classes (comparison groups). These features can be found by computing differentially abundant groups and applying relevant statistical analysis tools. Example tools include FIZZY [58] and Metagenomic prediction Analysis based on Machine Learning (metAML) [59].

4.3 Other Comparative Analyses

Researchers can compare microbial communities in terms of codon bias, as it can be used as a prediction tool for lifestyle-specific genes across the entire microbial community [60]. For a more in-depth review of this analysis and its implications, we refer readers to Quax et al. [61]. 16S-based analyses are often times hindered by limited taxonomic resolution; however, a high-resolution method termed oligotyping can overcome this limitation by evaluating individual nucleotide positions using Shannon entropy, identifying the most information-rich positions and defining oligotypes [62]. Such oligotypes can be used to investigate sub-OTU differences among different comparison groups [63, 63]. When dealing with poorly characterized microbiomes, researchers may have trouble completely determining the specific microbial species present. In light of this, Qin et al. [65] devised the generalized concept of a metagenomic linkage group (MLG), defined as "a group of genetic material in a metagenome that is probably physically linked as a unit rather than being independently distributed." In other words, they are groups of genes that co-exist among different individual samples and have consistent abundance levels and taxonomic assignments.

4.4 Statistical Analysis

Metagenomic sequencing data are compositional in nature and are constrained to sum to a constant. The total absolute abundances of bacteria are not recoverable from raw sequence counts, but the proportions of each taxon are. This type of data is subject to what is known as the "closure problem," which occurs when components necessarily compete to make the constant constraint sum [66]. This can cause great changes in the absolute abundance of one taxa that drives apparent changes in the abundances of other taxa, violating assumptions of sample independence, which can lead to bias and flawed inferences. Metagenomic sequence data also tends to be of high dimensionality (numerous categories), sparse (many zeros dominating all other values), under-determined (substantially fewer samples than taxa/variables), and with differing library sizes. Due to these characteristics, parametric statistical models may not be suitable. Nonparametric methods generally avoid variance estimates that can be skewed by sparse samples, however can lack power to perform inference on low-abundance taxa. In these cases, parametric methods can be a better choice, but researchers have to keep in mind the risk of data violating the assumptions of these models. For more information on compositional data analysis of the microbiome, we refer readers to the review by Tsilimigras and Fodor [67]. Researchers may opt for one or more of the statistical tests below:

Parametric tests: zero-inflated Gaussian (ZIG) mixture model [45] and DESeq negative binomial Wald test [68].

Nonparametric tests: Kruskall-Wallis, Wilcoxon Rank Sum Test, and Analysis of Composition of Microbiomes (ANCOM) [69].

We close these sections by mentioning two web platforms that provide many tools for comparative metagenomics: IMG/M [70] and MG-RAST [50]. Both accept user-provided inputs and run sophisticated automated pipelines generating browsable results. In addition, users can run diverse comparative analyses using their own data and other public metagenomes available on each one of these sites.

5   Case Study Using Data from the Human Microbiome Project

In this section, we present results comparing microbial communities of 20 individuals obtained from the Human Microbiome Project (HMP). We downloaded 16S V3-V5 and shotgun preprocessed data from ten buccal mucosa (BM) and ten tongue dorsum (TD) samples using the HMP's data access browser. All scripts used in this analysis are available at (http://github.com/andrewmaltezthomas/comparativemetagenomics/blob/master/index.rmd). All the analysis steps shown here assume data to have undergone preprocessing steps that are not in the scope of this chapter, and that the researcher is working with a taxon and/or function table for shotgun data and an OTU table and a OTU phylogenetic tree for 16S data.

5.1   Alpha Diversity

Create a mapping file: Software such as *Qiime* require a mapping file which contains all metadata pertinent to the analysis, including which sample belongs to which comparison group.

Filter the OTU table: OTU tables generated by 16S rRNA data are generally sparse, so in order to remove spurious OTUs formed during the OTU picking process, it is common practice to filter out OTUs with a minimum abundance threshold (in this analysis the minimum requirement was three reads) and found in a minimum number of samples (25% in the results presented here).

Find out the minimum number of sequences: This number is used to rarefy samples to the same depth and to perform rarefaction analysis. However, researchers may opt for a different normalization approach.

Perform rarefaction analysis: We performed sampling rarefaction using vegan's *specaccum()* function and sequencing rarefaction using *Qiime*'s *alpha_rarefaction.py*. Sampling effort rarefaction analysis revealed that TD samples possessed, on average, a greater number of OTUs than BM samples. It also showed that the discovery of new OTUs when using ten samples per group tended to reach a plateau, where approximately 2000 distinct OTUs were found (Fig. 1a). Sequencing rarefaction analysis revealed that, again, TD samples had higher richness (seen by the number of distinct OTUs) than BM samples and that obtaining 1800 sequences was not enough to saturate the number of OTUs present in all the samples (Fig. 1b).

Perform multiple rarefactions at the same depth: Performing multiple rarefactions, as opposed to one, increases sensibility to

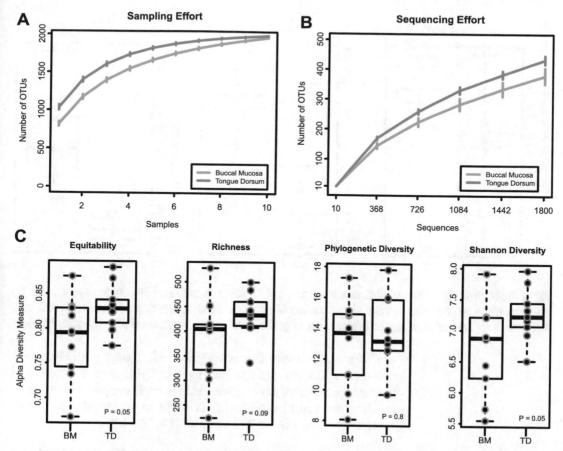

Fig. 1 Alpha diversity in buccal mucosa and tongue dorsum samples seen by 16S rRNA sequencing. (**a**) Sampling effort for both groups. *Lines* represent the mean number of OTUs and error bars represent ± standard error. (**b**) Sequencing effort for both groups. *Lines* represent the mean number of OTUs and error bars represent ± standard error. (**c**) Boxplots showing different alpha diversity metrics evaluated by 16S data. *Vertical lines* represent the median for each group and *dotted lines* represent the interquartile ranges between the 25th and 75th percentiles

detect differences in alpha diversity between groups and improves confidence in the results.

Calculate alpha diversity metrics on each of the rarefied tables: This step is aimed at calculating different alpha diversity metrics such as richness, evenness (or equitability), and diversity on each table and obtaining their mean. We used *Qiime*'s *alpha_diversity.py* and *collate_alpha.py* scripts. When we evaluated alpha diversity between both groups, we saw increases in evenness, Shannon diversity, and richness in TD samples compared to BM samples; however, these increases were not statistically significant (Fig. 1c).

Calculate the total number of genera: From the MetaPhlAn [71] and/or MG-RAST taxon table, count the number of genera (with abundances above a certain threshold, i.e., >0) for each sample.

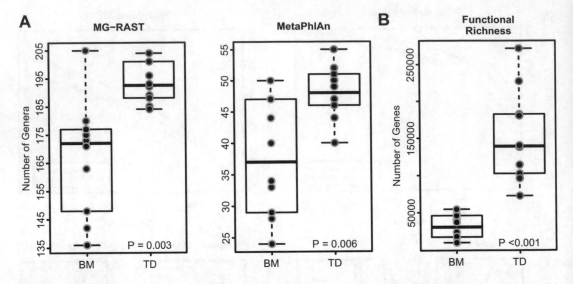

Fig. 2 Alpha diversity in buccal mucosa and tongue dorsum samples evaluated by shotgun sequencing. (**a**) Boxplots showing the total number of genera identified by shotgun sequencing by both MG-RAST and MetaPhlAn. (**b**) Boxplot showing the total number of genes identified by annotated shotgun sequencing data

Calculate the total number of genes. After gene prediction and gene annotation, researchers can parse the gff3 generated file and count the number of genes identified for each sample. Using shotgun data, we found significant increases in the total number of genera and genes among TD samples (Fig. 2a–b).

5.2   Beta Diversity

Calculate pairwise distances. The input is the OTU table containing the number of sequences observed in each OTU (rows) for each sample (columns) and a phylogenetic tree. The output is a symmetric distance matrix containing a dissimilarity value for each pairwise sample comparison (we used Bray-Curtis, Weighted UniFrac, and Unweighted UniFrac).

Compare pairwise distances. For each metric used in the previous step, a distance matrix is created which is used as input, along with a mapping file. Distances within all samples of a field category are compared (i.e., tongue dorsum vs buccal mucosa). When we analyzed differences in pairwise distances between both groups, we found that TD samples were significantly more similar amongst themselves both in terms of phylogenetic presence/absence (Unweighted UniFrac) and abundance (Weighted UniFrac), elucidating a phylogenetically more similar microbial community among these samples (Fig. 3a).

Ordination: Distance matrices can be read into R or generated using the vegan R package and used to create ordination plots using the *plot_ord()* function like in Fig. 3b.

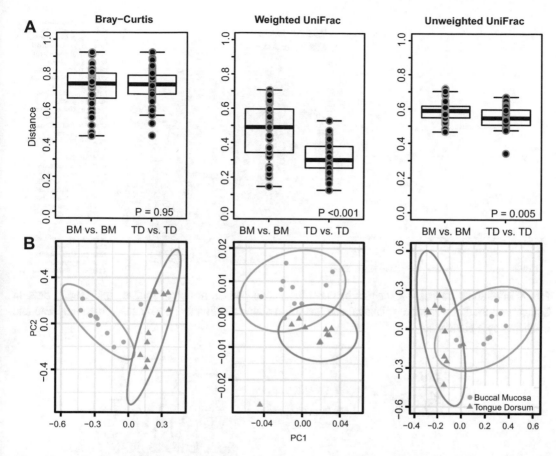

Fig. 3 Beta diversity comparisons between buccal mucosa and tongue dorsum samples using different distance metrics. (**a**) Inter group pairwise distance comparison seen by Bray-Curtis, Unweighted UniFrac, and Weighted UniFrac. (**b**) Principal Coordinate Analysis (PCoA) using three different distance metrics

5.3 Differential Abundance

Format the taxon table: Analysis using LEfSe requires researchers to format the MetaPhlAn generated taxon table in order to run the analysis. Using shotgun data, we investigated differences in genera abundance between both groups using the MetaPhlAn taxon table and LEfSe and found several taxa to be differentially abundant between both groups. We found significant increases of *Streptococcus*, *Gemella*, and *Proponiobacterium* in BM samples, whereas *Veillonella* and *Prevotella* were more abundant in TD samples (Fig. 4). Genera enriched in TD samples were primarily part of the *Proteobacteria* phylum, whereas genera enriched in BM samples were primarily part of the *Firmicutes* phylum (Fig. 4—cladogram).

Filter KEGG modules and pathways: After analyzing samples using HUMAnN, researchers should filter KEGG modules and pathways to keep those that were found in at least a predetermined number of samples (in this case study we used all) and with a coverage threshold for both modules and pathways as well (0.7 used here). When we investigated differences in KEGG modules, we found 16 to be significantly more abundant among TD samples compared to BM samples (Fig. 5). Among these, five modules were

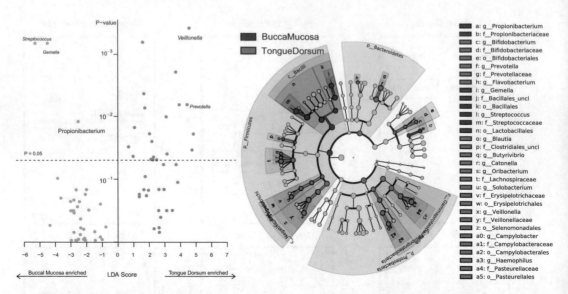

Fig. 4 Differential abundance analysis between taxonomic profiles of buccal mucosa and tongue dorsum samples analyzed by linear discriminant analysis (LDA) coupled with effect size measurements (LEfSe) and projected by a cladogram

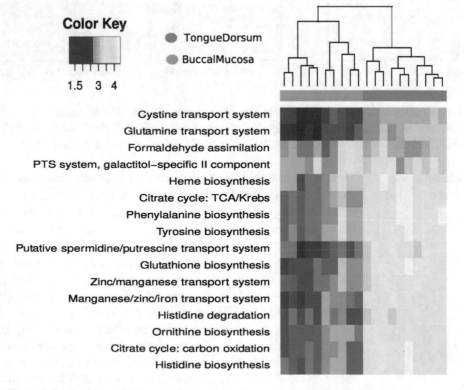

Fig. 5 Differentially abundant KEGG modules in buccal mucosa and tongue dorsum samples analyzed by HUMAnN

involved with transport systems and six with biosynthesis systems, accounting for more than half of the enriched modules. Readers should note that we discovered TD shotgun samples to have, on average, $1.4\times$ more sequences than BM samples, a fact that we accounted for when conducting this analysis. However, we found no KEGG modules or pathways significantly more abundant in BM samples, most probably caused by this difference in sequencing depth.

References

1. Whiteside SA, Razvi H, Dave S, Reid G, Burton JP (2015) The microbiome of the urinary tract—a role beyond infection. Nat Rev Urol 12:81–90. https://doi.org/10.1038/nrurol.2014.361

2. Costello EK, Lauber CL, Hamady M, Fierer N, Gordon JI, Knight R (2009) Bacterial community variation in human body habitats across space and time. Science 326:1694–1697. https://doi.org/10.1126/science.1177486

3. Nelson KE, Weinstock GM, Highlander SK, Worley KC, Creasy HH, Wortman JR, Rusch DB, Mitreva M, Sodergren E, Chinwalla AT, Feldgarden M, Gevers D, Haas BJ, Madupu R, Ward DV, Birren BW, Gibbs RA, Methe B, Petrosino JF, Strausberg RL, Sutton GG, White OR, Wilson RK, Durkin S, Giglio MG, Gujja S, Howarth C, Kodira CD, Kyrpides N, Mehta T, Muzny DM, Pearson M, Pepin K, Pati A, Qin X, Yandava C, Zeng Q, Zhang L, Berlin AM, Chen L, Hepburn TA, Johnson J, McCorrison J, Miller J, Minx P, Nusbaum C, Russ C, Sykes SM, Tomlinson CM, Young S, Warren WC, Badger J, Crabtree J, Markowitz VM, Orvis J, Cree A, Ferriera S, Fulton LL, Fulton RS, Gillis M, Hemphill LD, Joshi V, Kovar C, Torralba M, Wetterstrand KA, Abouellleil A, Wollam AM, Buhay CJ, Ding Y, Dugan S, FitzGerald MG, Holder M, Hostetler J, Clifton SW, Allen-Vercoe E, Earl AM, Farmer CN, Liolios K, Surette MG, Xu Q, Pohl C, Wilczek-Boney K, Zhu D, Zhu D (2010) A catalog of reference genomes from the human microbiome. Science 328:994–999. https://doi.org/10.1126/science.1183605

4. Grice EA, Segre JA (2012) The human microbiome: our second genome. Annu Rev Genomics Hum Genet 13:151–170. https://doi.org/10.1146/annurev-genom-090711-163814

5. Blaser M, Bork P, Fraser C, Knight R, Wang J (2013) The microbiome explored: recent insights and future challenges. Nat Rev Microbiol 11:213–217. https://doi.org/10.1038/nrmicro2973

6. Schmieder R, Edwards R (2012) Insights into antibiotic resistance through metagenomic approaches. Future Microbiol 7:73–89. https://doi.org/10.2217/fmb.11.135

7. Escobar-Zepeda A, Vera-Ponce de León A, Sanchez-Flores A (2015) The road to metagenomics: from microbiology to DNA sequencing technologies and bioinformatics. Front Genet 6:348. https://doi.org/10.3389/fgene.2015.00348

8. Huttenhower C, Gevers D, Knight R, Abubucker S, Badger JH, Chinwalla AT, Creasy HH, Earl AM, FitzGerald MG, Fulton RS, Giglio MG, Hallsworth-Pepin K, Lobos EA, Madupu R, Magrini V, Martin JC, Mitreva M, Muzny DM, Sodergren EJ, Versalovic J, Wollam AM, Worley KC, Wortman JR, Young SK, Zeng Q, Aagaard KM, Abolude OO, Allen-Vercoe E, Alm EJ, Alvarado L, Andersen GL, Anderson S, Appelbaum E, Arachchi HM, Armitage G, Arze CA, Ayvaz T, Baker CC, Begg L, Belachew T, Bhonagiri V, Bihan M, Blaser MJ, Bloom T, Bonazzi V, Paul Brooks J, Buck GA, Buhay CJ, Busam DA, Campbell JL, Canon SR, Cantarel BL, Chain PSG, Chen I-MA, Chen L, Chhibba S, Chu K, Ciulla DM, Clemente JC, Clifton SW, Conlan S, Crabtree J, Cutting MA, Davidovics NJ, Davis CC, DeSantis TZ, Deal C, Delehaunty KD, Dewhirst FE, Deych E, Ding Y, Dooling DJ, Dugan SP, Michael Dunne W, Scott Durkin A, Edgar RC, Erlich RL, Farmer CN, Farrell RM, Faust K, Feldgarden M, Felix VM, Fisher S, Fodor AA, Forney LJ, Foster L, Di Francesco V, Friedman J, Friedrich DC, Fronick CC, Fulton LL, Gao H, Garcia N, Giannoukos G, Giblin C, Giovanni MY, Goldberg JM, Goll J, Gonzalez A, Griggs A, Gujja S, Kinder Haake S, Haas BJ, Hamilton HA, Harris EL, Hepburn TA, Herter B, Hoffmann DE, Holder ME, Howarth C, Huang KH, Huse SM, Izard J, Jansson JK, Jiang H, Jordan C, Joshi V, Katancik JA, Keitel WA, Kelley ST, Kells C, King NB, Knights D, Kong HH, Koren O, Koren S, Kota KC, Kovar CL,

Kyrpides NC, La Rosa PS, Lee SL, Lemon KP, Lennon N, Lewis CM, Lewis L, Ley RE, Li K, Liolios K, Liu B, Liu Y, Lo C-C, Lozupone CA, Dwayne Lunsford R, Madden T, Mahurkar AA, Mannon PJ, Mardis ER, Markowitz VM, Mavromatis K, McCorrison JM, McDonald D, McEwen J, McGuire AL, McInnes P, Mehta T, Mihindukulasuriya KA, Miller JR, Minx PJ, Newsham I, Nusbaum C, O'Laughlin M, Orvis J, Pagani I, Palaniappan K, Patel SM, Pearson M, Peterson J, Podar M, Pohl C, Pollard KS, Pop M, Priest ME, Proctor LM, Qin X, Raes J, Ravel J, Reid JG, Rho M, Rhodes R, Riehle KP, Rivera MC, Rodriguez-Mueller B, Rogers Y-H, Ross MC, Russ C, Sanka RK, Sankar P, Fah Sathirapongsasuti J, Schloss JA, Schloss PD, Schmidt TM, Scholz M, Schriml L, Schubert AM, Segata N, Segre JA, Shannon WD, Sharp RR, Sharpton TJ, Shenoy N, Sheth NU, Simone GA, Singh I, Smillie CS, Sobel JD, Sommer DD, Spicer P, Sutton GG, Sykes SM, Tabbaa DG, Thiagarajan M, Tomlinson CM, Torralba M, Treangen TJ, Truty RM, Vishnivetskaya TA, Walker J, Wang L, Wang Z, Ward DV, Warren W, Watson MA, Wellington C, Wetterstrand KA, White JR, Wilczek-Boney K, Wu Y, Wylie KM, Wylie T, Yandava C, Ye L, Ye Y, Yooseph S, Youmans BP, Zhang L, Zhou Y, Zhu Y, Zoloth L, Zucker JD, Birren BW, Gibbs RA, Highlander SK, Methé BA, Nelson KE, Petrosino JF, Weinstock GM, Wilson RK, White O (2012) Structure, function and diversity of the healthy human microbiome. Nature 486:207–214. https://doi.org/10.1038/nature11234

9. Gilbert JA, Jansson JK, Knight R (2014) The earth microbiome project: successes and aspirations. BMC Biol 12:69. https://doi.org/10.1186/s12915-014-0069-1

10. MetaSUB International Consortium (2016) The metagenomics and metadesign of the subways and urban biomes (MetaSUB) international consortium inaugural meeting report. Microbiome 4:24. https://doi.org/10.1186/s40168-016-0168-z

11. Feng Q, Liang S, Jia H, Stadlmayr A, Tang L, Lan Z, Zhang D, Xia H, Xu X, Jie Z, Su L, Li X, Li X, Li J, Xiao L, Huber-Schönauer U, Niederseer D, Xu X, Al-Aama JY, Yang H, Wang J, Kristiansen K, Arumugam M, Tilg H, Datz C, Wang J, Jemal A, Brenner H, Kloor M, Pox CP, Vogelstein B, Kinzler KW, Grivennikov SI, Iida N, Belcheva A, Kostic AD, Castellarin M, Gevers D, Kostic AD, Qin J, Li J, Willett W, Yang K, Qin J, Sanapareddy N, Chen L, Xiong Z, Sun L, Yang J, Jin Q, Arumugam M, Ding T, Schloss PD, Knights D, Greene FL, Imperiale TF,

Smith E, Macfarlane G, Narushima S, Jaeggi T, Ma Y, Hwa V, Salyers AA, Raman R, Myette JR, Ulmer JE, Viaud S, Wu S, Arthur JC, Arthur JC, Dicksved J, Baxter NT, Zackular JP, Chen GY, Schloss PD, Weir TL, Smith EA, Macfarlane GT, Robrish SA, Oliver C, Thompson J, Robrish SA, Oliver C, Thompson J, Islam KB, Sayin SI, Devkota S, Yang F, Yoshimoto S, Jones RM, Okada T, Stadlmayr A, Bond JH, Winawer SJ, AG Z, Craig CL, Luo R, Kent WJ, Chao A, BH MA, Anderson MJ, Zapala MA, Schork NJ, Patil KR, Nielsen J (2015) Gut microbiome development along the colorectal adenoma–carcinoma sequence. Nat Commun 6:6528. https://doi.org/10.1038/ncomms7528

12. Thomas AM, de Jesus EC, Lopes A, Aguiar Junior S, Begnami MD, Rocha RM, Carpinetti PA, Camargo AA, Hoffmann C, Freitas HC, da Silva IT, Nunes DN, Setubal JC, Dias-Neto E (2016) Tissue-associated bacterial alterations in rectal carcinoma patients revealed by 16S rRNA community profiling. Front Cell Infect Microbiol 6:179. https://doi.org/10.3389/FCIMB.2016.00179

13. David LA, Maurice CF, Carmody RN, Gootenberg DB, Button JE, Wolfe BE, Ling AV, Devlin AS, Varma Y, Fischbach MA, Biddinger SB, Dutton RJ, Turnbaugh PJ (2014) Diet rapidly and reproducibly alters the human gut microbiome. Nature 505:559–563. https://doi.org/10.1038/nature12820

14. Pflughoeft KJ, Versalovic J (2012) Human microbiome in health and disease. Annu Rev Pathol 7:99–122. https://doi.org/10.1146/annurev-pathol-011811-132421

15. Lloyd-Price J, Abu-Ali G, Huttenhower C (2016) The healthy human microbiome. Genome Med 8:51. https://doi.org/10.1186/s13073-016-0307-y

16. Bashiardes S, Zilberman-Schapira G, Elinav E, Elinav E (2016) Use of metatranscriptomics in microbiome research. Bioinform Biol Insights 10:19–25. https://doi.org/10.4137/BBI.S34610

17. Hettich RL, Pan C, Chourey K, Giannone RJ (2013) Metaproteomics: harnessing the power of high performance mass spectrometry to identify the suite of proteins that control metabolic activities in microbial communities. Anal Chem 85:4203–4214. https://doi.org/10.1021/ac303053e

18. Yilmaz P, Kottmann R, Field D, Knight R, Cole JR, Amaral-Zettler L, Gilbert JA, Karsch-Mizrachi I, Johnston A, Cochrane G, Vaughan R, Hunter C, Park J, Morrison N, Rocca-Serra P, Sterk P, Arumugam M, Bailey M, Baumgartner L, Birren BW, Blaser

MJ, Bonazzi V, Booth T, Bork P, Bushman FD, Buttigieg PL, Chain PSG, Charlson E, Costello EK, Huot-Creasy H, Dawyndt P, DeSantis T, Fierer N, Fuhrman JA, Gallery RE, Gevers D, Gibbs RA, San Gil I, Gonzalez A, Gordon JI, Guralnick R, Hankeln W, Highlander S, Hugenholtz P, Jansson J, Kau AL, Kelley ST, Kennedy J, Knights D, Koren O, Kuczynski J, Kyrpides N, Larsen R, Lauber CL, Legg T, Ley RE, Lozupone CA, Ludwig W, Lyons D, Maguire E, Methé BA, Meyer F, Muegge B, Nakielny S, Nelson KE, Nemergut D, Neufeld JD, Newbold LK, Oliver AE, Pace NR, Palanisamy G, Peplies J, Petrosino J, Proctor L, Pruesse E, Quast C, Raes J, Ratnasingham S, Ravel J, Relman DA, Assunta-Sansone S, Schloss PD, Schriml L, Sinha R, Smith MI, Sodergren E, Spo A, Stombaugh J, Tiedje JM, Ward DV, Weinstock GM, Wendel D, White O, Whiteley A, Wilke A, Wortman JR, Yatsunenko T, Glöckner FO (2011) Minimum information about a marker gene sequence (MIMARKS) and minimum information about any (x) sequence (MIxS) specifications. Nat Biotechnol 29:415–420. https://doi.org/10.1038/nbt.1823

19. Weiss SJ, Xu Z, Amir A, Peddada S, Bittinger K, Gonzalez A, Lozupone C, Zaneveld JR, Vazquez-Baeza Y, Birmingham A, Knight R (2015) Effects of library size variance, sparsity, and compositionality on the analysis of microbiome data. Peer J PrePrints 3:e1157v1. https://doi.org/10.7287/PEERJ.PREPRINTS.1157V1

20. Kembel SW, Wu M, Eisen JA, Green JL (2012) Incorporating 16S gene copy number information improves estimates of microbial diversity and abundance. PLoS Comput Biol 8: e1002743. https://doi.org/10.1371/journal.pcbi.1002743

21. Angly FE, Dennis PG, Skarshewski A, Vanwonterghem I, Hugenholtz P, Tyson GW (2014) CopyRighter: a rapid tool for improving the accuracy of microbial community profiles through lineage-specific gene copy number correction. Microbiome 2:11. https://doi.org/10.1186/2049-2618-2-11

22. Wang Q, Garrity GM, Tiedje JM, Cole JR (2007) Naive Bayesian classifier for rapid assignment of rRNA sequences into the new bacterial taxonomy. Appl Environ Microbiol 73:5261–5267. https://doi.org/10.1128/AEM.00062-07

23. Nayfach S, Pollard KS (2015) Average genome size estimation improves comparative metagenomics and sheds light on the functional ecology of the human microbiome. Genome Biol 16:51. https://doi.org/10.1186/s13059-015-0611-7

24. Angly FE, Willner D, Prieto-Davó A, Edwards RA, Schmieder R, Vega-Thurber R, Antonopoulos DA, Barott K, Cottrell MT, Desnues C, Dinsdale EA, Furlan M, Haynes M, Henn MR, Hu Y, Kirchman DL, McDole T, McPherson JD, Meyer F, Miller RM, Mundt E, Naviaux RK, Rodriguez-Mueller B, Stevens R, Wegley L, Zhang L, Zhu B, Rohwer F (2009) The GAAS metagenomic tool and its estimations of viral and microbial average genome size in four major biomes. PLoS Comput Biol 5:e1000593. https://doi.org/10.1371/journal.pcbi.1000593

25. Quail MA, Smith M, Coupland P, Otto TD, Harris SR, Connor TR, Bertoni A, Swerdlow HP, Gu Y (2012) A tale of three next generation sequencing platforms: comparison of ion torrent, Pacific biosciences and Illumina MiSeq sequencers. BMC Genomics 13:341. https://doi.org/10.1186/1471-2164-13-341

26. Nayfach S, Pollard KS (2016) Toward accurate and quantitative comparative metagenomics. Cell 166:1103–1116. https://doi.org/10.1016/j.cell.2016.08.007

27. Wu D, Hugenholtz P, Mavromatis K, Pukall R, Dalin E, Ivanova NN, Kunin V, Goodwin L, Wu M, Tindall BJ, Hooper SD, Pati A, Lykidis A, Spring S, Anderson IJ, D'haeseleer P, Zemla A, Singer M, Lapidus A, Nolan M, Copeland A, Han C, Chen F, Cheng J-F, Lucas S, Kerfeld C, Lang E, Gronow S, Chain P, Bruce D, Rubin EM, Kyrpides NC, Klenk H-P, Eisen JA (2009) A phylogeny-driven genomic encyclopaedia of bacteria and Archaea. Nature 462:1056–1060. https://doi.org/10.1038/nature08656

28. Sunagawa S, Mende DR, Zeller G, Izquierdo-Carrasco F, Berger SA, Kultima JR, Coelho LP, Arumugam M, Tap J, Nielsen HB, Rasmussen S, Brunak S, Pedersen O, Guarner F, de Vos WM, Wang J, Li J, Doré J, Ehrlich SD, Stamatakis A, Bork P (2013) Metagenomic species profiling using universal phylogenetic marker genes. Nat Methods 10:1196–1199. https://doi.org/10.1038/nmeth.2693

29. Nayfach S, Rodriguez-Mueller B, Garud N, Pollard KS (2016) An integrated metagenomics pipeline for strain profiling reveals novel patterns of bacterial transmission and biogeography. Genome Res 26:1612–1625. https://doi.org/10.1101/gr.201863.115

30. Caporaso JG, Kuczynski J, Stombaugh J, Bittinger K, Bushman FD, Costello EK, Fierer N, Peña AG, Goodrich JK, Gordon JI, Huttley GA, Kelley ST, Knights D, Koenig JE, Ley RE, Lozupone CA, McDonald D, Muegge BD, Pirrung M, Reeder J, Sevinsky JR, Turnbaugh PJ, Walters WA, Widmann J,

Yatsunenko T, Zaneveld J, Knight R (2010) QIIME allows analysis of high-throughput community sequencing data. Nat Methods 7:335–336. https://doi.org/10.1038/nmeth.f.303

31. McMurdie PJ, Holmes S (2013) Phyloseq: an R package for reproducible interactive analysis and graphics of microbiome census data. PLoS One 8:e61217. https://doi.org/10.1371/journal.pone.0061217

32. Jari Oksanen, Guillaume Blanchet F, Michael Friendly, Roeland Kindt, Pierre Legendre, Dan McGlinn, Peter R. Minchin, O'Hara R.B, Gavin L. Simpson, Peter Solymos, M. Henry H. Stevens, Eduard Szoecs and Helene Wagner (2017). vegan: Community Ecology Package. R package version 2.4–3. https://CRAN.R-project.org/package=vegan

33. Finotello F, Mastrorilli E, Di Camillo B (2016) Measuring the diversity of the human microbiota with targeted next-generation sequencing. Brief Bioinform:bbw119. https://doi.org/10.1093/bib/bbw119

34. Anderson MJ, Crist TO, Chase JM, Vellend M, Inouye BD, Freestone AL, Sanders NJ, Cornell HV, Comita LS, Davies KF, Harrison SP, Kraft NJB, Stegen JC, Swenson NG (2011) Navigating the multiple meanings of β diversity: a roadmap for the practicing ecologist. Ecol Lett 14:19–28. https://doi.org/10.1111/j.1461-0248.2010.01552.x

35. Lozupone C, Knight R (2005) UniFrac: a new phylogenetic method for comparing microbial communities. Appl Environ Microbiol 71:8228–8235. https://doi.org/10.1128/AEM.71.12.8228-8235.2005

36. Tuomisto H (2010) A diversity of beta diversities: straightening up a concept gone awry. Part 1. Defining beta diversity as a function of alpha and gamma diversity. Ecography 33:2–22. https://doi.org/10.1111/j.1600-0587.2009.05880.x

37. Ondov BD, Treangen TJ, Melsted P, Mallonee AB, Bergman NH, Koren S, Phillippy AM (2016) Mash: fast genome and metagenome distance estimation using MinHash. Genome Biol 17:132. https://doi.org/10.1186/s13059-016-0997-x

38. Thomas AM, Gleber-Netto FO, Fernandes GR, Amorim M, Barbosa LF, Francisco ALN, Guerra de Andrade A, Setubal JC, Kowalski LP, Nunes DN, Dias-Neto E (2014) Alcohol and tobacco consumption affects bacterial richness in oral cavity mucosa biofilms. BMC Microbiol 14:250. https://doi.org/10.1186/s12866-014-0250-2

39. Friedman J, Alm EJ (2012) Inferring correlation networks from genomic survey data. PLoS Comput Biol 8:e1002687. https://doi.org/10.1371/journal.pcbi.1002687

40. Deng Y, Jiang Y-H, Yang Y, He Z, Luo F, Zhou J (2012) Molecular ecological network analyses. BMC Bioinformatics 13:113. https://doi.org/10.1186/1471-2105-13-113

41. Kurtz ZD, Müller CL, Miraldi ER, Littman DR, Blaser MJ, Bonneau RA (2015) Sparse and compositionally robust inference of microbial ecological networks. PLoS Comput Biol 11:e1004226. https://doi.org/10.1371/journal.pcbi.1004226

42. Xia LC, Ai D, Cram J, Fuhrman JA, Sun F (2013) Efficient statistical significance approximation for local similarity analysis of high-throughput time series data. Bioinformatics 29:230–237. https://doi.org/10.1093/bioinformatics/bts668

43. Mehdi Layeghifard, David M.Hwang, and David S.Guttman (2017). Disentangling Interactions in the Microbiome: A Network Perspective. Trends in Microbiology 25:3, pp. 217–228

44. Segata N, Izard J, Waldron L, Gevers D, Miropolsky L, Garrett WS, Huttenhower C (2011) Metagenomic biomarker discovery and explanation. Genome Biol 12:R60. https://doi.org/10.1186/gb-2011-12-6-r60

45. Paulson JN, Stine OC, Bravo HC, Pop M (2013) Differential abundance analysis for microbial marker-gene surveys. Nat Methods 10:1200–1202. https://doi.org/10.1038/nmeth.2658

46. White JR, Nagarajan N, Pop M (2009) Statistical methods for detecting differentially abundant features in clinical metagenomic samples. PLoS Comput Biol 5:e1000352. https://doi.org/10.1371/journal.pcbi.1000352

47. Kanehisa M, Goto S (2000) KEGG: Kyoto encyclopedia of genes and genomes. Nucleic Acids Res 28:27–30

48. Tringe SG, von Mering C, Kobayashi A, Salamov AA, Chen K, Chang HW, Podar M, Short JM, Mathur EJ, Detter JC, Bork P, Hugenholtz P, Rubin EM (2005) Comparative metagenomics of microbial communities. Science 308:554–557. https://doi.org/10.1126/science.1107851

49. Abubucker S, Segata N, Goll J, Schubert AM, Izard J, Cantarel BL, Rodriguez-Mueller B, Zucker J, Thiagarajan M, Henrissat B, White O, Kelley ST, Methé B, Schloss PD, Gevers D, Mitreva M, Huttenhower C (2012) Metabolic reconstruction for metagenomic data and its application to the human microbiome. PLoS Comput Biol 8:e1002358.

https://doi.org/10.1371/journal.pcbi.
1002358

50. Meyer F, Paarmann D, D'Souza M, Olson R, Glass EM, Kubal M, Paczian T, Rodriguez A, Stevens R, Wilke A, Wilkening J, Edwards RA (2008) The metagenomics RAST server–a public resource for the automatic phylogenetic and functional analysis of metagenomes. BMC Bioinformatics 9:386. https://doi.org/10.1186/1471-2105-9-386

51. Manor O, Borenstein E (2015) MUSiCC: a marker genes based framework for metagenomic normalization and accurate profiling of gene abundances in the microbiome. Genome Biol 16:53. https://doi.org/10.1186/s13059-015-0610-8

52. Kim J, Kim MS, Koh AY, Xie Y, Zhan X (2016) FMAP: functional mapping and analysis pipeline for metagenomics and metatranscriptomics studies. BMC Bioinformatics 17:420. https://doi.org/10.1186/s12859-016-1278-0

53. Kaminski J, Gibson MK, Franzosa EA, Segata N, Dantas G, Huttenhower C (2015) High-specificity targeted functional profiling in microbial communities with ShortBRED. PLoS Comput Biol 11:e1004557. https://doi.org/10.1371/journal.pcbi.1004557

54. Taxis TM, Wolff S, Gregg SJ, Minton NO, Zhang C, Dai J, Schnabel RD, Taylor JF, Kerley MS, Pires JC, Lamberson WR, Conant GC (2015) The players may change but the game remains: network analyses of ruminal microbiomes suggest taxonomic differences mask functional similarity. Nucleic Acids Res 43:9600–9612. https://doi.org/10.1093/nar/gkv973

55. Weimann A, Mooren K, Frank J, Pope PB, Bremges A, McHardy AC (2016) From genomes to phenotypes: traitar, the microbial trait analyzer. mSystems 1:e00101–e00116. https://doi.org/10.1128/mSystems.00101-16

56. Holmes I, Harris K, Quince C (2012) Dirichlet multinomial mixtures: generative models for microbial metagenomics. PLoS One 7:e30126. https://doi.org/10.1371/journal.pone.0030126

57. Maechler M, Rousseeuw P, Struyf A, Hubert M, Hornik K (2015) Cluster analysis basics and extensions. R package version 2.0.1. CRAN

58. Ditzler G, Morrison JC, Lan Y, Rosen GL (2015) Fizzy: feature subset selection for metagenomics. BMC Bioinformatics 16:358. https://doi.org/10.1186/s12859-015-0793-8

59. Pasolli E, Truong DT, Malik F, Waldron L, Segata N (2016) Machine learning meta-analysis of large metagenomic datasets: tools

and biological insights. PLoS Comput Biol 12:e1004977. https://doi.org/10.1371/journal.pcbi.1004977

60. Roller M, Lucić V, Nagy I, Perica T, Vlahovicek K (2013) Environmental shaping of codon usage and functional adaptation across microbial communities. Nucleic Acids Res 41:8842–8852. https://doi.org/10.1093/nar/gkt673

61. Quax TEF, Claassens NJ, Söll D, van der Oost J (2015) Codon bias as a means to fine-tune gene expression. Mol Cell 59:149–161. https://doi.org/10.1016/j.molcel.2015.05.035

62. Eren AM, Maignien L, Sul WJ, Murphy LG, Grim SL, Morrison HG, Sogin ML (2013) Oligotyping: differentiating between closely related microbial taxa using 16S rRNA gene data. Methods Ecol Evol 4:1111–1119. https://doi.org/10.1111/2041-210X.12114

63. Eren AM, Zozaya M, Taylor CM, Dowd SE, Martin DH, Ferris MJ (2011) Exploring the diversity of gardnerella vaginalis in the genitourinary tract microbiota of monogamous couples through subtle nucleotide variation. PLoS One 6:e26732. https://doi.org/10.1371/journal.pone.0026732

64. Eren AM, Borisy GG, Huse SM, Mark Welch JL (2014) Oligotyping analysis of the human oral microbiome. Proc Natl Acad Sci 111:E2875–E2884. https://doi.org/10.1073/pnas.1409644111

65. Qin J, Li Y, Cai Z, Li S, Zhu J, Zhang F, Liang S, Zhang W, Guan Y, Shen D, Peng Y, Zhang D, Jie Z, Wu W, Qin Y, Xue W, Li J, Han L, Lu D, Wu P, Dai Y, Sun X, Li Z, Tang A, Zhong S, Li X, Chen W, Xu R, Wang M, Feng Q, Gong M, Yu J, Zhang Y, Zhang M, Hansen T, Sanchez G, Raes J, Falony G, Okuda S, Almeida M, LeChatelier E, Renault P, Pons N, Batto J-M, Zhang Z, Chen H, Yang R, Zheng W, Li S, Yang H, Wang J, Ehrlich SD, Nielsen R, Pedersen O, Kristiansen K, Wang J (2012) A metagenome-wide association study of gut microbiota in type 2 diabetes. Nature 490:55–60. https://doi.org/10.1038/nature11450

66. Aitchison J (1982) The statistical analysis of compositional data. J R Stat Soc Ser B 44:139–177

67. Tsilimigras MCB, Fodor AA (2016) Compositional data analysis of the microbiome: fundamentals, tools, and challenges. Ann Epidemiol 26:330–335. https://doi.org/10.1016/j.annepidem.2016.03.002

68. Love MI, Huber W, Anders S (2014) Moderated estimation of fold change and dispersion

for RNA-seq data with DESeq2. Genome Biol 15:550. https://doi.org/10.1186/s13059-014-0550-8

69. Mandal S, Van Treuren W, White RA, Eggesbø M, Knight R, Peddada SD (2015) Analysis of composition of microbiomes: a novel method for studying microbial composition. Microb Ecol Health Dis 26:27663

70. Chen I-MA, Markowitz VM, Chu K, Palaniappan K, Szeto E, Pillay M, Ratner A, Huang J, Andersen E, Huntemann M, Varghese N, Hadjithomas M, Tennessen K, Nielsen T, Ivanova NN, Kyrpides NC (2017) IMG/M: integrated genome and metagenome comparative data analysis system. Nucleic Acids Res 45:D507–D516. https://doi.org/10.1093/nar/gkw929

71. Truong DT, Franzosa EA, Tickle TL, Scholz M, Weingart G, Pasolli E, Tett A, Huttenhower C, Segata N. MetaPhlAn2 for enhanced metagenomic taxonomic profiling. Nat Methods. 2015 12(10):902–3

Chapter 9

Genome Rearrangement Analysis: Cut and Join Genome Rearrangements and Gene Cluster Preserving Approaches

Tom Hartmann, Martin Middendorf, and Matthias Bernt

Abstract

Genome rearrangements are mutations that change the gene content of a genome or the arrangement of the genes on a genome. Several years of research on genome rearrangements have established different algorithmic approaches for solving some fundamental problems in comparative genomics based on gene order information. This review summarizes the literature on genome rearrangement analysis along two lines of research. The first line considers rearrangement models that are particularly well suited for a theoretical analysis. These models use rearrangement operations that cut chromosomes into fragments and then join the fragments into new chromosomes. The second line works with rearrangement models that reflect several biologically motivated constraints, e.g., the constraint that gene clusters have to be preserved. In this chapter, the border between algorithmically "easy" and "hard" rearrangement problems is sketched and a brief review is given on the available software tools for genome rearrangement analysis.

Key words Gene order analysis, Genome rearrangements, Cut and join, Gene cluster

1 Introduction

During evolution the gene content and also the arrangement of the genes within the genomes of species have been modified by various kinds of mutations. A genome consists of a set of chromosomes and each chromosome contains a set of genes. A chromosome represents a linear or circular string of DNA where the genes are located. Each gene of a chromosome has an orientation depending on which of the two strands of the DNA it is located. Mutations that change the arrangement of the genes on the chromosome are called rearrangement mutations (or rearrangements). Examples are inversions that reverse the order and orientation of a subsequence of genes on a chromosome and transpositions which move a subsequence of genes from one chromosome to another location on the same chromosome or to another chromosome. Other examples are fissions which split a chromosome into two chromosomes and fusions which merge two chromosomes to form a single

João C. Setubal et al. (eds.), *Comparative Genomics: Methods and Protocols*, Methods in Molecular Biology, vol. 1704,
https://doi.org/10.1007/978-1-4939-7463-4_9, © Springer Science+Business Media LLC 2018

chromosome. In addition to such rearrangement mutations which do not change the gene content of a genome, and there exist also rearrangements that change the gene content of a genome. However, the latter type of rearrangements are not considered in this chapter.

Gene order analysis aims to explain the differences of the gene arrangement (and gene content) between the genomes of extant species and to reconstruct their phylogenetic evolution. The most common approach for gene order analysis is maximum parsimony. This approach tries to explain the differences within a set of genomes by the minimum possible number of changes. For example, one might ask for a shortest sequence of (allowed) rearrangement mutations that transforms one given genome into another given genome. This problem is called the sorting problem. The corresponding problem that asks only for the smallest number of such mutations is called distance problem. Such distance information between genomes of species can be used, e.g., to reconstruct the phylogenetic relationships between the species, e.g., [1].

The exploration of the combinatorial and computational problems that occur in gene order analysis started with the pioneering works of Sankoff and Blanchette [2] and Watterson et al. [3]. Early breakthroughs have been obtained with respect to the sorting problem where polynomial time algorithms have been developed for the problem of sorting with inversions [4] and for sorting with inversions plus fission and fusion [5]. However, many other related problems have been shown to be NP-hard which makes it unlikely that they can be solved optimally in polynomial time. Examples are the problem of sorting with inversions for unsigned genomes (i.e., the orientations of the genes are ignored) [6], the inversion median problem (i.e., the problem to find a parsimonious common ancestral gene order for more than two given gene orders) [7], and the problem of sorting by transpositions [8]. Hence, one focus of the research in gene order analysis is to develop heuristics and approximation algorithms. Examples of such algorithms are the frequently used MGR algorithm for solving the inversion median problem [9] and approximation algorithms for the sorting by transpositions problem [10].

This chapter gives an overview on the different gene rearrangement problems and reviews the corresponding literature. We also give a brief review of the available software tools and web services for rearrangement analysis (see, e.g., Table 1). The chapter is organized along two lines of research in gene order analysis.

The first line of research tries to find models of rearrangement mutations which are well suited for a theoretical analysis. These models are based on two operations: (1) to cut a chromosome into fragments and (2) to rejoin such fragments (into new chromosomes). The differences between the models are the number of cut points of an operation and the different ways how the fragments

Table 1
List of resources and web services which are thematically related; sorting problem (SP), distance problem (DP), median problem (MP), small parsimony problem (SPP), large parsimony problem (LPP), transpositions ($\mathcal{TR}$), inverse transpositions ($\mathcal{ITR}$), inversions ($\mathcal{INV}$), double-cut and joins ($\mathcal{DCJ}$), model including inversions, translocations, fusions, and fissions ($\mathcal{HP}$), duplications and deletions ($\mathcal{IND}$), block-interchanges ($\mathcal{BI}$), restricted $\mathcal{DCJ}$ events ($\mathcal{RDCJ}$), tandem-duplications ($\mathcal{TD}$), duplications ($\mathcal{D}$), weighted inversions ($\mathcal{WINV}$)

Resource	Reference	Features/note
Web services		
CEGeD	[30, 31]	DP under $\mathcal{INV}$, $\mathcal{TR}$, and $\mathcal{DCJ}$
CREx	[32, 33]	SP under $\mathcal{INV}^{\ell} \cup \mathcal{TR}^{\ell} \cup \mathcal{ITR}^{\ell}$ and TDRL
GEvolutionS	[34]	simulates scenarios under $\mathcal{TR} \cup \mathcal{DCJ} \cup \mathcal{HP}$
GRIMM[a]	[35, 36]	SP under $\mathcal{HP}$ and $\mathcal{INV}$
MGR[a]	[9, 37]	LPP under $\mathcal{INV}$ and $\mathcal{HP}$
MGRA	[38, 39]	SPP and LPP under $\mathcal{DCJ}$
MLGO	[40, 41]	SPP and LPP under $\mathcal{DCJ} \cup \mathcal{IND}$
Roci	[42, 43]	SPP including $\mathcal{INV} \cup \mathcal{TR} \cup \mathcal{ITR}$ while preserving conserved intervals
SORT[2]	[44, 45]	SP under $\mathcal{INV}$, $\mathcal{BI}$, $\mathcal{HP} \cup \mathcal{BI}$, and $\mathcal{INV} \cup \mathcal{BI}$; infers phylogenetic trees based on distances
SBBI[a]	[46, 47]	SP under $\mathcal{BI}$
UniMoG[a]	[48]	DP and SP under $\mathcal{RDCJ}$, $\mathcal{INV}$, $\mathcal{TR}$, and $\mathcal{HP}$
Software for download		
baobabLUNA	[49, 50]	DP and SP under $\mathcal{INV}$; builds breakpoint graphs
dcjdDist	[51, 52]	phylogenetic reconstruction under $\mathcal{INV} \cup \mathcal{BI} \cup \mathcal{TD} \cup \mathcal{D}$
EMRAE	[53, 54]	LPP for synteny blocks under $\mathcal{INV} \cup \mathcal{HP} \cup \mathcal{TR}$
GENESIS	[55, 56]	SP under $\mathcal{WINV}$, $\mathcal{WINV} \cup \mathcal{TR}$, $\mathcal{WINV} \cup \mathcal{HP}$, and $\mathcal{WINV} \cup \mathcal{HP} \cup \mathcal{TR}$
GRAPPA	[23, 57]	LPP under $\mathcal{INV}$
GREDU	[58, 59]	DP under $\mathcal{DCJ} \cup \mathcal{IND}$
Mauve	[60, 61]	multiple alignment tool; DP of synteny blocks under $\mathcal{DCJ}$
median	[62, 63][b]	MP under $\mathcal{INV}$, $\mathcal{TR}$, and $\mathcal{WINV} \cup \mathcal{TR}$
minswrt	[62, 63][b]	DP under $\mathcal{WINV} \cup \mathcal{TR}$
MSOAR	[64, 65]	calculates orthologous genes of genomic sequences involving genome rearrangements ($\mathcal{HP} \cup \mathcal{IND}$)
PATHGROUPS	[66, 67]	SPP under $\mathcal{DCJ}$
phylo	[62, 63]	phylogenetic reconstruction under $\mathcal{WINV} \cup \mathcal{TR}$
revDis	[62, 63][b]	DP under $\mathcal{INV}$
weightedbb	[62, 63][b]	branch and bound algorithm for DP under $\mathcal{WINV} \cup \mathcal{TR}$

[a] Also available for download and local use
[b] And included references

can be rejoined. Thereby, most of the (classical) rearrangement operations are directly covered and a few others, e.g., transpositions, can be emulated by a combination of such cut and join operations. One focus is to sketch the border between easy problems, i.e., problems that are polynomial time solvable, and difficult problems, i.e., problems that are NP-hard.

The second line of research tries to identify biologically motivated constraints on the applicability of gene rearrangement mutations. One particular important type of constraints are conserved gene clusters, i.e., subsets of the genes that are observed in close proximity on all given genomes. Such gene clusters might form due to functional constraints or evolutionary inertia. The idea is to consider such conserved gene clusters in the reconstructions, i.e., no genome rearrangement is allowed that breaks a gene cluster. Even if a rearrangement problem might become or remain NP-hard with such additional restrictions, e.g., the preserving inversion sorting problem [11], the search space becomes more structured such that many problem instances can be solved efficiently [12–14]. It is worth to mention that in addition to the preservation of gene clusters, other biologically motivated constraints have been introduced, e.g., positional constraints on gene adjacencies motivated on chromosome conformation information [15, 16].

This chapter is organized as follows. In the next Subheading 2 a formal background on gene arrangements and rearrangement mutations is given. In addition, the basic problems of gene order analysis are introduced. An overview on the literature on cut and join models of rearrangement mutations is presented in Subheading 3. An overview on gene order analysis with conserved gene clusters is given in Subheading 4. The chapter ends with a conclusion in Subheading 5.

2   Preliminaries

A formal background on gene arrangements, rearrangement mutations, and basic problems of gene order analysis is given in this section.

2.1   Gene Orders

A *genome* is a set of linear or circular DNA sequences which are called *chromosomes*. Genomes are called *unichromosomal* if they consist of only a single chromosome and *multichromosomal* otherwise. If all chromosomes of a genome are linear (resp. circular), then the genome is called *linear* (resp. *circular*) and *mixed* otherwise.

A *gene* is a unit of genetic information that encodes a specific function. It is assumed here that each gene has a unique identifier and that it can be identified whether a gene occurs in a genome or not. If a gene occurs in a genome, it can be located and it corresponds to an oriented sequence of DNA. In this chapter we consider only the case that genes within a genome do not intersect. If not stated otherwise, it is assumed that a gene occurs at most once in a genome. The set of genes of a genome α is denoted by $\mathcal{G}(\alpha)$. A gene g can be represented by its *extremities*: the *tail* g^t, and the *head* g^h, i.e., the 5' and 3' end of the gene. A linear (resp. circular) chromosome can be represented by the linear (resp. circular) sequence of the extremities of its genes.

Given a genome α, an *adjacency* is an unordered pair $\{p, q\}$ of extremities p and q, $p \neq q$, of genes of $\mathcal{G}(\alpha)$ that are adjacent on a chromosome of α. The endpoints of linear chromosomes are called *telomeres*. A telomere is denoted by the pair $\{p, \circ\}$, where p is the extremity that is closest to the telomere and therefore p is not adjacent to the extremity of another gene. The set of all telomeres of a genome α is denoted by $\mathcal{T}(\alpha)$. The set of extremities $\mathcal{E}(\alpha)$ of a genome α consists of all extremities of the genes, i.e., $\mathcal{E}(\alpha) = \{g^h, g^t : g \in \mathcal{G}(\alpha)\}$. A genome α can be characterized by the set of adjacencies of its genes and its telomeres. In that case α denotes this set. Furthermore, $\mathcal{I}(\alpha)$ denoted the set of all adjacencies (without the telomeres) of a genome, i.e., $\mathcal{I}(\alpha) = \alpha \backslash \mathcal{T}(\alpha)$. Note that $\mathcal{I}(\alpha)$ uniquely determines the set of telomeres. For a set of genes $\mathcal{G}$, the set of all possible genomes is denoted by $\mathbb{G}(\mathcal{G})$ (or simply $\mathbb{G}$ if the context is clear).

A genome α can be represented by an undirected graph—the *genome graph*—which contains the extremities as vertices and an edge connects two vertices x and y if and only if either $\{x, y\}$ is an adjacency in α or x and y are head and tail of the same gene. *Linear* and *circular* chromosomes correspond to linear and circular connected components in the genome graph. Figure 1 illustrates an example of a genome graph.

An alternative representation of a genome α is a set of signed strings S_α, where each string lists the genes of one chromosome as if read from one telomere to the other (or in the case of circular chromosomes starting from an arbitrary gene), *see* Fig. 1. If the head of a gene x appears before its tail, the gene in the string gets a negative sign (represented by $-x$), otherwise a positive sign is assigned to the gene (a positive sign is omitted). The sign represents the (relative) strandedness of the genes. Note that both strings of the two reading directions of a linear chromosome and also all strings generated from different start points in circular chromosomes are considered to be equivalent. For unichromosomal genomes with n genes this representation is equivalent to a *signed permutation* of length n. Such a permutation π is denoted by

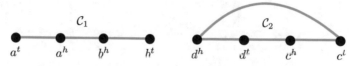

Fig. 1 Genome graph of the mixed multichromosomal genome $\alpha = \{\{a^t, \circ\}, \{a^h, b^h\}, \{b^t, \circ\}, \{c^t, d^h\}, \{d^t, c^h\}\}$ consisting of the linear chromosome $C_1 = \{\{a^t, \circ\}, \{a^h, b^h\}, \{b^t, \circ\}\}$ and the circular chromosome $C_2 = \{\{c^t, d^h\}, \{d^t, c^h\}\}$. The set of telomeres of α is $\mathcal{T}(\alpha) = \{\{a^t, \circ\}, \{b^t, \circ\}\}$. Genome α can also be represented by $S_\alpha = \{(a-b), (-d-c)^\circ\}$, where $^\circ$ marks the chromosome as *circular*

$(\pi(1)\ \pi(2)\ldots\pi(n))$, where $\pi(i)$ denotes the i-th element. The identity permutation $(1\ 2\ldots\ n)$ is denoted by ι. For differentiation the string corresponding to a circular chromosome is enclosed between $()^{\circ}$. In the following the two representations of unichromosomal genomes are used interchangeably, where π and σ denote genomes as permutations, and α and β denote genomes as sets of adjacencies and telomeres. The considered genomes are always assumed to consist of the same set of genes throughout this chapter.

Often in nature a subset of genes is found in close proximity in the genomes of many different species. Such a set of genes is called gene cluster [17]. A simple formal model for gene clusters are *common intervals* [18]. An *interval I* of a permutation π of length n is a subset of elements of π which form a consecutive segment, i.e., there exists a pair (i, j), with $1 \le i \le j \le n$, such that $\{|\pi(x)|: i \le x \le j\} = I$. For a set of signed permutations Π a common interval is a subset of the elements of the permutations that is an interval in each permutation in Π. Singleton sets $\{i\}$ with $i \in [1: n]$ as well as $\{1, \ldots, n\}$ are called *trivial common intervals*. The set of all common intervals of a set of permutations Π is denoted by $C(\Pi)$. A set of permutations Σ is *consistent* with the common intervals of a set of permutations Π if $C(\Pi) = C(\Pi \cup \Sigma)$.

2.2 Rearrangement Model

Different types of rearrangement mutations are of interest for rearrangement analysis. *See* Fig. 2 for a selection of such rearrangement mutations. The set of possible rearrangement mutations that is of interest is called a rearrangement model.

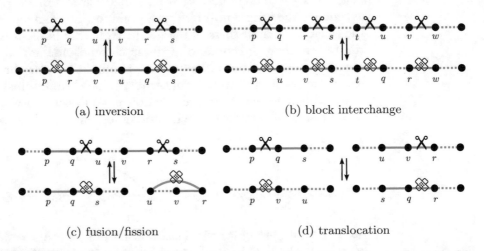

(a) inversion

(b) block interchange

(c) fusion/fission

(d) translocation

Fig. 2 Rearrangement events visualized on the genome graph. (**a**) An inversion reverses the order of the genes between two cut points (a cut is indicated by a scissor, a join is indicated by a plaster) and inverses the orientation of the affected genes. (**b**) A block interchange swaps two intervals. If the two intervals are adjacent, i.e., the middle cut points coincide, it is a transposition. (**c**) A fission cuts out an interval and creates a circular chromosome. A fusion inverts this operation. (**d**) A translocation swaps the ends of two chromosomes

Along the lines of [19] a *rearrangement model* M is defined as a binary relation over the set of all possible genomes, i.e., $M \subseteq \mathbb{G} \times \mathbb{G}$. A pair of genomes $R = (\alpha, \alpha')$ is a *rearrangement event* in M if and only if $R \in M$. The event R can be considered as a rearrangement that transforms α into α', we write $\alpha' = \alpha \circ R$. Given two genomes α and α' and a (rearrangement) model M, a *scenario* is a sequence $R_1, \ldots, R_k$ of rearrangement events in M with $\alpha' = \alpha \circ R_1 \circ \ldots \circ R_k$. The set of all possible scenarios for two given genomes α and α' is denoted by $S_M(\alpha, \alpha')$. The most famous rearrangement model for unichromosomal genomes is the inversion—or reversal—model $(\mathcal{INV})$. This model consists of all inversion operations and was studied first in [2, 3].

For each rearrangement model M a corresponding preserving variant, denoted by M^p, can be defined as the set of rearrangement operations of M which do not destroy any common interval of the two given gene orders in any of its intermediate gene orders. Formally, an event $\rho = (\pi, \pi')$ of a model M is called *preserving* with respect to a set of permutations Π if $C(\Pi) = C(\Pi \cup \{\pi, \pi'\})$, i.e., π as well as π' are consistent with Π.

2.3 Genome Rearrangement Analysis

There exist several approaches to extract phylogenetic information from gene arrangement data, *see* [20] for a comprehensive overview. One example is the computation of rearrangement distances between genomes. Another example is the joint reconstruction of a phylogenetic tree for a set of genomes and the corresponding rearrangement events along its edges. In the following the central combinatorial problems that need to be solved for such approaches are formally defined.

Given a rearrangement model M and two genomes α and α' the *distance problem* for M is to find the minimum number $d_M(\alpha, \alpha')$ of events from M to transform α into α'. That is, $d_M(\alpha, \alpha') = \min_{S \in S_M(\alpha, \alpha')} |S|$. To find a corresponding reconstruction, i.e., a corresponding scenario that transforms one genome into the other is called *sorting problem*. By relabeling the elements of α and α', we can always assume that α' is the identity permutation ι. For a rearrangement model M that includes events which involve a constant number of cuts it holds that for every $\alpha \in \mathbb{G}$ the set $\{(\alpha, \alpha') \in M : \alpha' \in \mathbb{G}\}$ has polynomial size. These are in particular all models involving a subset of the rearrangement operations that are shown in Fig. 2. For such models it holds that the sorting problem can be solved in polynomial time if a polynomial time algorithm solves the distance problem, e.g., [4, 19]. Due to the close connection between the sorting problem and the distance problem this chapter is focused on the distance problem. However, the sorting problem can sometimes be solved faster than by testing all possible rearrangement events, e.g., the sorting problem for the $\mathcal{INV}$ model can be solved in sub-quadratic time [21]. It should be mentioned that the distance problem was studied for the first time in [2] for the case of the $\mathcal{INV}$ model. In [4] a polynomial time algorithm for the sorting problem of signed permutations was given for the $\mathcal{INV}$ model. Examples of software tools which can solve this problem are SORT², UniMoG, and baobabLUNA. In addition, the software tool revDis can be used to solve the distance problem under $\mathcal{INV}$. *See* Table 1 for a summary.

Two central problems of gene order analysis for more than two genomes are the small and the large parsimony problem for gene orders. The *small parsimony problem* for a rearrangement model $\mathcal{M}$ and a given binary tree T, where every leaf is associated to a genome, asks for one ancestral genome α_i for every inner vertex i of T such that the sum of the distances between the two genomes of an edge of the tree is minimized, i.e., $\sum_{(u,v)\in E(T)} d_{\mathcal{M}}(\alpha_u, \alpha_v)$ has to be minimized, where $E(T)$ is the set of edges of T. For the *large parsimony problem* (also known as multiple genome rearrangement problem) the tree itself is sought in addition to the ancestral genomes at its inner vertices. The small and the large parsimony problem for gene orders were both studied, e.g., in [22].

A special case of the parsimony problems for a rearrangement model $\mathcal{M}$ is the *median problem* which asks for a gene order α that minimizes the sum of the distances to given genomes $\alpha_1, \ldots, \alpha_k$, i.e., to find a α with $\min_{\alpha\in\mathbb{G}}\sum_{i=1}^{k} d_{\mathcal{M}}(\alpha, \alpha_i)$. Mostly, the case of $k = 3$ is considered. The solution of this case is often used in algorithms for solving larger multiple genome rearrangement problems [9, 23, 24]. With a few notable exceptions [25–27] the small parsimony problem has been proven to be NP-hard for most rearrangement models. For example, the median problem with $k = 3$ is NP-hard for inversions [6] and for transpositions [28]. However, the software tools median and GRAPPA provide solver for both of these problems, *see* Table 1.

Genome rearrangement problems that are defined for preserving rearrangement models are called *preserving genome rearrangement problems*. For a discussion of further rearrangement models and problems, *see* [29]. In the following sections several basic algorithms for rearrangement models with and without the preserving property are studied.

3 Cut and Join Genome Rearrangement Models

This section reviews results for unconstrained rearrangement analysis, i.e., without additional constraints, e.g., to preserve gene cluster. The focus is on the so-called *cut and/or join* models. In particular, these are the single-cut or join model, the single-cut and join model, the double-cut and join model, and the multi-cut and join model. Since many of the results are based on particular graph structures these are introduced first in the following subheading.

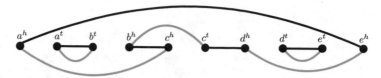

Fig. 3 Breakpoint graph for the circular genomes $S_\alpha = \{(-a\ b-c-d\ e)^\circ\}$ and $S_{\alpha'}$ $= \{(a-c-b)^\circ, (-d\ e)^\circ\}$. Adjacencies of α (resp. α') are represented by black (resp. gray) edges. Note that the edges of $BP(\alpha, \alpha')$ form a partition into alternating cycles and adjacencies that are common to both genomes form one-cycles

3.1 Genome Rearrangement Graphs

The *breakpoint graph* for signed genomes is a key element of efficient algorithms for the calculation of the distance between genomes under the $\mathcal{INV}$ model [4]. For a source genome α and a target genome α' the breakpoint graph $BP(\alpha, \alpha') = G(V, E_b \cup E_g)$ is defined as follows (*see* also Fig. 3). The vertices correspond to the extremities of the genes, i.e., $V = \mathcal{E}(\alpha)$. *Black edges* connect adjacent extremities of the source genome, i.e., $E_b = \alpha$ and *gray edges* connect adjacent extremities of the target genome, i.e., $E_g = \alpha'$.

For linear genomes two auxiliary vertices are added that are assumed to be adjacent to the first, respectively, the last extremity of the two genomes. Since each vertex has degree two the breakpoint graph can be partitioned into cycles, each of them with alternating black and gray edges. If both genomes are equal the breakpoint graph consists of a partition into color-alternating cycles of length two. Such cycles are called *one-cycles*. An extension of the breakpoint graph for more than two genomes has been introduced in [7] to solve the median problem for $\mathcal{INV}$. The software tool baobabLUNA provides a function which builds the breakpoint graph for two given genomes, *see* Table 1.

The *adjacency graph* $AG(\alpha, \alpha')$ is the line graph of the breakpoint graph of two genomes α and α' [31], *see* Fig. 4. Hence, the vertices of the adjacency graph are the adjacencies and telomeres of both genomes and edges connect two adjacencies if and only if they share one extremity, i.e., the edge multi-set is given by $\{\{u, v\}: u \in \alpha, v \in \alpha', u \cap v \neq \emptyset\}$. As for the breakpoint graph, shared adjacencies form cycles of the length two. But in contrast to the breakpoint graph, these cycles consist of color alternating vertices instead of color alternating edges. Since this is only a cosmetic difference, both cycles of length two are referred to as one-cycles. The degree of a vertex is one if it is a telomere and two otherwise. Since the adjacency graph is bipartite every cycle has an even length. Hence, the adjacency graph consists of cycles, *even paths* which connect telomeres of the same genome, and *odd paths* which connect telomeres of different genomes. An even path which starts and ends at an adjacency that belongs to the same genome α is called α-*path*.

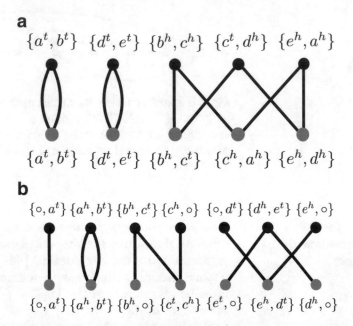

Fig. 4 (**a**) Adjacency graph for the circular genomes of Fig. 3. The adjacency graph contains three cycles. To visualize that $AG(\alpha, \alpha')$ is the line graph of $BP(\alpha, \alpha')$ gray (resp. black) vertices of $AG(\alpha, \alpha')$ correspond to gray (resp. black) edges of $BP(\alpha, \alpha')$ and the edges of $AG(\alpha, \alpha')$ correspond to the vertices of $BP(\alpha, \alpha')$. (**b**) Adjacency graph for mixed genomes $S_\beta = \{(a\ b\ c), (d\ e)\}$ and $S_{\beta'} = \{(-b-a), (c)^\circ, (e\ d)\}$. $AG(\beta, \beta')$ consists of one cycle, two odd paths, and two even paths

The breakpoint graph and the adjacency graph can both be constructed in linear time and require linear space [31]. The adjacency graph has the potential advantage that the genes of the two genomes are separated whereas they are tangled in the breakpoint graph which complicates the interpretation [68].

3.2 Single-Cut or Join Model

The *single-cut or join* model $SCOJ$ [25] includes two types of rearrangements (*see* Fig. 5a): A *cut* breaks an adjacency which creates two telomeres and a *join* forms a new adjacency by connecting two telomeres. Formally, a pair of genomes (α, α') is in $SCOJ$ if and only if there exist different extremities p and q such that either $\alpha \cup \{\{p, \circ\}, \{\circ, q\}\} = \alpha' \cup \{p, q\}$ (cut) or $\alpha \cup \{p, q\} = \alpha' \cup \{\{p, \circ\}, \{\circ, q\}\}$ (join) holds. The single-cut or join model is a simplistic approximation of genome rearrangement evolution since all genome rearrangements can be represented by compositions of cuts and joins. However, this model has the advantage to allow for an efficient solution of some core problems of genome rearrangement analysis as explained in the following. More realistic models are described in the next sections.

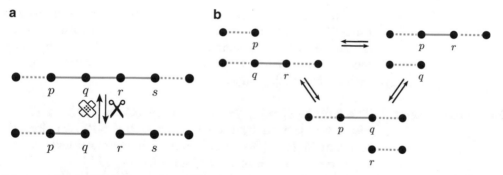

Fig. 5 Genome graphs representing rearrangement events. Dots indicate the existence of additional edges. (**a**) Events of the $\mathcal{SCOJ}$ model: cut event and join event. (**b**) Cut-and-join event of the $\mathcal{SCAJ}$ model. Together, both figures display the events of the $\mathcal{SCAJ}$ model

3.2.1 Polynomial Time Solvable Problems

For the $\mathcal{SCOJ}$ model efficient algorithms are known for the distance problem, the sorting problem, the median problem, and the small parsimony problem [25].

Under $\mathcal{SCOJ}$ a parsimonious scenario for two genomes α and α' is obtained by cutting all adjacencies which are in α but not in α' and joining all extremities which are in α' but not in α. Hence, $d_{\mathcal{SCOJ}}(\alpha, \alpha') = |\mathcal{I}(\alpha) \triangle \mathcal{I}(\alpha')|$, where $\triangle$ denotes the symmetric difference, i.e., for two sets X and Y it holds $X \triangle Y := (X \backslash Y) \cup (Y \backslash X)$.

This also solves the sorting problem under $\mathcal{SCOJ}$ in linear time. For details *see* [69]. The distance $d_{\mathcal{SCOJ}}(\alpha, \alpha')$ can also be interpreted in terms of the adjacency graph $AG(\alpha, \alpha')$. It holds that $d_{\mathcal{SCOJ}}(\alpha, \alpha') = 2N - 2C_2 - P$, where N is the number of genes, C_2 is the number of one-cycles, and P is the number of paths in AG (α, α'). This is because $|\mathcal{I}(\alpha)| = N - t_\alpha/2$, where t_α is the number of telomeres of α (analogously this holds for α'), $|\mathcal{I}(\alpha) \cap \mathcal{I}(\alpha')| = C_2$ and the fact that a path always connects two telomeres.

The median problem under $\mathcal{SCOJ}$ can also be solved in linear time [25]. The corresponding algorithm includes each adjacency into the median if it is an adjacency in the majority of the given genomes. That is, for input genomes $\alpha_1, \ldots, \alpha_k$ the median α consists of the adjacencies $\{p, q\} \in \bigcup_{i=1}^{k} \mathcal{I}(\alpha_i)$ with $|\{i \in [1 : k] : \{p, q\} \in \mathcal{I}(\alpha_i)\}| \geq \frac{k}{2}$. Note that the median for $\mathcal{SCOJ}$ is unique for an odd number of genomes whereas for an even number of genomes the inclusion or exclusion of adjacencies that are present in half of the genomes gives a parsimonious solution. For example, for $\alpha_1 = \{\{a^t, \circ\}, \{a^h, b^t\}, \{b^h, c^t\}, \{c^h, \circ\}\}$, $\alpha_2 = \{\{c^t, \circ\}, \{c^h, a^t\}, \{a^h, b^t\}, \{b^h, \circ\}\}$, and $\alpha_3 = \{\{a^t, \circ\}, \{a^h, c^t\}, \{b^h, c^h\}, \{b^t, \circ\}\}$ the median is $\mathcal{I}(\alpha) = \{\{a^h, b^t\}\}$. Since $\mathcal{I}(\alpha)$ is uniquely determined by $\mathcal{I}(\alpha)$, it follows that α is exactly the set $\{\{a^t, \circ\}, \{a^h, b^t\}, \{b^h, \circ\}, \{c^t, \circ\}, \{c^h, \circ\}\}$ with $\sum_{i=1}^{3} d_{\mathcal{SCOJ}}(\alpha, \alpha_i) = 1 + 1 + 3 = 5$. For more details and variants of the problem, *see* [25].

The small parsimony problem can also be solved in polynomial time [25]. The idea is to encode the presence/absence of the adjacencies as binary characters. The ancestral adjacencies can be reconstructed with a variant of Fitch's algorithm [70] which resolves conflicting adjacencies.

3.2.2 NP-Hard Problems

The large parsimony problem for $\mathcal{SCOJ}$ is NP-hard [25]. This result was proven by reduction from the NP-hard Steiner tree problem in $\{1, 0\}^N$ where binary characters are used to encode the presence or the absence of an adjacency [71].

Note that the $\mathcal{SCOJ}$ distance is effectively identical to the breakpoint distance [25], i.e., the number of adjacencies that are not common to both genomes. Hence, the polynomial time result for the breakpoint median problem for multichromosomal genomes [27] is consistent with the linear time result for the median problem under $\mathcal{SCOJ}$. The breakpoint median problem is NP-hard for unichromosomal genomes [72].

3.3 Single-Cut and Join Model

The *single-cut and join* model [19], denoted by $\mathcal{SCAJ}$, is an extension of the $\mathcal{SCOJ}$ model, i.e., $\mathcal{SCAJ} \supset \mathcal{SCOJ}$. Additionally to the cut and join operations of the $\mathcal{SCOJ}$ model, the $\mathcal{SCAJ}$ model allows for a *cut-and-join* operation which cuts an adjacency and connects two (potentially different) telomeres. A pair of genomes (α, α') is an event in $\mathcal{SCAJ}$ if and only if $(\alpha, \alpha') \in \mathcal{SCOJ}$ or there exist different extremities p, q, and r such that $\alpha \cup \{\{ p, r\}, \{q, \circ\}\} = \alpha' \cup \{\{ p, q\}, \{r, \circ\}\}$ (cut-and-join).

The cut-and-join event realizes the following new rearrangement events (*see* Fig. 5b): (1) a linear chromosome can be transformed into a circular chromosome and a linear chromosome (fission), (2) a starting sequence (prefix) or an ending sequence (suffix) of a linear chromosome is either inverted (affix inversion) or joined to another linear chromosome, and (3) a circular chromosome can be cut and joined with a linear chromosome yielding a linear chromosome (fusion).

3.3.1 Polynomial Time Solvable Problems

The sorting problem and the distance problem under $\mathcal{SCAJ}$ can be solved in linear time [19]. The distance of two genomes α and α' under $\mathcal{SCAJ}$ can be computed by $d_{\mathcal{SCAJ}}(\alpha, \alpha') = N - I/2 - C_2 + C_{\geq 3}$, where N is the number of genes, C_2 is the number of one-cycles, $C_{\geq 3}$ is the number of cycles of length at least three, and I is the number of odd paths in the adjacency graph $AG(\alpha, \alpha')$. The sorting algorithm as given in [19] is sketched in the following. For two genomes α and α' with $\alpha \neq \alpha'$ it holds that $AG(\alpha, \alpha')$ contains at least one path of length greater than one or a cycle of length greater than two (since otherwise both genomes would be equal). For each path and cycle one of the following events is used to reduce the distance between both genomes by one (*see* Fig. 6): (a) a one-cycle is detached from an α-path of length

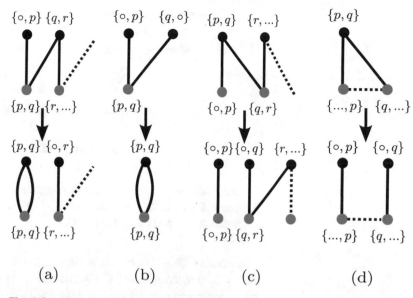

Fig. 6 Cases (**a**)–(**d**) of the algorithm for sorting α into α' under $\mathcal{SCAJ}$ shown on the adjacency graph. (Top) components of $AG(\alpha, \alpha')$ and (bottom) resulting components of $AG(\alpha \circ \rho, \alpha')$, where ρ is either a cut, a join, or a cut-and-join with $(\alpha, \alpha \circ \rho) \in \mathcal{SCAJ}$ and $d_{SCAJ}(\alpha, \alpha') > d_{SCAJ}(\alpha \circ \rho, \alpha')$

greater than two (cut-and-join), (b) an α-path of length two is replaced by a one-cycle (join), (c) an α'-path is split into two odd paths (cut), or (d) a cycle of length greater than two is replaced by an even path (cut). The algorithm terminates after $d_{SCAJ}(\alpha, \alpha')$ steps, because each of these operations reduces the distance by one. *See* [19] for a detailed analysis and a formal proof.

3.3.2 Open Problems

The complexity of other rearrangement problems and the distance problem where only linear chromosomes are allowed remain open.

3.4 Double-Cut and Join Model

The $\mathcal{DCJ}$ model acts on mixed genomes. This is the case, e.g., for genomes that contain plasmids in addition to the linear chromosomes [73–75] or in tumor genomes [76]. In the $\mathcal{DCJ}$ model an event cuts two adjacencies and forms two new adjacencies by joining four telomeres, *see* Fig. 7. More formally, a pair of genomes (α, α') is an event in $\mathcal{DCJ}$ if and only if $(\alpha, \alpha') \in \mathcal{SCAJ}$ or there exist $p, q, r, s \in \mathcal{E}(\alpha)$ such that $\alpha \cup \{\{p, s\}, \{r, q\}\} = \alpha' \cup \{\{p, q\}, \{r, s\}\}$ (double-cut and join). Translocations, fusions, fissions, and inversions are represented directly in $\mathcal{DCJ}$. The operations block-interchange and transposition are included indirectly via two $\mathcal{DCJ}$ operations: the excision of a circular intermediate and the reinsertion at a different position. This can be implemented naturally by assigning a weight of two to block-interchanges and transpositions and a weight of one to translocations, fusions, fissions, and inversions [77]. The occurrence of such implicit transpositions, i.e., two

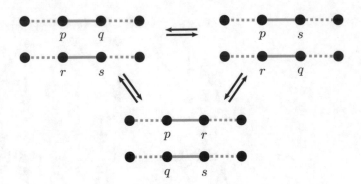

Fig. 7 Application of double-cut and join operation to adjacencies visualized on the genome graph. Note that the events of the submodel $\mathcal{SCAJ}$ which are illustrated in Fig. 5 are also events of $\mathcal{DCJ}$

consecutive $\mathcal{DCJ}$ rearrangements that are equivalent to a transposition, in parsimonious $\mathcal{DCJ}$ scenarios was estimated to 17 % of the rearrangement mutations for mammalian genomes [78].

3.4.1   *Polynomial Time Solvable Problems*

The distance problem under $\mathcal{DCJ}$ can be computed in linear time using the breakpoint graph [77]. The $\mathcal{DCJ}$ distance for two genomes α, α' can be computed by $d_{\mathcal{DCJ}}(\alpha,\alpha') = b - c$, where b is the number of breakpoints and c is the number of cycles in BP (α,α'). The web service CEGeD can be used to solve the distance problem under $\mathcal{DCJ}$, *see* Table 1. In order to apply the breakpoint graph for multichromosomal genomes so called capping, i.e., the addition of auxiliary end elements, and the concatenation of linear chromosomes is needed [77].

By using the adjacency graph a linear time algorithm was presented which has the advantage that also multichromosomal genomes are covered naturally [31]. With respect to the adjacency graph the $\mathcal{DCJ}$ distance is computed as $d_{\mathcal{DCJ}}(\alpha,\alpha') = N - (C + I/2)$ for two genomes α, α' with N genes, where C is the number of cycles and I is the number of odd paths in $AG(\alpha,\alpha')$.

The equivalence of the two distance formulas follows from the following facts: (1) the number of breakpoints b equals $N + t_{\alpha}/2 + E_{\alpha'} = N + t_{\alpha'}/2 + E_{\alpha}$, where t_{β} is the number of telomeres of a genome β and E_{β} is the number of β-paths, (2) $t_{\alpha}/2 + t_{\alpha'}/2 = I + E$ and $E = E_{\alpha} + E_{\alpha'}$, and (3) $c = C + I + E$. In the following a sketch of the proof of correctness of the $\mathcal{DCJ}$ distance formulas is given, for details *see* [31]. An alternative derivation is presented in [79]. The adjacency graph of two equal genomes consists of one-cycles (C_2)—one such cycle for each adjacency—and odd paths of length one (I_1)—one such path for each telomere. Hence sorting is equivalent to choosing $\mathcal{DCJ}$ events which increase the number of C_2 or I_1. Since a $\mathcal{DCJ}$ operation can: (1) not modify the number of cycles and odd paths simultaneously, (2) increase the

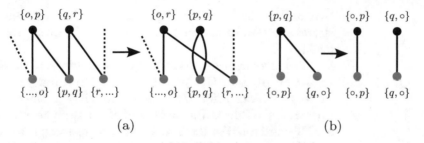

$$\{o,p\} \quad \{q,r\} \qquad\qquad \{o,r\} \quad \{p,q\} \qquad\qquad \{p,q\} \qquad\qquad \{o,p\} \quad \{q,o\}$$

$$\{...,o\} \ \{p,q\} \ \{r,...\} \qquad \{...,o\} \ \{p,q\} \ \{r,...\} \qquad \{o,p\} \quad \{q,o\} \qquad \{o,p\} \quad \{q,o\}$$

(a)   (b)

Fig. 8 The two cases of the $\mathcal{DCJ}$ sorting algorithm [31] shown for the adjacency graph. (**a**) Case 1. (**b**) Case 2

number of cycles at most by one, and (3) increase the number of odd paths at most by two it follows that $d_{\mathcal{DCJ}}(\alpha, \alpha') \geq N - (C + I/2)$ holds. The tightness of this bound was shown by giving a greedy algorithm that always attains the bound. In each step the greedy algorithm can apply one of the following two cases, *see* Fig. 8. Case 1: In the presence of the adjacencies $\{p, q\} \in \alpha'$ and $\{o, p\}, \{q, r\} \in \alpha$ the $\mathcal{DCJ}$ event is $(\alpha, \{\alpha \backslash \{\{o, p\}, \{q, r\}\}\} \cup \{\{p, q\}, \{o, r\}\})$. This creates a new one-cycle and reduces the size of a path by two. Case 2: For telomeres $\{p, \circ\}, \{q, \circ\} \in \alpha'$ and an adjacency $\{p, q\} \in \alpha$ the $\mathcal{DCJ}$ event is $(\alpha, \{\alpha \backslash \{p, q\}\} \cup \{\{p, \circ\}, \{q, \circ\}\})$. This replaces an even path of length two by two odd paths of length one. Observe that the second event uses only one cut.

In [31] a linearization of a circular genome is modeled by an additional cut of a vestigial adjacency $\{\circ, \circ\}$ and two joins of the resulting telomeres to telomere adjacencies, *see* [68] for a detailed description.

3.4.2 NP-Hard Problems

Many experimental studies do not determine the strandedness of the genes [80]. In such cases genomes are commonly represented by *unsigned permutations*. This motivates the *sorting problem for unsigned genomes (SUG)* under $\mathcal{DCJ}$ which was studied for the first time in [80]. The NP-hardness of this problem for unichromosomal unsigned genomes was shown by a reduction from the NP-hard *breakpoint graph decomposition (BGD)* problem [81]. The BGD problem is to find a decomposition of a breakpoint graph into a maximum number of edge-disjoint alternating cycles. Note that in contrast to the case of signed genomes in the breakpoint graph for unsigned genomes each gene corresponds to a single vertex. An approximation algorithm for solving the SUG problem for multi-chromosomal mixed genomes was presented in [80]. The algorithm is based on a modification of the approximation algorithm of [82] for the BGD problem.

Recall that similar to $\mathcal{DCJ}$ also for $\mathcal{INV}$ the distance problem for signed genomes is polynomial time solvable [4] whereas it is NP-hard for unsigned genomes [6]. This suggests that the complexity of the distance problem for rearrangements that cut and join two adjacencies is rather dependent on the availability of gene strandedness information than on the set of allowed rearrangement events.

The median problem under $\mathcal{DCJ}$ was shown to be NP-hard by reduction of the BGD problem [27]. Note that also this result holds analogously for the $\mathcal{INV}$ model [7]. Since the median problem is NP-hard the small and the large parsimony problem are NP-hard too. For the median problem exact algorithms [24, 83] and also heuristics [84, 85] have been presented in the literature. Based on the heuristic median solver an algorithm for the small phylogeny problem has been developed in [84]. Examples of software tools which can be used to solve the small parsimony problem under $\mathcal{DCJ}$ are MGRA and PATHGROUPS, *see* Table 1.

3.4.3 *Applications*

In [19] the distance problems under $\mathcal{SCAJ}$ and $\mathcal{DCJ}$ have been calculated for 281 synteny blocks of the human-mouse comparison from [86] and for 1359 synteny blocks of the genomes of chimp, rhesus monkey, mouse, rat, and dog from [87] with respect to the human genome. The results show that the obtained distances under $\mathcal{SCAJ}$ are much larger than the distances under $\mathcal{DCJ}$. The authors stress that the goal of the $\mathcal{SCAJ}$ model is rather an indicator for evaluating results under the $\mathcal{DCJ}$ model than being a realistic evolutionary model. Based on their results, the authors suggest that single-cut operations are more important in the mouse-human evolution than in the chimp-human evolution. The pairwise $\mathcal{DCJ}$ distance between synteny blocks from genomes of *Shigella boydii*, *Shigella dysenteriae*, *Shigella flexneri*, and *Escherichia coli* have been calculated in [68]. The generation of the synteny blocks and the calculation of the $\mathcal{DCJ}$ distances have been made by Mauve, *see* Table 1 for more information.

The algorithm for the small phylogeny problem which has been developed in [84] was used to analyze 13 chloroplast DNAs of genomes of *Campanulaceae* and the mammalian dataset from [88] (including the presented phylogenetic tree) which consists of the genomes of human, rat, mouse, cat, dog, pig, and cow. The results show that the reconstructed ancestral genomes contain between 1 and 5 circular chromosomes that occur in immediate ancestors of the seven mammalian species. The total number of used $\mathcal{DCJ}$ operations is 486 and the total number of restricted $\mathcal{DCJ}$ operations, i.e., $\mathcal{DCJ}$ operations that do not produce any circular chromosomes, is 487. This result strengthens the conjecture that there is no biological evidence of circular chromosomes in the nuclear genomes of higher eukaryotes [89].

Many software tools are based on the $\mathcal{DCJ}$ model, *see* Table 1 for an overview. For instance, GEvolutionS can be used to simulate evolutionary genome rearrangement scenarios and MLGO and GREDU can be used for the case that the input genomes do not have the same gene content.

3.5 Multi-Cut and Join Model

Rearrangement operations like inversions, fusions, fissions, and translocations can easily be modeled by cutting a genome at two positions before applying rejoin operations. However, rearrangement operations that create three breakpoints, e.g., transpositions and inverse transpositions, i.e., transpositions where in addition the orientation of the transposed genes is changed, can be modeled only indirectly when at most two cuts are allowed, e.g., by using a pair of $\mathcal{DCJ}$ operations or three $\mathcal{SCAJ}$ operations. Therefore, a generalized rearrangement model has been suggested [90] which cuts a genome at $k \in \mathbb{N}$ positions followed by rejoining the resulting fragments into new order. The resulting model is called *multi-cut and join* model ($\mathcal{MCJ}$) and for a specific $k \in \mathbb{N}$ we refer to it as *k-cut and join* model ($\mathcal{KCJ}$).[1] Formally, a pair of genomes (α, α') is an event in $\mathcal{KCJ}$ if and only if $(\alpha, \alpha') \in (\mathcal{K} - 1)\mathcal{CJ}$ or there exists a set of k adjacencies $K \subset \alpha$ such that $\alpha' \cup K = \alpha \cup X$, where X is a subset of $\{\{x, y\} : x, y \in \mathcal{E}(K), x \neq y\} \cup \{\{p, \circ\} : p \in \mathcal{E}(K)\}$ such that $\mathcal{E}(X) \cup \{p : \{p, \circ\} \in \mathcal{T}(X)\} = \mathcal{E}(K) \cup \{p : \{p, \circ\} \in \mathcal{T}(K)\}$, $|X| = k$, $X \cap K = \emptyset$, $1\mathcal{CJ} = \mathcal{SCAJ}$, and $2\mathcal{CJ} = \mathcal{DCJ}$. Note that for all $i \in [1: k-1]$ this definition implies that a $(\mathcal{K} - i)\mathcal{CJ}$ event is a particular event of $\mathcal{KCJ}$ which can be understood as a k-cut and join event which leaves exactly i of the k adjacencies unchanged.

3.5.1 Polynomial Time Solvable Problems

The distance problem under $\mathcal{KCJ}$ can be solved in polynomial time by computing $d_{\mathcal{KCJ}}(\alpha, \alpha') = \lceil (N - C_s(\alpha, \alpha'))/(k-1) \rceil$ for genomes α and α', where $k \geq 2$ is the number of cuts and $C_s(\alpha, \alpha')$ is the size of the maximum partition of the cycles in $BP(\alpha, \alpha')$ where the total number of black edges in each subset of cycles is equal to 1 mod $(k-1)$ [90]. For instance, $C_2(\alpha, \alpha')$ equals the number of cycles in $BP(\alpha, \alpha')$ (since for any number c of cycles $(c \equiv 1)$ mod 1) and $C_3(\alpha, \alpha')$ gives the number of odd cycles in $BP(\alpha, \alpha')$. Hence for $k = 2$, the formula equals the $\mathcal{DCJ}$ distance formula presented in [77]. Further, two algorithms for computing the distance formula between two genomes—a dynamic programming algorithm which is practical for small values of k and a linear time algorithm with exponential (in k) time preliminary computations—were presented in [90].

3.5.2 Open Problems

The distance problem under $\mathcal{KCJ}$ for linear multichromosomal genomes was studied in [91] resulting in lower bounds for the rearrangement distance. To the best of our knowledge no additional polynomial time algorithms have been published for the median problem and the small/large parsimony problem.

---

[1] In [90] these rearrangements are called *multi-break* rearrangements.

4   Preserving Genome Rearrangement Models

This section discusses the sorting problem, the median problem, and the small parsimony problem under $\mathcal{INV}^p$. Some results for related preserving rearrangement models are discussed at the end of the section.

The sorting problem under $\mathcal{INV}^p$ has been introduced in [11] with the objective to produce biologically more relevant results. Unfortunately, the sorting problem under $\mathcal{INV}^p$ is NP-hard [11]. But, it is fixed-parameter tractable [92] and there exist linear run time algorithms for many relevant instances [12, 93], and algorithms with a polynomial average run time [92]. Algorithms for the median problem and the small parsimony problem under $\mathcal{INV}^p$ that have a polynomial run time for many relevant data sets have been proposed in [94, 95], *see* Subheading 4.2.

4.1 Strong Interval Tree

The strong interval tree (SIT)[2] is the central data structure for efficient preserving rearrangement analysis. The main reason is that the SIT can be computed in linear time and represents the common intervals (which can be quadratic in number) in linear space [12].

Let Π be a set of k genomes that are represented by signed permutations and λ be a consistent reference permutation (typically $\lambda \in \Pi$). A common interval $I \in C(\Pi)$ is *strong* if every other common interval in $C(\Pi)$ is either included in I or it includes I. By definition the strong intervals of Π form a hierarchy which is captured by the *strong interval tree* (SIT). The SIT of Π with respect to λ, denoted by $T^\lambda(\Pi)$, is an ordered tree where each vertex represents a strong common interval of Π and the edges represent the minimum inclusion relation. The order of the children of a vertex in the SIT are without loss of generality given by their order in the reference permutation λ. For every inner vertex I of a SIT with children $I_1, \ldots, I_l$ that are ordered according to the reference permutation λ the *quotient permutation* associated with I for $\pi \in \Pi$ is the permutation π_I^λ which satisfies that $_I^\lambda(i)$ precedes $_I^\lambda(j)$ if and only if I_i is to left of I_j for $i \neq j$. A quotient permutation is called *linear increasing* if it is equal to ι, *linear decreasing* if it is $(l\ (l-1)\ldots 1)$, and *prime* otherwise. A vertex I of a SIT is called *linear* if all k quotient permutations are either linear increasing or linear decreasing. Otherwise it is called *prime*. It holds that a vertex of a SIT is linear if and only if every union of consecutive children is a common interval, whereas for a prime vertex only the union of all children is a common interval [12].

A so-called *k-sign* $\{+1, -1\}^k$ is assigned to the vertices to represent the orientation of linear quotient permutations and the

---

[2] Note that strong interval trees are similar to PQ-trees [96].

orientation of the elements in the case of leaf vertices. For a vertex I the i-th element of a k-sign, denoted by $s(i)$, is determined based on the following rules: (1) A leaf I has $s(i) = +1$ if the corresponding element has the same sign in π_i as in λ and $s(i) = -1$ otherwise. (2) A linear inner vertex I has $s(i) = +1$ if π_{iI}^λ is the identity permutation and -1 otherwise. (3) A prime vertex with linear parent inherits the $k - sign$ of the parent. A SIT is *unambiguous* if every prime vertex has a linear parent and *ambiguous* otherwise. SITs without prime vertices are called *definite*. In the *signed quotient permutation* each element is assigned the sign of the corresponding child node, i.e., $\pi_{iI}^\lambda(j)$ is assigned the i-th component of the k-sign of the j-th child. For a linear vertex I of the SIT a sign $s_I(i)$ contains the same information as the quotient permutation π_{iI}^λ, i.e., there is a bijective relation between signs of linear vertices of definite SITs and consistent permutations. Note that these rules uniquely determine the signs of every vertex of unambiguous and definite SITs, but the signs of a prime root vertex and prime vertices with prime parent in ambiguous trees are not determined. An example illustrating a SIT for a set of permutations is shown in Fig. 9.

4.2 Algorithms for the Preserving Inversion Model

Algorithms for the sorting problem under $\mathcal{INV}^p$ for signed unichromosomal linear genomes and a partition of the set of problem instances into instances that can be solved in linear time, polynomial time, or exponential time have been presented in [12]. More precisely, problem instances with a definite SIT can be solved in

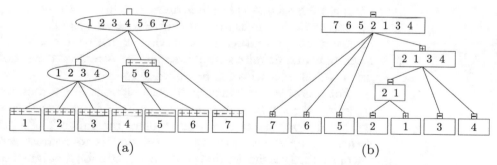

(a)   (b)

Fig. 9 (a) Strong common interval tree of $\Pi = \{(1\ldots7), (-7\,1\,3\,2\,4\,6\,-5), (6\,-5\,-4\,3\,-1\,2\,7), (-5\,-6\,7\,3\,4\,2\,-1)\}$ where the trivial common intervals, $\{5, 6\}$, and $\{1, 2, 3, 4\}$ are the strong common intervals of Π. Prime vertices and linear vertices are represented by ellipses and rectangles, respectively. The root vertex and vertex $\{1, 2, 3, 4\}$ are prime and vertex $\{5, 6\}$ is linear increasing with respect to $(1\ldots7)$. **(b)** Definite SIT $T^\iota(\Sigma)$ for $\Sigma = \{(7\,6\,5\,-2\,1\,-3\,-4), \iota\}$. Note that every vertex is linear since every union of consecutive children of each vertex is a common interval of Σ. The signs of the vertices are shown at the top of the rectangles. The signs with respect to ι are omitted since it is $+$ for all vertices. Vertex $\{2, 1\}$ is linear decreasing since its quotient permutation is $(2\ 1)$ and the quotient permutation $(1\ 2\ 3)$ of vertex $\{2, 1, 3, 4\}$ implies that it is linear increasing. A scenario sorting $\pi_1 = (7\,6\,5\,-2\,1\,-3\,-4)$ to $(-7\,-6\,-5\,-4\,-3\,-2\,-1)$ is obtained by applying inversions $\{7\}, \{6\}, \{5\}, \{4\}, \{3\}, \{1\}, \{1, 2\}$, and $\{1, 2, 3, 4\}$ to π_1. Recall that ι and $(-7\ \ 6\,-5\,-4\,-3\,-2\,-1)$ are considered to be equal

linear time, those with an unambiguous SIT can be solved in sub-quadratic time, and instances with an ambiguous SIT have a worst case exponential run time.

In the following we will identify inversions by the interval that they reverse. Consider a signed permutation π that is to be transformed into ι. Note that arbitrary pairs of signed permutations can be reduced to this case by renaming the elements of the permutations. Let $T^\iota(\Pi)$ be the strong interval tree of $\Pi = \{\pi, \iota\}$. Instead of the 2-sign at each prime vertex with linear parent and each linear vertex a 1-sign (or just sign for short) is stored at the vertices. The sign is equal to the 2-sign component that corresponds to π. This is because the sign of the target permutation ι is $+$ for all vertices with a sign. Therefore, we can call a vertex linear increasing (resp. decreasing) if the quotient permutation is linear increasing (resp. decreasing).

The key for solving the sorting problem under $\mathcal{INV}^p$ is that an inversion is preserving if and only if it is a vertex of the SIT or a union of children of a prime vertex [12]. Thus, linear vertices can only be reversed as a whole whereas the children of prime vertices can be freely rearranged. With respect to the SIT the problem of sorting by preserving inversions is to apply rearrangements such that all quotient permutations are transformed into the identity permutation, i.e., the vertices become linear increasing. Hence, if a vertex I of $T^\iota(\pi)$ has a different sign than its parent vertex, it holds that the inversion defined by I is always part of any optimal sorting scenario [12] (Lemma 2), i.e., the inversions that correspond to vertices with a sign different to the one of their parent define a parsimonious scenario [12] (Theorem 2). This can easily be implemented to run in linear time, *see* Fig. 9b for an example. Since the inversions in parsimonious preserving scenarios for a problem instance with a definite strong interval tree commute the set of all parsimonious scenarios can be obtained easily.

For a problem instance with unambiguous SIT a method to transform the signed quotient permutation of prime vertices into the identity permutation is needed. Since the children of a prime vertex can be freely rearranged a solution is to reconstruct an unconstrained parsimonious inversion scenario for the signed quotient permutation. That is, for every prime vertex I a parsimonious scenario from π_I^λ to ι is computed if I has a positive sign. If it has a negative sign a scenario from π_I^λ to $(-n \ldots -1)$ is computed. Applying the corresponding inversions to π results in a definite SIT which can be processed as explained beforehand. The run time of the algorithm for unambiguous SITs is dominated by solving the sorting problem for prime vertices which is done by the algorithm presented in [97]. The algorithm from [97] solves the sorting problem under $\mathcal{INV}$ for signed permutations in sub-quadratic run time $O(n\sqrt{n}\log(n))$. An example for sorting an unambiguous SIT under $\mathcal{INV}^p$ is given in Fig. 10a.

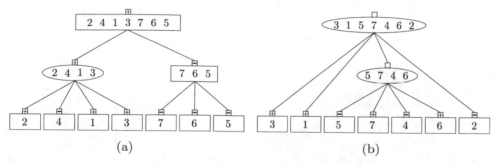

(a)   (b)

Fig. 10 (a) Unambiguous SIT $T'(\Pi)$ for $\Pi = \{\ \pi = (2-4\ 1\ 3-7-6-5),\ \iota\}$. Vertex $\{2\ 4\ 1\ 3\}$ is prime since its quotient permutation is $(2\ 4\ 1\ 3)$. Its parent vertex is linear increasing which results in an unambiguous SIT. A parsimonious scenario sorting $(2-4\ 1\ 3)$ to ι is given by the inversions $\{1, 3, 4\}$, $\{2, 3\}$, $\{3\}$, and $\{1, 2, 3\}$. Applying the scenario to π yields $\pi' = (1\ 2\ 3\ 4-7-6-5)$ which has a definite SIT $T'(\pi', \iota)$. For π' the inversion $\{5, 6, 7\}$ is a parsimonious scenario. Both scenarios together are a parsimonious scenario for the unambiguous SIT $T'(\Pi)$. **(b)** Example of an ambiguous SIT. Here, the signs of prime vertices of $T'(\{(3\ 1-5\ 7-4\ 6-2),\ \iota\})$ are not uniquely determined. A parsimonious scenario is obtained by a negative sign for the root vertex and a positive sign for its child prime vertex

For ambiguous SITs the signs of prime vertices with prime parent are unknown, *see* Fig. 10b. By trying every combination of sign assignments and applying the algorithm for unambiguous SITs an exact solution can be obtained. An improvement is possible by applying dynamic programming separately for every component of connected prime vertices. Assume that $u \in \mathbb{N}$ unsigned prime vertices exist, in this case the described algorithm for ambiguous SITs (which uses the algorithm from [97]) has an exponential run time of $O(2^u n \sqrt{n}\log(n))$ in the worst case.

In the following the algorithm of [94] for the small parsimony problem under $\mathcal{INV}^p$ for sets of genomes with a definite SIT is presented. The algorithm runs in polynomial time. The basis of the approach is an extension of the results of [98] which was first used in an approach for solving the preserving inversion median problem [95]. The idea of the algorithm is to extract binary characters from the SIT which are then processed by Fitch's algorithm [70] for maximum parsimony. Figure 11 illustrates the algorithm which is described below.

Again, the foundation of the algorithm is the insight that an inversion is preserving with respect to a set of permutations Π if and only if it is either a vertex of $T(\Pi)$ or a union of consecutive child vertices of a prime vertex. This result from [94] is a generalization of a result of [12]. Hence, for a linear vertex preserving inversions can only change its order. Therefore, for each linear vertex it needs to be determined in which of the permutations it has to be inverted or not. For a set of permutations $\Pi = \{\pi_1, \ldots, \pi_k\}$ the Parity Lemma [12] and its reformulation for SITs with k-signs [94] states that a vertex I has to be inverted in permutation π_i in a parsimonious preserving scenario if and only if its sign $s_I(i)$ differs from the

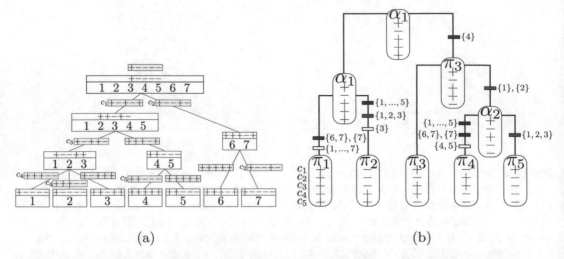

(a)   (b)

Fig. 11 (a) SIT $T'(\Pi)$ with k-signs for $\pi_1 = \iota$, $\pi_2 = (6{-}7\ 3{-}2{-}1\ 4\ 5)$, $\pi_3 = (6{-}7{-}5\ 4{-}3{-}2{-}1)$, $\pi_4 = (-7{-}6{-}1{-}2\ 3{-}5\ 4)$, and $\pi_5 = (6{-}7{-}5\ 4{-}1{-}2\ 3)$. The character state of a vertex is placed on the edge to its parent. Character state assignments of vertex {1} is $(+++--)$ because the k-signs of vertex {1} and vertex {1, 2, 3} are equal in the first three positions and unequal in positions four and five. SIT $T'(\Pi)$ shows five unique, nontrivial characters which are denoted by $c_1, \ldots, c_5$. The permutation π_2 is uniquely determined by character states and k-signs since the signs of all vertices in pre-order are $-1, +1, -1, -1, -1, +1,$ $+1, +1, +1, +1, +1, -1$. (b) Optimal solution of the small parsimony problem under $\mathcal{INV}^p$ which is obtained by Fitch's algorithm [70] for T and nontrivial, unique characters $c_1, \ldots, c_5$. Ancestral permutations $\alpha_1 = (6{-}7{-}5{-}4{-}3{-}2{-}1)$ and $\alpha_2 = (6{-}7{-}5\ 4{-}\ 3\ 2\ 1)$ are determined by preserving inversions represented on the edges. Root permutation α_1 is constructed from π_3 by reverting element {4}. This information is obtained since the character state assignment of both vertices differs only in one sign of c_5 which corresponds to vertex {4} in the SIT

sign $s_J(i)$ of its parent vertex J. Hence, the essential information is the difference of the k-signs of the vertices and their respective parents. To capture these differences every vertex of the SIT $T^\lambda(\Pi)$ is assigned to a binary character representing the information on the equality or inequality of its k-signs and the k-signs of its parent. Formally, consider a non-root vertex I and its parent vertex J of $T^\lambda(\Pi)$ with k-signs s_I and s_J. The binary *character state assignment* of I is a k-tuple c_I such that $c_I(i) = s_I(i) \cdot s_J(i)$ for $i \in [1: k]$. The character state assignment for the root vertex is defined by comparing its k-sign with $\{+1\}^k$. Note that a character state assignment for every vertex of $T^\lambda(\Pi)$ uniquely determines Π since π_i is determined by multiplying $c_I(i)$ and parents sign $s_J(i)$ from top to bottom starting at root vertex with $+1$. Hence, each assignment of character states to the nodes of the SIT uniquely determines a consistent permutation, *see* Fig. 11a for an example.

Due to the bijective relation between consistent permutations, character state assignments, and preserving inversions, the small parsimony problem for a set of permutations Π with definite SIT and phylogenetic tree T can be solved exactly and efficiently by solving the small parsimony problem for the character states for the vertices of $T^\lambda(\Pi)$. Consider a set of permutations Π with a definite SIT $T^\lambda(\Pi)$, the character state assignments of its vertices, and a given tree T. Solving the small parsimony problem for T and the binary characters defined for the vertices yields a reconstruction of ancestral character states of T. Given the ancestral character states of a vertex of T, the signs for the vertices of the SIT and the corresponding permutations are constructed by the following procedure. Starting with the identity permutation all strong common intervals need to be inverted for which the sign differs from the one of its parent. *See* Fig. 11b for an example. This algorithm runs in $O(kn)$ time for a set Π of k permutations of length n if $T^\lambda(\Pi)$ is definite. Because of the one-to-one relation between the characters defined by the SIT and parsimonious inversions the large parsimony problem for binary characters under $\mathcal{INV}^p$ is *NP*-hard as well—even for sets of permutations with definite SIT [94].

In [95] an exact algorithm—called TCIP—for the median problem under $\mathcal{INV}^p$ was presented. TCIP uses the bijective relations between consistent permutations, character state assignments, and preserving inversions which yields a linear run time for definite SITs. For ambiguous SITs different unconstrained versions of the median problem have to be solved for the quotient permutations of prime vertices considering different k-sign assignments which significantly increases the run time of TCIP. However, it has been shown empirically that median problems of random gene orders as well as organellar gene orders often have a definite SIT and then TCIP has a good performance.

4.2.1 Application

In [94] the small phylogeny problem has been analyzed under $\mathcal{INV}^p$ for 4 unique *γ-Proteobacteria* gene orders from [99] and for a set of *Burkholderia* gene orders. Pairwise scenarios under $\mathcal{INV}^p$ between 16 synteny blocks of the X Chromosome of the human, mouse, and rat genomes from [100] have been constructed in [12]. The results show that the SIT for the rat and mouse comparison is definite and that a parsimonious preserving scenario contains 11 inversion. The comparison between human and rat (resp. mouse) shows an unambiguous SIT which results into a preserving scenario with 13 inversions (resp. 12 inversions).

4.3 Related Preserving Problems

Phylogenetic reconstructions should consider all relevant rearrangement operations. Mitochondrial gene orders, for instance, evolve by inversions, (inverse) transpositions, and tandem-duplication-random-loss (TDRL) events (i.e., a tandem duplication of a continuous sequence of genes followed by the loss of one copy of each duplicated gene [101]). In particular TDRLs are important rearrangement events in mitochondrial genomes [102–104]. The algorithm CREx which solves the preserving sorting problem heuristically under these four rearrangement operations has been presented in [33]. The basic principle of CREx is the detection of patterns in the SIT that determine corresponding rearrangement events: (1) An inversion corresponds to a vertex with a different sign as its parent, (2) a transposition is represented by a vertex that has two children and its sign differs from the one of its children and its parent, (3) an inverse transposition corresponds to a vertex whose sign is different to its parents signs and the signs of all but the first (or last) children, and (4) a TDRL corresponds to a prime vertex whose quotient permutation has only positive or only negative elements. CREx uses a step wise approach which identifies (inverse) transposition patterns and inversion patterns in linear vertices of SITs. In the second step prime vertices are heuristically solved by combining TDRL and inversion events. For a detailed description of CREx, the reader is referred to [13].

The sorting problem under $\mathcal{DCJ}^p$ was studied in [98, 105]. In this study a version of the preserving property was applied which allows to cut out circular intermediates consisting of a subset of common intervals. Polynomial time algorithms for multichromosomal mixed genomes with SIT consisting of prime vertices and linear vertices with two children only, e.g., ambiguous SITs, were given. The sorting problem under $\mathcal{DCJ}^p$ turns out to be *NP*-hard for definite and unambiguous SITs [98]. The problem is already difficult for linear vertices with three children, because it is impossible to decide for a parsimonious sorting direction. However, Bérard et al. presented a fixed parameter polynomial time algorithm which uses a specific pattern of common intervals as a parameter to solve the sorting problem for definite SITs [98]. The average-time complexity of their algorithm is still open. Interestingly, the results of [98] for the sorting problem imply the first case where the models $\mathcal{INV}^p$ and $\mathcal{DCJ}^p$ differ in complexity.

4.3.1 Application

CREx has been used in [106] to study the phylogeny of 185 Metazoa mitochondrial gene orders. In particular, the gene orders of Arthropod species and the Chordata species have been studied. A comprehensive analysis of the results is given in [13]. Furthermore, CREx has been used in several publications for the analysis of mitochondrial gene orders. A recent example is [107], where the mitochondrial genome of *Aglaiogyrodactylus forficulatus* was compared with the genomes of other monogenoidean flatworm species.

5   Conclusion

In this chapter we have given an overview on genome rearrangement analysis. The focus was on the following two approaches. The first approach is the development of models for rearrangement mutations that are well suited for a theoretical analysis. In particular, models that use the two operations cut, i.e., to split a chromosome into fragments, and join, i.e., to merge fragments of chromosomes to new chromosomes. The second approach is to identify biologically motivated constraints on the applicability of gene rearrangement mutations. In particular, constraints that model conserved gene clusters have been considered. Several open problems for genome rearrangement analysis have been mentioned.

References

1. Wang L-S, Warnow T, Moret BME, Jansen RK, Raubeson LA (2006) Distance-based genome rearrangement phylogeny. J Mol Evol 63(4):473–483

2. Sankoff D (1992) Edit distance for genome comparison based on non-local operations. In: Proceedings of the 3rd annual symposium on combinatorial pattern matching (CPM '92). Lecture Notes in Computer Science, vol 644, pp 121–135

3. Watterson GA, Ewens WJ, Hall TE, Morgan A (1982) The chromosome inversion problem. J Theor Biol 99(1):1–7

4. Hannenhalli S, Pevzner PA (1999) Transforming cabbage into turnip: polynomial algorithm for sorting signed permutations by reversals. J ACM 46(1):1–27

5. Hannenhalli S, Pevzner PA (1995) Transforming men into mice (polynomial algorithm for genomic distance problem). In: Proceedings of the 36th annual symposium on foundations of computer science (FOCS '95), pp 581–592

6. Caprara A (1997) Sorting by reversals is difficult. In: Proceedings of the 11th annual international conference on computational molecular biology (RECOMB '97), pp 75–83

7. Caprara A (2003) The reversal median problem. INFORMS J Comput 15(1):93–113

8. Bulteau L, Fertin G, Rusu I (2012) Sorting by transpositions is difficult. SIAM J Discrete Math 26(3):1148–1180

9. Bourque G, Pevzner PA (2002) Genome-scale evolution: reconstructing gene orders in the ancestral species. Genome Res 12(1):26–36

10. Elias I, Hartman T (2006) A 1.375-approximation algorithm for sorting by transpositions. IEEE/ACM Trans Comput Biol Bioinform 3(4):369–379

11. Figeac M, Varré J-S (2004) Sorting by reversals with common intervals. In: Proceedings of the 4th international workshop algorithms in bioinformatics (WABI '04). Lecture Notes in Computer Science, vol 3240, pp 26–37

12. Bérard S, Bergeron A, Chauve C, Paul C (2007) Perfect sorting by reversals is not always difficult. IEEE/ACM Trans Comput Biol Bioinform 4(1):4–16

13. Bernt M (2009) Gene order rearrangement methods for the reconstruction of phylogeny. PhD thesis, University Leipzig

14. Bernt M, Merkle D, Middendorf M (2007) A fast and exact algorithm for the perfect reversal median problem. In: Proceedings of the 3rd international symposium on bioinformatics research and applications (ISBRA '07). Lecture Notes in Computer Science, vol 4463, pp 305–316

15. Swenson KM, Simonaitis P, Blanchette M (2016) Models and algorithms for genome rearrangement with positional constraints. Algorithm Mol Biol 11(1):1–10

16. Véron AS, Lemaitre C, Gautier C, Lacroix V, Sagot M-F (2011) Close 3D proximity of evolutionary breakpoints argues for the notion of spatial synteny. BMC Genomics 12(1):1–13

17. Graham GJ (1995) Tandem genes and clustered genes. J Theor Biol 175(1):71–87

18. Heber S, Stoye J (2001) Finding all common intervals of k permutations. In: Proceedings of the 12th annual symposium on combinatorial pattern matching (CPM '01). Lecture Notes in Computer Science, vol 2089, pp 207–218

19. Bergeron A, Medvedev P, Stoye J (2010) Rearrangement models and single-cut operations. J Comput Biol 17(9):1213–1225

20. Felsenstein J, Felenstein J (2004) Inferring phylogenies, vol 2. Sinauer Associates, Sunderland

21. Tannier E, Sagot M-F (2004) Sorting by reversals in subquadratic time. In: Proceedings of the 15th annual symposium on combinatorial pattern matching (CPM '04). Lecture Notes in Computer Science, vol 3109, pp 1–13

22. Sankoff D, Blanchette M (1998) Multiple genome rearrangement and breakpoint phylogeny. J Comput Biol 5(3):555–570

23. Moret BME, Wang L-S, Warnow T, Wyman SK (2001) New approaches for reconstructing phylogenies from gene order data. Bioinformatics 17(9):165–173

24. Zhang M, Arndt W, Tang J (2009) An exact solver for the DCJ median problem. In: Proceedings of the pacific symposium on biocomputing (PSB '09), pp 138–149

25. Feijão P, Meidanis J (2011) SCJ: a breakpoint-like distance that simplifies several rearrangement problems. IEEE/ACM Trans Comput Biol Bioinform 8(5):1318–1329

26. Ohlebusch E, Abouelhoda M, Hockel K (2007) A linear time algorithm for the inversion median problem in circular bacterial genomes. J Discrete Algorithms 5(4):637–646

27. Tannier E, Zheng C, Sankoff D (2009) Multichromosomal median and halving problems under different genomic distances. BMC Bioinform 10(1):1–15

28. Bader M (2011) The transposition median problem is NP-complete. Theor Comput Sci 412(12–14):1099–1110

29. Fertin G, Labarre A, Rusu I, Tannier E, Vialette S (2009) Combinatorics of genome rearrangements, 1st edn. The MIT Press, Cambridge

30. Bergeron A, Mixtacki J, Stoye J (2006) CEGeD. http://bibiserv.techfak.uni-bielefeld.de/ceged

31. Bergeron A, Mixtacki J, Stoye J (2006) A unifying view of genome rearrangements. In: Proceedings of the 6th international workshop algorithms in bioinformatics (WABI '06). Lecture Notes in Computer Science, vol 4175, pp 163–173

32. Bernt M, Merkle D, Ramsch K, Fritzsch G, Perseke M, Bernhard D, Schlegel M, Stadler PF, Middendorf M (2007) CREx. http://pacosy.informatik.uni-leipzig.de/crex

33. Bernt M, Merkle D, Ramsch K, Fritzsch G, Perseke M, Bernhard D, Schlegel M, Stadler PF, Middendorf M (2007) CREx: inferring genomic rearrangements based on common intervals. Bioinformatics 23(21):2957–2958

34. Krell P (2014) GEvolutionS. http://bibiserv.techfak.uni-bielefeld.de/gevolutions

35. Tesler G (2002) GRIMM: genome rearrangements web server. Bioinformatics 18 (3):492–493

36. Tesler G, Yu Y, Pevzner P (2002) GRIMM. http://grimm.ucsd.edu/GRIMM/

37. Bader M, Abouelhoda MI, Ohlebusch E (2002) MGR. http://grimm.ucsd.edu/MGR/

38. Alekseyev MA, Pevzner PA (2009) Breakpoint graphs and ancestral genome reconstructions. Genome Res 19(5):943–957

39. Alekseyev MA, Pevzner PA (2009) MGRA. http://mgra.cblab.org/

40. Hu F, Lin Yu, Tang J (2014) MLGO. http://www.geneorder.org/server.php

41. Hu F, Lin Yu, Tang J (2014) MLGO: phylogeny reconstruction and ancestral inference from gene-order data. BMC Bioinform 15 (1):1–6

42. Stoye J, Wittler R (2009) A unified approach for reconstructing ancient gene clusters. IEEE/ACM Trans Comput Biol Bioinform 6(3):387–400

43. Wittler R (2004) Roci. http://bibiserv.techfak.uni-bielefeld.de/roci

44. Huang Y-L, Huang C-C, Tang CY, Lu CL (2009) SoRT². http://genome.cs.nthu.edu.tw/SORT2/

45. Huang Y-L, Lu CL (2010) Sorting by reversals, generalized transpositions, and translocations using permutation groups. J Comput Biol 17(5):685–705

46. Christie DA (1996) Sorting permutations by block-interchanges. Inf Process Lett 60 (4):165–169

47. Martin M (2007) SBBI. http://bibiserv.techfak.uni-bielefeld.de/sbbi

48. Hilker R, Sickinger C, Friesen R, Mixtacki J, Stoye J (2005) UniMoG. http://bibiserv.techfak.uni-bielefeld.de/dcj

49. Braga MDV (2008) baobabLUNA. http://doua.prabi.fr/software/luna#perm

50. Braga MDV (2009) baobabluna: the solution space of sorting by reversals. Bioinformatics 25(14):1833–1835

51. Bader M (2009) dcjdDist. http://www.uni-ulm.de/in/theo/m/alumni/bader/

52. Bader M (2009) Sorting by reversals, block interchanges, tandem duplications, and deletions. BMC Bioinform 10(Suppl 1):S9

53. Zhao H, Bourque G (2009) EMRAE. http://www.gis.a-star.edu.sg/~bourque/software.html

54. Zhao H, Bourque G (2009) Recovering genome rearrangements in the mammalian phylogeny. Genome Res 19(5):934–942

55. Gog S, Bader M, Ohlebusch E (2008) Genesis: genome evolution scenarios. Bioinformatics 24(5):711–712

56. Gog S, Bader M, Ohlebusch E (2009) GEN-ESIS. http://www.uni-ulm.de/en/in/insti tute-of-theoretical-computer-science/m/ alumni/bader/

57. Bader DA, Moret BME, Warnow T, Wyman SK, Yan M, Tang J, Siepel AC, Caprara A (2004) GRAPPA. https://www.cs.unm.edu/ ~moret/GRAPPA/

58. Shao M (2015) GREDU. https://github. com/shaomingfu/gredu

59. Shao M, Lin Yu, Moret B (2014) An exact algorithm to compute the DCJ distance for genomes with duplicate genes. In: Proceedings of the 18th annual international conference on computational molecular biology (RECOMB '14). Lecture Notes in Computer Science, vol 8394, pp 280–292

60. Darling AC, Mau B, Blattner FR, Perna NT (2004) Mauve: multiple alignment of conserved genomic sequence with rearrangements. Genome Res 14(7):1394–1403

61. Darling ACE, Mau B, Blattner FR, Perna NT (2015) Mauve. http://darlinglab.org/ mauve/mauve.html

62. Bader M, Abouelhoda MI, Ohlebusch E (2008) A fast algorithm for the multiple genome rearrangement problem with weighted reversals and transpositions. BMC Bioinform 9(1):1–13

63. Bader M, Abouelhoda MI, Ohlebusch E (2008) phylo. http://www.uni-ulm.de/ in/theo/m/alumni/bader/

64. Fu Z, Chen X, Vacic V, Nan P, Zhong Y, Jiang T (2007) MSOAR: a high-throughput ortholog assignment system based on genome rearrangement. J Comput Biol 14(9):1160–1175

65. Fu Z, Chen X, Vacic V, Nan P, Zhong Y, Jiang T (2009) MSOAR. http://msoar.cs.ucr.edu/ index.php

66. Zheng C, Sankoff D (2011) On the pathgroups approach to rapid small phylogeny. BMC Bioinform 12(1):1–9

67. Zheng C, Sankoff D (2011) Pathgroups. http://albuquerque.bioinformatics.uottawa. ca/lab/software.html

68. Friedberg R, Darling AE, Yancopoulos S (2008) Genome rearrangement by the double cut and join operation. Methods in molecular biology, vol 452, pp 385–416. Humana Press, New York

69. Feijão P, Meidanis J (2009) SCJ: a variant of breakpoint distance for which sorting, genome median and genome halving problems are easy. In: Proceedings of the 9th international workshop algorithms in bioinformatics (WABI '09). Lecture Notes in Computer Science, vol 5724, pp 85–96

70. Fitch WM (1971). Toward defining the course of evolution: minimum change for a specific tree topology. Syst Biol 20 (4):406–416

71. Foulds LR, Graham RL (1982) The steiner problem in phylogeny is NP-complete. Adv Appl Math 3(1):43–49

72. Pe'er I, Shamir R (1998) The median problems for breakpoints are NP-complete. Elec Colloq Comput Complexity 5(71)

73. Casjens S, Palmer N, van Vugt R, Huang WM, Stevenson B, Rosa P, Lathigra R, Sutton G, Peterson J, Dodson RJ, Haft D, Hickey E, Gwinn M, White O, Fraser CM (2000) A bacterial genome in flux: the twelve linear and nine circular extrachromosomal DNAs in an infectious isolate of the Lyme disease spirochete *Borrelia burgdorferi*. Mol Microbiol 35(3):490–516

74. Qiu WG, Schutzer SE, Bruno JF, Attie O, Xu Y, Dunn JJ, Fraser CM, Casjens SR, Luft BJ (2004) Genetic exchange and plasmid transfers in Borrelia burgdorferi sensu stricto revealed by three-way genome comparisons and multilocus sequence typing. Proc Natl Acad Sci USA 101(39):14150–14155

75. Volff JN, Altenbuchner J (2000) A new beginning with new ends: linearisation of circular chromosomes during bacterial evolution. FEMS Microbiol Lett 186(2):143–150

76. Raphael BJ, Pevzner PA (2004) Reconstructing tumor amplisomes. Bioinformatics 20 (Suppl 1):265–273

77. Yancopoulos S, Attie O, Friedberg R (2005) Efficient sorting of genomic permutations by translocation, inversion and block interchange. Bioinformatics 21(16):3340–3346

78. Jiang S, Alekseyev MA (2015) Implicit transpositions in shortest DCJ scenarios. In: Proceedings of the 2nd international conference on algorithms for computational biology (AlCoB '15). Lecture Notes in Computer Science, vol 9199, pp 13–24

79. Bergeron A, Stoye J (2013) The genesis of the DCJ formula. Computational biology, vol 19, pp 63–81. Springer, New York

80. Chen X (2010) On sorting permutations by double-cut-and-joins. In: Proceedings of the 16th annual international computing and combinatorics conference (COCOON '10).

Lecture Notes in Computer Science, vol 6196, pp 439–448

81. Kececioglu J, Sankoff D (1995) Exact and approximation algorithms for sorting by reversals, with application to genome rearrangement. Algorithmica 13(1–2):180–210

82. Lin Y, Moret BM (2008) Estimating true evolutionary distances under the DCJ model. Bioinformatics 24(13):114–122

83. Xu AW, Sankoff D (2008) Decompositions of multiple breakpoint graphs and rapid exact solutions to the median problem. In: Proceedings of the 8th international workshop algorithms in bioinformatics (WABI '08). Lecture Notes in Computer Science, vol 5251, pp 25–37

84. Adam Z, Sankoff D (2008) The ABCs of MGR with DCJ. Evol Bioinform Online 4:69–74

85. Lenne R, Solnon C, Stützle T, Tannier E, Birattari M (2008) Reactive stochastic local search algorithms for the genomic median problem. In: Proceedings of the 8th European conference on evolutionary computation in combinatorial optimisation (EvoCOP '08). Lecture Notes in Computer Science, vol 4972, pp 266–276

86. Pevzner P, Tesler G (2003) Transforming men into mice: the Nadeau-Taylor chromosomal breakage model revisited. In: Proceedings of the 7th annual international conference on computational molecular biology (RECOMB '03), pp 247–256

87. Ma J, Zhang L, Suh BB, Raney BJ, Burhans RC, Kent WJ, Blanchette M, Haussler D, Miller W (2006) Reconstructing contiguous regions of an ancestral genome. Genome Res 16(12):1557–1565

88. Murphy WJ, Larkin DM, Everts-van der Wind A, Bourque G, Tesler G, Auvil L, Beever JE, Chowdhary BP, Galibert F, Gatzke L, Hitte C, Meyers SN, Milan D, Ostrander EA, Pape G, Parker HG, Raudsepp T, Rogatcheva MB, Schook LB, Skow LC, Welge M, Womack JE, O'Brien SJ, Pevzner PA, Lewin HA (2005) Dynamics of mammalian chromosome evolution inferred from multispecies comparative maps. Science 309 (5734):613–617

89. Brown TA (2006) Genomes. Garland Science, New York

90. Alekseyev MA, Pevzner PA (2008) Multi-break rearrangements and chromosomal evolution. Theor Comput Sci 395(2):193–202

91. Alekseyev MA (2008) Multi-break rearrangements and breakpoint re-uses: from circular to linear genomes. J Comput Biol 15 (8):1117–1131

92. Bouvel M, Chauve C, Mishna M, Rossin D (2011) Average-case analysis of perfect sorting by reversals. Discrete Math Algorithms Appl 3(3):369–392

93. Bérard S, Chauve C, Paul C (2008) A more efficient algorithm for perfect sorting by reversals. Inf Process Lett 106(3):90–95

94. Bernt M, Chao K-M, Kao J-W, Middendorf M, Tannier E (2012) Preserving inversion phylogeny reconstruction. In: Proceedings of the 12th international workshop algorithms in bioinformatics (WABI '12). Lecture Notes in Computer Science, vol 7534, pp 1–13

95. Bernt M, Merkle D, Middendorf M (2008) Solving the preserving reversal median problem. IEEE/ACM Trans Comput Biol Bioinform 5(3):332–347

96. Booth KS, Lueker GS (1976) Testing for the consecutive ones property, interval graphs, and graph planarity using PQ-tree algorithms. J Comput Syst Sci 13(3):335–379

97. Tannier E, Bergeron A, Sagot M-F (2007) Advances on sorting by reversals. Discrete Appl Math 155(6):881–888

98. Bérard S, Chateau A, Chauve C, Paul C, Tannier E (2009) Computation of perfect DCJ rearrangement scenarios with linear and circular chromosomes. J Comput Biol 16 (10):1287–1309

99. Belda E, Moya A, Silva FJ (2015) Genome rearrangement distances and gene order phylogeny in γ-proteobacteria. Mol Biol Evol 22 (6):1456–1467

100. Gibbs RA, Weinstock GM, Metzker ML, Muzny DM, Sodergren EJ, Scherer S, Scott G, Steffen D, Worley KC, Burch PE, et al (2004) Genome sequence of the Brown Norway rat yields insights into mammalian evolution. Nature 428(6982):493–521

101. Chaudhuri K, Chen K, Mihaescu R, Rao S (2006) On the tandem duplication-random loss model of genome rearrangement. In: Proceedings of the 17th annual ACM-SIAM symposium discrete algorithm (SODA '06), pp 564–570

102. Boore JL (2000) The duplication/random loss model for gene rearrangement exemplified by mitochondrial genomes of deuterostome animals, pp 133–147. Springer, New York

103. Inoue JG, Miya M, Tsukamoto K, Nishida M (2003) Evolution of the deep-sea gulper eel mitochondrial genomes: large-scale gene rearrangements originated within the eels. Mol Biol Evol 20(11):1917–1924

104. San Mauro D, Gower DJ, Zardoya R, Wilkinson M (2006) A hotspot of gene order rearrangement by tandem duplication and random loss in the vertebrate mitochondrial genome. Mol Biol Evol 23(1):227–234

105. Bérard S, Chateau A, Chauve C, Paul C, Tannier E (2008) Perfect DCJ rearrangement. In: Proceedings of the RECOMB international workshop comparative genomics (RCG '08). Lecture Notes in Computer Science, vol 5267, pp 158–169

106. Bernt M, Middendorf M (2011) A method for computing an inventory of metazoan mitochondrial gene order rearrangements. BMC Bioinform 12(9):1

107. Bachmann L, Fromm B, Patella de Azambuja L, Boeger WA (2016) The mitochondrial genome of the egg-laying flatworm Aglaiogyrodactylus forficulatus (Platyhelminthes: Monogenoidea). Parasit Vectors 9(1):1–8

Chapter 10

Whole Genome Duplication in Plants: Implications for Evolutionary Analysis

David Sankoff and Chunfang Zheng

Abstract

The recurrent cycle of whole genome duplication (WGD) followed by massive duplicate gene loss (fractionation) differentiates plant evolutionary history from that of most other phylogenetic domains, where WGD has occurred relatively rarely, even on an evolutionary time scale. We discuss the mechanism of WGD and its biological consequences. We survey the prevalence of WGD in the flowering plants. We outline some of the major kinds of combinatorial optimization problems arising in computational biology for analyzing WGD. Fractionation and its consequences are the subject of mathematical modeling questions and further combinatorial algorithms. A strong connection is made between WGD in phylogenetic context and the theory of gene trees and species trees. We illustrate the analysis of WGD with studies involving a large number of sequenced plant genomes, including grape, the crucifers and other rosids, the asterid tomato, the eudicot *Nelumbo nucifera* and pineapple, a monocot.

Key words Angiosperm, Genome halving, Genome aliquoting, Fractionation, Rearrangement, Consolidation, Phylogeny, Gene trees, Core eudicots, *Nelumbo*, Pineapple, Tomato, Brassica

1 Introduction

In nature, the genomes of most eukaryote species are diploid, in that the cell nucleus contains a single maternal and a single paternal copy of each chromosome. Polyploidization arises as an accident, or series of accidents, of meiosis, whereby a viable zygote emerges containing two or more intact genomes, called *subgenomes*, in a single nucleus. The subgenomes in an *allopolyploid* must be highly compatible, similar enough to allow coherent cellular function to proceed, but should be sufficiently different so that subsequent meioses proceed without mistaken alignment of maternal and paternal chromosomes from different subgenomes (*homeologous chromosomes*). The two or more subgenomes in an *autopolyploid* are identical, at least in initial generations, containing two (or more) copies of maternal and paternal chromosomes. Meiosis in this case is risky due to the potential alignment not of pairs of

João C. Setubal et al. (eds.), *Comparative Genomics: Methods and Protocols*, Methods in Molecular Biology, vol. 1704, https://doi.org/10.1007/978-1-4939-7463-4_10, © Springer Science+Business Media LLC 2018

parental chromosomes, but of three or four chromosomes at a time, setting up a high probability of failure of segregation and of the production of functional gametes.

Despite the accidental nature of either an allo- or autopolyploidy event, and the great likelihood that, if one occurs, it will not lead to a population of fertile and hardy descendants, it is nevertheless known to have occurred in certain species, especially plant species, where the sheer number of seeds that can be produced compensates for the low probability of successful individual polyploidization occurrences. Indeed, many plant species remain polyploids over long periods of time, with double, triple, etc. the number of chromosomes as the ancestral diploid, and maintaining the separation between home-ologous sets of chromosomes during meiosis. Some polyploids can coexist with diploid forms of the same species in the same or neigh-boring populations, and great variability in ploidy characterizes certain plants. Human activity has resulted in the induction or maintenance of polyploidy in some species because of the desirable agricultural or horticultural properties they may have.

On the evolutionary timescale polyploids may transition back to diploidy. The initially identical or nearly identical DNA sequences of pairs or triplets of genes on homeologous chromosomes diverge by random mutation and selection, while non-coding sequences may diverge even faster. The two, three or more copies may diverge in function (*neofunctionalization* or *subfunctionalization*) or some copies (but not all) may be lost completely through pseudogeniza-tion or excision. This loss process, called *fractionation*, affects all subgenomes though generally one retains more genes than the other(s), a tendency known as *subgenome dominance*. A slower process, *genome rearrangement*, results in fusions of chromosomes from the same or different subgenomes and transfer of large chro-mosomal fragments from one chromosome to another, irrespective of the subgenome identity of the donor or receiving chromosome. It becomes meaningless to say that such-and-such a chromosome belongs to one subgenome rather than the other, and the only trace of the polyploidization is the presence of a small set of duplicate gene pairs with the same degree of divergence, suggesting an early event creating many duplicate pairs. We say the genome has *rediploidized* or simply *diploidized*.

For historical reasons, the term *Whole Genome Duplication* (WGD) is generally applied in the context of studying an extant species that is thought to have originated in polyploidization fol-lowed by rediploidization. Though cumbersome as a term, it is not less preferable than the tongue-twisting coinage *paleopolyploid*. WGD is sometimes used to refer to a true (not rediploidized) polyploid or to refer to ancient triplications and higher order polyploidization.

In this chapter, we first discuss the prevalence of WGD in the angiosperms, the flowering plants, in Subheading 2.

This establishes the great importance of analyzing WGD in any chromosome-level study of genome evolution.

Next, we review a number of theoretical topics inspired by WGD. These are mostly, but not exclusively, framed in terms of the theory of genome rearrangements, and deal with evolution on the level of karyotypes and gene order on chromosomes, rather than DNA sequences or proteins. One problem is that of *genome halving* (Subheading 3), the problem of reconstructing the gene order on the chromosomes of an ancient tetraploid (two subgenomes), based on an extant genome containing the same pairs of genes, but scattered in any order and orientation on some set of chromosomes. The solution to this is outlined in Subheading 3.1. The potential of non-uniqueness of genome halving solutions prompted the *guided halving* approach, which we sketch briefly in Subheading 3.2. For higher order polyploids—hexaploid, octaploid, etc.—genome halving becomes *genome aliquoting* and this non-trivial extension to halving is described in Subheading 3.3.

In the next section, we propose some models and inference questions involving whole genome duplication and fractionation. In Subheading 4.2 we set up a purely mathematical question about the statistical properties of alternating "visible" and "invisible" line segments, inspired by the deletion of chromosomal fragments by fractionation. In Subheading 4.3, we address the problem of recovering some of the gene order information lost during fractionation, in trying to answer questions about genome rearrangement.

Subheading 5 introduces the notion of "event trees." The idea is to use the distribution of similarities among duplicated gene pairs as they are generated by speciation and WGD to reconstruct phylogenies.

In Subheading 6, we survey empirical treatments of various flowering plants. Since real genomes are far more complex than the models assumed by the combinatorial algorithms presently available, analyses of plant genomes tend to be more robust but less generalizable and less ambitious in their goals.

2   Prevalence of WGD in the Angiosperms

The hypothesis that a given species has been subject to a whole genome duplication event during its evolution is based on the discovery of numerous pairs of syntenic regions on two different chromosomes (or regions of a single chromosome) within the same genome, covering a high proportion of the genome. Such evidence for WGD events has shown up across the whole eukaryote spectrum, from the protist *Paramecium* [1] to brewer's yeast [2], all flowering plant lineages [3], several insects [4, 5], early vertebrates [6], fish [7, 8], and amphibians [9]. In mammals, reports of WGD

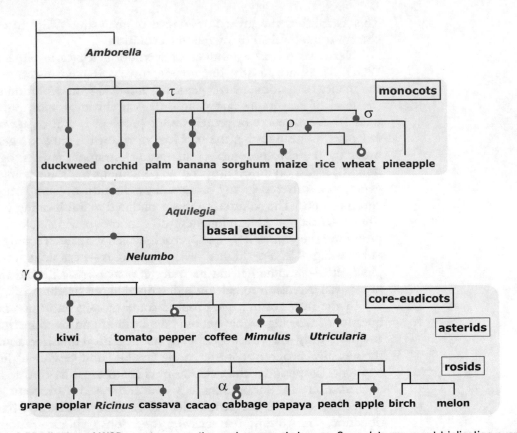

Fig. 1 Distribution of WGD events across the angiosperm phylogeny. Open dots represent triplication events (hexaploidization). The α, γ, ρ, σ, and τ events mentioned in the text are labelled

in the octodontids [10] remain controversial [11], pending genome sequencing [12]. The widespread distribution of WGD in the flowering plants is illustrated in Fig. 1. Indeed two instances of WGD occurred in the plant lineage leading up to the angiosperms, one just before the emergence of these flowering plants, and an earlier one pre-dating all the seed plants [13]. The first angiosperms sequenced all showed evidence of WGD events: the *Arabidopsis thaliana* genome [14–16], the rice genome [17, 18], and the poplar [19]. The fourth sequenced plant, the grapevine [20], revealed a whole genome triplication, called "γ, that engendered a far-reaching radiation of the "core eudicots" that includes over 150,000 extant species. Moreover, the rice genome turns out to share three WGD events in its ancestry in common with the other cereals [21], the earliest of which, the "τ" event, is also ancestral to most other monocots, some 60,000 in number.

In fact, as illustrated in Fig. 1, WGD events occur scattered across the entire angiosperm phylogeny. Though the earliest branching flowering plant, *Amborella trichopoda* [22], escaped any subsequent WGD, all the sequenced monocots, and both of the sequenced basal eudicots, have at least one WGD since branching off from the other angiosperms, while all sequenced genomes within the core eudicot asterid clade, except coffee, also have at least one WGD. The rosid clade contains many genomes with no WGD since γ, but each of these is also closely related to genomes that have experienced one, two, three, or more since that event. The selection of genomes in Fig. 1 is not a random choice, but was deliberately configured to reflect the intermingling of lineages with and without WGD.

3   Genome Halving and Related Problems

3.1   The Halving Problem

The *Genome Halving* problem asks, given a genome T with two copies of each gene, distributed in any manner among the chromosomes, to find the ancestral "perfectly duplicated" genome, written $A \oplus A$, consisting of two identical halves, i.e., two identical sets of chromosomes with one copy of each gene in each half, such that the rearrangement distance $d(T, A \oplus A)$ between T and $A \oplus A$ is minimal. Note that part of this problem is to find a labelling as "1" or "2" of the two genes in a pair of copies of T, so that all n copies labelled "1" are in one half of $A \oplus A$ and all those labelled "2" are in the other half. The genome A represents the ancestral genome at the moment immediately preceding the WGD event giving rise to $A \oplus A$.

For reversal and translocation distance, a linear-time solution was discovered in 1999 [23]. For reversal distance, these results have been reformulated [24] using an alternative representation of the breakpoint graph. There are also versions for DCJ [25, 26] and for breakpoint distance [27].

Generalizations of the algorithms to doubled genomes with missing gene copies have also been developed [28, 29].

A harder problem is to find the distance between a tetraploid with no rearrangements and an arbitrarily rearranged genome with the same doubled set of genes—the *Double Distance problem* [27].

3.2   Guided Halving

A problem with genome halving is that there are usually many, very different, perfectly duplicated genomes $A \oplus A$ leading to a minimum distance with T. For biological purposes it would be preferable to be able to use some additional, or external, information to choose amongst these solutions. Thus the *Guided Genome Halving* problem [29–31] asks, given a genome T, as well as another genome R containing only one copy of each of the n genes (a non-duplicated outgroup), find A so that $d(T, A \oplus A) + d(A, R)$ is minimal. The solution A need not be a solution to the original halving problem. The reversals and translocations version and the DCJ version of this problem are NP-hard [27].

Guided halving using the heuristic pathgroups approach [32] extends naturally to gene order reconstruction in phylogenies containing WGD events [33].

3.3 Aliquoting

The *Genome Aliquoting* problem [34] is the problem of finding a genome with one copy of every gene given a genome with exactly k copies of every gene, where $k \geq 3$, such that the distance between the given and resulting genomes is minimized according to some distance metric. More precisely, given a genome T with k copies of each gene, distributed in any manner among the chromosomes, we wish to find the ancestral "perfectly k-tupled" genome, written $A \oplus \cdots A$, consisting of k identical disjoint parts, i.e., "k" identical sets of chromosomes with one copy of each gene in each part, such that the rearrangement distance $d(T, A \oplus \cdots A)$ between T and $A \oplus \cdots A$ is minimal. Note that part of this problem is to find a labelling as "1", "2", …,"k" of the k genes in the k copies of T, so that all n gene copies labelled "1" are in one part of $A \oplus \cdots A$, all those labelled "2" are in another part, and so on. The genome A represents the ancestral genome at the moment immediately preceding the polyploidization event giving rise to $A \oplus \cdots A$. If we allow $k = 2$, this becomes the Genome Halving problem.

The *breakpoint distance* version of Genome Aliquoting has a polynomial time algorithm, while it remains an open problem whether or not a polynomial time algorithm for the case of DCJ distance exists.

4   Modeling Fractionation

4.1 The Fractionation Process

The repeated alternation of WGD and periods of fractionation in the flowering plants necessitates the excision of excess non-coding DNA [35, 36], including genes that have been inactivated by pseudogenization or other processes. Fractionation, the process following WGD, whereby one of the genes in most duplicate pairs is lost, in a random or partly random manner, is thus the focus in this section. This process may cause more gene order disruption than classical chromosomal rearrangements such as reversal or reciprocal translocation, as illustrated in Fig. 2. In genomics, this process was hypothesized by Wolfe and Shields, who discovered the ancient tetraploidization of *Saccharomyces cerevisiae* [2], and further studied through the comparison of the *S. cerevisiae* gene order with that of related diploid yeasts [37, 38].

In general, fractionation inflates the apparent number of reciprocal translocations, greatly seriously exaggerating the overall amount of chromosomal rearrangement that has taken place in two sister genomes, one of which has undergone a WGD, as illustrated in Fig. 3.

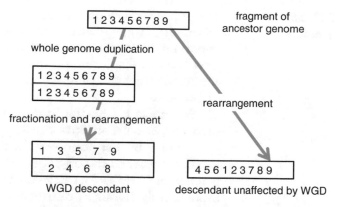

Fig. 2 Fractionation leading to different adjacencies in WGD descendant and unaffected genome. All the adjacencies in the WGD descendant are not found in the ancestor and are caused by fractionation. The adjacencies between 6 and 1 and between 3 and 7 in the unaffected genome are caused by three reversal rearrangements, but because of the fractionation in the WGD descendant the rearrangement distance (DCJ) between the two descendant is actually seven—a combination of reversals, fission, fusions, and translocations. Ignoring fractionation would thus lead to the inference of more than twice as many rearrangements as actually occurred to account for the different sets of adjacencies in the two genomes

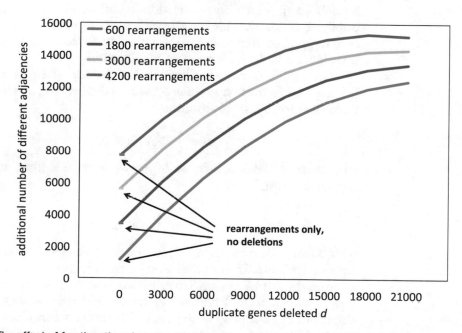

Fig. 3 The effect of fractionations in terms of extra adjacencies (a proxy for rearrangement distances) in both genomes of length n. For each fixed level of rearrangement r, the number of extra adjacencies (over the $n + 2r$ expected) increases dramatically as the number of genes deleted during fractionation increases. Original number of genes $n = 24,000$

4.2   A Model
for Fractionation

The process of fractionation gives rise to an interesting mathematical model. Though not very realistic, it nevertheless captures important biological aspects of fractionation. Mathematically, it gives rise to a simple, but previously unexplored way of generating alternating black and white segments as continuous analogs of runs of 1s and 0s.

We model the fractionation process in terms of a number of successive sweeps, at times $t = 1, 2, \ldots$, of a point process with parameter ν on the positive reals, representing one copy of the WGD genome. At the origin, $t = 0$, we say that all points of this genome are "visible." A deletion event, rendering a segment of exponentially (mean μ) distributed length "invisible," occurs at each point determined by the point process. Though our description will be in terms of the three parameters, only $\frac{\mu}{\nu}$ and t are meaningful for purposes of inference.

The second copy of the genome remains undisturbed throughout and retains a 1-to-1, length preserving, correspondence with the fractionating copy, without regard to any disruption caused by invisibility. This biologically inspired property is what makes the model more than just a curiosity. The origins of the construction lie in more realistic discrete models, whose mathematical development is still incomplete [39–42]. Still more realistic are "two-sided" models [43], which allow deletion to affect either of the two duplicate genomes. This is more difficult because the exponential deletion process sometimes has to be truncated to avoid two-sided invisibility, a biologically undesirable situation.

During the first sweep, illustrated at the top of Fig. 4 at time (or step) $t = 1$, the first *deletion point* x_1 is determined by sampling from the exponential distribution

$$\rho(x) = \frac{1}{\nu} e^{-\frac{x}{\nu}}, \quad x \geq 0, \tag{1}$$

with mean ν. Then a *deletion length* a_1 is chosen from another exponential distribution

$$\gamma(a) = \frac{1}{\mu} e^{-\frac{a}{\mu}}, \quad a \geq 0, \tag{2}$$

with mean μ. The segment $(x_1, x_1 + a_1)$ is "deleted," or is designated as invisible. The next deletion point x_2 is chosen by sampling x_2' from the first exponential distribution (mean ν), so that $x_2 = x_2' + x_1 + a_1$. Then the length a_2 of the second deleted segment is determined by sampling from γ again. The process continues in this way to find $x_3, a_3, \ldots$ Concatenating only those segments that are still visible, we see that $x_1, x_2, \ldots$ are points determined by a point process with parameter ν. Associated with each of these points x is an "event counter" $C(x)$. Initially, each $C(x) = 1$. We define a function $\pi_t(i)$, $i = 1, \ldots$ measuring the proportion of event

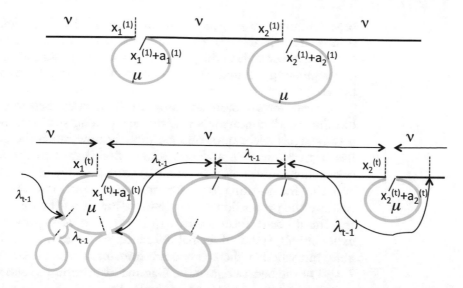

Fig. 4 Processes pertinent to first sweep and t-th sweep. Solid horizontal bars represent the visible regions of the genome. Grey curves represent invisible regions. Dashed markers represent deletion points, solid markers represent end of deletion segments. ν and μ are the means of the deletion point spacing and deletion segment length variables, while λ_{t-1} is the mean space between visible deletion points after the $t-1$-st sweep

counters registering i events at time $t \geq 1$. Thus $\pi_1(1) = 1$ and $\pi_1(j) = 0$, for all $j > 1$.

At times $t = 1, 2, \ldots$, the second, third, $\ldots$ sweeps begin, all independent of the first sweep and each other, and each applied to the concatenated visible segments only. We sample $x_1^{(t)}$ and $a_1^{(t)}$ in the same way as x_1 and a_1 according to ρ and γ, respectively, to determine a deletion interval $[x_1^{(t)}, x_1^{(t)} + a_1^{(t)})$.

If the interval $[x_1^{(t)}, x_1^{(t)} + a_1^{(t)})$ contains no previously defined deletion point, a new event counter at $C(x_1^{(t)})$ is set at 1. If $[x_1^{(t)}, x_1^{(t)} + a_1^{(t)})$ already contains $j > 1$ deletion points $z_1, \ldots, z_j$, the event counter at $C(x_1^{(t)})$ is set at $1 + \Sigma_{i=1}^{j} C(z_i)$. The j deletion points $z_1, \ldots, z_j$ become invisible, along with the rest of the segment $[x_1^{(t)}, x_1^{(t)} + a_1^{(t)})$ that contains them.

We find the next deletion point by sampling $x_2^{(t)'}$ from ρ, and setting $x_2(t) = x_1^{(t)} + a_1^{(t)} + x_2^{(t)'}$. We continue the t sweep, adding visible deletion points and making others invisible. Some deletion points from the earlier sweep will remain unchanged, i.e. are still visible. The $x_i^{(t)}$ by themselves define a point process with parameter ν on the concatenated visible segments. But the $x_i^{(t)}$ and the additional deletion points remaining from the earlier sweep define a process with mean λ_t, a parameter that decreases with t, as the undeleted segments are interrupted by more and more deletions. This parameter is important as it is directly inferable from the observed genome at time t.

Extensive simulations reveal λ_t to follow an exponential distribution, while the total accumulated lengths of invisible segments at time t follows a more general Gamma distribution [44]. Analytical results are available on $C(t)$, but this does not correspond to anything observable in the genome; nothing distinguishes an invisible segment generated by five deletion events from one generated by ten.

At each sweep, more and more of the genome becomes invisible. Since each concatenation of visible segments still extends to the positive reals, we cannot observe directly how much the genome has been reduced in absolute terms. But thanks to the length-preserving isomorphism between the second copy of the genome and the fractionating one, for any large finite interval we can observe the proportion of the genome that is left by time t. Since this should be of form similar to $\left(1 + \frac{\mu}{\nu}\right)^{-t}$, involving quotients of exponentials, standard formal inference processes may be unavailable, but whether there is enough information in the statistics of λ_t and of the parameters of the Gamma distribution to allow some inference about $\frac{\mu}{\nu}$ and t is an open question.

4.3 The Consolidation Problem

As mentioned in Subheading 4.1, fractionation inflates the apparent amount of chromosomal rearrangement that has actually taken place in two sister genomes one of which has undergone a WGD. Here we discuss how to computationally detect, characterize, and correct for this impediment to the study of evolution [45, 46].

The method is based on the identification and isolation of "fractionation intervals," regions in both the WGD descendant and its unaffected sister genome that may have been rearranged internally, but have (so far) been unaffected by rearrangements exchanging genes from within the interval and genes external to the interval. This is followed by a procedure for the *consolidation* of the two fractionated regions in the WGD descendant that correspond to a single region in the unaffected genome. These are then represented by a single "virtual" gene, identical in the unaffected genome and in two copies in the WGD descendant, removing the cause of excess rearrangement in the comparison of the two genomes. Figure 5 shows how this completely corrects for effect of fractionation in inflating the rearrangement estimates (cf. Fig. 3).

The running time of the latest version of the algorithm [46] is asymptotically linear in the genome size. It can handle whole genome triplication (ancient hexaploidy) and higher multiplicity events.

5 Species Trees and Events Trees

The investigation of gene trees and species trees furnishes a genuinely genomic perspective on evolution insofar as it requires a complete inventory of the paralogs of the orthologously related

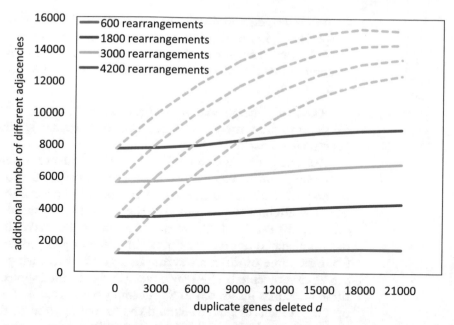

Fig. 5 Solid lines: Apparent amount of rearrangements after application of consolidation algorithm and taking into account adjacencies within fractionation regions. Dashed lines: Before algorithm

genes in the species under study. However, gene trees and species trees are each based on a tiny portion of the genome.

In the context of WGD in flowering plants, we can take the gene-tree/species tree approach to another level, to a more comprehensive kind of genomic data than the usual one-gene-at-a-time focus. Specifically, we can study the set of $\binom{N}{2} + N$ gene similarity distributions within and across N species where WGD has affected one or more of these species. This typically involves many thousands of genes in finding a single "events tree," rather than finding a compromise among thousands of single-gene gene trees.

Though there are statistically more elaborate ways of identifying the distributions [47], we can nonetheless proceed with our gene-tree approach by simply identifying local modes or "peaks" in all the $\binom{N}{2} + N$ similarity distributions, and translating these into phylogenetically related paralogous and orthologous entities. We have developed a rapid algorithm to resolve these in the case of ideal instances where no data are missing and all data are mutually compatible [48].

There are two principles underlying our method for reconstructing the species tree and the events tree from a perfect set (i.e., no events are undetected in any distribution where they "should" be visible) of inter- and intra-genome comparisons:

- each intra-genome distribution of similarities only has peaks due to all the WGD in its direct lineage, and

- each inter-genome distribution contains only one peak due to speciation, i.e., at the date of the most recent common ancestor of the two species, as well as all the peaks due to the WGDs in common to the two species, i.e., WGDs pre-dating the speciation event.

The first principle may be seen as a special case of the second, considering that there are zero speciation events separating a genome from itself.

Assuming that we can infer the age of an event simply by identifying one or more "peaks" of the similarity distribution it engenders, without recourse to other estimation procedures, foregoes any attempt to pick out events only visible as "shoulders" of other events on the similarity distribution. It also makes it potentially difficult to test whether peaks in different comparisons result from the same or different event. In practice these two problems can be circumvented. This may be seen in the detailed application of these principles illustrated in Subheading 6.5 below. And it opens up the problem of how to extend the formal method to data less than perfect, which our algorithm currently requires.

6   A Survey of Some WGD Events

Among the techniques used to detect and characterize WGD events in practice are syntenic dot plots, distributions of gene duplicate similarities (including all-position similarities, K_s, and 4dTv [49, 50]) and aliquoting based on frequent paralogy between subgenomes but not within subgenomes. We illustrate these general approaches to a number of flowering plant genomes.

6.1   Core Eudicots

The core eudicots are all descendants of an ancestral hexaploidization approximatively 125 Mya, leading within a few million years to a remarkably diverse radiation into many orders, most of which are grouped into the rosid and asterid subclasses. Among the sequenced core eudicot genomes that have been published, the grapevine *Vitis vinifera* [20], a rosid, is perhaps the most conservative, from the viewpoints both of sequence mutation rates and gross chromosomal structure. From the latter, the original hexaploid structure can be inferred to have involved the tripling of seven chromosomes, the grapevine conserving most of this with a handful of chromosomal fusions and fissions reducing the 21 ancestral chromosomes to 19. Figure 6 shows the results of applying a "practical aliquoting" algorithm to grapevine genome paralogy data [51].

Syntenic dot-plots (omitted here) for the self-comparison of both grapevine and of cacao clearly show a pattern of pairwise homologies falling largely into 21 groups according to the

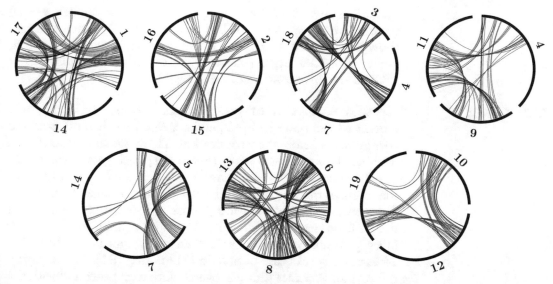

Fig. 6 Partitioning of grape genome into three subgenomes by the aliquoting algorithm. Arcs making up the circumference of each circle represent grape chromosomes. Lines within circles represent paralogies established at the time of hexaploidization. Note that between circles defined by the algorithm, hypothesized to reflect the seven pre-hexaploid core eudicot chromosomes, there are virtually no paralogies, and within circles, no paralogies within subgenomes, and many paralogies between subgenomes. Note also that chromosomes 4, 7, and 14 appear in two circles each, reflecting chromosomal fusions in the grape lineage, while one circle is labeled by four chromosomes: 3, 4, 7, 18 because of the incorporation of fissioned parts of an ancient chromosome into chromosome 4 and 7

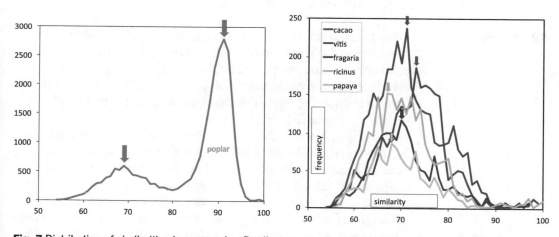

Fig. 7 Distribution of similarities in gene pairs. Duplicate genes in seven genomes, showing triplication peaks between 67% and 73%. Poplar WGD peak at 91%

chromosomal location of the two homologs [20, 52]. This is also true to a lesser extent for peach and is even more obscured in strawberry and other more highly rearranged genomes.

Turning to the detection of WGD through duplicate gene similarity distributions, Fig. 7 shows how intra-genome duplicate similarities are distributed in seven rosids in a parallel way all showing strong evidence of the triplication. All of the genomes show a clear peak at $70 \pm 3\%$ sequence similarity. In addition, poplar showed a larger peak at 91%, reflecting the more recent WGD it underwent as indicated in Fig. 1.

6.2 Nelumbo

Nelumbo nucifera is of great interest because it is the only sequenced and published [53] eudicot that branched off from the core eudicots before the γ triplication. There was some question of whether the γ event was really two events, since geneticists do not usually observe hexaploidization as a single step. It was thought that perhaps the first step, a tetraploidization, occurred before the divergence from *Nelumbo* and the second step, a combination of the doubled genome with a closely related diploid, soon after. To investigate this possibility, we carried out a "practical halving" of *Nelumbo*, a special case of practical aliquoting [54]. In comparing the two subgenomes thus discovered with each other and with the three subgenomes of grape (*see* Fig. 8), we could discard the possibility that there was any WGD before the speciation giving rise to the two genomes.

Both grape and *Nelumbo* have rather conservative genomes, so that it is relatively easy to pair chromosomal regions in *Nelumbo* and to match triple of regions in grape. This gives rise to a reconstruction of the ancestral form of each before γ and before the *Nelumbo* WGD. This is depicted in Fig. 9, which suggests elements of a common eudicot ancestor.

6.3 Tomato

The publication of the tomato genome [55] included the first evidence and affirmation of a triplication in the Solanaceae lineage. The data and analysis presented, however, was difficult to decipher as proof that the entire ancestral genome had been triplicated. We used an aliquoting algorithm to confirm this in tomato and in the genus *Capsicum* [51, 56].

In Fig. 10, we have colored each set of tripled regions red, blue, and green according to which contained the largest, second largest, and smallest number of genes. The differential between the red regions and the others is far too great to be attributed to multinomial sampling with equal probabilities, and is reminiscent of the situation of other flowering plant WGD descendants [57], where subgenome dominance survives despite rearrangements breaking up and reassembling the chromosomes irrespective of their WGD origins. Thus the red regions in Fig. 10 would all or mostly originate in the same subgenome at the time of hexaploidization. The dominant subgenome, early in this process, by means of regulatory and epigenetic mechanisms, depresses the expression level of the genes in the other subgenomes and facilitates their loss during fractionation (cf. the discussion in [57]).

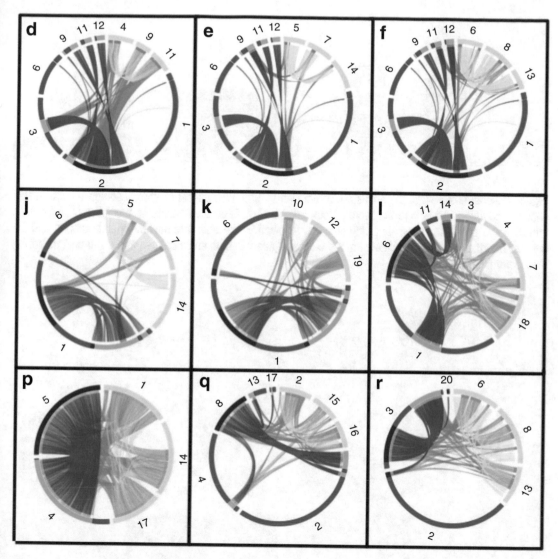

Fig. 8 Comparison of inferred pre-duplication chromosomes in *Nelumbo* ancestor and pre-triplication regions in the core eudicot ancestor. Yellow chromosomes and paralogy edges: *Vitis*. Violet chromosomes and paralogy edges: *Nelumbo*. Black edges: orthologies between three *Vitis* subgenomes and two *Nelumbo* subgenomes

This is a likely explanation, but does not account for another aspect of the pattern in Fig. 10. We might expect, all things being equal, that the largest region be distributed among more tomato chromosomes while the smallest regions be found on only one chromosome. In fact we observe the opposite, with the smallest regions, colored green, being spread over 1.8 chromosomes, on the average, with the regions colored red being confined to 1.4 chromosomes, and the blue-colored regions in between (1.53). This observation is consistent with the hypothesis that all the red regions originate with a single subgenome that joined an original tetraploid (reflected in the blue and green regions), already considerably

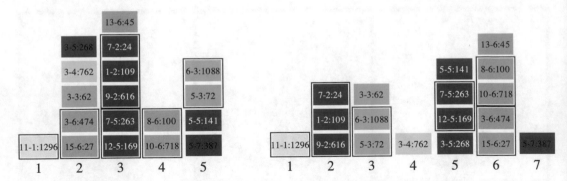

Fig. 9 Reconstructed *Nelumbo* ancestral chromosomes and *Vitis* ancestral chromosomes (not to scale), showing common blocks and conserved block adjacencies. Each block contains the label of a *Nelumbo* chromosome pair in the original halving solution, followed by the *Vitis* chromosome triplet number, and the number of orthologs. Heavy outline surround blocks adjacent in both ancestral genomes, and undoubtedly in their common eudicot ancestor

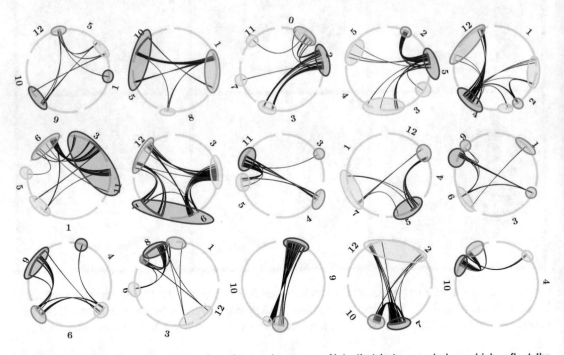

Fig. 10 Aliquoting of tomato genome into three subgenomes. Note that between circles, which reflect the 15 hypothesized pre-hexaploid Solanaceae chromosomes, there are virtually no paralogies, and within circles, no paralogies within subgenomes, and many paralogies between subgenomes. Note also that several chromosomes each appear in more than one circle, reflecting chromosomal fusions in the Solanaceae lineage, and that most circles are labeled by more than three chromosomes because of the assorted amalgamation of fissioned parts of ancient chromosomes

fractionated and rearranged. However, the blue-green tetraploidization would not have been an autopolyploidy event since the average sequence similarity blue-green paralogs is not significantly greater than that of red-blue or red-green paralogs.

6.4   Pineapple

Besides its intrinsic interest as an important food crop, pineapple offers an opportunity to study the early evolution of the order Poales, which also contains the Poaceae family, but whose early evolution has been obscured by the so-called ρ WGD. Since the family Bromeliaceae, containing pineapple, diverged from the Poaceae before ρ, it provides a window into the earlier σ and τ WGDs shared by all Poales. Fractionation reduces the number of WGD-generated paralogous pairs to single copy rapidly, so that while it is often straightforward how to do genome reconstruction after a WGD, it is relatively difficult to study evolution prior to a WGD based only on paralogs. Since there is a built-in redundancy in the orthologous pairs generated by speciation, before or after a WGD in either or both of two genomes, more orthologous pairs are available for reconstruction. To take maximum advantage of this fact, and to optimize the amount of information input to the reconstruction of an ancestral Poales genome, we looked for multiple orthologous syntenic regions in pineapple to a published outgroup genome, *pirodela polyrhiza* (duckweed), or to overlapping Spirodela regions. Within each set of pineapple regions thus produced, we then searched for quadruples of paralogous regions made up of two pairs or regions. Each pair was required to have average similarities clustered around a recent mode of the distribution. The similarities across the two pairs of regions had to be clustered around an earlier mode of the similarity distribution. The quadruples that emerge from this search should correspond to the chromosomes produced by each round of WGD, though this may be obscured by rearrangement and fractionation. Figure 11 shows the remarkably clear pattern that was derived by this method applied to the pineapple genome [58], with duckweed providing the outgroup genome. This result was of special interest because the two WGD σ and τ are shared by the Poaceae crops wheat, rice, maize, etc., but the early history of these is scrambled by the more recent WGD ρ. Thus the pineapple analysis allowed us to resolve the controversial ancient history of the Poaceae.

6.5   The Brassicaceae

In Subheading 5, we introduced the systematic study of peaks of $\binom{N}{2} + N$ distributions of duplicate gene similarity in the context of gene trees and event trees.

To illustrate this discussion, we draw on six published genomes in the Brassicaceae family, three in the genus *Brassica*: *B. rapa* (turnip, Chinese cabbage) [59], *B. oleracea* (cabbage, cauliflower) [60] and *Raphanus sativus* (radish) [61], two in the genus *Arabidopsis*: *A. lyrata* (rock cress) [62] and *A. thaliana* (thale cress, mouse-ear cress) [14], and one in the genus *Sisymbrium*: *S. irio* (London rocket) [63]. Figure 12 shows the phylogenetic relationship among the six species:

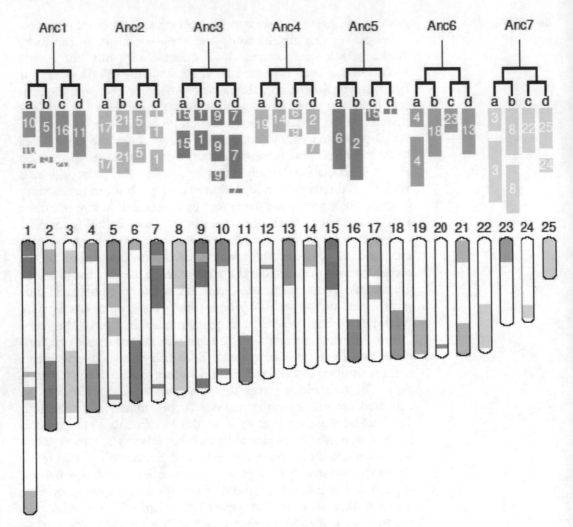

Fig. 11 Accessing the cereal ancestral genome through analysis of pineapple WGD

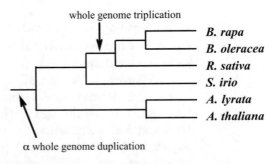

Fig. 12 Phylogenetic relationship of six species in the family Brassicaceae, showing lineages affected by WGD and triplication events

We extracted genomic data from these species using the database in CoGe [64, 65]. We then used the SynMap routine (with default parameters) on this platform to compare the gene orders of each of the $\binom{6}{2} = 15$ pairs of genomes. This procedure implicitly validates the identification of orthologs produced by speciation by detecting collinear arrays of several duplicate pairs in two species with approximately the same divergence: "syntenic blocks." Similarly, we did a self-comparison of five of the six genomes; the sixth one, the *Sisymbrium* genome, not having enough closely spaced duplicate pairs for SynMap to produce paralogous syntenic blocks. The distributions of similarities calculated are shown in Fig. 13. The peaks found in each genome are tabulated in Table 1.

From Fig. 13 and Table 1, we note that the data are not quite "perfect"; the earliest duplication, detected at 79–80% in the *Arabidopsis* self-comparisons, shows no peaks in the other self-comparisons—there is a shoulder or heavy tail in the appropriate place in the *Brassica* self-comparisons, but this is swamped by the later triplication. The triplication itself is visible in all three *Brassica* self-comparisons and in the comparison of *B. oleracea* and *B. rapa*. In the comparison of the latter two with Raphanus, this peak is barely visible as a shoulder to the Raphanus speciation distribution.

More interesting is that the peaks at 90% reflecting the *Sisymbrium* speciation, known to occur before the *Brassica* triplication, suggest that speciation is more recent, since the triplication peak is at 89%. This apparent conflict is clearly ascribable to a slower rate of evolution (lower λ), since the divergence of *Arabidopsis* from *Sisymbrium* also seems to occur more recently (88%) than the divergence of *Arabidopsis* from the *Sisymbrium* sister genus *Brassica* (86%). Note that the small differences between peak similarities are not insignificant, given the many thousands of gene pairs involved in these comparisons.

Were we to fill in the missing "α" peaks, and correct the *Sisymbrium* times to account for slower evolution, the data set would be perfect and our algorithm would convert it to a species tree with duplication times indicated. This could be then displayed in the form of Fig. 14. This events tree represents a general template for gene families evolving through WGD and fractionation-based gene loss only. The gene tree for any particular gene family would have exactly the same form, but with losses of various lineages.

7   Conclusion

In the history of extant flowering plants, there are many whole genome duplications and triplications, and these are not confined to one or two phylogenetic domains. This presents a challenge for

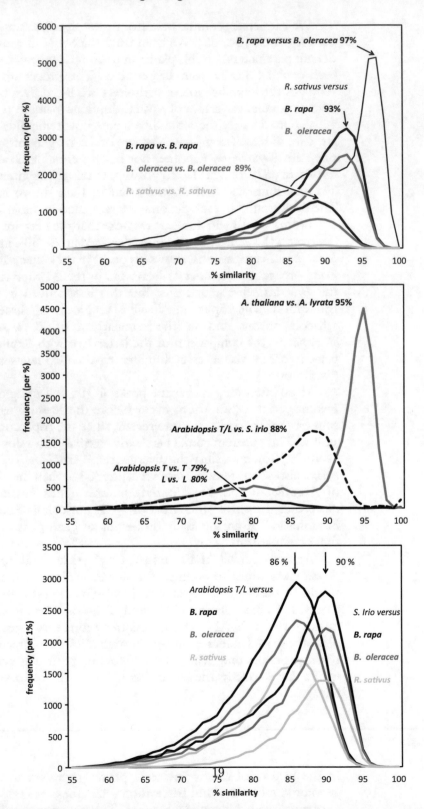

Fig. 13 Gene similarity distribution between 15 pairs of genomes in the Brassicaceae and 5 self comparisons. Local modes ("peaks") are indicated. Only one of each comparison is shown for *Arabidopsis*, the other is superimposed and indistinguishable

Table 1
Peak similarity level, by genome

Peak number	Description	Genome					
		BR	BO	RS	SI	AL	AT
1	*α* duplication [66]	np	np	np	np	80	80,79
2	Divergence of genus *Arabidopsis*	86	86	86,87	88	88–86	88–86
3	Whole genome triplication	89	89	87	–	–	–
4	Divergence of genus *Sisymbrium*	90	90	90	90	–	–
5	Divergence of genus *Raphanus*	93	93	93	–	–	–
6	Speciation of *Arabidopsis T & L*	–	–	–	–	95	95
7	Speciation of *B. rapa & B. oleracea*	97	97	–	–	–	–

np: no peak, but one could be found by mixtures of distribution methods. –: no peak expected. Note peak 3 occurring before peak 4 due to slow evolutionary rate (*λ*) of *Sisymbrium*

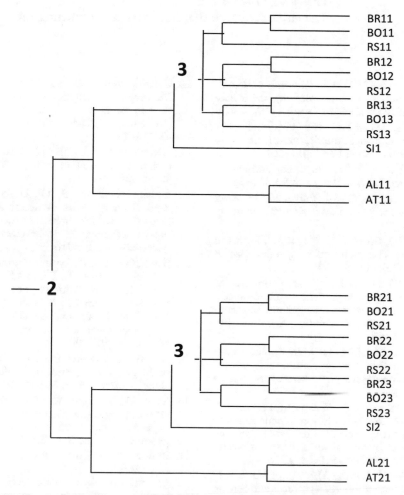

Fig. 14 Event tree for the Brassicaceae. Boldface numbers indicate WGD or triplication. All families of genes descended from the various genome WGD or WGT without any additional duplications must be formed from this tree with truncations of appropriate lineages

the combinatorial analysis of evolution and phylogeny in the angiosperms. We survey a series of new combinatorial optimization problems and models proposed to investigate WGD, and the fractionation process that WGD engenders. This is illustrated through a description of a diverse set of genomes whose evolution we have studied. In particular, we have pointed out connections between gene-tree/species-tree theory and the study of whole genome duplications in a phylogeny.

Acknowledgements

Research supported in part by grants from the Natural Sciences and Engineering Research Council of Canada (NSERC) and by National Science Foundation IOS −1339156. DS holds the Canada Research Chair in Mathematical Genomics.
Competing Interests
The authors declare that they have no competing interests.

References

1. Aury J-M et al (2006) Global trends of whole-genome duplications revealed by the ciliate *Paramecium tetraurelia*. Nature 444:171–178

2. Wolfe KH, Shields DC (1997) Molecular evidence for an ancient duplication of the entire yeast genome. Nature 387:708–713

3. Soltis DE et al (2009) Polyploidy and angiosperm diversification. Am J Bot 96:336–348

4. Lokki J, Saura A (1980) Polyploidy in insect evolution. In: Polyploidy. Springer, Boston, pp 277–312

5. Tsutsui ND, Suarez AV, Spagna JC, Johnston JS (2008) The evolution of genome size in ants. BMC Evol Biol 8:64

6. Nakatani Y, Takeda H, Kohara Y, Shinichi M (2007) Reconstruction of the vertebrate ancestral genome reveals dynamic genome reorganization in early vertebrates. Genome Res 17:1254–1265

7. Jaillon O et al (2004) Genome duplication in the teleost fish tetraodon nigroviridis reveals the early vertebrate proto-karyotype. Nature 431:946–957

8. Kassahn KS, Dang VT, Wilkins SJ, Perkins AC, Ragan MA (2009) Evolution of gene function and regulatory control after whole-genome duplication: comparative analyses in vertebrates. Genome Res 19:1404–1418

9. Mable BK, Alexandrou MA, Taylor MI (2011) Genome duplication in amphibians and fish: an extended synthesis. J Zool 284:151–182

10. Gallardo MH, Gonzalez CA, Cebrian I (2006) Molecular cytogenetics and allotetraploidy in the red vizcacha rat, *Tympanoctomys barrerae* (Rodentia, Octodontidae). Genomics 88:214–221

11. Lavrenchenko LA (2014) Hybrid speciation in mammals: illusion or reality? Biol Bull Rev 4:198–209

12. Upham N, Evans B, Ojeda A (2015) The super-sized genomes of desert vizcacha rats. https://crowd.instrumentl.com/campaigns/super-sized-genomes-desert-vizcacha-rats/. Accessed April 1, 2016

13. Jiao Y, Wickett NJ, Ayyampalayam S, Chanderbali AS, Landherr L, Ralph PE, Tomsho LP, Hu Y, Liang H, Soltis PS, Soltis DE, Clifton SW, Schlarbaum SE, Schuster SC, Leebens-Mack J, Ma H, dePamphilis CW (2011) Ancestral polyploidy in seed plants and angiosperms. Nature 473:97–100

14. Arabidopsis Genome Initiative (2000) Analysis of the genome sequence of the flowering plant *Arabidopsis thaliana*. Nature 408:796–815

15. Blanc G, Hokamp K, Wolfe KH (2003) A recent polyploidy superimposed on older large-scale duplications in the Arabidopsis genome. Genome Res 13:137–144

16. Bowers, JE, Chapman BA, Rong J, Paterson AH (2003) Unravelling angiosperm genome evolution by phylogenetic analysis of chromosomal duplication events. Nature 422:433–438

17. Goff S et al (2002) A draft sequence of the rice genome (oryza sativa l. ssp. japonica). Science 296:92–100

18. Yu J et al (2002) A draft sequence of the rice genome (oryza sativa l. ssp. indica). Science 296:79–92

19. Tuskan G, DiFazio S, Jansson S, Bohlmann J, Grigoriev I, Hellsten U, Putnam N, Ralph S, Rombauts S, Salamov A, Schein J, Sterck L, Aerts A, Bhalerao R, Bhalerao R, Blaudez D, Boerjan W, Brun A, Brunner A, Busov V, Campbell M, Carlson J, Chalot M, Chapman J, Chen G, Cooper D, Coutinho P, Couturier J, Covert S, Cronk Q, Cunningham R, Davis J, Degroeve S, Dejardin A, dePamphilis C, Detter J, Dirks B, Dubchak I, Duplessis S, Ehlting J, Ellis B, Gendler K, Goodstein D, Gribskov M, Grimwood J, Groover A, Gunter L, Hamberger B, Heinze B, Helariutta Y, Henrissat B, Holligan D, Holt R, Huang W, Islam-Faridi N, Jones S, Jones-Rhoades M, Jorgensen R, Joshi C, Kangasjarvi J, Karlsson J, Kelleher C, Kirkpatrick R, Kirst M, Kohler A, Kalluri U, Larimer F, Leebens-Mack J, Leple J, Locascio P, Lou Y, Lucas S, Martin F, Montanini B, Napoli C, Nelson D, Nelson C, Nieminen K, Nilsson O, Pereda V, Peter G, Philippe R, Pilate G, Poliakov A, Razumovskaya J, Richardson P, Rinaldi C, Ritland K, Rouze P, Ryaboy D, Schmutz J, Schrader J, Segerman B, Shin H, Siddiqui A, Sterky F, Terry A, Tsai C, Uberbacher E, Unneberg P, Vahala J, Wall K, Wessler S, Yang G, Yin T, Douglas C, Marra M, Sandberg G, Van de Peer Y, Rokhsar D (2006) The genome of black cottonwood, populus trichocarpa (torr. & gray). Science 313:1596–1604

20. Jaillon O et al (2007) The grapevine genome sequence suggests ancestral hexaploidization in major angiosperm phyla. Nature 449:463–467

21. McKain MR, Tang H, McNeal JR, Ayyampalayam S, Davis JI, dePamphilis CW, Givnish TJ, Pires JC, Stevenson DW, Leebens-Mack JH (2016) A phylogenomic assessment of ancient polyploidy and genome evolution across the poales. Genome Biol Evol 8:1150–1164

22. Amborella Genome Project (2013) The Amborella genome and the evolution of flowering plants. Science 342:1241089

23. El-Mabrouk, N, Sankoff D (2003) The reconstruction of doubled genomes. SIAM J Comput 32:754–792

24. Alekseyev MA, Pevzner PA (2007) Colored de Bruijn graphs and the genome halving

25. Mixtacki J (2008) Genome halving under DCJ revisited. In: Hu X, Wang J (eds) Computing and combinatorics (COCOON). 17th annual conference. Lecture notes in computer science, vol 5092. Springer, Berlin/Heidelberg, pp 276–286

26. Warren R, Sankoff D (2009) Genome halving with double cut and join. J Bioinforma Comput Biol 7:357–371

27. Tannier E, Zheng C, Sankoff D (2009) Multi-chromosomal median and halving problems under different genomic distances. BMC Bioinf 10:120

28. Gagnon Y, Tremblay-Savard O, Bertrand D, El-Mabrouk N (2010) Advances on genome duplication distances. In: Tannier E (ed) Comparative genomics (RECOMB CG '10). Lecture notes in computer science, vol 6398. Springer, Berlin/Heidelberg, pp 25–38

29. Sankoff D, Zheng C, Wall PK, dePamphilis C, Leebens-Mack J, Albert VA (2009) Towards improved reconstruction of ancestral gene order in angiosperm phylogeny. J Comput Biol 16:1353–1367

30. Gavranović H, Tannier E (2010) Guided genome halving: probably optimal solutions provide good insights into the preduplication ancestral genome of Saccharomyces cerevisiae. In: Pacific symposium on biocomputing, vol 15, pp 21–30

31. Zheng C, Zhu Q, Adam Z, Sankoff D (2008) Guided genome halving: hardness, heuristics and the history of the Hemiascomycetes. Bioinformatics 24:i96–i104

32. Zheng C (2010) Pathgroups, a dynamic data structure for genome reconstruction problems. Bioinformatics 26:1587–1594

33. Zheng C, Sankoff D (2011) On the Pathgroups approach to rapid small phylogeny. BMC Bioinf 12:S4

34. Warren R, Sankoff D (2010) Genome aliquoting revisited. In: Tannier E (ed) Comparative genomics (RECOMB CG). 8th annual workshop. Lecture notes in computer science, vol 6398. Springer, Berlin/Heidelberg, pp 1–12

35. Freeling M et al (2012) Fractionation mutagenesis and similar consequences of mechanisms removing dispensable or less-expressed DNA in plants. Curr Opin Plant Biol 15:131–139

36. Eckardt N (2001) A sense of self: the role of DNA sequence elimination in allopolyploidization. Plant Cell 13:1699–1704

37. Dietrich FS et al (2004): *Ashbya gossypii* genome as a tool for mapping the ancient

Saccharomyces cerevisiae genome. Science 304:304–307

38. Kellis M, Birren BW, Lander ES (2004) Proof and evolutionary analysis of ancient genome duplication in the yeast *Saccharomyces cerevisiae*. Nature 428:617–624

39. Byrnes JK, Morris GP, Li WH (2006) Reorganization of adjacent gene relationships in yeast genomes by whole-genome duplication and gene deletion. Mol Biol Evol 23:1136–1143

40. van Hoek MJ, Hogeweg P (2007) The role of mutational dynamics in genome shrinkage. Mol Biol Evol 24:2485–2494

41. Sankoff D, Zheng C, Zhu Q (2010) The collapse of gene complement following whole genome duplication. BMC Genomics 11:313–313

42. Wang B, Zheng C, Sankoff D (2011) Fractionation statistics. BMC Bioinf 12(S9):S5

43. Sankoff D, Zheng C, Wang B (2012) A model for biased fractionation after whole genome duplication. BMC Genomics 13(S1):S8

44. Yu Z, Sankoff D (2016) A continuous analog of run length distributions reflecting accumulated fractionation events. BMC Bioinf 17:412

45. Zheng C, Sankoff D (2012) Fractionation, rearrangement and subgenome dominance. Bioinformatics 28:i402–i408

46. Jahn K, Zheng C, Kováč J, Sankoff D (2012) A consolidation algorithm for genomes fractionated after higher order polyploidization. BMC Bioinf 13(S19):S8

47. McLachlan GJ, Peel D, Basford KE, Adams P (1999) The EMMIX software for the fitting of mixtures of normal and t-components. J Stat Softw 4(2):1–14

48. Sankoff D, Zheng C, Lyons E, Tang H (2016) The trees in the peaks. In: Algorithms for computational biology. Lecture notes in bioinformatics, vol 9702. Springer, Cham

49. Kimura M (1984) The neutral theory of molecular evolution. Cambridge University Press, Cambridge

50. Kumar S, Subramanian S (2002) Mutation rates in mammalian genomes. Proc Natl Acad Sci 99:803–808

51. Zheng C, Sankoff D (2013) Practical aliquoting of flowering plant genomes. BMC Bioinf 14(15):S8

52. Argout X et al (2011) The genome of *Theobroma cacao*. Nat Genet 43:101–108

53. Ming R, VanBuren R, Liu Y, Yang M, Han Y, Li L-T, Zhang Q, Kim M-J, Schatz MC, Campbell M, Li J, Bowers JE, Tang H, Lyons E, Ferguson AA, Narzisi G, Nelson DR, Blaby-Haas CE, Gschwend AR, Jiao Y, Der JP, Zeng F, Han J, Min XJ, Hudson KA, Singh R, Grennan AK, Karpowicz SJ, Watling JR, Ito K, Robinson SA, Hudson ME, Yu Q, Mockler TC, Carroll A, Zheng Y, Sunkar R, Jia R, Chen N, Arro J, Wai CM, Wafula E, Spence A, Han Y, Xu L, Zhang J, Peery R, Haus MJ, Xiong W, Walsh JA, Wu J, Wang M-L, Zhu YJ, Paull RE, Britt AB, Du C, Downie SR, Schuler MA, Michael TP, Long SP, Ort DR, Schopf JW, Gang DR, Jiang N, Yandell M, dePamphilis CW, Merchant SS, Paterson AH, Buchanan BB, Li S, Shen-Miller J (2013) Genome of the long-living sacred lotus (*Nelumbo nucifera* Gaertn.). Genome Biol 14(5):1–11

54. Zheng C, Sankoff D (2014) Practical halving; the *Nelumbo nucifera* evidence on early eudicot evolution. Comput Biol Chem 50:75–81

55. Tomato Genome Consortium et al (2012) The tomato genome sequence provides insights into fleshy fruit evolution. Nature 485:635–641

56. Denoeud F, Carretero-Paulet L, Dereeper A, Droc G, Guyot R, Pietrella M, Zheng C, Alberti A, Anthony F, Aprea G et al (2014) The coffee genome provides insight into the convergent evolution of caffeine biosynthesis. Science 345:1181–1184

57. Schnable JC, Springer NM, Freeling M (2011) Differentiation of the maize subgenomes by genome dominance and both ancient and ongoing gene loss. Proc Natl Acad Sci 108:4069–4074

58. Ming R, VanBuren R, Wai CM, Tang H, Schatz MC, Bowers JE, Lyons E, Wang M-L, Chen J, Biggers E et al (2015) The pineapple genome and the evolution of cam photosynthesis. Nat Genet 47:1435–1442

59. Wang X, Wang H, Wang J, Sun R, Wu J, Liu S, Bai Y, Mun J-H, Bancroft I, Cheng F, Huang S, Li X, Hua W, Wang J, Wang X, Freeling M, Pires JC, Paterson AH, Chalhoub B, Wang B, Hayward A, Sharpe AG, Park BS, Weisshaar B, Liu B, Li B, Liu B, Tong C, Song C, Duran C, Peng C, Geng C, Koh C, Lin C, Edwards D, Mu D, Shen D, Soumpourou E, Li F, Fraser F, Conant G, Lassalle G, King GJ, Bonnema G, Tang H, Wang H, Belcram H, Zhou H, Hirakawa H, Abe H, Guo H, Wang H, Jin H, Parkin IAP, Batley J, Kim J-S, Just J, Li J, Xu J, Deng J, Kim JA, Li J, Yu J, Meng J, Wang J, Min J, Poulain J, Hatakeyama K, Wu K, Wang L, Fang L, Trick M, Links MG, Zhao M, Jin M, Ramchiary N, Drou N, Berkman PJ, Cai Q, Huang Q, Li R, Tabata S, Cheng S, Zhang S, Zhang S, Huang S, Sato S, Sun S, Kwon S-J, Choi S-R, Lee T-H, Fan W, Zhao X, Tan X,

Xu X, Wang Y, Qiu Y, Yin Y, Li Y, Du Y, Liao Y, Lim Y, Narusaka Y, Wang Y, Wang Z, Li Z, Wang Z, Xiong Z, Zhang Z (2011) The genome of the mesopolyploid crop species *Brassica rapa*. Nat Genet 43:1035–1039

60. Liu S, Liu Y, Yang X, Tong C, Edwards D, Parkin IAP, Zhao M, Ma J, Yu J, Huang S, Wang X, J Wang, Lu K, Fang Z, Bancroft I, Yang T-J, Hu Q, Wang X, Yue Z, Li H, Yang L, Wu J, Zhou Q, Wang W, King GJ, Pires JC, Lu C, Wu Z, Sampath P, Wang Z, Guo H, Pan S, Yang L, Min J, Zhang D, Jin D, Li W, Belcram H, Tu J, Guan M, Qi C, Du D, Li J, Jiang L, Batley J, Sharpe AG, Park B-S, Ruperao P, Cheng F, Waminal NE, Huang Y, Dong C, Wang L, Li J, Hu Z, Zhuang M, Huang Y, Huang J, Shi J, Mei D, Liu J, Lee T-H, Wang J, Jin H, Li Z, Li X, Zhang J, Xiao L, Zhou Y, Liu Z, Liu X, Qin R, Tang X, Liu W, Wang Y, Zhang Y, Lee J, Kim HH, Denoeud F, Xu X, Liang X, Hua W, Wang X, Wang J, Chalhoub B, Paterson AH (2014) The *Brassica oleracea* genome reveals the asymmetrical evolution of polyploid genomes. Nat Commun 5:3930

61. Kitashiba H, Li F, Hirakawa H, Kawanabe T, Zou Z, Hasegawa Y, Tonosaki K, Shirasawa S, Fukushima A, Yokoi S, Takahata Y, Kakizaki T, Ishida M, Okamoto S, Sakamoto K, Shirasawa K, Tabata S, Nishio T (2014) Draft sequences of the radish (*Raphanus sativus* l.) genome. DNA Res 21(5):481–490

62. Hu TT, Pattyn P, Bakker EG, Cao J, Cheng J-F, Clark RM, Fahlgren N, Fawcett JA, Grimwood J, Gundlach H, Haberer G, Hollister JD, Ossowski S, Ottilar RP, Salamov AA, Schneeberger K, Spannagl M, Wang X, Yang L, Nasrallah ME, Bergelson J, Carrington JC, Gaut BS, Schmutz J, Mayer KFX, Van de Peer Y, Grigoriev IV, Nordborg M, Weigel D, Guo Y-L (2011) The *Arabidopsis lyrata* genome sequence and the basis of rapid genome size change. Nat Genet 43:476–481

63. Haudry A, Platts AE, Vello E, Hoen DR, Leclercq M, Williamson RJ, Forczek E, Joly-Lopez Z, Steffen JG, Hazzouri KM, Dewar K, Stinchcombe JR, Schoen DJ, Wang X, Schmutz J, Town CD, Edger PP, Pires JC, Schumaker KS, Jarvis DE, Mandakova T, Lysak MA, van den Bergh E, Schranz ME, Harrison PM, Moses AM, Bureau TE, Wright SI, Blanchette M (2013) An atlas of over 90,000 conserved noncoding sequences provides insight into crucifer regulatory regions. Nat Genet 45:891–898

64. Lyons E, Freeling M (2008) How to usefully compare homologous plant genes and chromosomes as DNA sequences. Plant J 53:661–673

65. Lyons E, Pedersen B, Kane J, Freeling M (2008) The value of nonmodel genomes and an example using SynMap within CoGe to dissect the hexaploidy that predates rosids. Trop Plant Biol 1:181–190

66. Kagale S, Robinson SJ, Nixon J, Xiao R, Huebert T, Condie J, Kessler D, Clarke WE, Edger PP, Links MG et al (2014) Polyploid evolution of the Brassicaceae during the cenozoic era. Plant Cell 26:2777–2791

Chapter 11

Sequence-Based Synteny Analysis of Multiple Large Genomes

Daniel Doerr and Bernard M. E. Moret

Abstract

Current methods for synteny analysis provide only limited support to study large genomes at the sequence level. In this chapter, we describe a pipeline based on existing tools that, applied in a suitable fashion, enables synteny analysis of large genomic datasets. We give a hands-on description of each step of the pipeline using four avian genomes for data. We also provide integration scripts that simplify the conversion and setup of data between the different tools in the pipeline.

Key words Genome comparison, Synteny analysis, Marker sequences, Large genomes

1   Introduction

The structural organization of genomes was studied long before the advent of genome sequencing technology, using chromosomal banding and other means, eventually leading to detailed chromosomal maps. Renwick [1] introduced the term *synteny* to denote close collocation of genomic elements on the same chromosome. With the advent of large-scale sequencing, synteny came to denote conserved collocation of genomic elements within large blocks of sequence and these blocks in turn became known as *syntenic blocks*.

Comparing the complete DNA sequences of large eukaryotic genomes for several species presents many challenges. The complexity of the necessary computations severely restricts the number of species and, even for three or four genomes, forces an undesirable trade-off between speed and accuracy. The large range of evolutionary changes, from sequence indels and point mutations through genome rearrangements and segmental duplications to deletions and insertions of entire blocks of sequence, serves to destroy collinearity and otherwise disguises similarities, thereby introducing ambiguities in the comparison. (This particular issue limits all syntenic analyses to collections of reasonably related

João C. Setubal et al. (eds.), *Comparative Genomics: Methods and Protocols*, Methods in Molecular Biology, vol. 1704,
https://doi.org/10.1007/978-1-4939-7463-4_11, © Springer Science+Business Media LLC 2018

genomes.) Multiway comparisons scale poorly, as the number of choices to be considered grows exponentially with the number of genomes to be compared. Finally, the genomes themselves are neither well defined (as they vary from one individual to the other within a population) nor perfectly sequenced and assembled (for instance, very few genomes are fully assembled, being given instead as contigs, with many poorly assembled genomes described with 10–100 times as many contigs as they have chromosomes), so that comparisons at the sequence level on a nucleotide-by-nucleotide basis are subject to many possible confounding factors.

The response to these challenges has been to compute a simplified representation of the genomes in terms of syntenic blocks and then carry out the multiway comparison at the level of syntenic blocks rather than at the level of base pairs. At first, researchers focused on genes as the base units, leading to studies of the gene content and gene order of genomes and mechanisms that affect these two representations. However, the vast majority of nucleotide bases in large genomes are not associated with genes, yet conservation across species is a powerful tool to identify functional elements and conduct meaningful comparisons among non-genic regions. Thus the focus shifted from genes to *genomic markers*, DNA segments that are well conserved across all or most of the given genomes. If each genome is found to have one (or more) contiguous region that contains the same markers (in the same order or in different orders), then each such region is a syntenic block and together these regions define a *syntenic block family*. (The similarity in terminology with genes and gene families is intentional and justified: genes are just very large markers.) The purpose of a synteny analysis is to produce families of syntenic blocks such that the blocks themselves are well conserved (have many shared markers and limited sequence variation overall) and the syntenic block families together cover much of each genome.

Syntenic blocks reduce the number of individual items to compare (in many analyses the length of these blocks varies from hundreds of thousands to as many as tens of millions of base pairs), afford some tolerance against missing or erroneous sequence data (from read calling errors to assembly errors) and against individual variation, and reduce the number of evolutionary events that must be considered when conducting a comparison (sequence-level events are no longer directly relevant), thus making comparison of multiple large genomes possible.

Because syntenic blocks and their families are just another representation of a collection of genomes, one would want to produce these blocks directly from sequence data, with as little prior knowledge as possible, and also produce blocks of various characteristics (coarser and larger blocks for quick analyses, fine-grained decompositions for accuracy and coverage, etc.). These two goals remain elusive, although much work is in progress for direct synteny analysis on unannotated genome sequences: tools such as Sibelia [2] and Satsuma [3] already provide solutions for bacterial genomes (Sibelia) or small datasets (Satsuma), but cannot handle a collection of large eukaryotic genomes.

In this chapter, we present a pipeline for synteny analysis of collections of large genomes. Our pipeline is based on several available tools. We provide scripts and give a hands-on description for each step of the pipeline, using four birds: *Gallus gallus* (chicken), *Meleagris gallopavo* (turkey), *Taeniopygia guttata* (zebra finch), and *Ficedula albicollis* (collared flycatcher). Our scripts are available for download on GitHub.[1] Our pipeline uses the whole-genome alignment tool Mauve [4] and the synteny detection tool i-ADHoRe [5]. We also use Circos [6] for creating a genome-wide visualization of syntenic blocks. Our scripts are written in Python 2 and require the Python library `Biopython` (and, optionally, `matplotlib`).

2   Preparing the Genomic Dataset

Careful selection of genome data is crucial to any synteny analysis. Many large genomes are only partially assembled, producing some modest number of contigs, alongside many short sequences of unknown or dubious origin. Such unassembled genomes pose some insurmountable difficulties to current synteny tools. While there exist other methods for scaffolding genomes based on comparative analyses [7], this task is not part of any synteny tool to date. (i-ADHoRe is able to identify syntenic blocks that are conserved across multiple contigs, but it only does so in the context of segmental or whole-genome duplication.) We therefore confine our workflow to fully or nearly assembled genomes.

As a first step, one should inspect the genome sequence files. First count the number and size of sequence records. Then, small or negligible sequences should be removed or assembled into larger sequences. The latter can be based on previous synteny analyses, comparative assembly, or simple sequential concatenation, so that in the end, each genome is represented by a manageable, clearly arranged set of sequences. Furthermore, each sequence should have a short but meaningful name by which it can be later identified when visually evaluating the outcome of the synteny discovery.

---

[1] https://github.com/danydoerr/large_syn_workflow.

The analysis described in the following is based on genomic sequences retrieved from NCBI[2]. We downloaded the following sequence files and computed their numbers of sequence records:

```
file name                                                #sequence records
GCA_000002315.3_Gallus_gallus-5.0_genomic.fna                        23474
GCA_000146605.3_Turkey_5.0_genomic.fna                              231286
GCA_000151805.2_Taeniopygia_guttata-3.2.4_genomic.fna               37095
GCA_000247815.2_FicAlb1.5_genomic.fna                               21428
```

Each of these files contains thousands of sequence records with all but few of no relevance to our analysis, because they are too short. As a first step, we therefore discard all sequences that are smaller than 1 Mbp. For this task, we provide a simple script called `extract_minlen_seq.py`, which takes as input a value for minimum sequence length and a FASTA file:

```
$ extract_minlen_seq.py 1000000 GCA_000002315.3_Gallus_gallus-\
    5.0_genomic.fna > C.min_1Mbp.fna
```

This task is repeated for the remaining sequence files, which are now labeled by a single character that identifies the corresponding species: C for chicken, T for turkey, Z for zebra finch, and F for collared flycatcher. The number of sequence records came down to a manageable few:

```
file name        #records   sequence record IDs
C.min_1Mbp.fna      31       CM000093.4..CM000107.4 CM000109.4.. \
                             CM000119.4 CM000121.4..CM000124.4 \
                             KQ759483.1
T.min_1Mbp.fna      30       CM000962.2..CM000978.2 CM000980.2.. \
                             CM000991.2 CM000993.2
Z.min_1Mbp.fna      39       CM000515.1..CM000532.1 CM000534.1.. \
                             CM000546.1 EQ832640.1 EQ832641.1 \
                             EQ832723.1 EQ832760.1 EQ832819.1 \
                             EQ832820.1 EQ833162.1 EQ833367.1
F.min_1Mbp.fna      39       CM001988.1..CM002017.1 CM002020.1 \
                             KE165308.1 KE165340.1..KE165342.1
```

With just a few exceptions, sequence records now correspond to chromosome scaffolds. Any remaining undesirable sequences can be individually removed from the sequence files.

Because the sequences have been downloaded from a public database, they are labeled with their database identifier. This label is necessary for bookkeeping, yet inconvenient for manual and visual analysis of the genomic dataset. Short labels, such as chromosome

---

[2] https://ncbi.nlm.nih.gov/genome.

numbers, would simplify the manual analysis and provide short identifiers that can be used in the visualization. Because the FASTA files are too large to edit comfortably in a text editor and because, in some datasets, the preprocessing could involve the concatenation of some sequence records, we provide a script to edit FASTA files based on a limited set of instructions:

```
JOIN <ID 1> (h|t) <ID 2> (h|t) INTO <ID 3>
RENAME <ID 1> TO <ID 2>
REMOVE <ID>
```

The *rename* and *remove* operations are straightforward. The *join* operation requires, next to the sequence IDs, the extremities ("*h*" for *head* and "*t*" for *tail*) of the sequences that will be joined to produce a concatenated sequence with a specified ID. (In our example, concatenation is not necessary.)

Our script, edit_sequences.py, requires a sequence file and an instruction file, where each line corresponds to one edit operation, as shown by the contents of the edit file C.edit for the chicken dataset below:

```
-- file: C.edit ----------------------------------------------
RENAME CM000093.4 TO 1
RENAME CM000094.4 TO 2
RENAME CM000095.4 TO 3
RENAME CM000096.4 TO 4
RENAME CM000097.4 TO 5
RENAME CM000098.4 TO 6
RENAME CM000099.4 TO 7
RENAME CM000100.4 TO 8
RENAME CM000101.4 TO 9
RENAME CM000102.4 TO 10
RENAME CM000103.4 TO 11
RENAME CM000104.4 TO 12
RENAME CM000105.4 TO 13
RENAME CM000106.4 TO 14
RENAME CM000107.4 TO 15
RENAME CM000109.4 TO 17
RENAME CM000110.4 TO 18
RENAME CM000111.4 TO 19
RENAME CM000112.4 TO 20
RENAME CM000113.4 TO 21
RENAME CM000114.4 TO 22
RENAME CM000115.4 TO 23
RENAME CM000116.4 TO 24
RENAME CM000124.4 TO 25
RENAME CM000117.4 TO 26
RENAME CM000118.4 TO 27
```

```
RENAME CM000119.4 TO 28
RENAME CM000123.4 TO 33
REMOVE KQ759483.1
RENAME CM000121.4 TO W
RENAME CM000122.4 TO Z
```

The final sequence files are obtained by calling `edit_sequences.py`:

```
$ edit_sequences.py C.min_1Mbp.fasta C.edit
```

Now, the sequence data of each genome in the dataset is purged from irrelevant content. Each dataset yields 30–31 sequence records, with 0. 97 Gbp to 1. 04 Gbp, as shown in Table 1.

3   Constructing Genomic Markers

We now provide a brief description on how to use the software tool progressiveMauve[3][4] to obtain a genomic marker set across multiple genome sequences. Further information can be found in Mauve's comprehensive online user guide[4] and in the archive of the active Mauve user mailing list.[5] progressiveMauve is a multiple genome alignment tool which exploits unique local alignments in the genomic dataset as anchor blocks for a multiple sequence

Table 1
Genomic dataset of the four birds

Species	ID	Version	Scfs.	Size (Gbp)	CDSs	Markers	%cov.
Gallus gallus (chicken)	C	5.0	30	1.02	46,393	643,043	40.4
Ficedula albicollis (collared flycatcher)	F	1.5	30	1.04	26,464	643,043	39.5
Meleagris gallopavoi (turkey)	T	5.0	30	0.97	26,423	643,043	42.3
Taeniopygia guttata (zebra finch)	Z	3.2.4	31	1.02	19,447	643,043	40.3

Columns from left to right: Species name and parenthesized colloquial name; short identifier; dataset version in NCBI; number of scaffolds after editing; genome size after editing; number of coding sequences (CDSs); number of markers identified by Mauve that are larger than 300 bp and have homologs in all four birds; the percentage of nucleotide bases covered by these markers in their respective genomes

---

[3] Available for download at http://darlinglab.org/mauve/download.html.

[4] http://darlinglab.org/mauve/user-guide.

[5] https://sourceforge.net/p/mauve/mailman/mauve-users.

alignment. Using a guide tree, the method progressively aligns genomic sequences, using a sum-of-pairs anchor score.

A decisive advantage of progressiveMauve in comparison with competing methods is its uncomplicated use. In most analyses, no adjustments to its default parameter settings are necessary. Should customization be needed, it usually suffices to adjust a single parameter, the *match seed weight* (command line parameter --seed-weight). The match seed weight defines a threshold that alignment scores of unique matches must surpass in order to be considered in the initial construction of anchor blocks. Lower values will increase the sensitivity of the alignment and thus permit the validation of a reasonable number of markers when analyzing divergent genomes. Adjusting this parameter also influences alignment blocks that are subsequently identified through positional conservation, because, by default, the *minimum locally collinear block weight* (command line parameter --weight) is set to three times the match seed weight. Without changing any default settings, we call the program as follows:

```
progressiveMauve --output-guide-tree=C_F_T_Z.tree \
    --backbone-output=C_F_T_Z.backbone --output=C_F_T_Z.xmfa \
    C.fna F.fna T.fna Z.fna 2>&1 | tee mauve.log
```

Next to the alignment guide tree and the *XMFA* file, which will store the whole-genome alignment data, Mauve also provides a *backbone* table specifying which genomic segments have been matched with each other in the alignment. We will use the backbone table to extract the genomic markers and their affiliations for the synteny analysis in the following section.

4 Synteny Analysis with i-ADHoRe

Most synteny analysis tools to date are only applicable to small genome datasets. i-ADHoRe [5] is one of the few tools that have been specifically designed to handle large eukaryotic genomes. It provides both fast algorithms and multithreading for the most time-consuming steps. The tool's configuration is defined through an input file containing the user's parameter settings. A comprehensive list of parameters and their options is provided in the manual included in the software package. Further, i-ADHoRe requires a proprietary format for its input files. Each contig/chromosome of any input genome must be represented by an individual file. For convenience, such files should be grouped in separate folders corresponding to their genome memberships. Relationships between markers must be provided in a further file, in one of two possible formats: either markers are associated with a family identifier (`table_type=family`) or pairwise relationships are individually provided, permitting also non-transitive relationships between markers (`table_type=blast`).

i-ADHoRe can be run in three different modes (parameter name `cluster_type`): `colinear`, `cloud`, and `hybrid`. The first mode detects collinear syntenic blocks in an iterative procedure, integrating marker content and order information from previous alignments into profiles for identifying further, more degenerate syntenic blocks. In doing so, each iteration leads to a higher level of syntenic block families with increasing size. The cloud mode intends to detect syntenic blocks that underwent internal rearrangements and so are better identified by their shared marker content than by ordering. How much the ordering can deviate from collinearity is bounded by a parameter (`q_value`). Lastly, the hybrid mode discovers collinear regions prior to performing synteny analysis in the cloud mode. Neither cloud nor hybrid mode supports the profile search performed in the collinear mode. For this reason, it is advisable to use the collinear mode due to its superior ability to identify degenerate syntenic blocks. In all three modes, i-ADHoRe allows gaps in syntenic blocks. Various parameters allow to fine-tune the size of these gaps in different contexts. In practice, it often suffices to control their setting through a shared value.

Processing the genome data and Mauve's backbone table into the input format required by i-ADHoRe is an elaborate task. Therefore, we provide a script which performs this conversion conveniently in one program call. Our script, called `mauve2iadhore.py`, offers a few parameter settings to adjust the most influential parameters of i-ADHoRe directly upon creating the input files. It can also filter segments of Mauve's backbone file that fall below a given minimum length. All options are listed in Table 2. Our script will also enable i-ADHoRe's multithreading feature by providing it with the number of cores that are available on the machine on which the script is executed.

For the analysis of the four avian genomes, we call `mauve2iadhore.py` as shown below. We require that segments in Mauve's backbone file that will be used as markers in subsequent analysis must be conserved across all four genomes (`-n4`) and have a minimum length of 300 bp (`-l300`). In our bird dataset, Mauve identifies many markers that fit our constraints (*see* Table 1), many more than the number of coding sequences in these genomes, enabling a more fine-grained synteny analysis. The price to pay: the gap size for syntenic blocks in the subsequent i-ADHoRe run must be set appropriately high (`-g300`).

```
$ mauve2iadhore.py -c colinear -n4 -l300 -g300 C_F_T_Z.backbone \
    C.fna F.fna T.fna Z.fna
```

Table 2
Command line options of conversion script `mauve2iadhore.py`

Options	Default value	Description
`-n INT, --quorum=INT`	2	Minimum number of species in which each marker must have a homologous counterpart.
`-l INT, --minlength=INT`	100	Minimum length a segment must have to be included in the output.
`-g INT, --max_gap_size=INT`	30	Maximum distance between markers in a cloud or collinear cluster.
`-c CLUSTERTYPE,` `--cluster_type=CLUSTERTYPE`	colinear	i-ADHoRe cluster type must be any of (colinear | hybrid | cloud).
`-q [0, 1], --q_value=[0, 1]`	0.5	Minimum r^2 distance for markers in a cloud cluster.
`-o OUTDIR, --outdir=OUTDIR`	"."	Directory to which the output files will be written.

The script produces then the following files and folders:

```
C/  C_F_T_Z.log  F/  T/  Z/  blast_table.txt  dataset.ini

./C: 1.1st 10.1st 11.1st 12.1st 13.1st 14.1st 15.1st 17.1st \
     18.1st 19.1st 2.1st 20.1st 21.1st 22.1st 23.1st 24.1st \
     25.1st 26.1st 27.1st 28.1st 3.1st 4.1st 5.1st 6.1st 7.1st \
     8.1st 9.1st W.1st Z.1st

./F: 1.1st 10.1st 11.1st 12.1st 13.1st 14.1st 15.1st 17.1st \
     18.1st 19.1st 1A.1st 2.1st 20.1st 21.1st 22.1st 23.1st \
     24.1st 25.1st 26.1st 27.1st 28.1st 3.1st 4.1st 4A.1st \
     5.1st 6.1st 7.1st 8.1st 9.1st Z.1st

./T: 1.1st 10.1st 11.1st 12.1st 13.1st 14.1st 15.1st 16.1st \
     17.1st 19.1st 2.1st 20.1st 21.1st 22.1st 23.1st 24.1st \
     25.1st 26.1st 27.1st 28.1st 29.1st 3.1st 30.1st 4.1st \
     5.1st 6.1st 7.1st 8.1st 9.1st Z.1st

./Z: 1.1st 10.1st 11.1st 12.1st 13.1st 14.1st 15.1st 17.1st \
     18.1st 19.1st 1A.1st 1B.1st 2.1st 20.1st 21.1st 22.1st \
     23.1st 24.1st 25.1st 26.1st 27.1st 28.1st 3.1st 4.1st \
     4A.1st 5.1st 6.1st 7.1st 8.1st 9.1st Z.1st
```

Finally, we call i-ADHoRe by passing it the created configuration file `dataset.ini`:

```
$ i-adhore dataset.ini
```

According to the configuration setup by our conversion script, i-ADHoRe deposits its output files in a folder named `output` below the current working directory. Among the various files that i-ADHoRe creates, `output/multiplicons.txt` and `output/segments.txt` contain the central information regarding the discovered syntenic block families.

5   Evaluation

We evaluate syntenic blocks based on synteny criteria suggested by Ghiurcuta and Moret [8] and provide a genome-wide visualization of synteny blocks between pairs of species of our dataset.

Ghiurcuta and Moret presented two measures for scoring a syntenic block family: the *relaxed score* represents the fraction of markers that are connected to any other markers within their syntenic block family; conversely, the *weighted score* is a stricter measure describing the fraction of markers that are connected to at least one marker in each syntenic block.

We provide a script, `synteny_score.py` that computes these scores from the output of an i-ADHoRe run. Our script prints for each syntenic block family its corresponding relaxed or weighted synteny score. Optionally, it is also able to directly create a plot that visualizes a histogram over all synteny scores. To this end, the script requires the python package `matplotlib` library, which must be installed on the system.

We can now evaluate the syntenic block families discovered by i-ADHoRe in the avian dataset. To visualize the histograms shown in Fig. 1, we call our script by providing the `-v` parameter as follows:

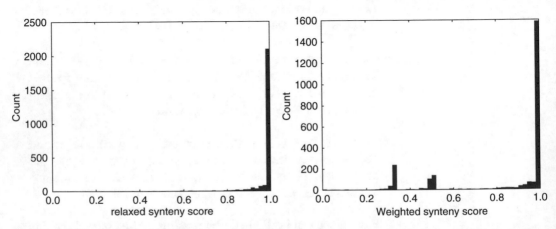

Fig. 1 Histogram of relaxed and weighted scores of syntenic blocks in the avian dataset identified by i-ADHoRe

```
$ synteny_scores.py -t relaxed -v dataset.ini output/segments.txt
$ synteny_scores.py -t weighted -v dataset.ini output/segments.txt
```

By default, the calls create two files containing the figures, `relaxed_scores.eps` and `weighted_scores.eps`, respectively, which will be located in the current working directory. However, an alternative output file name can be specified with the `-f` parameter.

Although i-ADHoRe provides its own graphical output, it does not produce plots to study the entire set of syntenic blocks across whole genomes. Therefore, we created an alternative genome-wide visualization, using the popular visualization tool Circos [6]. For each pair of genomes, we instruct Circos to draw all their synteny blocks and relationships. Our visualization permits a quick assessment of the segmentation of genomes into markers and syntenic blocks, of divergence in the arrangement of genomic markers, and of genome coverage.

We call script `iadhore2circos.py` on the avian dataset as follows:

```
$ iadhore2circos.py -c dataset.ini output/multiplicons.txt \
    output/segments.txt
```

The script creates for each genome pair an individual *Circos configuration file*, but also further configuration files. The `-c` parameter causes each link between syntenic blocks to be drawn in a different color. Otherwise, all links associated with the same chromosome are drawn in the same color. Further, our script provides the option `-l` to draw higher-level intervals identified by i-ADHoRe in `colinear` mode. It remains to call the Circos binary on each of these files, as exemplified below for the genome pair chicken and collared flycatcher.

```
$ circos -conf C_F.circos.conf
```

The plots thus created are shown in Fig. 2. In each plot, the outer circle shows the pair of genomes drawn in blue and green, respectively, partitioned into its contigs/chromosomes. Black bars drawn on top correspond to locations of markers. Lastly, as mentioned above, colored links indicate relations between syntenic blocks among the two species.

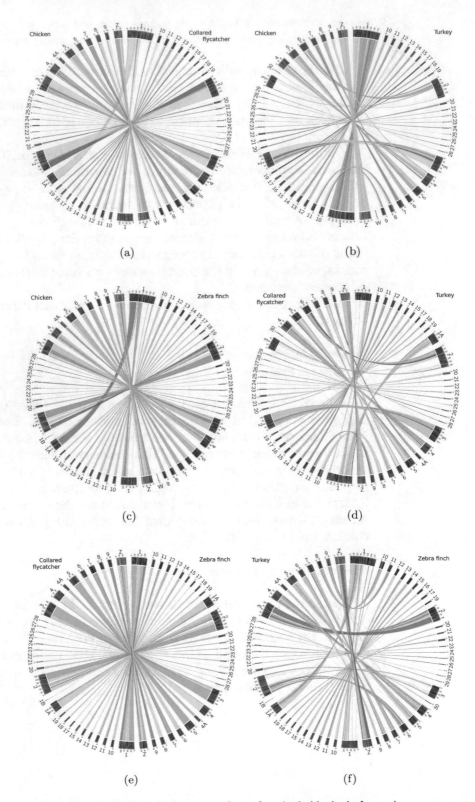

(a)

(b)

(c)

(d)

(e)

(f)

Fig. 2 Circos plots visualizing the pairwise comparison of syntenic blocks in four avian genomes

References

1. Renwick JH (1971) The mapping of human chromosomes. Annu Rev Genet 5(1):81–120
2. Minkin I, Patel A, Kolmogorov M, Vyahhi N, Pham S (2013) Sibelia: a scalable and comprehensive synteny block generation tool for closely related microbial genomes. In: Theory and applications of models of computation. Springer, Berlin/Heidelberg, pp 215–229
3. Grabherr MG, Russell P, Meyer M, Mauceli E, Alföldi J, Di Palma F, Lindblad-Toh K (2010) Genome-wide synteny through highly sensitive sequence alignment: Satsuma. Bioinformatics 26 (9):1145–1151
4. Darling AE, Mau B, Perna NT (2010) progressiveMauve: multiple genome alignment with gene gain, loss and rearrangement. PLoS One 5(6):e11147
5. Proost S, Fostier J, De Witte D, Dhoedt B, Demeester P, Van de Peer Y, Vandepoele K (2012) i-ADHoRe 3.0-fast and sensitive detection of genomic homology in extremely large data sets. Nucleic Acids Res 40(2):e11
6. Krzywinski MI, Schein JE, Birol I, Connors J, Gascoyne R, Horsman D, Jones SJ, Marra MA (2009) Circos: an information aesthetic for comparative genomics. Genome Res 19 (9):1639–1645
7. Husemann P, Stoye J (2010) r2cat: synteny plots and comparative assembly. Bioinformatics 26 (4):570–571
8. Ghiurcuta CG, Moret BME (2014) Evaluating synteny for improved comparative studies. Bioinformatics 30(12):i9–i18

Chapter 12

Family-Free Genome Comparison

Daniel Doerr, Pedro Feijão, and Jens Stoye

Abstract

The comparison of genome structures across distinct species offers valuable insights into the species' phylogeny, genome organization, and gene associations. In this chapter, we review the family-free genome comparison tool FFGC which provides several methods for gene order analyses that do not require prior knowledge of evolutionary relationships between the genes across the studied genomes. Moreover, the tool features a complete workflow for genome comparison, requiring nothing but annotated genome sequences as input.

Key words Gene family-free, Gene order analysis, Conserved adjacencies, Common intervals, Double-cut-and-join, Genome similarity, Genome distance

1 Introduction

A prominent branch in the field of computational comparative genomics is devoted to the study of the structural organization of genomes. Gene order analysis, i.e. the comparative study of genomic sequences that have been scrambled by genome rearrangement events, confers detailed insights into the species' evolutionary past helping to resolve their phylogenetic relationships, the structural organization of ancestral genomes, and functional dependencies of genes, only to name a few applications.

The gene order analyses subject to this work comprise not only the computation of various genomic distances, but also the detection of conserved gene adjacencies, gene clusters, or larger syntenic regions.

Comparing gene orders of distinct genomes presumes knowledge of relationships between their defining genes. Whereas initial methods were confined to one-to-one homology assignments between genes of distinct genomes, many of the current methods allow for general gene family assignments, thereby internally resolving (or at least tolerating) ambiguities in conserved gene order originating from gene duplicates or losses. Hereby, a gene family

João C. Setubal et al. (eds.), *Comparative Genomics: Methods and Protocols*, Methods in Molecular Biology, vol. 1704,
https://doi.org/10.1007/978-1-4939-7463-4_12, © Springer Science+Business Media LLC 2018

is an equivalence class of genes, leading to a partition of a studied dataset into disjoint homologous groups of genes.

Gene families are controversial: not only is the process of inferring homology error-prone, but also the term "gene family" itself is subject to various interpretations. This leads to wide disparities between the conspicuous number of available gene family databases. Errors originating from false gene family assignments are passed on and may become amplified in subsequent gene order analysis. Conversely, knowledge of gene neighborhoods allows to make more substantiated claims about homology. This leads to a classic circularity problem: gene families are a prerequisite of gene order analysis, yet the outcome of the latter can improve the inference of homology. The aim of *family-free* genome comparison is to break this circularity by developing methods for gene order analysis that, rather than depending on gene families, rely on the input data of gene family clustering, which are loosely constrained qualitative or quantitative measures of gene relationships.

Over the past years, several family-free methods have been proposed and developed [1–5]. In this work, we present a workflow encompassing many methods that have been published to date. The workflow is implemented and available as part of the tool FFGC, available for download at http://bibiserv.cebitec.uni-bielefeld.de/ffgc. FFGC provides functionality for all steps of a family-free analysis starting from annotated genome sequences. The following sections will guide through each step of the workflow, thereby explaining the objectives of the family-free methods available in FFGC.

2 Prerequisites of Family-Free Analysis

The workflow of family-free analysis, visualized in Fig. 1, is divided into three steps: (1) the computation of local sequence alignment scores between genes of two or more gene order sequences; (2) the construction of a gene relationship graph; and (3) the actual family-free gene order analysis. In the following, we will describe the first two steps that are prerequisite to all family-free analyses. Our tool FFGC is designed so that these prerequisite steps, which are often the most time consuming, only need to be carried out once. The outcome is a gene relationship graph that is then input to all subsequent family free analyses alike.

In FFGC, a genome is entirely represented by its set of chromosomes, whereby each chromosome corresponds to a linear or circular sequence of unique gene identifiers drawn from the universe of genes Σ. Each gene $g \in \Sigma$ is labeled with a *sign*, denoted $sgn(g)$, which is either positive $(+)$ or negative $(-)$, indicating the gene's orientation on its genomic sequence. In relating genes between different genomes, two basic data structures have been proposed in the past, which are the *gene connection graph* [5] and the *gene similarity graph* [1].

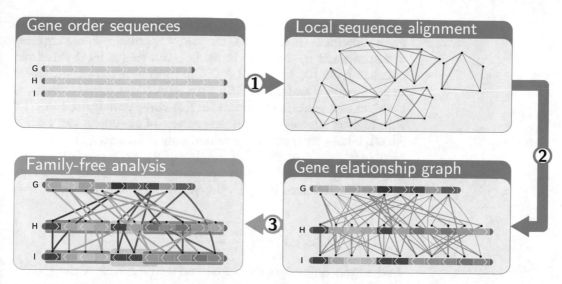

Fig. 1 Overview of family-free analysis workflow implemented in FFGC

Definition 1 (Gene Connection Graph, Gene Similarity Graph). Given two genomes $S_1, \ldots, S_k$, a *gene connection graph* $G(S_1, \ldots, S_k)$ of genomes $S_1, \ldots, S_k$ is a k-partite graph with one vertex for each gene in each of the k genomes. An edge between two genes of distinct genomes indicates that there is some *evolutionary connection* between these genes. If edges are additionally weighted by a strictly positive similarity value, the graph is called *gene similarity graph*.

The construction of gene connection graphs and gene similarity graphs requires the assessment of qualitative and quantitative relationships between genes, respectively. Different kinds of information can be used for this task, ranging from establishing relationships based on common cellular tasks, such as participation in the same metabolic pathways, to similarity in molecular function, to alignment scores. In this work, we confine ourselves entirely to alignment scores, thereby relying on the detection of significant hits in local sequence alignment.   FFGC constructs a gene similarity graph from the input set of genome sequences, subsequently ignoring its weights for those family-free analyses that require an (unweighted) gene connection graph. To establish similarities between genes, the tool relies on the BLAST+ [6] software package, which is used to identify significant hits in local sequence alignment (HSPs) between all pairs of genes originating from distinct genomes. The comparison (step 2 of the FFGC workflow) is performed either on the nucleotide or protein sequence level, depending on the user's initial choice when creating the project. FFGC allows to prune the gene similarity graph using two filter techniques. This step is performed iteratively until the graph remains either unchanged or a maximum number of iterations is exceeded.

On the one hand, FFGC can discard edges by identifying spurious similarities. In doing so, the tool implements the *stringency filter* proposed by Lechner et al. [7], utilizing a local threshold parameter $f \in [0, 1]$ and BLAST bitscores between genes. Given two genomes S and T, an HSP with BLAST bitscore $bitscore(s, t)$ between two genes, s in S and t in T, is compared against an HSP with highest bitscore between any gene s' of genome S and gene t. An edge between s and t is retained only if $bitscore(s, t) \geq f \cdot \max \{bitscore(s', t) \mid s' \text{ in } S\}$. Edge weights of the gene similarity graph between any two vertices corresponding to some genes s and t are then calculated according to the *relative reciprocal BLAST score* (RRBS) [8]:

$$\text{RRBS}(s, t) = \frac{bitscore(s, t) + bitscore(t, s)}{bitscore(s, s) + bitscore(t, t)} \ .$$

In doing so, only edges are established whose corresponding RRBS value is strictly positive.

On the other hand, FFGC can remove vertices if their corresponding genes are either (1) not similar to any other genes associated with at least a certain number of genomes or (2) not residing on contigs of minimum size. If a gene's corresponding vertex is no longer present in the pruned gene similarity graph, it will be omitted in its gene order sequence subject to any subsequently described family-free analysis.

The provided filters can improve the stability of family-free gene order analysis against disturbances originating from incorrect gene annotations or spurious sequence similarities.

3   Genomic Similarities and Distances

FFGC implements several pairwise measures of genome similarity which are described in the following. First, we discuss measures based on *gene adjacencies* that were proposed by Kowada et al. [5] for pairwise gene connection graphs and by Braga et al. [1] for pairwise gene similarity graphs. Subsequently, we study a family-free variant of the *double-cut-and-join* (DCJ) distance.

A pair of genes in a genome form an *adjacency* if no other gene lies in-between them on their common genomic sequence. A first measure corresponds to counting the number of *conserved adjacencies*:

Definition 2 (Conserved Adjacency). Given two genomes S and T and a gene connection graph $(V, E) = G(S, T)$, a pair of adjacencies (s, s') in S and (t, t') in T is called a *conserved adjacency*, if one of the following two holds:

(a) $(s, t) \in E, (s', t') \in E, sgn(s) = sgn(t)$ and $sgn_S(s') = sgn_T(t')$; or

(b) $(s, t') \in E, (s', t) \in E, sgn(s) \neq sgn(t')$ and $sgn(s') \neq sgn(t)$.

Problem 1 (Total Adjacencies [5]). Given two genomes S and T, enumerate all conserved adjacencies in their gene connection graph $G(S, T)$.

Since genes can be connected to many other genes, conserved adjacencies may overlap in either genome with those of others, resulting in *conflicts* between them. Hence this measure is less apt for some evolutionary studies. The next measure for gene adjacencies resolves these conflicts: **Problem 2 (Adjacency Matching [5]).** Given two genomes S and T and a gene connection graph $G(S, T)$, compute a maximum cardinality set of non-conflicting conserved adjacencies.

The following family-free measure integrates gene similarities, thereby establishing one-to-one homology assignments between genes of two genomes S and T. To this end, a *matching* $M \subseteq E$ in their corresponding gene similarity graph $(V, E) = G(S, T)$ is established. The measure tolerates gene duplication events by matching those duplicates that either have high similarity to each other or are contained in a conserved adjacency with high adjacency score in the M-induced genomes S^M and T^M. Thereby, the M-induced genome sequences S^M and T^M are the subsequences of S and T, respectively, that contain only those genes associated with vertices incident to edges of M. In constructing a matching, not only gene similarities are taken into account, but also adjacencies:

$$edg(M) = \sum_{e \in M} w(e) \tag{1}$$

$$adj_{ST}(M) = \sum_{\substack{e, f \in M \text{ form a} \\ \text{conserved adjacency} \\ \text{of } S^M, T^M}} \sqrt{w(e) \cdot w(f)} \tag{2}$$

Problem 3 (FF-Adjacencies [1]). Given two genomes S, T and some $\alpha \in [0, 1]$, find a matching M in gene similarity graph $G(S, T)$ such that the following formula is maximized:

$$\mathcal{F}_\alpha(M) = \alpha \cdot adj_{ST}(M) + (1 - \alpha) \cdot edg(M). \tag{3}$$

FFGC also implements a family-free variant for a genome rearrangement distance, namely the Double Cut and Join (DCJ) operation [9, 10]. A DCJ acts on a genome by cutting two adjacencies and reconnecting the free extremities in two possible ways. This results in a very simple model that is also comprehensive, since it includes most common rearrangement operations, such as reversals, translocations, and transpositions.

Given two genomes with the same genes, the DCJ distance is defined as the minimum number of DCJ operations to transform one genome into the other, and it is calculated in linear time [10]. In the family-free context, given genomes S and T, a gene similarity graph $G(S, T)$ and a matching $\mathcal{M}$, the $\mathcal{M}$-induced genome sequences $S^{\mathcal{M}}$ and $T^{\mathcal{M}}$ are essentially genomes with the same set of genes, where it is possible to derive a weighted DCJ distance $d_\sigma(S^{\mathcal{M}}, T^{\mathcal{M}})$, by combining the rearrangement distance $d_{\mathrm{DCJ}}(S^{\mathcal{M}}, T^{\mathcal{M}})$ between $S^{\mathcal{M}}$ and $T^{\mathcal{M}}$ and the gene dissimilarity in the form of edge weights $edg(\mathcal{M})$.

Problem 4 (FF-DCJ [4]). Given two genomes S, T and some $\alpha \in [0, 1]$, find a matching $\mathcal{M}$ in gene similarity graph $G(S, T)$ such that the weighted DCJ distance is minimized:

$$d_\alpha(\mathcal{M}) = \alpha \cdot d_{\mathrm{DCJ}}(S^{\mathcal{M}}, T^{\mathcal{M}}) + (1 - \alpha) \cdot (|\mathcal{M}| - edg(\mathcal{M})). \quad (4)$$

4 Gene Cluster Analysis

A peculiar feature of prokaryotic and fungal genomes appears in sets of functionally associated genes in so far as they are sometimes located physically close to each other on the organisms' chromosomal sequences. Such sets are called *gene clusters*. Most prominent gene clusters are *operons*, which are gene sets that are co-transcribed. Popular methods in gene cluster detection exploit local preservation of genes through comparative gene order studies of related species. To this end, broader notions of conserved gene order are employed that ignore gene orientation and tolerate local genome rearrangements. Hereby, the concept of *common intervals* is frequently used in comparative gene cluster studies [11–13]. Given two strings over a finite alphabet, a pair of intervals are called *common intervals* if the set of characters in both intervals is identical. In [3], Doerr et al. extended this concept to family-free analysis. In doing so, a pair of intervals in genomes S and T corresponds to a subgraph in their gene connection graph $(V, E) = G(S, T)$. That is, two intervals, $[i, j]$ in genome S and $[k, l]$ in genome T, induce a subgraph $(V', E') = G(S[i, j], T[k, l])$. Now, according to their model, $[i, j]$ and $[k, l]$ are called *weak common intervals* if each vertex of their induced subgraph is incident to at least one edge:

Definition 3 (Weak Common Intervals). Given a gene connection graph $G(S, T)$ of two genomes S and T, two intervals $[i, j]$ in S and $[k, l]$ in T are *weak common intervals* if and only if in the induced subgraph $(V', E') = G(S[i, j], T[k, l])$ each vertex $v \in V'$ has degree $deg(v) \geq 1$.

Further, Doerr et al. [3] studied a variant tolerating a limited number of insertions and deletions:

Definition 4 (Approximate Weak Common Intervals). Given a gene connection graph $G(S, T)$ of two genomes S and T, and *indel threshold* $\delta \geq 0$, two intervals, $[i, j]$ in S and $[k, l]$ in T are *δ-approximate weak common intervals* if and only if in the induced subgraph $(V', E') = G(S[i, j], T[k, l])$ no more than δ vertices $v_1, \ldots, v_\delta \in V'$ have degree $deg(v_1) = \cdots = deg(v_\delta) = 0$.

Both definitions can be straightforwardly generalized to gene connection graphs over more than two genomes giving rise to sets of (approximate-) weak common intervals. Many uninformative sets are ruled out by restricting to those that are *closed*:

Definition 5 (Closed Sets of Intervals). Given a gene connection graph $(V, E) = G(S_1, \ldots, S_k)$, a set of intervals $\mathcal{I}$ is *closed* if for each interval $I \in \mathcal{I}$ there exists no left or right neighboring vertex $u \in \{i - 1, j + 1\} \subset V$ such that for each interval $J \in \mathcal{I} \setminus I$ there exists an edge $(u, v) \in E$, with $v \in J$.

A set is *maximal* if it cannot be extended by including further valid members. We conclude with the following broadly-stated discovery problem:

Problem 5. Given a set of genomes $S_1, \ldots, S_k$ and their gene connection graph $G(S_1, \ldots, S_k)$, a quorum parameter $q \leq k$, and $\delta \geq 0$, find all maximal closed sets of δ-approximate weak common intervals that have members in at least q genomes.

---

5 Family-Free Analysis with FFGC

We now provide some technical details for performing family-free analysis with the tool FFGC. Whereas traditional gene order analysis requires an additional preprocessing step for gene family clustering, the family-free workflow not only reduces the expenditure of work for the user, but also gives them more control over their experiments by reducing the number of critical parameters. Although any set of genetic markers can be used for gene order analysis, most commonly, annotated gene sequences are utilized, often even restricted to protein coding genes. Because the large majority of publicly available genomes already provide gene annotations, the acquisition of gene order sequences is usually a trivial task.

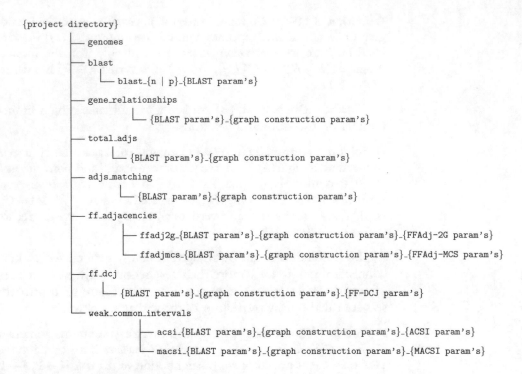

Fig. 2 Hierarchical organization of a project directory maintained by FFGC

The tool FFGC provides functionality for all steps of the family-free analysis workflow starting from annotated genome sequences. That is, supplied with two or more annotated genome sequences, the create_project command of FFGC creates an autarkic *project directory* in which all data generated in the course of analyzing the given genome sequences is stored. The thereby generated folder hierarchy is schematically represented in Fig. 2. In creating the directories, FFGC includes parameter values in folder names for all steps of the workflow, enabling the simultaneous execution, allocation, and simple maintenance of generated data from several analyses with varying parameter settings.

The create_project command of FFGC admits three alternative input variants: (1) files in *genbank* format, (2) pairs of *(multi-record) fasta* and *general feature format* (GFF) files, and (3) fasta files that are already in an anticipated formatting.

For input variant (2), each fasta file must be associated with a single organism, and each of its records must correspond to a contig or chromosome of the organism's genome. Further, their corresponding GFF files must share the same name—except for the file ending ".gff".

For input variant (3), each fasta record must correspond to an atomic unit of a gene order sequence, featuring a unique *record ID*

Table 1
Description of parameters used by tasks provided by FFGC

Task	Parameter	Description
Global settings	python2_bin	Path to python 2 binary, in case the *source* distribution is used
	threads	Limit of parallel threads in executing a single task
	cplex_memory	Memory limit (in *gigabytes*) for a single CPLEX thread
	cplex_time	Time limit for optimizer after which CPLEX returns best, but possibly suboptimal solution (in *minutes*)
BLAST	blast_params	Parameter string for blastn or blastp command, depending whether local blasthits are identified on nucleotide or protein sequence level
	blast_dir	Path to blast binaries, in case the *source* distribution is used
Gene relationships	pw_params	String of one or more of the following parameter options using in constructing and pruning the gene relationship graph
		-s < FLOAT > Local threshold parameter $f \in [0, 1]$ of stringency filter
		-n < INT > minimum number of genomes to which a gene must exhibit similarities
		-l < INT > minimum accepted size of a contig/chromosome, measured in numbers of "non-zero similarity" genes
		-i < INT > limit of number of iterations for pruning gene relationship graph
FF-Adjacencies	ff_alpha	Convex combination parameter $\alpha \in [0, 1]$ in solving problem FF-Adjacencies, used by both the exact algorithm and heuristic FFAdj-MCS
Weak common intervals	wci_delta	Approximate weak common intervals parameter, allowing for $\delta \geq 0$ indels, used for both pairwise and multi-way comparisons
	wci_min	Minimum number of genes with shared similarity in a weak common intervals pair, used for both pairwise and multi-way comparisons
	wci_quorum	Quorum of genomes in which a set of weak common intervals needs to occur; if set to zero, it must span all genomes; only used in multi-way comparisons
	wci_blocksize	Size of genomic segments that are computed in parallel; if set to zero, parallel computation is disabled; only used in multi-way comparisons

that indicates its association to a chromosome or contig as described in Table 1. Further, the order of the records in their corresponding fasta files must already correspond to the order of their anticipated gene order sequences.

For input variants (1) and (2), create_project allows annotated genomic features to be filtered by type. The selected annotations are then extracted and in further analysis considered as the atomic units of gene order sequences that are henceforth denoted by *genes*. FFGC enables the performance of family-free analysis on either the nucleotide or the protein sequence level.

After the project is created, the genome sequences, intermediary data, and outputs of the various family-free analyses are maintained by the *workflow management system* snakemake [14]. In doing so, each family-free method corresponds to a sequence of tasks, some of which are shared by more than one or even all family-free analyses. Tasks are phrased in snakemake as *rules* with specific input and output requirements. FFGC makes use of and produces files in various formats which are described in Table 2. Moreover, snakemake keeps track of file versions as well as parameter settings, only executing rules as necessary. This minimizes the time- and space-consuming computation of shared intermediary data. Both snakemake and FFGC support concurrent computing, which makes it possible to process large datasets in acceptable time when multi-processor compute cluster systems are available. The dependency tree of the snakemake workflow is shown in Fig. 3.

FFGC provides the following snakemake rules to for solving the above-described problems that can be individually executed by calling snakemake <rule> in an FFGC project directory. Rules all_total_adjs, all_adjs_matching, and all_ffadj_exact solve Problems 1, 2, and 3, for all pairs of genomes, respectively. Note that rule all_ffadj_exact relies on the proprietary optimization package CPLEX.[1] Additionally, the tool implements the heuristic method FFAdj-MCS described in [2] that has no external dependencies (rule all_ffadj_heuristic). Rule all_ffdcj_exact, which solves Problem 4, also has an dependency to CPLEX.

FFGC contains two methods for gene cluster detection. The first, ACSI, which is described in [3], solves Problem 5 for pairwise gene connection graphs (i.e. $k = 2$). The corresponding snakemake rule is all_weak_common_intervals_pw. The implemented method also computes a score for each discovered interval that can be subsequently used to identify promising gene cluster candidates. Hereby, ACSI relies on the edge weights of the genomes' gene similarity graph, combining them into a score that reflects both the intervals' sizes and the similarities between their contained genes.

The second method implemented in FFGC, called MACSI (snakemake rule all_weak_common_intervals_multi), supports gene cluster detection for multiple genomes. But rather than solving Problem 5 directly, MACSI returns a graph in which intervals are represented by vertices and two vertices are connected by an edge if their corresponding intervals are members of at least one common

---

[1] http://www.ibm.com/software/integration/optimization/cplex-optimizer/.

Table 2
Description of file types and their formatting used in FFGC

Filetype/-name	Description
Snakefile	The "*Makefile*" of snakemake containing the rules of the FFGC workflow. Format specifications can be found at http://snakemake.bitbucket.org
config.yaml	Configuration file in YAML format, containing the parameter settings of all tasks of the worfklow
< X > .*gos*	Gene order sequence file of a genome *X* in *multi-record fasta* format. Each file corresponds to a distinct genome. The ID of each record is a concatenated string of key/value pairs delimited by "|, the single most important being the chromosome| < chromosome ID > attribute. The succession of records corresponds to the genes" order in their corresponding gene order sequences
*.blasttbl	BLAST hits in tabular, default tab-delimited output format
genome_ map. cfg	File in Python's *ConfigParser* format containing additional information about the genomes in the dataset. Each *section* is associated with a distinct genome, and contains the following attributes: *name, fasta_file, active_genes*. The latter indicates the genes whose associated vertices are part of the gene similarity graph used in family-free gene order analyses
< X > _ < Y > . *sim*	Pairwise gene similarity file, describing a gene similarity graph between two genomes *X* and *Y*. The file adheres to a tab-separated tabular format, where each row corresponds to an edge in the gene similarity graph and the columns contain the following information: *chromosome ID in X, gene ID in X, chromosome ID in Y, gene ID in Y, relative orientation, gene similarity*. Hereby the *gene ID* corresponds to the gene's rank in the list of active genes of its gene order sequence
< X > _ < Y > . *adj*	File in tab-delimited tabular format describing pairwise conserved adjacencies between two genomes *X* and *Y*, where each row corresponds to one conserved adjacency pair and columns denote the following: *chromosome ID in X, gene ID 1 in X, gene ID 2 in X, chromosome ID in Y, gene ID 1 in Y, gene ID 2 in Y, relative orientation of adjacency*
< X > _ < Y > . *wci*	File in tab-delimited tabular format where each row corresponds to a closed pair of approximate weak common intervals between two genomes *X* and *Y*. The columns hold the following information: *chromosome ID in X, first gene ID in X, last gene ID in X, chromosome ID in Y, first gene ID in Y, last gene ID in Y, interval score as described in [3], number of indels, number of genes with shared similarity*
*.mwci	File in tab-delimited tabular format describing the interval graph output to program MACSI, where each row corresponds to one edge in the graph, and columns are as follows: *genome X, chromosome ID in X, first gene ID in X, last gene ID in X, genome Y, chromosome ID in Y, first gene ID in Y, last gene ID in Y*

maximal closed set of δ-approximate weak common intervals with members in at least q genomes. In doing so, the direct, but storage-consuming, solution of Problem 5 is traded for a compact format, at the expense of losing set membership information of δ-approximate weak common intervals.

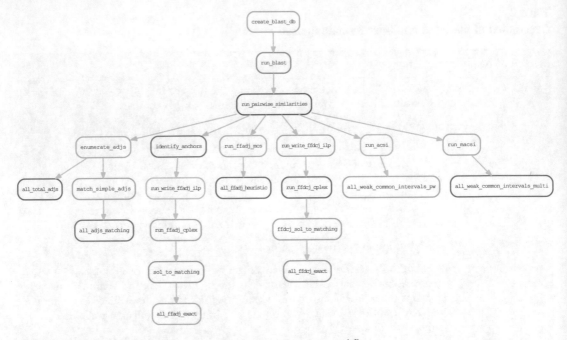

Fig. 3 Dependency hierarchy of `FFGC` rules in `snakemake` workflow

References

1. Braga MDV, Chauve C, Doerr D, Jahn K, Stoye J, Thévenin A, Wittler R (2013) The potential of family-free genome comparison. In: Models and algorithms for genome evolution. Computational biology, vol 19, Chapter 13. Springer, London, pp 287–323

2. Doerr D, Thévenin A, Stoye J (2012) Gene family assignment-free comparative genomics. BMC Bioinf 13(Suppl 19):S3

3. Doerr D, Stoye J, Böcker S, Jahn K (2014) Identifying gene clusters by discovering common intervals in indeterminate strings. BMC Genomics 15(Suppl 6):S2

4. Martinez FV, Feijão P, Braga MD, Stoye J (2015) On the family-free DCJ distance and similarity. Algorithms Mol Biol 10(1):1–10

5. Kowada LAB, Doerr D, Dantas S, Stoye J (2016) New genome similarity measures based on conserved gene adjacencies. In: Proceedings of RECOMB 2016. Lecture notes in bioinformatics, vol 9649. Springer, Berlin, pp 204–224

6. Camacho C, Coulouris G, Avagyan V, Ma N, Papadopoulos J, Bealer K, Madden TL (2008) BLAST+: architecture and applications. BMC Bioinf 10:421–421

7. Lechner M, Findeiß S, Steiner L, Marz M, Stadler PF, Prohaska SJ (2011) Proteinortho: detection of (co-)orthologs in large-scale analysis. BMC Bioinf 12:124

8. Pesquita C, Faria D, Bastos H, Ferreira AEN, Falcão AO, Couto FM (2008) Metrics for GO based protein semantic similarity: a systematic evaluation. BMC Bioinf 9(Suppl 5):S4

9. Yancopoulos S, Attie O, Friedberg R (2005) Efficient sorting of genomic permutations by translocation, inversion and block interchange. Bioinformatics 21(16):3340–3346

10. Bergeron A, Mixtacki J, Stoye J (2006) A unifying view of genome rearrangements. In: Lecture notes in computer science, vol 4175. Springer, Berlin/Heidelberg, pp 163–173

11. Schmidt T, Stoye J (2004) Quadratic time algorithms for finding common intervals in two and more sequences. In: Proceedings of CPM 2004. Lecture notes in computer science, vol 3109. Springer, Berlin/Heidelberg, pp 347–358

12. Rahmann S, Klau GW (2006) Integer linear programs for discovering approximate gene clusters. In: Proceedings of WABI 2006. Lecture notes in bioinformatics, vol 4175. Springer, Berlin/Heidelberg, pp 298–309

13. Jahn K (2011) Efficient computation of approximate gene clusters based on reference occurrences. J Comput Biol 18(9):1255–1274

14. Köster J, Rahmann S (2012) Snakemake-a scalable bioinformatics workflow engine. Bioinformatics 28(19):2520–2522

Chapter 13

Comparative Methods for Reconstructing Ancient Genome Organization

Yoann Anselmetti, Nina Luhmann, Sèverine Bérard, Eric Tannier, and Cedric Chauve

Abstract

Comparative genomics considers the detection of similarities and differences between extant genomes, and, based on more or less formalized hypotheses regarding the involved evolutionary processes, inferring ancestral states explaining the similarities and an evolutionary history explaining the differences. In this chapter, we focus on the reconstruction of the organization of ancient genomes into chromosomes. We review different methodological approaches and software, applied to a wide range of datasets from different kingdoms of life and at different evolutionary depths. We discuss relations with genome assembly, and potential approaches to validate computational predictions on ancient genomes that are almost always only accessible through these predictions.

Key words Comparative genomics, Paleogenomics, Ancient genomes, Ancestral genomes

1 Introduction

Rearrangements were the first discovered genome mutations [1], long before the discovery of the molecular structure of DNA. Molecular evolutionary studies started with the reconstruction of the organization of ancient *Drosophila* chromosomes, from the comparison of extant ones [2]. However, it took almost 30 more years before the formal introduction of *paleogenetics*, as the field of reconstructing ancient genes [3]. Since then, the development of sequencing technologies and the availability of sequenced genomes has led to the introduction of *paleogenomics*, a field that aims at reconstructing ancient whole genomes using computational methods. The term paleogenomics can be understood in two ways: ancient genome sequencing [4], or the computational reconstruction of ancestral genome features, given extant sequences, offspring, and relatives [5]. We take it in the latter meaning, though we highlight several links between both interpretations.

João C. Setubal et al. (eds.), *Comparative Genomics: Methods and Protocols*, Methods in Molecular Biology, vol. 1704, https://doi.org/10.1007/978-1-4939-7463-4_13, © Springer Science+Business Media LLC 2018

Despite its early start as a molecular evolution problem, paleogenomics is still in its infancy. Whereas evolution by substitutions has been studied extensively from the 1960s, and has now well established mathematical and computational foundations, evolution by genome scale events such as rearrangements looks almost like a fallow field. Two reasons can be invoked. First, rearrangement studies require having fully assembled genomes, and genome assembly is still an extremely challenging problem, resulting in a small number of available genomes, compared to gene sequences for example. Second, the state space of sequence evolution is very small (4 possible nucleotides or 20 possible amino acids per ancestral locus), leading to computational problems that are much easier than the rearrangement ones, which work on the basically infinite discrete space of possible chromosomal organizations (gene orders for example). However, none of these reasons is biological, and recent progresses in technology and methodology are susceptible to quickly change this situation.

There have been tremendous methodological developments over the last 10–15 years. Standard and principled computational methods are now able to propose reconstructions of the organization of ancestral genomes over all kingdoms of life: mammals [6, 7], insects [8, 9], fungi [10], plants such as monocotyledons [11–13] (reviewed in [14]) and dicotyledons [13–16], bacteria [17–19]. Prospective ad hoc methods have attempted the reconstruction of more ancient animal proto karyotypes: amniotes [20–22], bony fishes [23–25], vertebrates [20, 21, 26], chordates [27], or even eumetazoa [28].

Here, we review some of the existing methods for reconstructing ancient gene orders, focusing on their methodological principles, strengths, and weaknesses. We detail the data preprocessing steps that are necessary to use these methods. We finally review the available software and give an insight on the possible validations of ancestral genomes.

2 Preliminaries: Material and Preprocessing

The starting material of comparative paleogenomics is composed of extant genome sequences and assemblies. These are often available in public databases such as Ensembl and the UCSC Genome Browser [29, 30]. A genome assembly is a set of linear or circular DNA sequences (we refer the reader to [31] for a recent review on genome assembly). Depending on the combination of the properties of the sequenced genomes (repeats in particular), the sequencing technology, and the assembly algorithm, the assembled sequences can be at various levels of completion, from full chromosomes (in which case the genome is said to be fully assembled) to scaffolds or contigs (fragmented assembly); for the sake of exposition, we use here the term chromosome for an assembled contiguous DNA sequence. The fragmentation of extant genome assemblies has a significant impact on the quality of reconstructed ancestral genomes, which will be discussed in Subheading 3.4.

To reconstruct the organization of ancient genomes from the comparison of extant ones, it is first necessary to define sets of *markers* on extant genomes, that is, DNA segments defined by their coordinates on the genomes (chromosome or scaffold or contig, start position, end position, reading direction). Markers are clustered into families with the desired property that two markers in the same family are homologous over their whole length, and two markers from a different family show no or limited homology.

Gene families, available in some databases [29, 32], are good candidates for being markers, though intersecting genes and partial homologies can be a problem for certain methods. Markers can also be obtained by constructing synteny blocks from whole genome multiple alignments [33], Chapter 11, or by segmenting genomes according to pairwise alignments [34], or searching *ultra-conserved elements (UCEs)* [35] or virtual probes [36]. These methods are useful for example when considering genomes that exhibit low gene density.

Whether the considered markers are genes or other genomic markers, the identification of genomic marker families is both a fundamental initial step toward reconstructing ancestral genomes and a challenging computational biology problem, with links to sequence clustering, whole genome alignment, and phylogenetics, among others. There is currently no standard method or tool that is universally used and many applied works rely on ad hoc methods for this important preprocessing step.

Depending on combinatorial properties of the algorithms used to infer ancient genome organization from the comparison of extant genomes, several restrictions might need to be applied on families of genomic markers. Most methods require that no two markers overlap on a genome, as this might induce some ambiguity regarding their relative order along their chromosome. Other methods might also require that every genome contains at most one marker per family (*unique markers*) or at least one marker per family (*universal markers*), or both (unique and universal markers). Enforcing such constraints requires extra preprocessing of an initial marker set. Nevertheless, we consider now that we have obtained, for a set of extant genomes of interest, a dataset of genomic markers, that will serve as input to reconstruct the organization of one or several ancient genomes.

Eventually, a comparative approach requires phylogenetic information relating one or several ancestral species of interest to a set of extant species whose genome data are available. This information can range from a fully resolved *species phylogeny* with branch lengths [6, 7], to a partition of the extant species in three non-empty groups that define a single ancestral species (two groups of descendant species and one group of outgroup species). So in the extreme case of considering a single ancestral species, a minimal dataset is composed of genome information for a set of three extant species, composed of two species whose last common ancestor is the ancestral species of interest and one outgroup [37].

3   Ancestral Reconstruction Methods

All methods consider a genome as a set of circular or linear orderings of markers, representing chromosomes or chromosomal segments. This implies that the exact markers' physical coordinates are transformed into a relative ordering of markers. It induces a loss of information which can have an influence on the result [38] but it is universally used. Then methods differ in their strategies: either they model the evolution of these arrangements of markers by evolutionary events such as duplications, losses, rearrangements, or they model the evolution of more local syntenic features/characters such as the physical proximity of sets of markers. In the following, we call *adjacency* (resp. *interval*) a pair of (resp. a set of at least three) markers that either occur contiguously along an extant genome or are assumed to occur contiguously along an ancestral genome.

The first strategy (evolution of whole genomes) quickly leads to computational tractability issues. The second strategy (evolution of local syntenic characters such as adjacencies and intervals) benefits from a standard evolutionary toolbox modeling the evolution of presence or absence of a character, and tractability issues are postponed to a final linearization step where local characters are assembled into chromosome scale arrangements of markers. Linearization procedures then benefit from standard algorithms originating from algorithms for computing physical maps of extant genomes [39].

3.1   Whole Genome Evolution

We first describe the approach that considers the evolution of genomes seen as sets of linear or circular orders of markers, i.e., roughly permutations that can possibly be separated into several chromosomes. Evolutionary events like inversions, translocations, transpositions, fissions, and fusions, all subsumed in the now standard Double Cut and Join (DCJ) model [40], are susceptible to alter these genomes. The reconstruction of ancestral genomes then aims, given marker orders representing extant genomes at the leaves of a species phylogeny, at assigning marker orders for all ancestral nodes, maximizing a mathematical criterion according to the chosen evolutionary model. Most of the time this criterion is the parsimony score, which is the minimum number of events transforming a permutation into another [41], also called the distance, although some methods consider a likelihood criterion.

For most rearrangement models that do not include duplications, the distance between two genomes can be computed efficiently. But even the simplest non-pairwise ancestral genome reconstruction problem, the median problem reconstructing a genome minimizing the distance in a tree with only three leaves, is already NP hard [42]. Adding duplications makes all problems hard even for the comparison of two genomes [41]. Hence, with duplications considered, reconstructing rearrangement events that happened along the branches of a tree is not tractable either.

Heuristics for the ancestral genome reconstruction problem usually follow the strategy of assigning an initial genome arrangement to each internal node of the tree and then iteratively refining the solution by solving the median problem for internal nodes until no further improvement in the overall tree distance can be achieved. The implementation of GASTS [43] improves over previous methods applying this strategy by trying to find a good initial arrangement avoiding local optima. Using adequate subgraphs for heuristic assignment of the median, this method can handle multi chromosomal data with unique and universal markers. Another approach is based on the Pathgroup data structure [44] storing partially completed cycles in a breakpoint graph [41] for each branch in the phylogeny. Graphs are greedily completed and eventually form genomes at all internal nodes. This solution can be used as an initialization prior to local iterative improvements based on the median again using the Pathgroup approach. An interesting property of Pathgroup is that it can handle whole genome duplications. The method MGRA [45] on the other hand relies on a multiple breakpoint graph combining all extant genome organizations into one structure. MGRA then searches for breaks in agreement with the species tree structure transforming the breakpoint graph into an identity breakpoint graph. While MGRA requires unique and universal markers, it has recently been extended to handle unequal marker content [46]. More complex models of evolution have been considered, which include duplications for example [47, 48], but are tractable only under some specific condition, such as the hypothesis that rearrangement breakpoints are not re-used [47].

Some methods adopt a probabilistic point of view, like Badger [49], a software using Bayesian analysis under a model where circular genomes can evolve by reversals. It samples phylogenetic trees and rearrangement scenarios from the joint posterior distribution under this model by MCMC implementing different proposal methods in the Metropolis–Hastings algorithm. It is a similar local search to the heuristic on the minimization problem, but instead of giving a single solution without guarantee as an output, it provides a sample of solutions from a mathematically grounded distribution. However, it faces the same tractability issues concerning the convergence time.

Finally, a simpler rearrangement distance is the Single-Cut-or-Join (SCJ) distance [50] that models cuts and joins of adjacencies. With this model the ancestral reconstruction becomes tractable. Ancestral genomes that minimize the SCJ distance can be computed efficiently using a variant of the Fitch algorithm [51] in polynomial time; however, constraints required to ensure linear or circular ancestral marker orders result in mostly fragmented ancestral genomes. In [52], a Gibbs sampler for sampling rearrangement scenarios under the SCJ model has been described. It starts with an optimal fragmented scenario obtained as described above and then explores the space of co-optima by repeatedly changing the scenarios of single adjacencies.

3.2 Genomes as Sets of Adjacencies and Intervals: Mapping Approaches

The linear or circular orders of markers can be seen as sets of adjacencies and intervals, instead of permutations. Then each adjacency or interval can be considered independently, as a separate syntenic feature, which evolves within the larger context of whole genomes. This independence assumption allows computing quickly ancestral states for adjacencies and intervals. The main problem is that the collection of ancestral adjacencies and intervals is not guaranteed to be compatible with a linear or circular ordering.

We describe here a family of approaches that focus on a single-ancestral genome and consist of two main steps, which are inspired by the methods initially developed to compute physical maps of extant genomes:

1. Genomes of related extant species are compared to detect common local syntenic features, such as marker adjacencies or intervals, that are then considered candidate ancestral features for the ancestral genome of interest. Common features are not necessarily conserved from an ancestor due to convergent evolution or assembly errors for example, so this method generates false positives. In some methods, each local syntenic feature is weighted, according to its pattern of presence/absence in extant species genomes, to represent a confidence measure in the hypothesis it is indeed an ancestral syntenic feature.

2. A maximum weight subset of the potentially ancestral local syntenic features (detected in the first step) is selected that is compatible with the genome structure of the considered ancestral species (linear/circular chromosomes, ancestral copy number of markers, etc.) and is then assembled into a more detailed ancestral genome map.

The case of unique markers. The initial applications [6, 7] of these physical mapping principles to ancestral genome organization reconstruction considered unique markers, i.e., markers that are assumed to occur once and exactly once in the ancestral genome of interest.

In several methods [7, 10, 22, 53] step 1, the detection of common adjacencies and intervals and the inference of ancestral adjacencies and intervals, is implemented using a Dollo parsimony principle: any group of markers that are colocalized in two genomes of extant species whose evolutionary path in the species phylogeny contains the ancestral species of interest is deemed to be a potential ancestral syntenic feature. Here by *colocalized* we mean that the group of markers occur contiguously in both extant genomes regardless of their relative orders but without any other marker occurring in between; so the marker content of both occurrences of the colocalized group of markers in the extant genomes is identical while the marker orders can differ. Groups of two markers are adjacencies, while groups of more than two markers are intervals. Variations on the principle outlined above can be considered, such as relaxing the Dollo parsimony criterion or considering only adjacencies (*see* [6] for example) or considering probabilistic inference of ancestral adjacencies [54, 55].

Given a set of local ancestral syntenic groups, the second step aims at selecting a maximum weight subset of these groups that is compatible with the considered genome structure and does not contain any syntenic conflict, defined as a marker that is deemed adjacent to more than two other markers. Several methods such as Infercars [6] and MLGO [54] consider only marker adjacencies; these adjacencies define a graph whose vertices are markers and weighted edges represent adjacencies, and aim at computing a maximal set of weighted adjacencies that form a set of paths, each such path being then a linear order of markers called a *Contiguous Ancestral Region* (CAR). This problem is equivalent to a Traveling Salesman Problem (TSP) and is NP hard. It is addressed in [6] through a greedy heuristic and in [54] using a standard TSP solver. However, as shown in [56], if the linearity of CARs is relaxed and circular CARs are allowed, the optimization problem of selecting a maximum weight subset of adjacencies that forms a mix of linear and circular CARs is tractable and can be solved by reduction to a Maximum Weight Matching (MWM) problem.

When intervals are considered in addition to adjacencies, ancestral adjacencies and intervals can be encoded by a binary matrix, in the same way as hybridization experiments are encoded by binary matrices in physical mapping algorithms. The problem of extracting a conflict free maximum weight subset of adjacencies is then NP hard in all cases, i.e., even if a mix of circular and linear CARs is allowed. Traditionally, it is solved using either greedy heuristics or branch and bound algorithms (ensuring an optimal solution when they terminate). Moreover, when intervals are considered, CARs might not be completely defined and are represented using a PQ tree data structure that has been widely used in physical mapping algorithms [39] and is related to the classical combinatorial concept of Consecutive Ones Property (C1P) (*see* [7] and references there). The software ANGES [53] and ROCOCO [57] are, so far, the only ancestral genome reconstruction methods that consider intervals of markers and encode CARs using PQ trees.

Last, when markers are assumed to be unique in the ancestral genome of interest but are subject to insertion or loss during evolution, the model of common adjacencies and intervals might be too stringent. In this case, the notions of *gapped adjacencies and intervals* were introduced that allows for some flexibility in the definition of conserved group of markers. However, this implies also that the C1P model is too stringent and needs to be relaxed into a *gapped C1P* model, in which optimization problems are NP hard [58, 59].

These approaches have been used on various datasets, including mammalian genomes [6, 7, 60], the amniote ancestor [22], fungi genomes [10], insect genomes [8], plant genomes [12, 16].

Non-unique markers. If markers exhibit varying copy numbers in extant genomes, they cannot be assumed to all occur once and only once in the considered ancestral genome. The first issue is then, for a given marker, to infer its ancestral copy numbers. This is a classical evolutionary genomics problem, for example to infer the gene content of an extinct genome. Given a model of gains and losses of markers, it is possible to compute a more likely ancestral content [61, 62], or content that minimizes the number of gains and losses [63], by a Dynamic Programming (DP) algorithm following the general pattern of the Sankoff-Rousseau algorithm [64].

Once copy numbers of ancestral markers, or bounds on such copy numbers, have been obtained, the two-steps approach outlined in the previous paragraphs can be applied: first, local syntenies (adjacencies and intervals) are detected using similar notions of adjacencies and intervals (we refer the reader to [65] for an overview of interval models when duplicated markers can occur) and are weighted according to their conservation pattern, and, in a second step, a maximum weight subset of local syntenies is computed that is compatible with the marker copy numbers. This second problem is known as the C1P with multiplicity (*mC1P*) and has been shown to be NP hard in general; the only tractable case requires considering only adjacencies and allowing an unbounded number of circular CARs [56, 66]. Moreover, when markers have a copy number higher than one and only adjacencies are considered, a conflict free set of adjacencies does not define unambiguously a set of CARs; this issue is similar to the well-identified problem of determining the location and context of repeats in genome assembly [67]. This issue can be addressed, at least partially, by considering intervals framed by non-repeats (*repeat spanning intervals*) as described in [68, 69]. Finally, when variation of copy numbers can be attributed to Whole-Genome Duplications (WGD), specific methods based on a combination of gapped adjacencies and TSP algorithms have been proposed and applied to fungi and plant data [70].

3.3 Adjacency Evolution along Gene Phylogenies

We now discuss a variant of the approach described in the previous section, which still considers genomes as sets of adjacencies between markers, but assumes that evolutionary scenarios for marker families are also available and focuses on all ancestral genomes of the species phylogeny at once. Due to its similarity with traditional character-based phylogenetics, we rely on the standard phylogenetic vocabulary and call genomic markers *genes*. To summarize this approach, ancestral adjacencies are inferred, as previously, but using an optimization criterion and the available gene phylogenies both as a guide and a constraint.

Input: gene trees and adjacencies. This phylogeny-based approach requires as main input a fully binary rooted species phylogeny, and *reconciled phylogenies* for all gene families. This means that for all gene families, a rooted and annotated phylogenetic tree is required, depicting the whole history of the marker in ancestral and extant species in terms of speciations (S), duplications (D), transfers (T), or losses (L), where a transfer is the event of a species acquiring a genomic segment from another species (horizontal/lateral transfer). These reconciled gene trees can be obtained by several methods and software, depending on the set of evolutionary events one wants to consider (DTL or DL only), on the models and methods (parsimony or probabilistic approaches, joint or sequential reconstruction of the tree topology and reconciliation) [71–73]. Some databases also provide gene trees or reconciled gene trees [29, 32]. A reconciliation yields a presence pattern of ancestral genes in ancestral species. The leaves of these trees are the extant genes, and its internal nodes and events define ancestral genes.

The other information needed by the methods is the list of the gene adjacencies in the extant genomes. As defined above, we usually consider that two genes are adjacent if there is no other gene in that dataset between them, although here again relaxed notions of adjacencies can be considered.

Adjacency evolution: As genes and species, gene adjacencies also evolve. They can be gained, lost, duplicated, and transferred for example. The core element of the phylogeny-based methods we describe in this section is to infer the evolution of these adjacencies along the gene phylogenies, which themselves evolve within the species phylogeny. This leads to the inference of adjacencies between ancestral genes, i.e., ancestral adjacencies, and thus provides elements of the organization of genes in ancestral species. The currently available methods compute an evolutionary history of the adjacencies by either minimizing a discrete parsimony criterion or

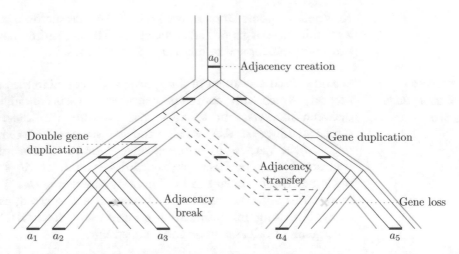

Fig. 1 Propagation of adjacencies (*red*) along gene phylogenies (*black* and *blue*) reconciled with a species phylogeny (*green*). This figure represents the evolutionary history of five extant adjacencies a_1 to a_5 sharing a common ancestor a_0 in agreement with the history of the genes present at their extremities. The double gene duplication on the *left side* induces an adjacency duplication, whereas the single-gene duplication on the *right side* does not. Events such as gene losses or rearrangements make adjacencies lost or broken

maximizing a likelihood within a probabilistic framework. The main difficulty in such methods is to infer adjacencies evolution scenarios that are consistent with the evolutionary history of the considered genes, encoded in their respective reconciled gene trees (*see* Fig. 1). The result of this approach, which considers each adjacency independently of all other adjacencies (like in the methods described in Subheading 3.2 but unlike those in Subheading 3.1), is a set of ancestral adjacencies for each ancestral species. As it is not guaranteed that these adjacencies are compatible with a linear structure, linearization methods such as [56] or global evolution methods such as [74] can be applied to infer valid ancestral gene arrangements, for each individual ancestor. This approach was followed in DupCAR [75], which imposes some constraints on the gene trees, and in the family of DeCo algorithms that we describe below.

DeCo algorithm family: The inference of adjacency histories is computed by Dynamic Programming techniques, implementing the rules of transmission of an adjacency from an ancestor to a descendant. As in the previous methods, at any point, a rearrangement can break or form an adjacency. But in addition, when a gene undergoes an event (Birth, Duplication, Loss, Transfer), an adjacency that has this gene as extremity necessarily changes: it can be gained, lost, duplicated, or transferred according to the evolutionary pattern of its extremities. The algorithm proceeds in three steps. A first step is to group adjacencies that may share a common ancestor in classes. Then, each class is examined independently using a DP algorithm that generalizes the Sankoff–Fitch parsimony algorithms on binary alphabets; here the binary character is the presence or absence of an adjacency that evolves along pairs of reconciled gene phylogenies. Last, a backtrack step infers an unambiguous parsimonious evolutionary scenario for each adjacency.

This principle has been first implemented in parsimony when gene trees are reconciled in a duplication/loss model [76]. Following this initial model, several extensions have been proposed, which we outline briefly now. DeCoLT is an extension of DeCo that allows modeling the lateral transfers of genes between species, a frequent evolutionary event in bacterial evolution [18]. Two probabilistic extensions were recently introduced: in [9], the optimization criterion is a maximum likelihood criterion, while DeClone [77] implements a probabilistic approach to parsimony by allowing sampling evolutionary scenarios according to a Boltzmann-Gibbs probability distribution. Last, Art DeCo [78] has been introduced to handle fragmented extant genome assemblies (*see* the next section). DeCo and its variants all run in polynomial time allowing using them on large-scale datasets such as 69 eukaryotic genomes [76, 79].

3.4 Handling Fragmented Extant Genomes

Ideally, to reconstruct an accurate and complete organization of one (or several) ancestral genome(s) with a comparative approach, one would like to rely on the complete chromosomal organization of the considered related extant genomes. However, currently, most genome assemblies are incomplete and can even be highly fragmented[1]. This fact is due to the prevalence of sequencing technologies producing short and accurate reads that do not allow assembling repeated regions [67]. Recent improvements in sequencing technologies (for example long read sequencing protocols), as well as advances in processing methods (for example hybrid assemblies [80, 81] and gap closing methods [82–84]), make it possible to obtain the complete genome organization of microbial genomes [85]; however, the problem of genome assembly is still hard for large eukaryotic genomes [86].

Fragmented extant genome assemblies are characterized by the fact that chromosomes are split into several contigs or scaffolds, whose relative order and orientation is not known. This missing information on order and orientation of these scaffolds might hide conserved syntenies such as marker adjacencies, which leads to similarly fragmented ancestral genome organization. One can see the problem of reconstructing the organization of ancestral genomes as similar to genome mapping or scaffolding problems, in which case ancestral genome reconstruction and extant genome assembly can be considered a unique problem that consists in ordering genomic markers whether ancient or extant. The

---

[1] see the GOLD database for example https://gold.jgi.doe.gov/statistics.

algorithmic similarity between these two problems has been remarked [87] by noting a similarity between the breakpoint graph [41], used for the reconstruction of gene order in ancestral genomes, and the de Bruijn graph [88], used in genome assembly. This observation has led to the recent development of approaches aiming at improving extant genome assembly in an evolutionary framework that reconstructs jointly ancient genome organization.

This similarity was first exploited by Munoz et al. [89], to give an order and an orientation to scaffolds by contig fusion with the construction of the breakpoint graph of a reference genome and a target genome to assemble. The concept was taken further by Aganezov et al. [90]. They considered several related extant genomes (possibly at various levels of fragmentation) and applied simultaneous co-scaffolding of all extant genomes, under the hypothesis that fragmentation breakpoints are not the same (i.e., between the same markers) in all species and conserved syntenies can thus be detected, although with a weaker conservation signal. The core of their method is an extension of the classical breakpoint graph to more than two genomes [45, 46] and follows the parsimony principle on permutations (*see* Subheading 3.1). In consequence the method is limited to a small number of species (less than 10) and does not handle duplications.

Another alternative is an extension of the DeCo algorithm (*see* Subheading 3.3), called Art DeCo [77]. The method scaffolds several fragmented-related genomes by reconstructing gene adjacencies evolution. The method is based on a parsimony principle that considers gains and breaks of adjacencies, but also the cost of creating scaffolding adjacencies in extant genomes but is applied independently to each adjacency, thus avoiding the computational tractability issue of a parsimony approach on permutations. Art DeCo can handle a large number of species (several dozens) as well as gene duplications. The linearization issue however propagates to extant genomes: neither extant nor ancestral genomes are guaranteed to be compatible with a linear or circular structure, and linearization algorithms are needed as a post process.

3.5   Using Ancient DNA

In addition to extant genomes, ancient DNA (aDNA) extracted from archaeological or paleontological remains can provide direct evidence about the contents and structure of an ancient genome. Early works using aDNA concentrated on mitochondrial DNA not older than a few 1000 years, recovered for example from quagga [91], extinct moa [92], cave bears [93], or Neanderthal [94]. Later, advances in sequencing technologies and in aDNA recovery protocols [95] opened the way to the sequencing of nuclear aDNA in even older samples of bacteria like *Yersinia pestis* [96, 97] or mammals like the extinct woolly mammoth [98] or ancient horses [99].

However due to postmortem DNA decay and degradation by nucleases, only short fragments of aDNA can be recovered. Subsequently, the retrieved sequences are usually aligned to references and variants are identified keeping aDNA damage patterns in mind, precluding the analysis of more complex rearrangements between the ancient and extant genomes [100]. While a contig assembly based on such data can be expected to be quite fragmented, classical scaffolding approaches can often not be applied to aDNA data, due to the nature of the aDNA capture process for example. Hence, comparative phylogenetic methods following principles similar to the ancestral reconstruction methods described above have to be used to order and orient the obtained contigs. Combining aDNA sequencing data with comparative methods is therefore useful in two ways: scaffolding of a fragmented aDNA assembly while improving the reconstruction of other, probably older ancient genomes in the phylogeny. We outline this approach below.

Given sets of contigs from aDNA assemblies assigned to internal nodes of the species phylogeny, one first needs to define a common set of markers between the ancient contigs and extant genome sequences. Each family of markers should then consist of at least one ancient contig fragment and its occurrences in several extant genomes. An iterative segmentation approach based on mappings of ancient contigs to extant genomes is described in FPSAC [69] although other fragmentation or synteny blocks construction algorithms can also be applied [34, 101].

Once marker families have been obtained using aDNA and extant DNA data, the methods outlined in the previous sections can be applied directly. For example, the FPSAC method [69] computes copy numbers for markers using discrete parsimony, infers potential ancestral adjacencies using the Dollo parsimony principle, linearizes these adjacencies using the MWM algorithm introduced in [56], and clears ambiguities due to repeated markers using the algorithms of [68]. Moreover, as the set of markers is likely not covering the whole ancient genome, gaps between adjacent markers in scaffolds need to be filled. In FPSAC, the corresponding extant gaps are identified and their sequences are aligned. Then, for each column of the alignment, the parsimonious ancestral state is reconstructed with the Fitch algorithm [51]. This approach has been successfully applied to a set of aDNA contigs from the human pathogen *Yersinia pestis*, which was obtained from remains of victims of the Black Death pandemic in the fourteenth century [102].

3.6 Software	We review in Table 1 below the main existing software implementing the principles described in the previous sections.
3.7 Validation	Validation is a constant concern in evolutionary studies. Different hypotheses, different methods, and different types of data may lead to different results [103], and their quality is difficult to quantify.

Table 1
Main methods publicly available for ancient genome reconstruction

Name	Adjacencies Intervals Permutations	Parsimony (Pa) Probabilistic (Pr)	Insertions and losses	Duplications	Transfers	Exploration of alternative solutions and/or support of solutions
ANGES	A/I	Pa	Y	N	N	Y
FPSAC	A/I	Pa	Y	Y	N	N
DeCo*	A	Pa/Pr	Y	Y	Y	Y
DupCAR	A	Pa	Y	Y	N	N
ROCOCO	A/I	Pa	N	N	N	N
MGRA2	P	Pa	Y	N	N	N
MGLO	A	Pr	Y	Y	N	N
Badger	P	Pr	N	N	N	Y
GASTS	P	Pa	N	N	N	Y
Pathgroup	P	Pa	N	N	N	N
Infercars	A	Pa	N	N	N	Y

Col. 1 records the name of the method. Col. 2 indicates which type of method it implements, either genomes as permutations (Subheading 3.1), or genomes as sets of adjacencies and intervals (Subheadings 3.2 and 3.3). Col. 3 records if it uses a parsimony assumption or a probabilistic approach. Col. 4 indicates if the method allows unequal marker content in extant and ancestral species. Col. 5 indicates if the underlying evolution model considers gene duplication. Col. 6 indicates if the underlying evolution model considers gene transfers. Col. 7 indicate if alternative solutions can be provided (through sampling for example) or if there is a measure of support for features of the provided solution. References of the listed methods: ANGES [53], FPSAC [69], DeCo and variants [9, 18, 76–78], DupCAR [75], ROCOCO [57], MGRA2 [45, 46], MGLO [54], Badger [49], GASTS [43], Pathgroup [44], infercars [6]

Predictions concern events that can be up to 4 billion years old, and no DNA molecule is preserved, even in exceptional conditions, more than 1 million years. And even for the rare cases when ancient DNA is available, it is often not for ancestral genomes, and assembly issues make it hard to use it for validation purposes (*see* Subheading 3.5).

Theoretical considerations about the models and methods can help to assess the validity of the results. Agreement with widely accepted biological hypotheses, statistical consistency, computational complexity, clarity, and validity of the underlying hypotheses have to be discussed [104]. For example, a majority of the methods presented in this chapter are based on parsimony, which assumes that the possibility of convergence or reversion is negligible, while all statistical studies tended to show that it was not the case [105]. Models have to find a good balance between realism, consistency, and complexity. An important feature of a methodology is whether it is able to provide several alternative equivalent solutions

[43] (most of the time an optimal or a likely solution is not unique), or better, a sampling of possible solutions according to a likelihood [49]. At least, if this is not possible, statistical supports of local features such as ancestral adjacencies can provide a robustness [77] (*see* Col. 7 in Table 1).

Though it is not possible to travel in time, nor to replay the tape of evolution [106], it is possible to experimentally generate some lineages and test reconstruction methods on them [107, 108]. It has been realized for ancestral sequence reconstruction purposes, but it is very expensive, time consuming, and usually generates easy instances where all methods perform equally well. It has never been done for chromosome organization, although some experiments could theoretically be used as benchmarks [109].

Another validation technique is to compare the results with similar ones produced by independent data and techniques. For example, molecular evolutionary studies can compare their results with fossil data [110, 111]. Bioinformatics ancestral genome reconstructions have, for example, been compared with reconstructions from cytogenetics data [103]. But as for ancient sequences, each kind of protocol has caveats, and none can be considered as the truth.

The main validation tool remains simulation. Genome evolution can be simulated in silico for a much higher number of generations than in experimental evolution, at a lower cost. There are at least two issues that need to be considered for the simulation, where no general consensus exists: the set of operations applied, and the parameters (e.g., relative frequencies) of the different operations, if more than one type is used. Moreover, they are often designed by the team developing the inference method, and even if they are designed to be used by another team for inference [112, 113], they originate from a community interested in proving the validity of inference methods and are based on similar models that underly the reconstruction methods. Situations where the teams developing the inference methods and testing them arc separated from the start are very rare [114] and, in their current state, existing testing schemes are not complex enough to be used for ancestral genome organization reconstruction yet. Nevertheless, this is likely an important aspect of ancient genome reconstruction methods that needs to be developed.

4   Conclusion—a Short User Guide

There has been an important effort, mostly over the last 10 years, in the development of computational methods for the reconstruction of ancestral genome organizations. Choosing a method among the many that are available requires considering several variables, such as the nature of available data, evolutionary properties of the considered lineages, computational infrastructures.

If a dataset is large (more than ~10 species), or if it contains many duplications that are deemed important to consider, it is better to look at methods that consider genomes as sets of adjacencies or intervals rather than permutations. The latter is appropriate for a small number of small genomes, provided duplicate markers can be ignored and a reasonable amount of computing power is available. In that case probabilistic methods as Badger should be preferred, because it proposes a sample of solutions based on grounded statistical principles, instead of a unique solution of a heuristic, but it is the most computationally intensive.

In all other cases, in our opinion, a local approach with adjacencies and intervals should be favored. If duplicates can be ignored (unique markers), ANGES is the most flexible tool, which allows retrieving most information (common intervals in addition to adjacencies). Otherwise, assuming duplicated markers are important and need to be considered, if good gene or marker phylogenies are available, the DeCo method and its variants are a natural choice providing the most comprehensive evolutionary scenarios. The choice of the variant depends if lateral transfers are considered, or the considered genomes are poorly assembled. In the absence of good reliable gene phylogenies, MGLO and FPSAC (used without aDNA data) are the only available methods.

Acknowledgment

C.C. is funded by the Natural Sciences and Engineering Research Council of Canada (NSERC) Discovery Grant 249834. E.T., S.B., and Y.A. are funded by the French Agence Nationale pour la Recherche (ANR) through PIA Grant ANR-10-BINF-01-01 "Ancestrome". N.L. is funded by the International DFG Research Training Group GRK 1906/1.

References

1. Sturtevant AH (1921) A case of rearrangement of genes in drosophila. Proc Natl Acad Sci U S A 7:235–237

2. Dobzhansky T, Sturtevant AH (1938) Inversions in the chromosomes of drosophila pseudoobscura. Genetics 23:28–64

3. Pauling L, Zuckerkandl E (1963) Chemical paleogenetics. Acta Chem Scand 17:S9–S16

4. Poinar HN, Schwarz C, Qi J et al (2006) Metagenomics to paleogenomics: large–scale sequencing of mammoth DNA. Science 311:392–394

5. Muffato M, Roest Crollius H (2008) Paleogenomics in vertebrates, or the recovery of lost genomes from the mist of time. Bioessays 30:122–134

6. Ma J, Zhang L, Suh BB et al (2006) Reconstructing contiguous regions of an ancestral genome. Genome Res 16:1557–1565

7. Chauve C, Tannier E (2008) A methodological framework for the reconstruction of contiguous regions of ancestral genomes and its application to mammalian genomes. PLoS Comput Biol 4:e1000234

8. Neafsey DE, Waterhouse RM, Abai MR et al (2015) Mosquito genomics. Highly evolvable malaria vectors: the genomes of 16 anopheles mosquitoes. Science 347:1258522

9. Semeria M, Tannier E, Guéguen L (2015) Probabilistic modeling of the evolution of gene synteny within reconciled phylogenies. BMC Bioinformatics 16(Suppl 14):S5

10. Chauve C, Gavranovic H, Ouangraoua A et al (2010) Yeast ancestral genome reconstructions: the possibilities of computational methods II. J Comput Biol 17:1097–1112

11. Sankoff D, Zheng C, Wall PK et al (2009) Towards improved reconstruction of ancestral gene order in angiosperm phylogeny. J Comput Biol 16:1353–1367

12. Murat F, Xu JH, Tannier E et al (2010) Ancestral grass karyotype reconstruction unravels new mechanisms of genome shuffling as a source of plant evolution. Genome Res 20:1545–1557

13. Ming R, VanBuren R, Wai CM et al (2015) The pineapple genome and the evolution of CAM photosynthesis. Nat Genet 47:1435–1442

14. Salse J (2016) Ancestors of modern plant crops. Curr Opin Plant Biol 30:134–142

15. Murat F, Louis A, Maumus F et al (2015) Understanding Brassicaceae evolution through ancestral genome reconstruction. Genome Biol 16:262

16. Murat F, Zhang R, Guizard S et al (2015) Karyotype and gene order evolution from reconstructed extinct ancestors highlight contrasts in genome plasticity of modern rosid crops. Genome Biol Evol 7:735–749

17. Wang Y, Li W, Zhang T et al (2006) Reconstruction of ancient genome and gene order from complete microbial genome sequences. J Theor Biol 239:494–498

18. Patterson M, Szöllősi G, Daubin V et al (2013) Lateral gene transfer, rearrangement, reconciliation. BMC Bioinformatics 14(Suppl 15):S4

19. Darling AE, Miklós I, Ragan MA (2008) Dynamics of genome rearrangement in bacterial populations. PLoS Genet 4:e1000128

20. Kohn M, Högel J, Vogel W et al (2006) Reconstruction of a 450–my–old ancestral vertebrate protokaryotype. Trends Genet 22:203–210

21. Nakatani Y, Takeda H, Kohara Y et al (2007) Reconstruction of the vertebrate ancestral genome reveals dynamic genome reorganization in early vertebrates. Genome Res 17:1254–1265

22. Ouangraoua A, Tannier E, Chauve C (2011) Reconstructing the architecture of the ancestral amniote genome. Bioinformatics 27:2664–2671

23. Jaillon O, Aury JM, Brunet F et al (2004) Genome duplication in the teleost fish Tetraodon nigroviridis reveals the early vertebrate proto–karyotype. Nature 431:946–957

24. Woods IG, Wilson C, Friedlander B et al (2005) The zebrafish gene map defines ancestral vertebrate chromosomes. Genome Res 15:1307–1314

25. Catchen JM, Conery JS, Postlethwait JH (2008) Inferring ancestral gene order. Methods Mol Biol 452:365–383

26. Naruse K, Tanaka M, Mita K et al (2004) A medaka gene map: the trace of ancestral vertebrate proto–chromosomes revealed by comparative gene mapping. Genome Res 14:820–828

27. Putnam NH, Butts T, Ferrier DEK et al (2008) The amphioxus genome and the evolution of the chordate karyotype. Nature 453:1064–1071

28. Putnam NH, Srivastava M, Hellsten U et al (2007) Sea anemone genome reveals ancestral eumetazoan gene repertoire and genomic organization. Science 317:86–94

29. Herrero J, Muffato M, Beal K et al (2016) Ensembl comparative genomics resources. Database 2016:bav096. https://doi.org/10. 1093/database/bav096

30. Speir ML, Zweig AS, Rosenbloom KR et al (2016) The UCSC genome browser database: 2016 update. Nucleic Acids Res 44: D717–D725

31. Nagarajan N, Pop M (2013) Sequence assembly demystified. Nat Rev Genet 14:157–167

32. Penel S, Arigon AM, Dufayard JF, Sertier AS, Daubin V, Duret L, Gouy M, Perrière G (2009) Databases of homologous gene families for comparative genomics. BMC Bioinformatics 10(Suppl 6):S3

33. Sankoff D, Nadeau JH (2003) Chromosome rearrangements in evolution: from gene order to genome sequence and back. Proc Natl Acad Sci U S A 100:11188–11189

34. M. Višnovská, T. Vinar, and B. Brejová (2013) DNA sequence segmentation based on local similarity. In: ITAT 2013 Proceedings, pp. 36–43

35. Dousse A, Junier T, Zdobnov EM (2016) CEGA–a catalog of conserved elements from genomic alignments. Nucleic Acids Res 44: D96–D100

36. M. Belcaid, A. Bergeron, A. Chateau, et al. (2007) Exploring genome rearrangements using virtual hybridization. In: APBC'07: 5th Asia–Pacific bioinformatics conference, Imperial College Press 2007, pp. 205–214

37. Kim J, Larkin DM, Cai Q et al (2013) Reference–assisted chromosome assembly. Proc Natl Acad Sci U S A 110:1785–1790

38. Biller P, Gueguen L, Knibbe C, Tannier E (2016) Breaking good: accounting for the fragility of genomic regions in rearrangement distance estimation. Genome Biol Evol 8 (5):1427–1439

39. Alizadeh F, Karp RM, Weisser DK et al (1995) Physical mapping of chromosomes using unique probes. J Comput Biol 2:159–184

40. Yancopoulos S, Attie O, Friedberg R (2005) Efficient sorting of genomic permutations by translocation, inversion and block interchange. Bioinformatics 21:3340–3346

41. Fertin G (2009) Combinatorics of genome rearrangements. MIT Press, Cambridge

42. Tannier E, Zheng C, Sankoff D (2009) Multichromosomal median and halving problems under different genomic distances. BMC Bioinformatics 10:120

43. Xu AW, Moret BME (2011) GASTS: parsimony scoring under rearrangements. In: Algorithms in bioinformatics. Springer, Berlin Heidelberg, pp 351–363

44. Zheng C, Sankoff D (2011) On the PATHGROUPS approach to rapid small phylogeny. BMC Bioinformatics 12(Suppl 1):S4

45. Alekseyev MA, Pevzner PA (2009) Breakpoint graphs and ancestral genome reconstructions. Genome Res 19:943–957

46. Avdeyev P, Jiang S, Aganezov S et al (2016) Reconstruction of ancestral genomes in presence of gene gain and loss. J Comput Biol 23:150–164

47. Ma J, Ratan A, Raney BJ et al (2008) The infinite sites model of genome evolution. Proc Natl Acad Sci U S A 105:14254–14261

48. Paten B, Zerbino DR, Hickey G et al (2014) A unifying model of genome evolution under parsimony. BMC Bioinformatics 15:206

49. D. Simon and B. Larget (2004) Bayesian analysis to describe genomic evolution by rearrangement (BADGER), version 1.02 beta, Department of Mathematics and Computer Science, Duquesne University

50. Feijao P, Meidanis J (2011) SCJ: a breakpoint–like distance that simplifies several rearrangement problems. IEEE/ACM Trans Comput Biol Bioinform 8:1318–1329

51. Fitch WM (1971) Toward defining the course of evolution: minimum change for a specific tree topology. Syst Biol 20:406–416

52. Miklós I, Smith H (2015) Sampling and counting genome rearrangement scenarios. BMC Bioinformatics 16(Suppl 14):S6

53. Jones BR, Rajaraman A, Tannier E et al (2012) ANGES: reconstructing ANcestral GEnomeS maps. Bioinformatics 28:2388–2390

54. Hu F, Zhou J, Zhou L et al (2014) Probabilistic reconstruction of ancestral gene orders with insertions and deletions. IEEE/ACM Trans Comput Biol Bioinform 11:667–672

55. J. Ma (2010) A probabilistic framework for inferring ancestral genomic orders. In: Bioinformatics and biomedicine (BIBM), pp. 179–184

56. Maňuch J, Patterson M, Wittler R et al (2012) Linearization of ancestral multichromosomal genomes. BMC Bioinformatics 13(Suppl 19): S11

57. Stoye J, Wittler R (2009) A unified approach for reconstructing ancient gene clusters. IEEE/ACM Trans Comput Biol Bioinform 6:387–400

58. Maňuch J, Patterson M, Chauve C (2012) Hardness results on the gapped consecutive–ones property problem. Discrete Appl Math 160:2760–2768

59. Maňuch J, Patterson M (2011) The complexity of the gapped consecutive–ones property problem for matrices of bounded maximum degree. J Comput Biol 18:1243–1253

60. Gavranović H, Chauve C, Salse J et al (2011) Mapping ancestral genomes with massive gene loss: a matrix sandwich problem. Bioinformatics 27:i257–i265

61. Csurös M (2010) Count: evolutionary analysis of phylogenetic profiles with parsimony and likelihood. Bioinformatics 26:1910–1912

62. De Bie T, Cristianini N, Demuth JP et al (2006) CAFE: a computational tool for the study of gene family evolution. Bioinformatics 22:1269–1271

63. Csűrös M (2013) How to infer ancestral genome features by parsimony: dynamic programming over an evolutionary tree. In: Models and algorithms for genome evolution. Springer, London, pp 29–45

64. Sankoff D, Rousseau P (1975) Locating the vertices of a steiner tree in an arbitrary metric space. Math Prog 9:240–246

65. Bergeron A, Chauve C, Gingras Y (2008) Formal models of gene clusters. In: Bioinformatics algorithms. John Wiley & Sons, Inc, Hoboken, pp 175–202

66. Wittler R, Maňuch J, Patterson M et al (2011) Consistency of sequence–based gene clusters. J Comput Biol 18:1023–1039

67. Treangen TJ, Salzberg SL (2012) Repetitive DNA and next–generation sequencing:

computational challenges and solutions. Nat Rev Genet 13:36–46

68. Rajaraman A, Zanetti J, Manuch J et al (2016) Algorithms and complexity results for genome mapping problems. IEEE/ACM Trans Comput Biol Bioinform 14 (2):418–430. https://doi.org/10.1109/TCBB.2016.2528239

69. Rajaraman A, Tannier E, Chauve C (2013) FPSAC: fast phylogenetic scaffolding of ancient contigs. Bioinformatics 29:2987–2994

70. Gagnon Y, Blanchette M, El Mabrouk N (2012) A flexible ancestral genome reconstruction method based on gapped adjacencies. BMC Bioinformatics 13(Suppl 19):S4

71. Nakhleh L (2013) Computational approaches to species phylogeny inference and gene tree reconciliation. Trends Ecol Evol 28:719–728

72. Szöllősi GJ, Tannier E, Daubin V et al (2015) The inference of gene trees with species trees. Syst Biol 64:42–62

73. Jacox E, Chauve C, Szöllősi GJ et al (2016) ecceTERA: comprehensive gene tree-species tree reconciliation using parsimony. Bioinformatics 32(13):2056–2058. https://doi.org/10.1093/bioinformatics/btw105

74. Luhmann N, Thévenin A, Ouangraoua A et al (2016) The SCJ small parsimony problem for weighted gene adjacencies. In: Bioinformatics research and applications. Springer, Berlin Heidelberg

75. Ma J, Ratan A, Raney BJ et al (2008) DUPCAR: reconstructing contiguous ancestral regions with duplications. J Comput Biol 15:1007–1027

76. Bérard S, Gallien C, Boussau B et al (2012) Evolution of gene neighborhoods within reconciled phylogenies. Bioinformatics 28: i382–i388

77. Chauve C, Ponty Y, Zanetti J (2015) Evolution of genes neighborhood within reconciled phylogenies: an ensemble approach. BMC Bioinformatics 16(Suppl 19):S6

78. Anselmetti Y, Berry V, Chauve C et al (2015) Ancestral gene synteny reconstruction improves extant species scaffolding. BMC Genomics 16(Suppl 10):S11

79. Duchemin W, Anselmetti Y, Patterson M et al (2017) DeCoSTAR: reconstructing the ancestral organization of genes or genomes using reconciled phylogenies. Genome Biol Evol 9:1312–1319

80. Koren S, Schatz MC, Walenz BP et al (2012) Hybrid error correction and de novo assembly of single–molecule sequencing reads. Nat Biotechnol 30:693–700

81. Antipov D, Korobeynikov A, McLean JS et al (2015) hybridSPAdes: an algorithm for hybrid assembly of short and long reads. Bioinformatics 32:1009–1015

82. Paulino D, Warren RL, Vandervalk BP et al (2015) Sealer: a scalable gap–closing application for finishing draft genomes. BMC Bioinformatics 16:230

83. Salmela L, Sahlin K, Mäkinen V et al (2016) Gap filling as exact path length problem. J Comput Biol 23:347–361

84. English AC, Richards S, Han Y et al (2012) Mind the gap: upgrading genomes with Pacific biosciences RS long read sequencing technology. PLoS One 7:e47768

85. Koren S, Phillippy AM (2015) One chromosome, one contig: complete microbial genomes from long–read sequencing and assembly. Curr Opin Microbiol 23:110–120

86. Rhoads A, Au KF (2015) PacBio sequencing and its applications. Genomics Proteomics Bioinformatics 13:278–289

87. Lin Y, Nurk S, Pevzner PA (2014) What is the difference between the breakpoint graph and the de Bruijn graph? BMC Genomics 15 (Suppl 6):S6

88. Compeau PEC, Pevzner PA, Tesler G (2011) How to apply de Bruijn graphs to genome assembly. Nat Biotechnol 29:987–991

89. Muñoz A, Zheng C, Zhu Q et al (2010) Scaffold filling, contig fusion and comparative gene order inference. BMC Bioinformatics 11:304

90. Aganezov S, Sitdykova N, AGC Consortium et al (2015) Scaffold assembly based on genome rearrangement analysis. Comput Biol Chem 57:46–53

91. Higuchi R, Bowman B, Freiberger M et al (1984) DNA sequences from the quagga, an extinct member of the horse family. Nature 312:282–284

92. Cooper A, Lalueza-Fox C, Anderson S et al (2001) Complete mitochondrial genome sequences of two extinct moas clarify ratite evolution. Nature 409:704–707

93. Stiller M, Baryshnikov G, Bocherens H et al (2010) Withering away–25,000 years of genetic decline preceded cave bear extinction. Mol Biol Evol 27:975–978

94. Krings M, Stone A, Schmitz RW et al (1997) Neandertal DNA sequences and the origin of modern humans. Cell 90:19–30

95. Marciniak S, Klunk J, Devault A et al (2015) Ancient human genomics: the methodology behind reconstructing evolutionary pathways. J Hum Evol 79:21–34

96. Rasmussen S, Allentoft ME, Nielsen K et al (2015) Early divergent strains of Yersinia Pestis in Eurasia 5,000 years ago. Cell 163:571–582

97. Wagner DM, Klunk J, Harbeck M et al (2014) Yersinia Pestis and the plague of Justinian 541–543 AD: a genomic analysis. Lancet Infect Dis 14:319–326

98. Miller W, Drautz DI, Ratan A et al (2008) Sequencing the nuclear genome of the extinct woolly mammoth. Nature 456:387–390

99. Orlando L, Ginolhac A, Zhang G et al (2013) Recalibrating Equus evolution using the genome sequence of an early middle pleistocene horse. Nature 499:74–78

100. Peltzer A, Jäger G, Herbig A et al (2016) EAGER: efficient ancient genome reconstruction. Genome Biol 17:1–14

101. Minkin I, Patel A, Kolmogorov M et al (2013) Sibelia: a scalable and comprehensive synteny block generation tool for closely related microbial genomes. In: Algorithms in bioinformatics. Springer, Berlin Heidelberg, pp 215–229

102. Bos KI, Schuenemann VJ, Golding GB et al (2011) A draft genome of Yersinia Pestis from victims of the black death. Nature 478:506–510

103. Froenicke L, Caldés MG, Graphodatsky A et al (2006) Are molecular cytogenetics and bioinformatics suggesting diverging models of ancestral mammalian genomes? Genome Res 16:306–310

104. Steel M, Penny D (2000) Parsimony, likelihood, and the role of models in molecular phylogenetics. Mol Biol Evol 17:839–850

105. Durrett R, Nielsen R, York TL (2004) Bayesian estimation of genomic distance. Genetics 166:621–629

106. Gould SJ (1990) Wonderful life: the burgess shale and the nature of history. Norton, New York

107. Hillis DM, Bull JJ, White ME et al (1992) Experimental phylogenetics: generation of a known phylogeny. Science 255:589–592

108. R.N. Randall (2012) Experimental phylogenetics: a benchmark for ancestral sequence reconstruction. https://smartech.gatech.edu/handle/1853/48998

109. Barrick JE, Yu DS, Yoon SH et al (2009) Genome evolution and adaptation in a long-term experiment with Escherichia Coli. Nature 461:1243–1247

110. Romiguier J, Ranwez V, Douzery EJP et al (2013) Genomic evidence for large, long-lived ancestors to placental mammals. Mol Biol Evol 30:5–13

111. Szöllosi GJ, Boussau B, Abby SS et al (2012) Phylogenetic modeling of lateral gene transfer reconstructs the pattern and relative timing of speciations. Proc Natl Acad Sci U S A 109:17513–17518

112. Beiko RG, Charlebois RL (2007) A simulation test bed for hypotheses of genome evolution. Bioinformatics 23:825–831

113. Dalquen DA, Anisimova M, Gonnet GH et al (2012) ALF–a simulation framework for genome evolution. Mol Biol Evol 29:1115–1123

114. Biller P, Knibbe C, Beslon G, Tannier E (2016) Comparative genomics on artificial life. In: Computability in Europe, to appear. Springer, Cham

Chapter 14

Comparative RNA Genomics

Rolf Backofen, Jan Gorodkin, Ivo L. Hofacker, and Peter F. Stadler

Abstract

Over the last two decades it has become clear that RNA is much more than just a boring intermediate in protein expression. Ancient RNAs still appear in the core information metabolism and comprise a surprisingly large component in bacterial gene regulation. A common theme with these types of mostly small RNAs is their reliance of conserved secondary structures. Large scale sequencing projects, on the other hand, have profoundly changed our understanding of eukaryotic genomes. Pervasively transcribed, they give rise to a plethora of large and evolutionarily extremely flexible noncoding RNAs that exert a vastly diverse array of molecule functions. In this chapter we provide a—necessarily incomplete—overview of the current state of comparative analysis of noncoding RNAs, emphasizing computational approaches as a means to gain a global picture of the modern RNA world.

Key words Long noncoding RNA, RNA secondary structure, Chromatin, Alternative splicing, Evolution

1 Introduction

Protein-coding genes share the strong statistical patterns implied by the coding regions. Hence they are relatively easy to identify in genomic DNA and specialized methods can be used for their analysis that capitalize on the information amino acid sequences and their usually extensive sequence conservation. Noncoding transcripts and genes, on the other hand, are extremely heterogeneous and in general cannot be handled by a single computational approach.

A key result of systematic high-throughput sequencing studies [1–3] is that an overwhelmingly large fraction of a mammalian genome is transcribed in some cell type, tissue, or developmental stage. Many of these transcripts are expressed only at very low levels or in very specific circumstances [4]. The discussion whether these "dark matter transcripts" are biological reality or technical artifacts seems to have been (largely) settled in favor of the reality of pervasive transcription [3, 5]. Unexpectedly large numbers of noncoding transcripts have also been observed in many other organisms

João C. Setubal et al. (eds.), *Comparative Genomics: Methods and Protocols*, Methods in Molecular Biology, vol. 1704, https://doi.org/10.1007/978-1-4939-7463-4_14, © Springer Science+Business Media LLC 2018

including yeast [6–8], plants [9], protists [10], and even in procaryotes [11–13].

The genomic annotation of ncRNAs in general lacks behind the annotation of coding regions, at least in part owing to the diversity of ncRNAs and their often lineage-specific phylogenetic distribution. The classification and nomenclatures of the diverse groups of RNAs are still not a settled issue. *Long noncoding RNAs* (lncRNAs) are often defined as ncRNAs longer than 200 nt while lacking coding potential and essentially grouped into a *single* class of ncRNAs in spite of their apparent diversity [14]. This rather arbitrary definition of a 200 nt length cutoff originates from experimental protocols [15]. Its widespread and uncritical use unfortunately gives rise to some confusion and inconsistencies in the literature. For instance, *small* bacterial RNAs (e.g., ryfA RNA [16]) are often longer than 200 nt long, and ribosomal RNAs, telomerase RNAs, long snoRNAs [17], etc. are also usually considered as separated types of RNAs. We will use lncRNA here to refer to all those non-protein-coding RNAs that do not fall into one of the well-studied groups of structured RNAs. These in particular include long mRNA-like RNAs (mlncRNAs) that are processed in a similar way as mRNAs but lack coding capacity, and long intergenic ncRNAs, lincRNAs, which we understand as lncRNAs located outside protein coding genes and are not anti-sense or processed from introns of other annotated genes. The latter type of transcripts are included among the lncRNAs. Both mlncRNAs and lincRNA are thus subsumed here in the class of lncRNAs.

Some RNA classes, in particular transfer RNAs (tRNA), ribosomal RNAs (rRNAs), and the RNA components of RNAse P and the signal recognition particle date back to the last common ancestor of all extant life forms. Small nucleolar RNAs have been directing chemical modifications of rRNA since the common ancestor of Archaea and Eukarya. Eubacteria have evolved a plethora of regulatory RNAs, both independent small RNA genes (sRNAs) and genic RNA elements. In Eukarya, the RNA interference RNAi pathway has given rise to an ever increasing system of endogenous small RNAs. The biology and evolution of these RNA classes have been reviewed many times in the recent past, hence we will make no attempt to discuss these comparative well-understood entities in detail. Instead, we refer to reviews [18, 19] and some recent surveys of microRNAs [20] and snoRNAs [21–24] and the references therein.

This chapter intends to provide a broad overview of ncRNAs at genomic scales, with an emphasis on comparative aspects. We start with a discussion the different aspects of conservation in RNAs, which is both more diverse and more difficult to handle computationally than conservation of coding sequence. For details on the computational techniques and underlying algorithmic principles of the many bioinformatics tools mentioned throughout this chapter, we refer a recent book [25] and the list of references.

The distinct features of RNA conservation (Subheading 2) form the basis for homology search and homology based annotation of ncRNAs, discussed in Subheading 3. Subheading 4 is then devoted to de novo methods for detection of functional RNA elements and the associated difficulties. We finish with a short overview of RNA interactions, and recent advances in sequencing methods, and open questions.

2 Hallmarks of Conserved RNA

2.1 Structured RNAs

The best studied classes of ncRNAs heavily rely on their spatial structures. As a consequence, both the 3D structure and the underlying pattern of base pairs, that is, their secondary structure is highly conserved over evolutionary timescales. Extensive computer simulations have shown, on the other hand, that RNA secondary structures are very fragile against randomly placed mutations. About 15–20% of sequence divergence is sufficient to completely destroy similarities of secondary structures [26, 27]. The preservation of secondary structure in the presence of appreciable sequence divergence therefore is a highly efficient statistical predictor for negative selection and thus biological function of RNA (secondary) structure.

2.1.1 Secondary Structure Prediction

Since RNA function is so tightly coupled to its structure, structure prediction lies at the heart of many computational approaches. While some mechanisms, say the binding of a small molecule by a riboswitch, depend on the detailed three-dimensional RNA structure, it is often sufficient to consider *secondary* structure, i.e., the set of Watson-Crick base pairs. This is fortunate since secondary structure is computationally much easier to handle than tertiary structures. As early as 1978, Ruth Nussinov [28] noted that the RNA secondary structure with maximum number of base pairs can be found by an efficient dynamic programming algorithm, whose computational effort scales as $\mathcal{O}(n^3)$, i.e. with the cube of the sequence length. In 1981, Zuker and Stiegler [29] extended this algorithm to compute the minimum free energy structure with respect to a loop-dependent energy model of the type that is still in use today.

Many extensions and variation of this basic algorithm have been formulated over time. In order to deal with inherent inaccuracies of structure prediction, most practitioners advocate methods that do not rely on the prediction of a single optimal structure. Instead, one can predict a set of suboptimal structures [30, 31], or rigorously compute the partition function over all possible structures [32]. From the partition function one can derive the probability of individual base pairs, or even sample structures from the equilibrium ensemble [33].

Of particular interest for our purposes are methods that compute the common structure of a set of related sequences from an alignment. RNAalifold [34, 35], for example, is a straightforward extension of energy directed folding to an alignment, using the averaged energy as well as a simple covariance term for scoring. Pfold [36, 37] employs a simple stochastic context free grammar, but has a more sophisticated covariance score based on a phylogenetic tree. PETfold [38] uses the evolutionary framework of Pfold to constrain evolutionary supported base pairs in energy folding for each of the sequences to obtain a consensus structure. Given good input alignments these methods achieve much better accuracies than single sequence folding methods.

2.1.2 Sequence Biases

Organisms with AT-rich genomes exhibit substantially increased GC levels both in the exons of their protein-coding genes and in their structured ncRNAs. The effect can be exploited to find ncRNA candidates with the help of a simple Hidden Markov Model that distinguishes an AT-rich background from a GC-rich foreground [39]. While the background can be trained on the overall genomic nucleotide distribution, easy-to-find ncRNAs such as tRNAs and ribosomal rRNAs serve to parametrize the foreground. The approach was successful for both prokaryotes (*Pyrococcus*) [39] and eukaryotes (*Dictyostelium discoideum*) [40]. Recently, a detailed analysis of lncRNAs in mammals showed that their exons are also more GC-rich than their introns [41]. The relatively high GC content of many ncRNAs is presumably explained by the need to stabilize functionally important secondary structures.

2.1.3 Thermodynamic Stability

Selection pressures for increased stability not only affect sequence composition. There is good evidence that most RNAs with well-conserved secondary structures have free energies of folding that a significantly more negative than random RNAs of the same length and nucleotide composition [42–44]. The effect is conveniently quantified as a z-score $z(x) = (f(x) - \mu(x))/\sigma(x)$, where $f(x)$ is the observed folding energy for sequence x, and $\mu(x)$ and $\sigma(x)$ are the mean and standard deviation of the energy distribution obtained by randomizing the order of the nucleotides in x. As pointed out in [45], the values of $\mu(x)$ and $\sigma(x)$ depend on the definition of the shuffling procedure and for RNA are sensitive to dinucleotide content because of the energy contributions of stacked base pairs.

The Euler algorithm is very efficient algorithm for generating truly uniform random k-mer-preserving sequences [46–49]. It uses a random walk on the directed multigraph G whose vertices are the $(k-1)$-mers of the input and whose arcs two $(k-1)$-mers u and

v that appear as consecutive infixes of the input. A random k-mer preserving permutation of the input corresponds to a random Euler walk in G [48]. The Euler walks in turn correspond to the arborescences of G, i.e., the rooted directed spanning trees. Many efficient approaches to generate random arborescences are known, *see* [49] for a recent overview.

The computation of $\mu(x)$ and $\sigma(x)$ from shuffled sequences is demanding since it requires that each of the shuffled sequences be folded. Software tools that aim at genome-wide applications such as RNAz [43], RNAz 2.0 [50], and RNASurface [51] therefore replace the explicit computation of mean and variance by regression models for μ and σ as a function of sequence features such as nucleotide or di-nucleotide frequencies. Support vector regression has proved very efficient in this context.

A parameter that is closely related to the thermodynamic stability of an RNA secondary structure is the average base pair distance

$$D := \sum_{S', S''} d_{bp}\left(S', S''\right) \frac{e^{-\beta f(S')}}{Z} \frac{e^{-\beta f(S'')}}{Z} \tag{1}$$

within a Boltzmann-weighted ensemble of the secondary structures of a given sequence x. The base pair distance $d_{bp}(S', S'')$ of two structures S' and S'' formed by the same sequence is symmetric difference of their sets of base pairs. The sum over all pairs of secondary structures is of course infeasible in practice. A short computation shows, however, that it can also be expressed as $D = \sum_{i < j} p_{ij}(1 - p_{ij})$ in terms of the probabilities p_{ij} that bases i and j are paired, which are readily computed with McCaskill's algorithm [32]. In analogy to the folding energies, the D-values of functional RNAs can be compared to the expectation for randomized sequences using a z-score as normalized parameter, *see* Table 1.

2.1.4 Mutational Robustness

A more subtle indicator of functional RNAs is an increased level of robustness against mutations. On the one hand, one expects a second-order selective effect that increases neutrality whenever secondary structure is under stabilizing selection [53, 54], on the other hand there is also a correlation between thermodynamic stability and mutational robustness [55] in the sequence-structure map of RNAs [27]. A large number of indices of structural robustness have been proposed, many with the aim of identifying structurally disruptive mutations. To this end, structures may be encoded as minimum energy secondary structures, as the ensemble of secondary structures, or by means of the base pairing probabilities $p_{ij}(x)$. Among the commonly used measures of structural divergence are the average value of $|S(x) \triangle S(x')|$ [56], the number of disrupted base pairs in the reference $|S(x) \setminus S(x')|$ [57], the

Table 1
Many RNA classes are thermodynamically more stable and have structural ensembles that are less diverse than expected

ncRNA class	N	$z(\Delta G)$ Mono	Di	$z(D)$ Mono
tRNA	579	−1.84	−1.71	−0.5
5S rRNA	606	−1.62	−1.71	−0.7
Hammerhead III	251	−3.08	−3.17	−1.5
Group II−Intron	116	−3.88	−3.77	−1.2
SRP RNA	73	−3.37	−3.09	−
U5	199	−2.73	−2.38	−2.73

For samples of N sequences, z-scores computed for the folding energies ΔG (for both mono- and di-nucleotide shuffling) and for the ensemble diversity, Eq. 1 are listed. Data compiled from [42, 52]

Euclidean distance of base pairing probabilities $\Sigma_{i<j} \ (p_{ij}(x) - p_{ij}(x'))^2$ [58], the Kullback-Leibler distance between the Boltzmann-weighted ensembles of secondary structures [59], and the Pearson correlation of position-wise pairing probabilities [60]. A measure of overall robustness of the structure of x can then be obtained by averaging the divergence between x and all possible 1-error mutants. Recent work [57] shows that robustness parameters are indeed indicative of functional RNAs with conserved secondary structures.

2.1.5 Structural Conservation

The most successful indicator of functional RNAs remains, however, structural conservation. For a typical RNA structure about one third of mutations will be neutral [27]. At the same time, simulations suggest that with carefully selected mutations it is usually possible to change *all* positions in an RNA sequence without ever changing its structure [27]. Indeed, many ncRNA families exhibit highly conserved structures but surprisingly low sequence similarity, *see*, e.g., [61]. In helical regions one often observes so-called *compensatory* mutation: an AU pair in one sequence, for example, is replaced by a CG pair in another sequence. The terminology derives from the fact that the first of the two mutations (say A→C) would destroy the pairing, while the second (U→G) restores it again. When only one of the paired bases is changed, as in a GU to GC mutation, we speak of *consistent* mutations.

Compensatory mutations are often seen as the hallmark of conserved functional structures. Early attempts to decide whether a given alignment contains a conserved structures [62–64] relied mainly on counting such events. These methods, however, require a fairly large number of compensatory mutations, which limit their sensitivity.

In the context of the RNAz program, Washietl et al. [43] introduced a measure called *structure conservation index* (SCI) to quantify structural conservation. The SCI compares the folding energy of individual sequences with that of the consensus structure

$$SCI = E_{cons}/\overline{E}_{single} \tag{2}$$

Here, $\overline{E}_{single}$ is the arithmetic mean of the folding energies of each sequence in the alignment, while the consensus folding energy E_{cons} is obtained by RNAalifold [34].

The SCI only depends on folding energies, not on the structures themselves. While this may seem counterintuitive, it makes the measure less sensitive to errors in the predicted structures. A quite extensive comparison of different measures for structure conservation can be found in [58]. It confirmed the SCI as one of the best available measures for this purpose. In general, measures based on a predicted consensus structure performed better than those based on pairwise comparison of RNAs in the alignment. The SCI was recently extended from comparing individual MFE structures to consensus structures to comparing base pair probabilities of individual sequences to ensemble reliabilities as computed by PET-fold [38, 65]. This Structure Ensemble Conservation Index, SECI, is employed in the analysis of the full scale screen on vertebrates using CMfinder (see below) [66]. It is worth noting that measures of structural conservation, or equivalently, of structural diversity, are in themselves not an appropriate measure for the correctness of a structure prediction over an alignment. That is, conserved structures may also be predicted in a consistently incorrect manner. Still, at least for sequences with enough variation to support covariance patterns, one may expect that the SCI or similar measures are well correlated with the accuracy of the predicted structure.

Several approaches also exist to quantify the covariation of individual base pairs or helices. Mutual information (MI) between two columns of an alignment is perhaps the most natural thing to use. Since MI is agnostic of rules for secondary structure formation, it can detect tertiary interaction as well as canonical base pairs at the price of requiring a fairly large number of sequences. For smaller alignments, ad hoc scores such as the RNAalifold covariance score or modified Mutual Information scores that consider only canonical base pairs tend to perform better [67]. A further improvement of this measure was introduced with RIlogo, a tool for visualization of alignments and their RNA–RNA interactions [68].

Probabilistic models with an explicit phylogenetic tree can be employed as well. Here, one compares the likelihood to observe two columns of an alignment between two models of sequence evolution, one where columns evolve independently (characterized by a 4×4 rate matrix) and one trained on pairs of columns representing known conserved base pairs (16×16 rate matrix). Pfold uses this idea in the context of consensus structure prediction, while TRANSAT computes the log-likelihood score

$$\Lambda(h) = \frac{1}{L}\log_2 \frac{P(h \mid \theta_{paired})}{P(h \mid \theta_{unpaired})} \qquad (3)$$

for all potential helices h with length $L \geq 4$. PETfold extend Pfold [36, 37] by employing a two step approach where first the most reliable base pairs are found. These are then employed as constraints for the energy-based folding of the individual sequences.

Selective constraints on RNA structure can also be computed from explicit estimates of differences in substitution rates between paired and unpaired positions in structured RNAs relative to a background model of neutrally evolving DNA. For both hominids and drosophilids, substitution rates are drastically reduced. In fact, the estimated selection coefficients are significantly higher than for constraints at nonsynonymous sites of protein-coding genes [69]. A detailed model of the selective effects of compensatory mutations in RNA structures is discussed in [70].

2.2 Non-structured RNAs

Only a small subset of lncRNAs shows levels of sequence conservation comparable to protein-coding genes or the well-conserved families of structured ncRNAs. Nevertheless, a large fraction of lncRNAs is under measurable purifying selection [71–75]. As a consequence there is an ongoing discussion to what extent lncRNAs convey biological function or whether many or most of them are "Junk RNA" [76, 77]. Although important secondary structure elements have been suggested for several lncRNAs, the majority does not seem to be substantially enriched in evolutionary conserved RNA elements [78, 79]. In spite of this, it remains unclear which extent lncRNA might contain smaller RNA structures or domains to carry out essential functions [78, 80]. The methodology employed to conduct the RNA structure predictions is based on single sequence folding or structure predictions on sequence based alignments [75, 79]. Given the poor conservation of sequence in lncRNAs, significant conservation of secondary structures in non-aligned regions cannot be ruled out. Computational screens indeed report at least weak enrichments of conserved secondary structures overall [81]. The genome-wide screen for conserved RNA structures (CRSs) in vertebrate genomes using CMfinder for structural alignments revealed a slight enrichment of CRS towards the 5' end of lncRNAs [66]. Although there is no enrichment elsewhere and most lncRNA do not host CRSs there are still predicted many CRSs on lncRNAs, for example, 22% of lncRNAs in GENCODE (v25) [4] host a CRS [66].

LncRNAs exhibit notably higher degrees of tissue specificity when compared to protein-coding genes. These expression patterns are almost as well conserved among orthologous lncRNAs as among orthologous protein-coding transcripts [82, 83]. Other authors, however, reported a substantially higher divergence of expression [84, 85]. The discrepancy seems to be explained by more or less restrictive definitions of the corresponding genes, since many lncRNAs also rapidly adapt their gene structures [82, 86].

Among more distant species, orthology of lncRNAs cannot be established unambiguously due to rapid sequence divergence. Several authors noted that lncRNAs can often be found at syntenic positions [82, 87, 88]. These also seem to have significantly correlated expression patterns, which may hint at analogous functions.

2.2.1   Conservation of Splicing Patterns

Sequence patterns along multi-exonic lncRNA loci resemble protein-coding genes. These mRNA-like lncRNAs (mlncRNA) have exons that are more GC-rich than their introns. Furthermore there is good evidence for purifying selection preserving exonic splicing enhancers in both human and fruitfly [41]. Conservation of splicing, which may explain lncRNA function through the link between splicing and the recruitment of chromatin modifiers, indeed explains most of the purifying selection pressures acting on (m)lncRNAs [79].

Combining genome-wide multiple sequence alignments (MSAs) with carefully mapped transcriptome data readily yields a genome-wide comparative map of splice junctions. The available transcriptome data, however, are still concentrated on a few model organisms. The map is therefore plagued by very sparse data for most non-model organisms.

The propensity of a sequence interval to be a functional splice site can be evaluated computationally because both splice donors and splice acceptors features very well-defined sequence motives. A standard tool for this purpose is `MaxEntScan` [90]. It models the short donor and acceptor motives using a probabilistic model based on the "Maximum Entropy Principle." In contrast to position weight matrices or (inhomogeneous) Markov models, it accounts for both adjacent and non-adjacent dependencies in the motives thus achieving increased sensitivity. For each known splice site known from transcriptome data it is therefore possible to determine whether the homologous position in a related species is also a functional splice site or not.

The combined map of experimental and computationally predicted splice junctions is highly specific and makes it possible to quantify in detail the evolution of mlncRNA gene structures [89], *see* Fig. 1. Almost 40% of the individual splice sites and about 70–80% of human mlncRNA transcripts appear to be conserved across the major eutherian families according to the computational

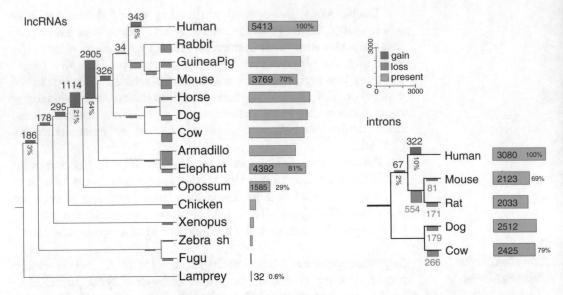

Fig. 1 Conservation of lncRNAs determined by conserved splice sites. L.h.s.: An lncRNA is considered as conserved if at least one perfectly conserved splice junction is observed. R.h.s.: Evolution of introns in the lncRNA subset conserved in all five species. Data are shown for a stringently filtered subset of GENCODE human lincRNAs, thus gains are measured only along the lineage leading to human and losses only along the sister lineages. Adapted and redrawn from [89]

analysis in [89]. These numbers are largely consistent with estimates based on the direct comparison of transcriptome datasets [83, 85] and the expression-based estimate mentioned above [75]. About 1/6 of the human lncRNAs has recognizable homologs in marsupials or even more distant, non-mammalian vertebrates [89]. These numbers have to be considered as lower bounds since they refer only to loci that are included in the genome-wide MSAs. The poor sequence conservation of most lncRNAs, however, severely limits the sensitivity of the MSAs at phylogenetic distances beyond family level.

2.3 Unspliced and Unstructured lncRNAs

With few exceptions, among them fungal U6 snRNAs [91], almost all of the well-structured ncRNAs are unspliced. There is, however, also a large class of other unspliced transcripts. In the human genome almost 5% of the protein-coding genes are not spliced [92]. It may not be a surprise that there is also large group of unspliced lncRNAs. These fall into at least four distinct classes: (1) intronic transcripts typically associated with protein-coding loci, (2) lncRNAs associated with long 3'-UTRs, (3) independent unspliced RNAs found in intergenic regions, and (4) an enigmatic class of very long macroRNAs.

Totally and partially intronic transcripts (TINs and PINs) that are usually unspliced and lack coding capacity have been reported in large numbers for both human and mouse [93–96]. This class includes many unspliced long anti-sense intronic RNAs [97, 98]. Very little is known about their biogenesis and function. Presumably the best-studied example is the TIN ANRASSF1 [99], a pol-II transcribed, capped, and polyadenylated lncRNA that regulates the expression of the tumor suppressor RASSF1A expression via epigenetic mechanisms involving PRC2. Intergenic examples include the MALAT-1 and MENβ RNAs [100–102], two unusually well-conserved RNAs [103], as well as disease-associated RNAs such as PRNCR1 [104].

MacroRNAs covering up to several hundred kb were recently observed as highly expressed RNAs in signaling pathways [105] and in cancer cells [106]. Very similar transcripts such as Airn [107, 108] and KCNQ1OT1 [109] are involved in the regulation of imprinted loci. These enigmatic RNAs are very poorly conserved. At least some of them presumably function by transcriptional interference. Almost nothing, finally, is known about 3'-UTR derived RNAs [110].

A survey of unspliced lncRNAs based on EST data reported that only 15–20% of the unspliced EST clusters are conserved between human and mouse. Nevertheless there are more than 5000 syntenically conserved loci expressing unspliced lncRNAs in both human and mouse [111].

3   Homology Search

Homology search is the task of finding one or more sequences that are related to a known query, in our context an ncRNA, in a target sequence, usually an (unannotated) genome. Despite the power of blast and substantial progress in recent years, this is still a nontrivial problem. There are several effects that conspire to make the task difficult [112]: many ncRNAs are short, thus limiting the available information from the outset; most lncRNAs and many structured RNAs evolve rapidly at sequence level, preserving their sequences much less than their functionally important secondary structure elements; and in contrast to protein-coding sequences, insertions, deletions, and structural rearrangements appear to be much more frequent in RNA genes compared to their protein-coding sisters. The Rfam database forms *the* starting for homology based annotation for a vast number of RNA families. It contains in its current version 12.0 [113] 2450 RNA families; nevertheless, there are many RNA families, in particular from procaryotes, that are not yet included and for which in practice only individual sequences are available as queries.

3.1   Sequence-Based Methods

By far the most widely used tool for homology search of nucleic acid sequences is blast [114]. Exact semiglobal sequence alignment methods such as gotohscan [115] can provide a noticeable increase in sensitivity albeit at substantial computational costs.

`maxAlike` [116] predicts a maximum likelihood estimate for the nucleotide probabilities of an unknown homolog given a sequence alignment and a phylogenetic tree. The estimated sequence can then be used as an improved query in a sequence- or pattern-based homology search.

A limiting factor for the accuracy of `blast` is the small alphabet size. As a consequence, relatively long, gap-less seeds are required. This, however, limits sensitivity for many ncRNAs because insertions and deletions are quite abundant. Telomerase RNA, for instance, is extremely hard to find in a genome sequence because it does not preserve longer gap-less sequence regions [117]. On the other hand, alignment quality can be improved by including local context information [118]. Translating the sequence to a 16-letter alphabet to account for dinucleotides makes it possible to use `blastp` as search engine in conjunction with a suitably defined scoring scheme [119]. This leads to a significant improvement in sensitivity.

Several classes of structured noncoding RNAs can be characterized by a pattern of short but well-conserved sequence elements that are separated by poorly conserved regions of sometimes highly variable lengths. This situation is difficult for alignment-based methods. The `fragrep` tool combines pattern search with a chaining algorithm to accommodate such situations [120].

A general strategy for homology search in complex cases is to use a multi-step filtering procedure employing consecutively more stringent but computationally more expensive filters on smaller and smaller sets of candidate sequences. The `fragrep` tool can serve as one such filter. Profile-HMMs are another option. Both exact, i.e., provably loss-less [121], and much faster, heuristic HMMs [122] have been developed to preprocess the input for covariance models (discussed below). Specialized filter steps are also included in tRNAscan-SE [123], which after nearly two decades is still the best search tool specifically for tRNAs.

3.2 Secondary Structure Descriptors

A series of software tools utilize constraints on secondary structures. These fall into two broad classes: `RNAMotif` [124], rnabob, or `Palingol` [125] provide descriptor languages to explicitly specify a search pattern. A different approach is taken by `infernal` and `erpin`, where the user input is a structure-annotated multiple sequence alignment from which the software itself computes a sequence-structure model that is suitable for search. Because of the practical and theoretical importance of covariance models we discuss the infernal approach separately in the following section.

One of the earliest descriptor-based search algorithms was `RNAMOT` [126]. It allowed the specification of stems and unpaired strands with variable lengths and primary sequence constraints. `rnabob` (Sean Eddy 1996, unpubl., http://selab.janelia.org/soft ware.html) provides an extension of this language and a more versatile handling of mis-pairing within stems. The `Palingol` [125] language was inspired by functional programming. `PatScan` [127] provided increased flexibility by incorporating position weight matrices to represent sequence constraints. The most widely used tool of this class is `RNAMotif` [124] since it combines most of the capabilities of the earlier programs and a procedural language for evaluating and scoring pattern matches. The main practical drawback of all descriptor-based approaches is the need to construct the search patterns by hand. The `Locomotif` tool [128] alleviates many of the technical issues. Still, a human researcher has to know in detail what to search for. In particular for less well-studied RNA families, however, this knowledge is in many cases quite limited even for experienced experts [112].

`erpin` [129] therefore transforms a training alignment into a set of weight matrices for each structural element and then matches this matrix set against a sequence database. The advantage of this strategy, which frees the user from the construction of the search pattern, is also its major disadvantage: The user has little chance to modify the search pattern. A benchmarking study covering several training set-based RNA search programs can be found in [130].

3.3 Covariance Models

Rather than using models that are more or less explicitly based on prior knowledge of the structure in question, a probabilistic model can be extracted from a given input alignment annotated with a consensus structure. Just as a probabilistic model over protein or DNA sequences can be extracted and subsequently used to align other sequences to it, as in the case of Pfam [131] using profile hidden Markov models (HMMs), a similar strategy can be employed for sequence and secondary structure of RNAs.

With Covariance Models (CMs) this is precisely what is aimed for. The sequence modeling in CMs is very similar to that of an HMM, while the structure is modeled as a stochastic context-free grammar (SCFG), *see*, e.g., [132, 133], by including compensating base pairs or covariance patterns in the modeling. Where an HMM builds a statistic profile that is position specific, the CM takes the statistics of the covariance patterns of the input alignment into account. In brief, the alignment is represented by a number of states: match states representing single positions or positions with covarying (base pairs), mismatches, insertions, and deletions. These states emit nucleotides or base pairs with some probabilities to model a structure. The states themselves are connected by various transitions between the states modeling positions in the alignment and positions modeling base pairs, which also come with probabilities. All these probabilities are estimated from observed frequencies in the input alignment.

CMs are implemented in `Infernal` that comes with a suite of tools, such as `cmbuild` to build a model from an alignment and `cmsearch` to screen for matches on novel sequences. Sequences are scored against the model to compute the most probable match over different states. This in turn determines exactly how the models' structure is projected onto the sequence. The most recent versions of Infernal [134] use an efficient, nearly loss-less HMM filter to quickly reject potential matches that cannot yield high CM scores. This avoids a large fraction of the computational efforts and has led to substantial speed-up of the method. The calibration of the probabilities emitted by the CMs with random sequences makes it possible to estimate match probabilities and to compute E-values for a given match. Infernal has been used to create CMs for each of the RNAs in Rfam [113], the main database of structured RNA families. The CMs over these families are also becoming increasingly used for genome-wide annotations, *see*, e.g., [135, 136].

CMs require a sufficient number of known examples from an RNA family to gain discriminatory power. A method to bootstrap and automate the process of building CMs is presented in RNA-lien [137]. In an iterative manner, new candidates sequences are found using blast, candidates are accepted or rejected after scoring with a CM, good hits are added to the alignment and the CM is rebuilt to make use of the new sequences.

4   Methods for Comparative RNA Structured Discovery

As discussed earlier, conservation of secondary structure is one of the hallmarks of functional RNAs. Many methods therefore target conserved RNA secondary structures, hence this topic takes center stage here. We deliberately ignore here the vast literature on transcript discovery from RNA-seq data and focus on approaches that are comparative and grounded in genomic data.

4.1   Sequence Alignment-Based Methods

4.1.1   Energy Directed Folding

Comparative methods require a set of homologous RNAs as input and it is natural to perform a multiple sequence alignment as the first step of the analysis. From this alignment a consensus structure can be predicted using several available methods. In particular RNAalifold [34] from the ViennaRNA package has been used as the basis for RNA gene finders. A nice property of RNAalifold is that it uses the same energy model employed for single sequence folding, making folding energies of alignment and single sequence folding comparable. Thus folding an alignment with only a single sequence, or identical sequences will give the same result as folding that sequence using RNAfold.

The perhaps first RNA gene finder based on consensus structure prediction was AlifoldZ [42]. It starts from the observation that folding energies, as assessed through z-scores, tend to be lower for RNAs with a functional structures than random RNAs. For single sequences the signal is, however, too weak for reliable classification. AlifoldZ therefore works with sequence alignments, replacing single sequence folding with consensus structure prediction. A z-score is computed by comparing the energy of the consensus structure of the alignment with folding energies of randomized alignments. This requires a procedure to shuffle alignments as discussed in Subheading 4.5. Even with alignments of just two sequences this gives a huge improvement over single sequence z-scores and allows for reliable separation of true ncRNAs from decoys.

As discussed above, shuffling alignments is tricky, and the `AlifoldZ` shuffling procedure is not always able to remove all signal from the randomized alignments. `SissiZ` [138] therefore proposes an alternative way to obtain randomized alignments: It estimates a phylogenetic tree and substitution rates from the input alignment and uses this to simulate random alignments that will on average exhibit the same sequence composition and local sequence conservation. Since the simulation initially produces gap-free alignments, gaps are inserted afterwards wherever the original alignment had gaps. Importantly, the sequence simulation framework allows for dependencies between sites, which is used here to produce sequences that preserve dinucleotide frequencies. By replacing the `AlifoldZ` shuffling procedure with these simulated alignments, `SissiZ` yields a significant improvement in classification accuracy, especially when the dinucleotide model is used.

One disadvantage of both `AlifoldZ` and `SissiZ` is speed, since typically about 1000 shuffled (or simulated) alignments are used for z-scores estimation. In `RNAz` [43, 50, 139] z-scores are computed for each individual sequence in the alignment and then averaged. Computing the z-score $z = \frac{E - \mu}{\sigma}$ requires the mean μ and standard deviation σ of folding energies for random sequences with the same composition. `RNAz` uses a regression SVM to predict μ and σ and thus avoids costly sampling. The second criterion used is the SCI as a measure of structure conservation, *see* Subheading 2.1.5. The combination of SCI and z-score leads to a clear separation of native ncRNA alignments and decoys (generated by shuffling). For classification `RNAz` uses an SVM that takes z-score, SCI, sequence identity, length of the alignment, and number of sequences as input. The SVM is trained on a large body of native RNA alignments derived from Rfam, as well as shuffled alignments as negative set.

In version `RNAz-2.0` the z-score computation was extended to use a dinucleotide shuffling as background. In addition, `RNAz-2.0` provides two decision SVMs, one trained on sequence alignment (generated by ClustalW), the other on structural alignments generated by LocARNA. The dinucleotide background model increases classification accuracy, while structural alignments extend the applicability of `RNAz` to alignments with low sequence conservation.

Any of the methods evaluating secondary structure content is applied to individual sequence windows with a typical size on the order of 100 nt. To conduct genome-wide screens, partially over-lapping windows covering the available genome-wide alignments are excised and processed individually. Typically predictions for overlapping or adjacent locations are then collated in a post-processing step.

The pipeline proposed in [81] integrates two of the methods to assess secondary structure conservation: RNAz and SissiZ [138]. The hybrid algorithm first processes genomic alignments to remove identical sequences and sequences with high gap content and then submits cleaned input to the "best" structure prediction tool, which is determined based on the alignment's sequence char-acteristics. The decision for a particular algorithm and scoring scheme was first trained on extensive benchmarking data.

4.1.2 Approaches Based on Covariance Models

One of the earliest methods to detect structured RNAs in aligned sequences was qRNA [140]. It takes a pair-wise sequence alignment, for example the output of BLAST [114], and predicts a conserved RNA structure of a pre-defined window of fixed sized length. Three scoring models are used. One model is a pair-SCFG that scores structure including evolutionary conversed compensating base changes. Another is an HMM model that scores coding sequencing including conserved codons. Finally a background or null model, a pair HMM model, accounts for evolving sequences without con-straints on the individual positions.

An alternative version to the energy based model RNAz is to employ an SCFG based scoring scheme as done with EvoFold [141]. In contrast the MFE based strategy in Alifold and along the strategy of qRNA, EvoFold employs a phylo-SCFG, that is an SCFG that takes the branch length of the evolutionary tree into account and thereby weigh the sequences to reflect their evolution-ary relationship. EvoFold employs a sliding window approach and in each window a structure is predicted using the Pfold phylo-SCFG while having two models one for single nucleotide and one for di-nucleotides describing non-pairing positions and base pair-ing positions in a stem, respectively. Two models are used, one scoring structured regions and one regions outside the structured regions and the final score is a log-likelihood under these two models. EvoFold was trained on the available sequences in Rfam at the time. The FDR of EvoFold was estimated to 62%. In subsequent work EvoFam was introduced as clustering of EvoFold predictions in 3′UTRs [142].

4.2 Structural Alignments

4.2.1 Computational Methods

The sensitivity of all methods that require sequence alignments as input is necessarily limited by the accuracy of the given sequence alignments. In fact, sequence-based whole-genome aligners regu-larly misalign structural ncRNAs [143]. Structure-based alignment, which could increase the sensitivity, has been prohibitive for genome-wide screens due to its high computational costs. While it is still infeasible to apply Sankoff-based structural aligners such as FoldAlign [144–146], dynalign [147, 148], or locarna [149, 150] to complete genomes, it has become feasible to screen homologous regions that have been identified as syntenic.

Both dynalign and FoldAlign follow the original Sankoff algorithm [151] and include both energy and alignment scoring in a objective function. In contrast, locarna takes pre-computed base pairing probability matrices of the individual sequences as input and then uses a Sankoff algorithm with a very simple scoring model and a restriction to the frequent base pairs present in the input. This allows for a reduction of computational complexity as the low chance pairs can be filtered on the fly [149]. In FoldAlign the Sankoff algorithm is explicitly made local while a forward dynamic programming allows for a heuristic pruning scheme to reduce the computational complexity. For more details, we refer to [152].

While FoldAlign computes local pairwise structural alignments, CMfinder can conduct local structural alignment of multiple sequences [153]. The core idea of CMfinder is to consider a set of related, but unaligned sequences. Initially, the sequences are folded single-wise using RNAfold [154] to generate putative RNA structures. Conversely, small stretches of identical sequences are found by BLAST [114]. These are subsequently used as anchors to build CMs (using the Infernal) and these are then used to screen the sequences for further matches. An EM (Expectation-Maximization) step is, in similar ways to the sequence based motifs search program MEME [155], then used to refine the CMs, screen the sequences again and so on until convergence is obtained. More details can also be found in [156]. Detailed benchmarking studies of RNA structure prediction methods are described in [157, 158].

4.2.2 Computational Methods Applied for Genome-Wide Discovery

A simple approach is to use available genome-wide MSAs and to realign local slices, that is sliding windows, using more expensive and accurate methods. This idea has been tested for RNAz 2.0 [50], leading to a substantial improvement in accuracy. More recently, the REAPR pipeline [159] introduced a very efficient banding technique for multiple RNA alignments making possible to apply an enhanced version of locarna [149] to improve MSAs on a genome-wide scale. Coupled with RNAz 2.0 the REAPR realignments also resulted in a substantial increase of sensitivity [159].

Whereas these screens explicitly make use of the sequence based alignment, free structural alignment screens have also been carried out, but under the constraint that the sequences are corresponding to one another in the genomic context. In that regard an early screen was made using an older version of FoldAlign, where alignable regions between human and mouse (as of UCSC genome browser) were used to anchor unaligned sequence [160] that are potential homologs. The borders of a block of sequence-based alignment were used to extend (sequence-wise) the corresponding unaligned sequences until reaching another block of sequence-wise alignment, gaps or repeat sequence. Hence on all the pair-wise regions not aligned in sequence, these were fed into FoldAlign. The resulting screen was subsequently analyzed experimentally including northern blots [160].

The CMfinder tool was applied to a bacteria over 5'UTRs extracted from genes with conserved domains [161]. Through a range filtering steps both of evolutionary and score-wise nature 22 resulting candidates were obtained. CMfinder was also employed on the early ENCODE project data covering 1% of the human genome [162] and in contrast to the combined RNAz and EvoFold ignored the multiple sequence based alignments and processed the sequences unaligned [163]. Thus corresponding genomic sequences between the mammalian/vertebrate genomes were structurally aligned from scratch. A *composite* score was employed that weighted two ratios, all multiplied by the number of species. The first is the ratio of sequence conservation and the average sequence identity, and the second is the ratio of the number of base pairs in the consensus sequence and the length of the obtained alignment. The FDR was estimated to 50%. Interestingly, the overlap to the RNAz and EvoFold is not large (*see* Fig. 2). At first glance this might appear as a surprise given that the methods are attempting to solve the same task. Obviously this shows that all methods can be improved, but given that the three methods employ three fairly disjoint strategies this is not a surprise and the full pictures should be seen as a complement of all three methods.

CMfinder was recently applied to a genome-wide screen of the human genome searching structurally aligned and thereby predicted conserved RNA structures (CRSs), using ~160 CPU years resulting in ~780,000 hits covering ~516,000 regions with an estimated FDR of about 14% [66]. The screen revealed enrichment for CRSs in several functionally defined classes of elements most notably transcribed regulatory regions. Compared to the screen of the 1% ENCODE regions, the scoring scheme has substantially been updated. Although this approach is similar to EvoFold's phylo-SCFG, it deviates in numerous ways including taking poorly conserved regions into account (neutral evolution or alignment errors), use a simpler model of base-pairs, indels and other gaps, and as indicated above takes folding energies into account.

4.3 Structured RNAs in Coding Regions

The worlds of protein-coding genes and those of noncoding RNAs (ncRNAs) are often seen as clearly separated. A small number of examples from both prokaryotes and eukaryotes, reviewed in [164], demonstrate that this is not strictly true, however: there are evolutionary conserved functional RNA structures that are superimposed on well-conserved, functional ORFs. Important examples are the mammalian steroid receptor activator gene SRA

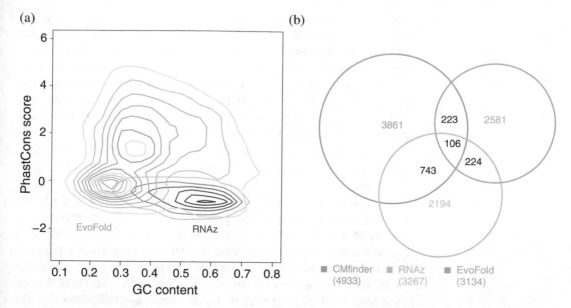

Fig. 2 (a) Comparison of EvoFold and RNAz predictions in the regions selected for the ENCODE pilot study [179]. **(b)** Overlap in prediction of CMfinder, RNAz and EvoFold on the 1% ENCODE regions (adapted from [163])

[165], although a recent study did not confirm significant covariation of the predicted base pairs [166], the fruitfly *oscar* RNA [167], or internal ribosome entry sites (IRES) of some viral coding genes [168]. Recent finding suggests the phenomenon of dual functions both as a coding mRNA and a structured ncRNAs may be much more common than previously thought [169, 170].

Computational approaches point in the same direction. At present RNAdecoder [171] is the only tool specifically designed to recognize evolutionary conserved RNA secondary that is superimposed on an ORF. With its help statistical evidence for a large number of such elements has been reported in [172]. More recently, it was shown that RNAz also functions on coding regions albeit with reduced specificity [173]. A screen of fruitfly genomes suggested that there should be at least hundreds of transcripts with dual functions. In an ORF-centered approach, strong evidence for large-scale superposition of additional functions, including RNA second structure, was reported for both fly [174] and mammalian genomes [175].

4.4 Evaluating Large Scale Screens

It is a common feature of all the classification tools for structured RNAs discussed in the previous section that they perform nearly perfectly in discriminating the well-conserved structured RNAs compiled by the Rfam database from random genomic locations or shuffled decoys. In genome-wide applications, however, the very large numbers of test are performed and, more crucially, many or most of the screened alignments blocks differ drastically in conservation and sequence composition from typical Rfam alignments. Such inputs, however, may be misclassified with much higher frequencies than those used for training. To a certain extent, this effect is reduced by training the classifiers on shuffled alignments that preserve important characteristic of the positive training data; still little can be said about regions of the feature space that are not populated by test or training instances.

Shuffling techniques can be used to destroy the secondary structure signal in an input alignment while at the same time preserving all other important features of the input. A "mock" (background) screen that evaluates a shuffled version of all input alignments from the real (foreground) screen yields an estimate of the number of false positive predictions. All classification tools also provide some scoring parameter λ that expresses each method's internal confidence into a particular prediction. For instance, RNAz reports the classification confidence of its support vector machine, EvoFold reports a length-normalized likelihood-ratio score, CMfinder computes a *pscore* by essentially adding a model for poorly conserved regions to the EvoFold scoring, and a heuristic P-score was developed for the FoldAlign approach. This parameter can then be used to control the false discovery rate by simply counting the number $F(\lambda)$ of predictions in the real (foreground) screen with a score not worse than λ and the number $B(\lambda)$ of predictions in the mock (background) screen with a score not worse than λ. The false discovery rate for cutoff λ is then FDR$(\lambda) = B(\lambda)/F(\lambda)$ [176]. It is important to keep in mind that this estimate of the FDR is only as good as the approximation of the true background by the shuffled alignments. The FDR(λ) can also be broken into bins of sequence identity and GC content, as these two covariates often impact prediction quality, e.g. [66].

Two distinct approaches are available for generating the background: (1) the selection of background data from the genome, or (2) the construction of artificial background data. For studies that focus their foreground on particular regions of the genome one may choose regions from the remainder of the genome as background. Ideally the background sample matches the foreground in as many potentially confounding factors as possible. Of course, one needs to have reason to believe that the feature of interest is really confined to foreground set. Because of the pervasive transcription of most genomes, it seems difficult to argue that some genomic regions will be devoid of evolutionary conserved functional RNAs. In such a setting, the background model has to be created artificially using an appropriate randomization technique.

4.5 Alignment Shuffling Techniques

Shuffling methods for alignments are conceptually based on shuffling approaches for sequences. Correspondingly, shuffled alignments correspond to permutations of alignment columns. In addition to the preservation of sequence composition and, in more modern approaches, dinucleotide patterns, however, it is also necessary to control gaps in the shuffled alignments [43].

The `Alifoldz` program [42] introduced a shuffling procedure that would swap columns of an alignment only if the two columns exhibit the same gap pattern and similar level of sequence conservation. This works well for smaller alignments, however, for alignments with many sequences of low similarity, often not enough pairs of columns eligible for swapping can be found, so that the randomization is incomplete. A standalone version `rnazRandomizeAln.pl` is available as part of the `RNAz` suite. `shufflepair.pl` [177] simultaneously preserves dinucleotide frequency, gaps, and local conservation in pairwise sequence alignments. `Multiperm` [178] preserves not only the gap and local conservation structure in alignments of arbitrarily many sequences, but also the approximate dinucleotide frequencies.

4.6 A Puzzling Lack of Consistency

Over the last decade genomic screens for conserved RNA structures have been conducted with different methods that evaluate blocks of aligned sequences. The results consistently showed disappointingly little overlap between the different methods. A closer inspection of the distributions of sequence conservation, GC content, and depth of the sequence alignment, however, reveals that the "sweet spots" of the different methods are very different, and times nearly mutually exclusive.

For example, `RNAz` 1.0 favors high GC content and rather moderate levels of sequence conservation, while `evofold` focuses on AU-rich sequences with substantially higher conservation, Fig. 2a. Similarly, `sissiz`, `sizziz` with ribosome-like scoring, and `RNAz` 2.0 clearly operate optimally in very different regimes [81]. The `FoldAlign`-based approach [160], which evaluates structural alignments, operates largely in a regime that is inaccessible to all methods that require sequence alignments as input.

Despite an excellent classification performance on benchmark sets of (mostly) structured RNAs taken from the `Rfam` database, estimates of FDR obtained from shuffled sequences remain as high as 50–80% for single classifiers such as `RNAz` [50]. Both the `FoldAlign` screen in [160] and the `CMfinder` screen in [163] had estimated false positive rates of 50%. More complex strategies as pursued in [81] can reduce the FDR to about 5–20% by choosing the most effective classifier as a function of GC content and sequence conservation in the alignment block. Improved scoring schemes including the GC content used in a recent `CMfinder`-based survey [66] also reduced the FDR to about 14%.

FDR estimates can differ dramatically depending on the shuffling method used to construct the background model. In particular, preservation of dinucleotide frequencies (a major difference between RNAz 1.0 and RNAz 2.0) has a major beneficial impact [50]. There seems to be also an influence of the phylogenetic group under consideration. FDR estimates for drosophilids, for example, are systematically smaller than for mammals (RNAz 1.0, for instance, reports 56 vs. 81% [50, 180]).

The inclusion of known 3D motifs may serve as an efficient filter for predicted RNA structures. For example, recently, it was shown that combining RNAz screens with searches for RNA 3D modules can lower the FDR of the RNAz [181]. This combination led to a decrease of the original FDR of 47% by down to a factor of 4 using sissiz shufflings. An issue with such methods is, of course, that they are restricted to previously cataloged 3D motifs such as K-turns and thus may introduced systematic biases towards certain ncRNA classes.

4.7 RNA Genes from Conserved Splice Sites

Spliceosomal splice sites are marked by highly conserved sequence motifs that can easily be recognized by position-specific weight matrices or similar statistical models [182]. It is possible, therefore, to identify evolutionary conserved splice donors and acceptors in multiple sequence alignments. In combination with additional machine learning techniques that evaluate the sequence between consecutive splice donor/acceptor pairs, either short introns [183] or short exons [184] can be identified with very high specificity from genome-wide MSAs alone. To increase the specificity for the large genomes of vertebrates, species specific PSSM models of splice site motives were extended to a full evolutionary model encapsulating the position-wise evolution of the sequence motifs [184]. The approach has led to the discovery of several evolutionary well-conserved mlncRNAs. It has been made obsolete, however, by the availability of cost-effective transcriptome data.

4.8 RNA Gene Finding in Procaryotes

The special structure of procaryotic genes has been employed to help identify sRNA genes. In particular, promoter and terminator elements are identifiable in many bacterial species. In particular rho-independent terminators, which feature a characteristic stem-loop structure can often, but not always, be identified directly from the genomic sequence [185, 186]. It is important to notice that some, and possibly many, bacterial clades do not seem to have this type of terminator elements [11]. In particular in extremophiles, functional RNAs are also distinguished by their base composition [39]. Pipelines such as ISI [187] and sRNAPredict2 [188] and their successors such as [189] integrate comparative genomics approaches with the search for procaryote-specific features. A recent study combines several secondary structure prediction tools and comparative approaches such as qrna and RNAz into a multi-objective meta-method, effectively capitalizing on the different sensitivities and specificities of the individual methods and their different optimal regimes [190].

A very different approach is taken by NAPP [191, 192]. It is based on the idea of phylogenetic profiling, i.e., the distribution of conserved elements non-protein coding RNA elements across a phylogenetically diverse set of bacterial genomes. Clusters of similar sequences with a phylogenetically coherent distribution, or whose presence/absence pattern match that of proteins, are likely candidates for noncoding RNAs. CMfinder has been applied to discover large (structured) bacterial ncRNAs, structured RNAs in general as well as ribozymes [161, 193–195].

As in eukaroytic systems, however, the importance of de novo gene identification is declining with the availability of large RNA-seq data sets for virtually all newly sequences genomes. Nevertheless it remains an important and non-trivial topic to distinguish functional ncRNA genes and regulatory RNA elements form other noncoding parts of the genome.

5 Target Prediction

5.1 General Principles

The search for an RNA target usually relies on the prediction of RNA–RNA interactions. A wide variety of methods have been developed for this task with a wide array of different application scenarios in mind. We refer the reader to [196–198] for comparisons of different methods in a benchmarking studies and focus on the underlying models and algorithmic ideas in the following.

Early approaches for RNA–RNA interaction prediction such as GUUGle [199] were based on the detection of complementary regions using modified alignment strategies. Individual basc pair models such as in TargetRNA [200] or RIsearch [201] follow a similar idea but introduced a simplified energy function for scoring inter-molecular base pairs. The optimal duplex under this model can be determined using a fast alignment-like algorithm. The first full thermodynamic model for the interaction duplex was provided by RNAhybrid [202], which implements a restricted version of the Zuker algorithm.

However, it soon turned out that the internal structure of the participating RNAs has to be taken into account, since the RNA–RNA interaction between complementary regions can be blocked by such internal structures. In principle, two different strategies for integrating internal structures have been pursued. The first one is to predict a common secondary structure for the two interacting RNAs. However, from the computational point of view, this corresponds to the problem of folding pseudoknotted structure and thus is NP-complete [203].

5.2 Restricted RNA-RNA Interaction Models

Thus, several simplifications of the problem have been considered. The first one are co-folding approaches [204, 205], which search for nested structures in the concatenation of the input sequences. However, due to the condition of a nested interaction structure, co-folding approaches exclude many possible interactions such as kissing hairpins. One solution to this problem is suited for the case that we have only one continuous interaction site and has been introduced with RNAup [206]. Here, the influence of intra-molecular base-pairs is summarized into an accessibility term as follows. To allow for an interaction between different RNAs, the interaction sites have to be free of intra-molecular base pairs (accessible). The probability of the sub-population of structures with accessible interaction sites can be calculated using a modified version of the McCaskill algorithm [207]. The log-transform of the accessibility probabilities, i.e., the corresponding ensemble energies, are then added to the duplex energy as a penalty for making the interaction sites accessible. Finally, the interaction with the minimal combined energy is the one predicted as the optimal one. RNAup, however, is too time consuming for genome-wide approaches as it has to store in the dynamic programming (DP) table the start *and* end for each putative interaction site to determine the correct accessibility. There have been two different approaches to reduce this complexity. The first one is IntaRNA [208], which uses a heuristic strategy that does not require to store the ends of interaction sites in the DP tables. In addition, IntaRNA enforces a *seed* region in the interaction, which is a short region (usually around 7 nucleotides) of perfect or near perfect complementarity. Albeit being a heuristic and faster version of RNAup, the seed requirement in IntaRNA seems to compensate for the heuristic choices as the prediction performance of IntaRNA and RNAup is essentially the same [209]. The other strategy is implemented in RNAplex [210]. Here, the calculation of the accessibility probability for the whole site is essentially approximated by a Markov-Chain with a limited history, which also avoids to store the end of interaction sites in the DP table.

5.3 RIP Model

RNAup, IntaRNA, and RNAplex can predict kissing hairpin interactions, but are restricted to one continuous interaction site. One possibility is to extend the idea of accessibility-based calculation of RNA–RNA interactions to more than one interaction sites by determining the joint accessibility of several sites [211–213]. The other possibility is to determine a full interacting structure in a restricted structure model that includes kissing hairpins but disallows so-called zig-zag conformations [203] to avoid NP-completeness. This has first been implemented in the IRIS software [214], and was later extended in [203] to a more general energy model, often referred to as the Alkan model. Partition function algorithms for this problem allow to calculate melting temperatures and interaction probabilities [215, 216].

5.4 Conserved Interaction Sites

Albeit these interaction prediction methods mentioned so far are successfully predicting true interactions, the false positive rates in genome-wide screens are usually too high. One possible solution is to search for conserved interactions, however, two different interpretations of conservation have been considered. The first extends the idea of alignment based folding approaches such as RNAalifold [34, 35] for searching conserved RNA structures to RNA–RNA interactions. They determine conserved interaction duplexes, which can be found by searching for conserved base pairs between the alignment of an sRNA and the alignment of a putative conserved target. Examples are Petcofold [65, 217] and ripalign [218]. The existence of a conserved duplex, if found, is a very strong signal for a true interaction. Specialized RNA-RNA interaction prediction tools have been developed for snoRNA target prediction that takes into account the highly specialized structural of the interaction regions [219–222].

However, as shown in [223], the interaction site itself, especially on the target mRNA, is oftentimes not significantly conserved in true interactions. This can be explained by asymmetric nature of sRNA or miRNA regulation, where a single small RNA has a large number of non-homologous targets. As a consequence the small RNA is under extreme selective constraint to maintain its interaction site or sites, while the population of targets, usually mRNAs, shows rapid turnover. To cope with this situation, CopraRNA [224] implements a relates notion of conserved interactions by dropping the requirement of a conserved duplex or interaction sites and instead requiring only the presence of a predicted interaction between homologous sRNA/mRNA pairs in different species. This is achieved by combining the scores of the interaction of a specific sRNA and its putative targets across different species. Technically, this is solved by determining p-values for all possible interactions in each of the considered species. The p-values for the same interaction across different species are then combined using an inverse normal method. CopraRNA yields a much lower false positive rate in comparison to single genome methods as discussed before.

5.5 Fast Genome-Wide Approaches

For large scale, genome or transcriptome-wide applications efficient filters for candidate interactions are required. In this context, index-based string search methods are of interest. The first application of this type was GUUGLE [199], dedicated to identify miRNA/mRNA interactions in plants. It employs a suffix array based search that accommodates G-U wobble pairs. In RIsearch a simplified energy model, neglecting intra-molecular interactions is implemented to increase speed [201]. In RIsearch2 the seed and extend paradigm is integrated directly in the same code, and a data index structures are made for both query and subject (database) sequences resulting in genome-wide applications [225]. This strategy was employed in other applications such as transcriptome-wide siRNA offtarget analysis allowing to siRNAs to be ranked by their offtarget volume, genome-wide calculations of clusters of miRNA targets and fast filtering of targets of the predicted structured RNAs in genomic sequence.

6   RNA Structure-Seq Methods

In the last few years several high-throughput methods have become available that use chemical and enzymatic probing coupled with next generation sequencing as readout. Computational analyses have focussed on integrating the measurements into RNA folding programs. This is typically achieved by interpreting SHAPE reactivity data measures to pseudoenergies [226–228]. Using different models of bonus energies, the same approach can also be used for chemical probing DMS [229] or enzymatic probing (PARS [230, 231]). The use of such "soft constraints" has been shown consistently to improve the accuracy of structure prediction [232]. The latest versions of the `ViennaRNA` package provides a generic handling of such external data [233, 234]. At present, very little comparative work has been done with this type of data. In principle, structure-seq data could be either compared directly between homologous species or used to first improve the structure predictions and then to use existing methods of RNA structure comparison.

7   Concluding Remarks

Despite the flood of RNA-seq data even the best studied genomes feature rather incomplete ncRNA annotations owing to both computational and experimental difficulties. Low expression levels and highly specific spatio-temporal expression patterns make it difficult to obtain exhaustive transcript catalaogs. Poor sequence conservation, on the other hand, makes it difficult to establish homology through the conservation of secondary structure or splicing patterns. The restriction of computational surveys to syntenic regions somewhat simplified the problem. The rapid evolution of the genomes themselves, however, leaves much territory hard to access. Recent surprising discoveries such as the highly structured large bacterial RNAs reported in [193] clearly demonstrate that our knowledge of the "RNome" is still far from complete.

A general concern affecting all studies of lncRNA evolution are potential ascertainment biases in the initial sets. Annotation efforts tend to favor well-characterized transcripts and appear to be biased against unspliced transcripts. In addition, 3′ ends of non-poly-A transcripts are often poorly determined, and even many gene models of protein-coding mRNAs are likely truncated. While it is likely that qualitative patterns summarized in this chapter hold true, specific quantitative statements maybe subject to change with more complete data sources.

Comparative genomics of RNA is still a rapidly evolving field with many exciting topics having received little or no attention from a comparative perspective. A rapidly growing field of research is the investigation of RNA–protein interactions at global scales. Experimental techniques such RIP, CLIP, and ChIRP coupled with high throughput sequencing as readout are starting to paint a comprehensive picture of the universe of RNA binding proteins. Their interaction with RNAs typically requires specific sequence patterns and in many cases also a preferred structural environment [235]. It remains an exciting question to what extent evolutionary conserved RNA–protein interactions contribute to the conservation of DNA sequence elements and the many conserved secondary structure features. A large fraction of well-annotated long noncoding RNAs is involved in chromatin-related processes. Many of them appear to target multiple specific chromosomal locations [236, 237]. As in the case of RNA–protein interactions, it remains to be seen to what extent such RNA–DNA interactions are maintained over large evolutionary times.

Recent advances in RNA biochemistry and high throughput methods have led to the discovery of systematic chemical modifications of many classes of RNA molecules beyond the classical example of tRNAs, spawning a new research field of *epitranscriptomics* [238–240]. The impact of the many post-transcriptional chemical modifications on RNA structure and functions is still largely an open question. Even less is known about their evolutionary computation.

Currently available model of RNA evolution assumes that RNA structures are conserved by maintaining exact patterns of base pairing. This is not necessarily the case however. It may suffice at time to maintain the overall show of a molecules. PKR, for example, recognized long co-linear stem structures [241], which may be realized by co-axial stacking in quite different secondary structures [242, 243]. Conceivably, large numbers of RNA structures escape detection because structural conservation and sequence homology are incongruent, as in the example of stem-sliding in Fig. 3. Attempts to model their 3D structure promise substantial advances in such cases.

```
. ( ( ( ( ( . . . . ) ) ) ) ) .
. ( ( ( ( ( . . . . - ) ) ) ) ) .
ACCCCCUCCGGGGGGA
ACCCCCUCCG-GGGGGA
CCCCCCUCCGGGGGGA
CCCCCCUCCG-GGGGGA
CCCCCCUCCCGGGGGA
-CCCCCCUCCCGGGGGA
( ( ( ( ( ( . . . . . ) ) ) ) ) .
- ( ( ( ( ( . . . . . ) ) ) ) ) .
```

Fig. 3 Evolutionary stem sliding. The two hairpins shown in "dot-parenthesis" notation have no base pair in common. The middle structure folds into both structures with similar energy, the mutants fix different alternatives. The best sequence and the best structure alignment are different in this case

Acknowledgements

This work was funded in part by the German Federal Ministry of Education and Research (BMBF; 031A538B) within the German Network for Bioinformatics Infrastructure (de.NBI), the Deutsche Forschungsgemeinschaft (DFG; BA 2168/11-2, BA2168/3-3, and STA 850/19) within the Priority Programme SPP 1738, the Innovation Fund Denmark (0603-00320B, 5163-00010B), The Danish Council for Independent Research (DFF-4005-00443).

References

1. Kapranov P, Willingham AT, Gingeras TR (2007) Genome-wide transcription and the implications for genomic organization. Nat Rev Genet 8:413–423

2. Carninci P, FANTOM Consortium (2005) The transcriptional landscape of the mammalian genome. Science 309:1559–1563

3. ENCODE Project Consortium (2012) An integrated encyclopedia of DNA elements in the human genome. Nature 489:57–74

4. Derrien T, Johnson R, Bussotti G, Tanzer A, Djebali S, Tilgner H, Guernec G, Martin D, Merkel A, Knowles DG, Lagarde J, Veeravalli L, Ruan X, Ruan Y, Lassmann T, Carninci P, Brown JB, Lipovich L, Gonzalez JM, Thomas M, Davis CA, Shiekhattar R, Gingeras TR, Hubbard TJ, Notredame C, Harrow J, Guigó R (2012) The GENCODE v7 catalog of human long noncoding RNAs: analysis of their gene structure, evolution, and expression. Genome Res 22:1775–1789

5. Clark MB, Amaral PP, Schlesinger FJ, Dinger ME, Taft RJ, Rinn JL, Ponting CP, Stadler PF, Morris KJ, Morillon A, Rozowsky JS, Gerstein M, Wahlestedt C, Hayashizaki Y, Carninci P, Gingeras TR, Mattick JS (2011) The reality of pervasive transcription. PLoS Biol 9:e1000625

6. Tisseur M, Kwapisz M, Morillon A (2011) Pervasive transcription – lessons from yeast. Biochimie 93:1889–1896

7. Wu J, Delneri D, O'Keefe RT (2012) Non-coding RNAs in *Saccharomyces cerevisiae*: what is the function? Biochem Soc Trans 40:907–911

8. Leong HS, Dawson K, Wirth C, Li Y, Wirth Y, Smith DL, Wilkinson CRM, Miller CJ (2014) A global non-coding RNA system

modulates fission yeast protein levels in response to stress. Nat Commun 5:3947

9. Xuan H, Zhang L, Liu X, Han G, Li J, Li X, Liu A, Liao M, Zhang S (2015) PLNlncRbase: a resource for experimentally identified lncRNAs in plants. Gene 573:328–332

10. Woehle C, Kusdian G, Radine C, Graur D, Landan G, Gould SB (2014) The parasite *Trichomonas vaginalis expresses* thousands of pseudogenes and long non-coding RNAs independently from functional neighbouring genes. BMC Genomics 15:906

11. Sharma CM, Hoffmann S, Darfeuille F, Reignier J, Findeiß S, Sittka A, Chabas S, Reiche K, Hackermüller J, Reinhardt RR, Stadler PF, Vogel J (2010) The primary transcriptome of the major human pathogen *Helicobacter pylori*. Nature 464:250–255

12. Lybecker M, Bilusic I, Raghavan R (2014) Pervasive transcription: detecting functional RNAs in bacteria. Transcription 5:e944039

13. Wade JT, Grainger DC (2014) Pervasive transcription: illuminating the dark matter of bacterial transcriptomes. Nat Rev Microbiol 12:647–653

14. Perkel JM (2013) Visiting "noncodarnia". BioTechniques 54(6):303–304

15. Mercer TR, Dinger ME, Mattick JS (2009) Long non-coding RNAs: insights into functions. Nat Rev Genet 10(3):155–159

16. Wassarman KM, Repoila F, Rosenow C, Storz G, Gottesman S (2001) Identification of novel small RNAs using comparative genomics and microarrays. Genes Dev. 15 (13):1637–1651

17. Marz M, Gruber AR, Siederdissen CH, Amman F, Badelt S, Bartschat S, Bernhart SH, Beyer S, Kehr W, Lorenz R, Tanzer A, Yusuf D, Tafer H, Hofacker IL, Stadler PF (2011) Animal snoRNAs and scaRNAs with exceptional structures. RNA Biol 8:938–946

18. Bompfünewerer AF, Flamm C, Fried C, Fritzsch G, Hofacker IL, Lehmann J, Missal K, Mosig A, Müller B, Prohaska SJ, Stadler BMR, Stadler PF, Tanzer A, Washietl S, Witwer C (2005) Evolutionary patterns of non-coding RNAs. Theory Biosci. 123:301–369

19. The Athanasius F. Bompfünewerer RNA Consortium, Backofen R, Flamm C, Fried C, Fritzsch G, Hackermüller J, Hertel J, Hofacker IL, Missal K, Mosig SJ, Prohaska A, Rose D, Stadler PF, Tanzer A, Washietl S, Sebastian W (2007) RNAs everywhere: genome-wide annotation of structured RNAs. J Exp Zool B: Mol Dev Evol 308B:1–25

20. Hertel J, Stadler PF (2015) The expansion of animal microRNA families revisited. Life 5:905–920

21. Brown JW, Echeverria M, Qu LH (2003) Plant snoRNAs: functional evolution and new modes of gene expression. Trends Plant Sci 8:42–49

22. Kehr S, Bartschat S, Tafer H, Stadler PF, Hertel J (2014) Matching of soulmates: coevolution of snoRNAs and their targets. Mol Biol Evol 31:455–467

23. Jorjani H, Kehr S, Jedlinski DJ, Gumienny R, Hertel J, Stadler PF, Zavolan M, Gruber AR (2016) An updated human snoRNAome. Nucleic Acids Res 44(11):5068–5082

24. Bhattacharya DP, Bartschat S, Kehr S, Hertel J, Grosse I, Stadler PF (2016) Phylogenetic distribution of plant snoRNA families. BMC Genomics 17:969

25. Gorodkin J, Ruzzo WL (2014) RNA sequence, structure, and function: computational and bioinformatic methods. In: Methods in molecular biology, vol 1097. Humana Press/Springer, New York

26. Fontana W, Stadler PF, Bornberg-Bauer EG, Griesmacher T, Hofacker IL, Tacker M, Tarazona P, Weinberger ED, Schuster P (1993) RNA folding landscapes and combinatory landscapes. Phys Rev E 47:2083–2099

27. Schuster P, Fontana W, Stadler PF, Hofacker IL (1994) From sequences to shapes and back: a case study in RNA secondary structures. Proc R Soc Lond B 255:279–284

28. Nussinov R, Pieczenik G, Griggs JR, Kleitman DJ (1978) Algorithms for loop matchings. SIAM J Appl Math 35(1):68–82

29. Zuker M, Stiegler P (1981) Optimal computer folding of large RNA sequences using thermodynamics and auxilary information. Nucleic Acids Res 9(1):133–147

30. Zuker M (1989) On finding all suboptimal foldings of an RNA molecule. Science 244:48–52

31. Wuchty S, Fontana W, Hofacker IL, Schuster P (1999) Complete suboptimal folding of RNA and the stability of secondary structures. Biopolymers 49:145–165

32. McCaskill JS (1990) The equilibrium partition function and base pair binding probabilities for RNA secondary structure. Biopolymers 29(6–7):1105–1119

33. Ding Y, Lawrence CE (2001) Statistical prediction of single-stranded regions in RNA secondary structure and application to

predicting effective antisense target sites and beyond. Nucleic Acids Res 29(5):1034–1046

34. Hofacker IL, Fekete M, Stadler PF (2002) Secondary structure prediction for aligned RNA sequences. J Mol Biol 319:1059–1066

35. Bernhart SH, Hofacker IL, Will S, Gruber AR, Stadler PF (2008) RNAalifold: improved consensus structure prediction for RNA alignments. BMC Bioinf 9:474

36. Knudsen B, Hein J (2003) Pfold: RNA secondary structure prediction using stochastic context-free grammars. Nucleic Acids Res 31 (13):3423–3428

37. Sükösd Z, Knudsen B, Kjems J, Pedersen CN (2012) PPfold 3.0: fast RNA secondary structure prediction using phylogeny and auxiliary data. Bioinformatics 28:2691–2692

38. Seemann SE, Gorodkin J, Backofen R (2008) Unifying evolutionary and thermodynamic information for RNA folding of multiple alignments. Nucleic Acids Res 36 (20):6355–6362

39. Klein RJ, Misulovin Z, Eddy SR (2002) Noncoding RNA genes identified in AT-rich hyperthermophiles. Proc Natl Acad Sci USA 99:7542–7547

40. Larsson P, Hinas A, Ardell DH, Kirsebom LA, Virtanen A, Söderbom F (2008) *De novo* search for non-coding RNA genes in the AT-rich genome of *Dictyostelium discoideum*: performance of Markov-dependent genome feature scoring. Genome Res 18:888–899

41. Haerty W, Ponting CP (2015) Unexpected selection to retain high GC content and splicing enhancers within exons of multiexonic lncRNA loci. RNA 21:333–346

42. Washietl S, Hofacker IL (2004) Consensus folding of aligned sequences as a new measure for the detection of functional RNAs by comparative genomics. J Mol Biol 342:19–30

43. Washietl S, Hofacker IL, Stadler PF (2005) Fast and reliable prediction of noncoding RNAs. Proc Natl Acad Sci USA 102:2454–2459

44. Clote P, Ferré F, Kranakis E, Krizanc D (2005) Structural RNA has lower folding energy than random RNA of the same dinucleotide frequency. RNA 11:578–591

45. Workman C, Krogh A (1999) No evidence that mRNAs have lower folding free energies than random sequences with the same dinucleotide distribution. Nucleic Acids Res 27:4816–4822

46. Altschul SF, Erickson BW (1985) Significance of nucleotide sequence alignment: a method for random sequence permutation that preserves dinucleotide and codon usage. Mol Biol Evol 2:526–538

47. Fitch WM (1983) Random sequences. J Mol Biol 163:171–176

48. Kandel D, Matias Y, Unger R, Winker P (1996) Shuffling biological sequences. Discr Appl Math 71:171–185

49. Jiang M, Anderson J, Gillespie J, Joel M (2008) uShuffle: a useful tool for shuffling biological sequences while preserving the *k*-let counts. BMC Bioinformatics 9:192

50. Gruber AR, Findeiß S, Washietl S, Hofacker IL, Stadler PF (2010) RNAz 2.0: improved noncoding RNA detection. Pac Symp Biocomput 15:69–79

51. Soldatov RA, Vinogradova SV, Mironov AA (2014) RNASurface: fast and accurate detection of locally optimal potentially structured RNA segments. Bioinformatics 30:457–463

52. Washietl S (2005) Prediction of structured non-coding RNAs by comparative sequence analysis. PhD thesis, Univsity of Vienna

53. van Nimwegen E, Crutchfield JP, Huynen M (1999) Neutral evolution of mutational robustness. Proc Natl Acad Sci USA 96:9716–9720

54. Wagner A, Stadler PF (1999) Viral RNA and evolved mutational robustness. J Exp Zool MDE 285:119–127

55. Ancel LW, Fontana W (2000) Plasticity, evolvability, and modularity in RNA. J Exp Zool MDE 288:242–283

56. Borenstein E, Ruppin E (2006) Direct evolution of genetic robustness in microRNA. Proc Natl Acad Sci USA 103:6593–6598

57. Pei S, Anthony JS, Meyer MM (2015) Sampled ensemble neutrality as a feature to classify potential structured RNAs. BMC Genomics 16:35

58. Gruber AR, Bernhart SH, Hofacker IL, Washietl S (2008) Strategies for measuring evolutionary conservation of RNA secondary structures. BMC Bioinf 9:122

59. Salari R, Kimchi-Sarfaty C, Gottesman MM, Przytycka TM (2013) Sensitive measurement of single-nucleotide polymorphism-induced changes of RNA conformation: application to disease studies. Nucleic Acids Res 41:44–53

60. Sabarinathan R, Tafer H, Seemann SE, Hofacker IL, Stadler PF, Gorodkin J (2013) RNAsnp: efficient detection of local RNA secondary structure changes induced by SNPs. Hum Mut 34:546–556

61. Gardner PP, Wilm A, Washietl S (2005) A benchmark of multiple sequence alignment

programs upon structural RNAs. Nucleic Acids Res 33:2433–2439

62. Parsch J, Braverman JM, Stephan W (2000) Comparative sequence analysis and patterns of covariation in RNA secondary structures. Genetics 154:909–921

63. Coventry A, Kleitman DJ, Berger B (2004) MSARI: multiple sequence alignments for statistical detection of RNA secondary structure. Proc Natl Acad Sci USA 101:12102–12107

64. di Bernardo D, Down T, Hubbard T (2003) ddbRNA: detection of conserved secondary structures in multiple alignments. Bioinformatics 19:1606–1611

65. Seemann SE, Richter AS, Gorodkin J, Backofen R (2010) Hierarchical folding of multiple sequence alignments for the prediction of structures and RNA-RNA interactions. Algorithms Mol Biol 5:22

66. Seemann SE, Mirza AH, Hansen C, Bang-Berthelsen CH, Garde C, Christensen-Dalsgaard M, Torarinsson E, Yao Z, Workman C, Pociot H, Nielsen F, Tommerup N, Ruzzo WL, Gorodkin J (2017) The identification and functional annotation of RNA structures conserved in vertebrates. Genome Res 27(8):1371–1383

67. Lindgreen S, Gardner PP, Krogh A (2006) Measuring covariation in RNA alignments: physical realism improves information measures. Bioinformatics 22:2988–2995

68. Menzel P, Seemann SE, Gorodkin J (2012) RILogo: visualizing RNA-RNA interactions. Bioinformatics 28(19):2523–2526

69. Piskol R, Stephan W (2011) Selective constraints in conserved folded RNAs of Drosophilid and Hominid genomes. Mol Biol Evol 28:1519–1529

70. Kusumi J, Ichinose M, Takefu M, Piskol R, Stephan W, Iizuka M (2016) A model of compensatory molecular evolution involving multiple sites in RNA molecules. J Theor Biol 388:96–107

71. Ponjavic J, Ponting CP, Lunter G (2007) Functionality or transcriptional noise? Evidence for selection within long noncoding RNAs. Genome Res 17:556–565

72. Pang KC, Frith MC, Mattick JS (2006) Rapid evolution of noncoding RNAs: lack of conservation does not mean lack of function. Trends Genet 22:1–5

73. Marques AC, Ponting CP (2009) Catalogues of mammalian long noncoding RNAs: modest conservation and incompleteness. Genome Biol 10:R124

74. Guttman M, Amit I, Garber M, French C, Lin MF, Feldser D, Huarte M, Zuk O, Carey BW, Cassady JP, Cabili MN, Jaenisch R, Mikkelsen TS, Jacks T, Hacohen N, Bernstein BE, Kellis M, Regev A, Rinn JL, Lander ES (2009) Chromatin signature reveals over a thousand highly conserved large non-coding RNAs in mammals. Nature 458:223–227

75. Managadze D, Lobkovsky AE, Wolf YI, Shabalina SA, Rogozin IB, Koonin EV (2013) The vast, conserved mammalian lincRNome. PLoS Comput Biol 9:e1002917

76. Hüttenhofer A, Schattner P, Polacek N (2005) Non-coding RNAs: hope or hype? Trends Genet 21:289–297

77. Palazzo AF, Lee ES (2015) Non-coding RNA: what is functional and what is junk? Front Genet 6:2

78. Johnsson P, Lipovich L, Grandér D, Morris KV (2014) Evolutionary conservation of long non-coding RNAs: sequence, structure, function. Biochim Biophys Acta 1840:1063–1071

79. Schüler A, Ghanbarian AT, Hurst LD (2014) Purifying selection on splice-related motifs, not expression level nor RNA folding, explains nearly all constraint on human lincRNAs. Mol Biol Evol 31:3164–3183

80. Mercer TR, Mattick JS (2013) Structure and function of long noncoding RNAs in epigenetic regulation. Nat Struct Mol Biol 20:300–307

81. Smith MA, Gesell T, Stadler PF, Mattick JS (2013) Widespread purifying selection on RNA structure in mammals. Nucleic Acids Res 41:8220–8236

82. Hezroni H, Koppstein D, Schwartz MG, Avrutin A, Bartel DP, Ulitsky I (2015) Principles of long noncoding RNA evolution derived from direct comparison of transcriptomes in 17 species. Cell 11:1110–1122

83. Washietl S, Kellis M, Garber M (2014) Evolutionary dynamics and tissue specificity of human long noncoding RNAs in six mammals. Genome Res 24:616–628

84. Kutter C, Watt S, Stefflova K, Wilson MD, Goncalves A, Ponting CP, Odom DT, Marques AC (2012) Rapid turnover of long noncoding RNAs and the evolution of gene expression. PLoS Genet 8:e1002841

85. Necsulea A, Soumillon M, Warnefors M, Liechti A, Daish T, Zeller U, Baker J, Grützner F, Kaessmann H (2014) The evolution of lncRNA repertoires and expression patterns in tetrapods. Nature 505:635–640

86. Ward M, McEwan C, Mill JD, Janitz M (2015) Conservation and tissue-specific transcription patterns of long noncoding RNAs. J Hum Transcr 1:2–9

87. Ulitsky I, Shkumatava A, Jan CH, Sive H, Bartel DP (2011) Conserved function of lincRNAs in vertebrate embryonic development despite rapid sequence evolution. Cell 147:1537–1550

88. Young RS, Marques AC, Tibbit C, Haerty W, Bassett AR, Liu JL, Ponting CP (2012) Identification and properties of 1,119 candidate lincRNA loci in the *Drosophila melanogaster* genome. Genome Biol Evol 4:427–442

89. Nitsche A, Rose D, Fasold M, Reiche K, Stadler PF (2015) Comparison of splice sites reveals that long non-coding RNAs are evolutionarily well conserved. RNA 21:801–812

90. Eng L, Coutinho G, Nahas S, Yeo G, Tanouye R, Babaei M, Dörk T, Burge C, Gatti RA (2004) Nonclassical splicing mutations in the coding and noncoding regions of the ATM gene: maximum entropy estimates of splice junction strengths. Hum Mutat 23:67–76

91. Canzler S, Stadler PF, Hertel J (2016) U6 snRNA intron insertion occurred multiple times during fungi evolution. RNA Biol 13:119–127

92. Louhichi A, Fourati A, Rebaï A (2011) IGD: a resource for intronless genes in the human genome. Gene 488:35–40

93. Nakaya HI, Amaral PP, Louro R, Lopes A, Fachel AA, Moreira YB, El-Jundi TA, da Silva AM, Reis EM, Verjovski-Almeida S (2007) Genome mapping and expression analyses of human intronic noncoding RNAs reveal tissue-specific patterns and enrichment in genes related to regulation of transcription. Genome Biol 8:R43

94. Louro R, Nakaya HI, Amaral PP, Festa F, Sogayar MC, da Silva AM, Verjovski-Almeida-S, Reis EM (2007) Androgen responsive intronic non-coding RNAs. BMC Biol 5:4

95. Louro R, El-Jundi T, Nakaya HI, Reis EM, Verjovski-Almeida S (2008) Conserved tissue expression signatures of intronic noncoding RNAs transcribed from human and mouse loci. Genomics 92:18–25

96. Engelhardt J, Stadler PF (2012) Hidden treasures in unspliced EST data. Theory Biosci 131:49–57.

97. Rinn JL, Euskirchen G, Bertone P, Martone R, Luscombe NM, Hartman S, Harrison PM, Nelson FK, Miller P, Gerstein M, Weissman S, Snyder M (2003) The transcriptional activity of human chromosome 22. Genes Dev 17:529–540

98. Reis EM, Nakaya HI, Louro R, Canavez FC, Flatschart AV, Almeida GT, Egidio CM, Paquola AC, Machado AA, Festa F, Yamamoto D, Alvarenga R, da Silva CC, Brito GC, Simon SD, Moreira-Filho CA, Leite KR, Camara-Lopes LH, Campos FS, Gimba E, Vignal GM, El-Dorry H, Sogayar MC, Barcinski MA, da Silva AM, Verjovski-Almeida S (2004) Antisense intronic non-coding RNA levels correlate to the degree of tumor differentiation in prostate cancer. Oncogene 23:6684–6692

99. Beckedorff FC, Ayupe AC, Crocci-Souza R, Amaral MS, Nakaya HI, Soltys DT, Menck CFM, Reis EM, Verjovski-Almeida S (2013) The intronic long noncoding RNA ANRASSF1 recruits PRC2 to the *RASSF1A* promoter, reducing the expression of *RASSF1A* and increasing cell proliferation. PLoS Genet 9:e1003705

100. Sasaki YTF, Ideue T, Sano M, Mituyama T, Hirose T (2009) MENε/β noncoding RNAs are essential for structural integrity of nuclear paraspeckles. Proc Natl Acad Sci USA 106:2525–2530

101. Sunwoo H, Dinger ME, Wilusz JE, Amaral PP, Mattick JS, Spector DL (2009) MEN ε/β nuclear-retained non-coding RNAs are up-regulated upon muscle differentiation and are essential components of paraspeckles. Genome Res 19:347–359

102. Mao YS, Sunwoo H, Zhang B, Spector DL (2011) Direct visualization of the co-transcriptional assembly of a nuclear body by noncoding RNAs. Nat Cell Biol 13:95–101

103. Stadler PF (2010) Evolution of the long non-coding RNAs MALAT1 and MENβ/ε. In: Ferreira CE, Miyano S, Stadler PF (eds.) Advances in bioinformatics and computational biology, 5th brazilian symposium on bioinformatics. Lecture notes in computer science, vol 6268. Springer, Heidelberg, pp 1–12

104. Chung S, Nakagawa H, Uemura M, Piao L, Ashikawa K, Hosono N, Takata R, Akamatsu S, Kawaguchi T, Morizono T, Tsunoda T, Daigo Y, Matsuda K, Kamatani N, Nakamura Y, Kubo M (2011) Association of a novel long non-coding RNA in 8q24 with prostate cancer susceptibility. Cancer Sci 102:245–252

105. Hackermüller J, Reiche K, Otto C, Hösler N, Blumert C, Brocke-Heidrich K, Böhlig L, Nitsche A, Kasack K, Ahnert P, Krupp W, Engeland K, Stadler PF, Horn F (2014) Cell cycle, oncogenic and tumor suppressor pathways regulate numerous long and macro non-protein coding RNAs. Genome Biol 15:R48

106. Kapranov P, St Laurent G, Raz T, Ozsolak F, Reynolds CP, Sorensen PH, Reaman G, Milos P, Arceci RJ, Thompson JF, Triche TJ (2010) The majority of total nuclear-encoded non-ribosomal RNA in a human cell is 'dark matter' un-annotated RNA. BMC Biol 8:149

107. Seidl CIM, Stricker SH, Barlow DP (2006) The imprinted Air ncRNA is an atypical RNA-PII transcript that evades splicing and escapes nuclear export. EMBO J 25:1–11

108. Stricker SH, Steenpass L, Pauler FM, Santoro F, Latos PA, Huang R, Koerner MV, Sloane MA, Warczok KE, Barlow DP (2008) Silencing and transcriptional properties of the imprinted Airn ncRNA are independent of the endogenous promoter. EMBO J 27:3116–3128

109. Redrup L, Branco MR, Perdeaux ER, Krueger C, Lewis A, Santos F, Nagano T, Cobb BS, Fraser P, Reik W (2009) The long noncoding RNA Kcnq1ot1 organises a lineage-specific nuclear domain for epigenetic gene silencing. Development 136:525–530

110. Mercer TR, Wilhelm D, Dinger ME, Soldà G, Korbie DJ, Glazov EA, Truong V, Schwenke M, Simons C, Matthaei KI, Saint R, Koopman P, Mattick JS (2011) Expression of distinct RNAs from 3' untranslated regions. Nucleic Acids Res 39:2393–2403

111. Engelhardt J, Stadler PF (2015) Evolution of the unspliced transcriptome. BMC Evol Biol 15:166

112. Menzel P, Gorodkin J, Stadler PF (2009) The tedious task of finding homologous non-coding RNA genes. RNA 15:2075–2082

113. Nawrocki EP, Burge SW, Bateman A, Daub J, Eberhardt RY, Eddy SR, Floden EW, Gardner PP, Jones TA, Tate J, Finn RD (2015) Rfam 12.0: updates to the RNA families database. Nucl Acids Res 43:D130–D137

114. Altschul SF, Gish W, Miller W, Myers EW, Lipman DJ (1990) Basic local alignment search tool. J Mol Biol 215:403–410

115. Hertel J, de Jong D, Marz M, Rose D, Tafer H, Tanzer A, Schierwater B, Stadler PF (2009) Non-coding RNA annotation of the genome of *Trichoplax adhaerens*. Nucleic Acids Res 37:1602–1615

116. Menzel P, Stadler PF, Gorodkin J (2011) maxAlike: maximum-likelihood based sequence reconstruction with application to improved primer design for unknown sequences. Bioinformatics 27:317–325

117. Xie M, Mosig A, Qi X, Li Y, Stadler PF, Chen J-L (2008) Size variation and structural conservation of vertebrate telomerase RNA. J Biol Chem 283:2049–2059

118. Lu Y, Sze S-H (2009) Improving accuracy of multiple sequence alignment algorithms based on alignment of neighboring residues. Nucl. Acids Res 37:463–472

119. Bussotti G, Raineri E, Erb I, Zytnicki M, Wilm A, Beaudoing E, Bucher P, Notredame C (2011) BlastR-fast and accurate database searches for non-coding RNAs. Nucleic Acids Res 39:6886–6895

120. Mosig A, Sameith K, Stadler PF (2005) fragrep: efficient search for fragmented patterns in genomic sequences. Geno Prot Bioinfo 4:56–60

121. Weinberg Z, Ruzzo WL (2004) Exploiting conserved structure for faster annotation of non-coding RNAs without loss of accuracy. Bioinformatics 20:i334–i341

122. Weinberg Z, Ruzzo WL (2006) Sequence-based heuristics for faster annotation of non-coding RNA families. Bioinformatics 22:35–39

123. Lowe TM, Eddy SR (1997) tRNAscan-SE: a program for improved detection of transfer RNA genes in genomic sequence. Nucleic Acids Res 25:955–964

124. Macke TJ, Ecker DJ, Gutell RR, Gautheret D, Case DA, Sampath R (2001) RNAMotif, an RNA secondary structure definition and search algorithm. Nucl Acids Res 29:4724–4735

125. Billoud B, Kontic M, Viari A (1996) Palingol: a declarative programming language to describe nucleic acids' secondary structures and to scan sequence database. Nucl Acids Res 24:1395–1403

126. Gautheret D, Major F, Cedergren R (1990) Pattern searching/alignment with RNA primary and secondary structures: an effective descriptor for tRNA. Comput Appl Biosci 6:325–331

127. Dsouza M, Larsen N, Overbeek R (1997) Searching for patterns in genomic data. Trends Genet 13:497–498

128. Reeder J, Reeder J, Giegerich R (2007) Locomotif: from graphical motif description to RNA motif search. Bioinformatics 23:1392–1400

129. Gautheret D, Lambert A (2001) Direct RNA motif definition and identification from multiple sequence alignments using secondary structure profiles. J Mol Biol 313:1003–1011

130. Freyhult EK, Bollback JP, Gardner PP (2007) Exploring genomic dark matter: a critical assessment of the performance of homology

search methods on noncoding RNA. Genome Res 17:117–125

131. Finn RD, Coggill P, Eberhardt RY, Eddy SR, Mistry J, Mitchell AL, Potter SC, Punta M, Qureshi M, Sangrador-Vegas A, Salazar GA, Tate J, Bateman A (2016) The Pfam protein families database: towards a more sustainable future. Nucleic Acids Res 44(D1): D279–D285

132. Giegerich R (2014) Introduction to stochastic context free grammars. Methods Mol Biol 1097:85–106

133. Sükösd Z, Andersen ES, Lyngsø R (2014) SCFGs in RNA secondary structure prediction RNA secondary structure prediction: a hands-on approach. Methods Mol Biol 1097:143–162

134. Nawrocki EP, Eddy SR (2013) Infernal 1.1: 100-fold faster RNA homology searches. Bioinformatics 29:2933–2935

135. Nawrocki EP (2014) Annotating functional RNAs in genomes using Infernal. Methods Mol Biol 1097:163–197

136. Anthon C, Tafer H, Havgaard JH, Thomsen B, Hedegaard J, Seemann SE, Pundhir S, Kehr S, Bartschat S, Nielsen M, Nielsen RO, Fredholm M, Stadler PF, Gorodkin J (2014) Structured RNAs and synteny regions in the pig genome. BMC Genomics 15:459

137. Eggenhofer F, Hofacker IL, Siederdissen CH (2016) RNAlien - unsupervised RNA family model construction. Nucl Acids Res 44:8433–8441

138. Gesell T, Washietl S (2008) Dinucleotide controlled null models for comparative RNA gene prediction. BMC Bioinf 9:248

139. Washietl S, Hofacker IL, Lukasser M, Hüttenhofer A, Stadler PF (2005) Mapping of conserved RNA secondary structures predicts thousands of functional non-coding RNAs in the human genome. Nat Biotech 23:1383–1390

140. Rivas E, Eddy SR (2001) Noncoding RNA gene detection using comparative sequence analysis. BMC Bioinf 2:8

141. Pedersen JS, Bejerano G, Siepel A, Rosenbloom K, Lindblad-Toh K, Lander ES, Kent J, Miller W, Haussler D (2006) Identification and classification of conserved RNA secondary structures in the human genome. PLoS Comput Biol 2(4):e33

142. Parker BJ, Moltke I, Roth A, Washietl S, Wen J, Kellis M, Breaker R, Pedersen JS (2011) New families of human regulatory RNA structures identified by comparative

analysis of vertebrate genomes. Genome Res 21(11):1929–1943

143. Wang AX, Ruzzo WL, Tompa M (2007) How accurately is ncRNA aligned within whole-genome multiple alignments? BMC Bioinf 8:417

144. Gorodkin J, Stricklin SL, Stormo GD (2001) Discovering common stem-loop motifs in unaligned RNA sequences. Nucleic Acids Res 29:2135–2144

145. Havgaard JH, Torarinsson E, Gorodkin J (2007) Fast pairwise structural RNA alignments by pruning of the dynamical programming matrix. PLoS Comput Biol 3 (10):1896–1908

146. Sundfeld D, Havgaard JH, de Melo AC, Gorodkin J (2016) Foldalign 2.5: multi-threaded implementation for pairwise structural RNA alignment. Bioinformatics 22:1238–1240

147. Mathews DH, Turner DH (2002) Dynalign: an algorithm for finding the secondary structure common to two RNA sequences. J Mol Biol 317:191–203

148. Fu Y, Sharma G, Mathews DH (2014) Dynalign II: common secondary structure prediction for RNA homologs with domain insertions. Nucleic Acids Res 42:13939–13948

149. Will S, Missal K, Hofacker IL, Stadler PF, Backofen R (2007) Inferring non-coding RNA families and classes by means of genome-scale structure-based clustering. PLoS Comput Biol 3:e65

150. Will S, Joshi T, Hofacker IL, Stadler PF, Backofen R (2012) LocARNA-P: accurate boundary prediction and improved detection of structured RNAs for genome-wide screens. RNA 18:900–914

151. Sankoff D (1985) Simultaneous solution of the RNA folding, alignment and protosequence problems. SIAM J Appl Math 45:810–825

152. Havgaard JH, Gorodkin J (2014) RNA structural alignments, part I: sankoff-based approaches for structural alignments. Methods Mol Biol 1097:275–290

153. Yao Z, Weinberg Z, Ruzzo WL (2006) CMfinder–a covariance model based RNA motif finding algorithm. Bioinformatics 22 (4):445–452

154. Hofacker IL, Fontana W, Stadler PF, Bonhoeffer LS, Tacker M, Schuster P (1994) Fast folding and comparison of RNA secondary structures. Monatsh Chem 125:167–188

155. Bailey TL, Elkan C (1994) Fitting a mixture model by expectation maximization to

discover motifs in biopolymers. Proc Int Conf Intell Syst Mol Biol 2:28–36

156. Ruzzo WL, Gorodkin J (2014) De novo discovery of structured ncRNA motifs in genomic sequences. Methods Mol Biol 1097:303–318

157. Puton T, Kozlowski LP, Rother KM, Bujnicki JM (2013) CompaRNA: a server for continuous benchmarking of automated methods for RNA secondary structure prediction. Nucleic Acids Res 41(7):4307–4323

158. Puton T, Kozlowski LP, Rother KM, Bujnicki JM (2014) CompaRNA: a server for continuous benchmarking of automated methods for RNA secondary structure prediction. Nucleic Acids Res 42(8):5403–5406

159. Will S, Yu M, Berger B (2013) Structure-based whole-genome realignment reveals many novel noncoding RNAs. Genome Res 23:1018–1027

160. Torarinsson E, Sawera M, Havgaard JH, Fredholm M, Gorodkin J (2006) Thousands of corresponding human and mouse genomic regions unalignable in primary sequence contain common RNA structure. Genome Res 16:885–889

161. Weinberg Z, Barrick JE, Yao Z, Roth A, Kim JN, Gore J, Wang JX, Lee ER, Block KF, Sudarsan N, Neph S, Tompa M, Ruzzo WL, Breaker RR (2007) Identification of 22 candidate structured RNAs in bacteria using the CMfinder comparative genomics pipeline. Nucleic Acids Res 35:4809–4819

162. The ENCODE Project Consortium (2007) Identification and analysis of functional elements in 1% of the human genome by the ENCODE pilot project. Nature 447:799–816

163. Torarinsson E, Yao Z, Wiklund ED, Bramsen JB, Hansen C, Kjems J, Tommerup N, Ruzzo WL, Gorodkin J (2008) Comparative genomics beyond sequence-based alignments: RNA structures in the ENCODE regions. Genome Res 18:242–251

164. Ulveling D, Francastel C, Hubé F (2011) When one is better than two: RNA with dual functions. Biochimie 93:633–644

165. Leygue E (2007) Steroid receptor RNA activator (SRA1): unusual bifaceted gene products with suspected relevance to breast cancer. Nucl Recept Signal 5:e006

166. Rivas E, Clements J, Eddy SR (2017) A statistical test for conserved RNA structure shows lack of evidence for structure in lncRNAs. Nat Methods 14(1):45–48

167. Jenny A, Hachet O, Závorszky P, Cyrklaff A, Weston MD, Johnston DS, Erdélyi M, Ephrussi A (2006) A translation-independent role of oskar RNA in early Drosophila oogenesis. Development 133:2827–2833

168. Weill L, James L, Ulryck N, Chamond N, Herbreteau CH, Ohlmann T, Sargueil B (2010) A new type of IRES within gag coding region recruits three initiation complexes on HIV-2 genomic RNA. Nucleic Acids Res 38:1367–1381

169. Kumari, P, Sampath K (2015) cncRNAs: bi-functional RNAs with protein coding and non-coding functions. Semin Cell Dev Biol 47–48:40–51

170. Neuhaus K, Landstorfer R, Simon S, Schober S, Wright PR, Smith C, Backofen R, Wecko R, Keim DA, Scherer S (2017) Differentiation of ncRNAs from small mRNAs in Escherichia coli O157:H7 EDL933 (EHEC) by combined RNAseq and RIBOseq - ryhB encodes the regulatory RNA RyhB and a peptide, RyhP. BMC Genomics 18(1):216

171. Pedersen JS, Meyer IM, Forsberg R, Simmonds P, Hein J (2004) A comparative method for finding and folding RNA secondary structures within protein-coding regions. Nucleic Acids Res 32:4925–4936

172. Meyer IM, Miklós I (2005) Statistical evidence for conserved, local secondary structure in the coding regions of eukaryotic mRNAs and pre-mRNAs. Nucleic Acids Res 33:6338–6348

173. Findeiß S, Engelhardt J, Prohaska SP, Stadler PF (2011) Protein-coding structured RNAs: a computational survey of conserved RNA secondary structures overlapping coding regions in drosophilids. Biochimie 93:2019–2023

174. Stoletzki N (2008) Conflicting selection pressures on synonymous codon use in yeast suggest selection on mRNA secondary structures. BMC Evol Biol 8:224

175. Lin MF, Kheradpour P, Washietl S, Parker BJ, Pedersen JS, Kellis M (2011) Locating protein-coding sequences under selection for additional, overlapping functions in 29 mammalian genomes. Genome Res 21:1916–1928

176. Benjamini Y, Hochberg Y (1995) Controlling the false discovery rate: a practical and powerful approach to multiple testing. J Roy Stat Soc Ser B 57:289–300

177. Babak T, Blencowe BJ, Hughes TR (2007) Considerations in the identification of functional RNA structural elements in genomic alignments. BMC Bioinf 8:33

178. Anandam P, Torarinsson E, Ruzzo WL (2009) Multiperm: shuffling multiple

sequence alignments while approximately preserving dinucleotide frequencies. Bioinformatics 25:668–669

179. Washietl S, Pedersen JS, Korbel JO, Gruber A, Hackermüller J, Hertel J, Lindemeyer M, Reiche K, Stocsits C, Tanzer A, Ucla C, Wyss C, Antonarakis SE, Denoeud F, Lagarde J, Drenkow J, Kapranov P, Gingeras TR, Guigó R, Snyder M, Gerstein MB, Reymond A, Hofacker IL, Stadler PF (2007) Structured RNAs in the ENCODE selected regions of the human genome. Gen Res 17:852–864

180. Rose DR, Hackermüller J, Washietl S, Findeiß S, Reiche K, Hertel J, Stadler PF, Prohaska SJ (2007) Computational RNomics of drosophilids. BMC Genomics 8:406

181. Theis C, Zirbel CL, Siederdissen CHZ, Anthon C, Hofacker IL, Nielsen H, Gorodkin J (2015) RNA 3D modules in genome-wide predictions of RNA 2D structure. PLoS ONE 10(10):e0139900

182. Zhang XH-F, Leslie CS, Chasin LA (2005) Computational searches for splicing signals. Methods 37:292–305

183. Hiller M, Findeiß S, Lein S, Marz M, Nickel C, Rose D, Schulz C, Backofen R, Prohaska SJ, Reuter G, Stadler PF (2009) Conserved introns reveal novel transcripts in *Drosophila melanogaster*. Genome Res 19:1289–1300

184. Rose D, Hiller M, Schutt K, Hackermüller J, Backofen R, Stadler PF (2011) Computational discovery of human coding and non-coding transcripts with conserved splice sites. Bioinformatics 27:1894–1900

185. Kingsford C, Ayanbule K, Salzberg SL (2007) Rapid, accurate, computational discovery of Rho-independent transcription terminators illuminates their relationship to DNA uptake. Genome Biol 8:R22

186. Naville M, Ghuillot-Gaudeffroy A, Marchais A, Gautheret D (2011) ARNold: a web tool for the prediction of Rho-independent transcription terminators. RNA Biol 8:11–13

187. Pichon C, Felden B (2003) Intergenic sequence inspector: searching and identifying bacterial RNAs. Bioinformatics 19:1707–1709

188. Livny J, Fogel MA, Davis BM, Waldor MK (2005) sRNAPredict: an integrative computational approach to identify sRNAs in bacterial genomes. Nucleic Acids Res 13:4096–4105

189. Pichon C, du Merle L, Caliot M, Trieu-Cuot P, La Bouguénec C (2012) An in silico model for identification of small RNAs in whole bacterial genomes: characterization of antisense RNAs in pathogenic *Escherichia coli* and *Streptococcus agalactiae* strains. Nucl Acids Res 40:2846–2861

190. Arnedo J, Romero-Zaliz R, Zwir I, del Val C (2014) A multiobjective method for robust identification of bacterial small non-coding RNAs. Bioinformatics 30:2875–2882

191. Marchais A, Naville M, Bohn C, Bouloc P, Gautheret D (2009) Single-pass classification of all noncoding sequences in a bacterial genome using phylogenetic profiles. Genome Res 19:1084–1092

192. Ott A, Idali A, Marchais A, Gautheret D (2012) NAPP: the nucleic acid phylogenetic profile database. Nucl Acids Res 40: D205–D209

193. Weinberg Z, Perreault J, Meyer MM, Breaker RR (2009) Exceptional structured noncoding RNAs revealed by bacterial metagenome analysis. Nature 462(7273):656–659

194. Roth A, Weinberg Z, Chen AG, Kim PB, Ames TD, Breaker RR (2014) A widespread self-cleaving ribozyme class is revealed by bioinformatics. Nat Chem Biol 10(1):56–60

195. Weinberg Z, Kim PB, Chen TH, Li S, Harris KA, Lunse CE, Breaker RR (2015) New classes of self-cleaving ribozymes revealed by comparative genomics analysis. Nat Chem Biol 11(8):606–610

196. Pain A, Ott A, Amine H, Rochat T, Bouloc P, Gautheret D (2015) An assessment of bacterial small RNA target prediction programs. RNA Biol 12(5):509–513

197. Lai D, Meyer IM (2016) A comprehensive comparison of general RNA-RNA interaction prediction methods. Nucleic Acids Res 44(7): e61

198. Umu SU, Gardner PP (2017) A comprehensive benchmark of RNA-RNA interaction prediction tools for all domains of life. Bioinformatics 33(7):988–996

199. Gerlach W, Giegerich R (2006) GUUGle: a utility for fast exact matching under RNA complementary rules including G-U base pairing. Bioinformatics 22(6):762–764

200. Tjaden B, Goodwin SS, Opdyke JA, Guillier M, Fu DX, Gottesman S, Storz G (2006) Target prediction for small, noncoding RNAs in bacteria. Nucleic Acids Res 34 (9):2791–802

201. Wenzel A, Akbasli E, Gorodkin J (2012) RIsearch: fast RNA-RNA interaction search using a simplified nearest-neighbor energy model. Bioinformatics 28(21):2738–2746

202. Rehmsmeier M, Steffen P, Höchsmann M, Giegerich R (2004) Fast and effective

prediction of microRNA/target duplexes. RNA 10(10):1507–1517

203. Alkan C, Karakoç E, Nadeau JH, Sahinalp SC, Zhang K (2006) RNA-RNA interaction prediction and antisense RNA target search. J Comput Biol 13(2):267–282

204. Dimitrov RA, Zuker M (2004) Prediction of hybridization and melting for double-stranded nucleic acids. Biophys J 87 (1):215–226

205. Bernhart SH, Tafer H, Muckstein U, Flamm C, Stadler PF, Hofacker IL (2006) Partition function and base pairing probabilities of RNA heterodimers. Algorithms Mol Biol 1(1):3

206. Mückstein U, Tafer H, Hackermuller J, Bernhart SH, Stadler PF, Hofacker IL (2006) Thermodynamics of RNA-RNA binding. Bioinformatics 22:1177–1182

207. Bernhart SH, Mückstein U, Hofacker IL (2011) RNA accessibility in cubic time. Algorithms Mol Biol 6(1):3

208. Busch A, Richter AS, Backofen R (2008) IntaRNA: efficient prediction of bacterial sRNA targets incorporating target site accessibility and seed regions. Bioinformatics 24 (24):2849–2856

209. Wright PR, Georg J, Mann M, Sorescu DA, Richter AS, Lott S, Kleinkauf R, Hess WR, Backofen R (2014) CopraRNA and IntaRNA: predicting small RNA targets, networks and interaction domains. Nucleic Acids Res 42 (Web Server issue):W119–W123. PRW, JG and MM contributed equally to this work.

210. Tafer H, Hofacker IL (2008) RNAplex: a fast tool for RNA-RNA interaction search. Bioinformatics 24(22):2657–2663

211. Chitsaz H, Backofen R, Sahinalp SC (2009) biRNA: fast RNA-RNA binding sites prediction. In: Salzberg S, Warnow T (eds) Proceedings of the 9th workshop on algorithms in bioinformatics (WABI). Lecture notes in computer science, vol. 5724. Springer, Berlin, pp 25–36

212. Salari R, Backofen R, Sahinalp SC (2009) Fast prediction of RNA-RNA interaction. In: Salzberg S, Warnow T (eds) Proceedings of the 9th Workshop on Algorithms in Bioinformatics (WABI). Lecture Notes in Computer Science, vol 5724. Springer, Berlin, pp 261–272

213. Salari R, Backofen R, Sahinalp SC (2010) Fast prediction of RNA-RNA interaction. Algorithms Mol Biol 5:5

214. Pervouchine DD (2004) IRIS: intermolecular RNA interaction search. Genome Inform 15(2):92–101

215. Chitsaz H, Salari R, Sahinalp SC, Backofen R (2009) A partition function algorithm for interacting nucleic acid strands. Bioinformatics 25(12):i365–i373

216. Huang FWD, Qin J, Reidys CM, Stadler PF (2009) Partition function and base pairing probabilities for RNA-RNA interaction prediction. Bioinformatics 25(20):2646–2654

217. Seemann SE, Richter AS, Gesell T, Backofen R, Gorodkin J (2011) PETcofold: predicting conserved interactions and structures of two multiple alignments of RNA sequences. Bioinformatics 27(2):211–219

218. Li AX, Marz M, Qin J, Reidys CM (2011) RNA-RNA interaction prediction based on multiple sequence alignments. Bioinformatics 27(4):456–463

219. Schattner P, Brooks AN, Lowe TM (2005) The tRNAscan-SE, snoscan and snoGPS web servers for the detection of tRNAs and snoRNAs. Nucl Acid Res 33: W686–W689

220. Freyhult E, Edvardsson S, Tamas I, Moulton V, Poole AM (2008) Fisher: a program for the detection of H/ACA snoRNAs using MFE secondary structure prediction and comparative genomics – assessment and update. BMC Res Notes 1:49

221. Kehr S, Bartschat S, Stadler PF, Tafer H (2011) PLEXY: efficient target prediction for box C/D snoRNAs. Bioinformatics 27:279–280

222. Tafer H, Kehr S, Hertel J, Stadler PF (2010) RNAsnoop: efficient target prediction for box H/ACA snoRNAs. Bioinformatics 26:610–616

223. Richter AS, Backofen R (2012) Accessibility and conservation: general features of bacterial small RNA-mRNA interactions? RNA Biol 9 (7):954–965

224. Wright PR, Richter AS, Papenfort K, Mann M, Vogel J, Hess WR, Backofen R, Georg J (2013) Comparative genomics boosts target prediction for bacterial small RNAs. Proc Natl Acad Sci USA 110(37): E3487–E3496

225. Alkan F, Wenzel A, Palasca O, Kerpedjiev P, Rudebeck AF, Stadler PF, Hofacker IL, Gorodkin J (2017) RIsearch2: suffix array-based large-scale prediction of RNA-RNA interactions and siRNA off-targets. Nucleic Acids Res. 45: e60

226. Deigan KE, Li TW, Mathews DH, Weeks KM (2009) Accurate SHAPE-directed RNA structure determination. Proc Natl Acad Sci USA 106:97–102

227. Zarringhalam K, Meyer MM, Dotu I, Chuang JH, Clote P (2012) Integrating chemical footprinting data into RNA secondary structure prediction. PLoS One 7:e45160

228. Hajdin CE, Bellaousov S, Huggins W, Leonard CW, Mathews DH, Weeks KM (2013) Accurate SHAPE-directed RNA secondary structure modeling, including pseudoknots. Proc Natl Acad Sci USA 110:5498–5503

229. Cordero P, Kladwang W, VanLang CC, Das R (2012) Quantitative dimethyl sulfate mapping for automated RNA secondary structure inference. Biochemistry 51:7037–7039

230. Kertesz M, Wan Y, Mazor E, Rinn JL, Nutter RC, Chang HY, Segal E (2010) Genome-wide measurement of RNA secondary structure in yeast. Nature 467:103–107

231. Wan Y, Qu K, Zhang QC, Flynn RA, Manor O, Ouyang Z, Zhang J, Spitale RC, Snyder MP, Segal E, Chang HY (2014) Landscape and variation of RNA secondary structure across the human transcriptome. Nature 505:706–709

232. Sükösd Z, Swenson MS, Kjems J, Heitsch CE (2013) Evaluating the accuracy of SHAPE-directed RNA secondary structure predictions. Nucleic Acids Res 41:2807–2816

233. Lorenz R, Luntzer D, Hofacker IL, Stadler PF, Wolfinger MT (2016) SHAPE directed RNA folding. Bioinformatics 32:145–147

234. Lorenz R, Hofacker IL, Stadler PF (2016) RNA folding with hard and soft constraints. Algorithms Mol Biol 11:8

235. Ray D, Kazan H, Cook KB, Weirauch MT, Najafabadi HS, Li X, Gueroussov S, Albu M, Zheng H, Yang A, Na H, Irimia M, Matzat LH, Dale RK, Smith SA, Yarosh CA, Kelly SM, Nabet B, Mecenas D, Li W, Laishram RS, Qiao M, Lipshitz HD, Piano F, Corbett AH, Carstens RP, Frey BJ, Anderson RA, Lynch KW, Penalva LO, Lei EP, Fraser AG, Blencowe BJ, Morris QD, Hughes TR (2013) A compendium of RNA-binding motifs for decoding gene regulation. Nature 499:172–177

236. Chu C, Qu K, Zhong FL, Artandi SE, Chang HY (2011) Genomic maps of long noncoding RNA occupancy reveal principles of RNA-chromatin interactions. Mol Cell 44:667–678

237. Simon MD (2016) Insight into lncRNA biology using hybridization capture analyses. Biochim Biophys Acta 1859:121–127

238. Birkedal U, Christensen-Dalsgaard M, Krogh N, Sabarinathan R, Gorodkin J, Nielsen H (2015) Profiling of ribose methylations in RNA by high-throughput sequencing. Angew Chem Int Ed Engl 54(2):451–455

239. Liu N, Pan T (2016) N^6-methyladenosine-encoded epitranscriptomics. Nat Struct Mol Biol 23:98–102

240. Sibbritt T, Shafik A, Clark SJ, Preiss T (2016) Nucleotide-level profiling of m^5C RNA methylation. Methods Mol Biol 1358:269–284

241. Husain B, Hesler S, Cole JL (2015) Regulation of PKR by RNA: formation of active and inactive dimers. Biochemistry 54:6663–6672

242. Osman F, Jarrous N, Ben-Asouli Y, Kaempfer R (1999) A cis-acting element in the 3'-untranslated region of human TNF-alpha mRNA renders splicing dependent on the activation of protein kinase PKR. Genes Dev 13:3280–3293

243. Cohen-Chalamish S, Hasson A, Weinberg D, Namer LS, Banai Y, Osman F, Kaempfer R (2009) Dynamic refolding of IFN-gamma mRNA enables it to function as PKR activator and translation template. Nat Chem Biol 5:896–903

Chapter 15

Bioinformatic Approaches for Comparative Analysis of Viruses

Deyvid Amgarten and Chris Upton

Abstract

The field of viral genomic studies has experienced an unprecedented increase in data volume. New strains of known viruses are constantly being added to the GenBank database and so are completely new species with little or no resemblance to our databases of sequences. In addition to this, metagenomic techniques have the potential to further increase the number and rate of sequenced genomes. Besides, it is important to consider that viruses have a set of unique features that often break down molecular biology dogmas, e.g., the flux of information from RNA to DNA in retroviruses and the use of RNA molecules as genomes. As a result, extracting meaningful information from viral genomes remains a challenge and standard methods for comparing the unknown and our databases of characterized sequences may need to be modified. Thus, several bioinformatic approaches and tools have been created to address the challenge of analyzing viral data. In this chapter, we offer descriptions and protocols of some of the most important bioinformatic techniques for comparative analysis of viruses. We also provide comments and discussion on how viruses' unique features can affect standard analyses and how to overcome some of the major sources of problems. Topics include: (1) Clustering of related genomes, (2) Whole genome multiple sequence alignments for small RNA viruses, (3) Protein alignments for marker genes, (4) Analyses based on ortholog groups, and (5) Taxonomic identification and comparisons of viruses from environmental datasets.

Key words Comparative analysis, Viral genomes, Virus, Genomics, Metagenomics, Viromes, Bioinformatics, Multiple sequence alignment, VOCs, BLAST, Ortholog groups

1 Introduction

In the last decade, Next-Generation Sequencing (NGS) techniques have been revolutionizing the study of genomes in all domains of life. Due to their unique features, viral genomes are a special case in this context. Most viruses have relatively small genomes if compared with bacteria and eukaryotes and these small genomes often lack extensive repeated regions, which are a major problem with assembly and analysis of eukaryotic genomes [1]. On the other hand, viruses are extremely diverse and only a small fraction have been sequenced; therefore, new genomes are often completely different from all the others in our databases. This is exacerbated

João C. Setubal et al. (eds.), *Comparative Genomics: Methods and Protocols*, Methods In Molecular Biology, vol. 1704, https://doi.org/10.1007/978-1-4939-7463-4_15, © Springer Science+Business Media LLC 2018

when we consider new uncultured viruses obtained from environmental communities by metagenomic approaches [2, 3].

Furthermore, a whole new layer of complexity is added to the analyses of viruses as they are the only organisms known for carrying genomic information as RNA molecules. RNA viruses, which are probably present in all environments, have small genomes (usually <20 kb) and maintain a strict gene complement among viruses within a given species [4]. This contrasts with large DNA viruses, which are much more variable. Whereas all HIV isolates contain the same set of genes (although may be subject to recombination), different vaccinia viruses (200 kb DNA genome, used to vaccinate against smallpox) have a common set of essential genes and a variable set of host range/virulence genes [5]. This situation can be much more extreme among the DNA phages that infect bacteria. The diversity among these viruses is so great that sometimes only a few genes in a genome show any similarity to other genomes in the same taxonomic family [6]. This is in part because historically, structural similarity has been used by the *International Committee on Taxonomy of Viruses* (ICTV) to group viruses instead of genome sequence comparisons.

New strains of known virus species are constantly being added to the GenBank database, and so are completely new species with little or no similarity to previously characterized viruses. Keeping up with the analysis of this data is a serious challenge due to the complex nature of viral genomes and ever-increasing amount of data. Comparative analyses allow a mechanism for characterizing and extracting meaningful information from novel sequences, often through pairwise sequence alignments. Thus, alignments have been successfully used to retrieve functional similarities and homolog information in all different kinds of species, including viruses.

It is worth mentioning that standard algorithms may present some limitations concerning the analysis of viral sequences and, for this purpose, specific approaches and tools have been created to address this matter [7, 8]. Also, bioinformatics resources, such as the Viral Bioinformatics Resource Center (http://virology.ca), the Virus Pathogen Resource (ViPR) [9], and PhagesDB (http://phagesdb.org), have been responsible for processing and storing information so that analyses can be easily repeated or modified in later research.

This chapter aims to survey some of the comparative methods and the currently available resources (databases and analysis software) for dealing with viral data. Topics include comparisons of genomes and proteins from related viruses and methods to compare sequences from environmental samples in a microbial community perspective. More specifically, examples explored in this chapter include: (1) Grouping related genomes based on similarity searches of a new double-stranded DNA phage, (2) Investigation of genomic multiple sequence alignments (MSA) for RNA flaviviruses, (3) Study of a marker gene in the *Myoviridae* family, and (4) Taxonomy identification and comparisons of viral sequences from a composting microbial community.

2   Materials

There are many bioinformatics resources to help virologists in the task of characterizing viruses [7]. Some are specific to a type of genome (e.g., large double-stranded DNA or RNA genomes), whereas others are specific to a bioinformatics task, such as the detection of horizontal gene transfer (HGT) or gene predictions. This chapter tries to be as comprehensive as possible, but keep in mind that this section only lists those tools and resources used for the examples described. There are many different bioinformatics tools currently available, with ongoing development of new ones.

1. To work on most bioinformatics projects, researchers need an up-to-date desktop or laptop computer. The cost of investing in a new computer will be minimal compared to the time and effort wasted struggling with old hardware and out-dated software. Regardless of the operating system (OS), make sure the last version of Java Runtime Environment (JRE) is installed and that web browser is up-to-date.

2. Most of the programs discussed here run as Java clients in Java Web Start format, which only require JRE to be executed and are OS independent. They work by automatically downloading a copy of the Java software from the developers' servers onto the user's computer; thus they are always updated to the last version present on the servers.

3. Key online platforms:

   (a) *National Center for Biotechnology Information (NCBI)*: This widely used web platform provides access to general biomedical and genomic information and hosts a suite of databases and tools such as GenBank, NCBI BLAST [10] and Conserved Domain search (CDD-search) [11]. NCBI tools do not require registration and can be accessed by the address: http://www.ncbi.nlm.nih.gov/.

   Additionally, NCBI provides the *Viral Genomes Resource* [12], which collects all the viral genome sequence data and related information in one web resource (http://www.ncbi.nlm.nih.gov/genome/viruses/).

   (b) *Viral Bioinformatics Resource Center (VBRC)*: The VBRC, which is accessed via a web page, provides access to a database of large DNA viruses and a series of bioinformatic tools for the comparison and analysis of these viruses. The tools can also be used with genome data from other sources.

In order to obtain access to VBRC tools, it is necessary to create a free account. Just go to the website (http://virology.uvic.ca), click on the "register" button and fill out the requested data. It is easy and simple.

(c) *Metavir Analysis of Viromes*: This web server is designed to annotate viral metagenomic sequences and to provide user-friendly analyses and comparisons with other public virome datasets [13].

Metavir requires a simple and free user registration. Just go to the website (http://metavir-meb.univ-bpclermont.fr/), select "Register new user" and fill out requested data.

4. Key software:

(a) *Viral Orthologous Clusters (VOCs)*: VOCs [14] is the GUI client used to access a SQL database that stores gene, protein, and genome sequences along with gene ortholog information from large DNA viruses. VOCs also include a variety of comparative analysis tools. For example, it is simple to (1) send selected sequences to an alignment tool such as ClustalO [15], MUSCLE [16], or MAFFT [17] and have the results returned in a MSA editor, and (2) select gene families present in one virus but not in another.

VOCs is part of the VBRC suite of programs: http://virology.uvic.ca/virology-ca-tools/vocs/.

(b) *Base-By-Base (BBB)* [18]: Software for generating, visualizing, and editing MSAs. Standard alignment tools are embedded into the program and there are a variety of unique functions to manipulate and analyze MSAs.

BBB is part of the VBRC suite of programs: http://virology.uvic.ca/virology-ca-tools/base-by-base/.

3   Methods

3.1   First Things First: Grouping Genomes

Establishing a group of similar genomes is the starting point in comparative analysis and a variety of different methods can be used for this purpose, such as alignments, dotplots, and Average Nucleotide Identity (ANI) [19, 20]. Similarity searches are widely used by the scientific community to compare new viral genomes against a database of all known sequences in order to identify related genomes. Although the sequence alignments they produce are the golden standard in bioinformatics analysis, the algorithms used may have some limitations in the study of viral genomes. We discuss how the unique features of viruses can affect accuracy of alignments, *see* **Note 1**.

In this section, we use alignments to identify similarity between sequences and construct a group of related genomes. A new *Pseudomonas* phage isolated from composting is used as an illustrative example for the procedures, which can be summarized as follows: *Step 1*–Select a genome of interest, *Step 2*–BLAST query genome against NCBI database, and *Step 3*–Select similar genomes to compose the group.

3.1.1 Step 1: Select a Genome of Interest

Different researchers are likely to have different goals regarding comparative analysis of a new genome, usually depending on its relationship to known genomes. Thus, investigations of a novel poxvirus will be different from those on a new tailed phage or an old pathogen such as Zika virus that is emerging again in new epidemics. Therefore, the genome of interest will be the basis of every comparative analysis and it is important to take a time to study and understand its unique features.

Check for genome structure, genome ends, repeats, noncoding regions, quality of the assembly, and other relevant information.

3.1.2 Step 2: BLAST Query Genome

1. Open the web browser and go to the NCBI BLAST webpage http://blast.ncbi.nlm.nih.gov/.

2. Choose BLASTN algorithm and upload the genome of interest as query.

3. Set the database to nr/nt only viruses (taxid:10239) and word size in "General parameters" to 7 nt. A smaller word size parameter increases algorithm sensitivity, which helps when looking for distant homologous sequences in viral databases. Other parameters can be left as default. Run the BLAST search.

3.1.3 Step 3: Select Similar Genomes to Compose the Group

Many viruses have high frequency of HTG and for this reason they may present genomes composed of "pieces," or mosaic genomes [21]. This feature has some implications in BLAST searches as the one performed in this section. For instance, hits with high identity but very low coverage are likely to be reported; however, this does not necessarily mean that they should be considered as related genomes for further comparative analyses.

Use "query cover" and "identity" parameters to identify which genomes have greatest similarity, since these parameters give the researcher an idea of how local alignments are covering the entire query sequence. As a rule of thumb, multiply (coverage × identity) and select genomes with values higher than 20% (as this is not a strict rule, values may vary). Pay special attention to hits with less than 30% of coverage, because they might be due to mosaicism in viral genomes.

BLASTN results for our example with phage ZC01 are shown in Table 1. We have selected the first 11 genomes to create our group of similar genomes, while the last two hits are probably due

Table 1
Table of best hits for phage ZCO1 whole genome BLASTN search against NCBI nr/nt only viruses database. First 11 genomes were selected to create a group of related genomes

Description	Query cover	E value	Identity	Accession
Pseudomonas phage vB_PaeS_PAO1_Ab19	95%	0	97%	LN610584.1
Pseudomonas phage vB_PaeS_PAO1_Ab20	97%	0	97%	LN610585.1
Pseudomonas phage vB_PaeS_PAO1_Ab18	97%	0	96%	LN610577.1
Pseudomonas phage PaMx11	98%	0	86%	JQ067087.2
Pseudomonas phage PaMx74	28%	0	71%	JQ067093.2
Pseudomonas phage AAT-1	28%	0	73%	KU204984.1
Pseudomonas phage PAE1	32%	0	70%	KT734862.1
Pseudomonas phage LKO4	32%	0	69%	KC758116.1
Bacteriophage M6	32%	0	69%	DQ163916.1
Pseudomonas phage YuA	31%	0	69%	AM749441.1
Pseudomonas phage MP1412	31%	0	69%	JX131330.1
Bacteriophage phi JL001	10%	2e-62	67%	AY576273.1
Ralstonia phage RSL1	1%	1e-34	75%	AB366653.2

to the mosaicism of phage genomes and were not selected. The group of related genomes should be used for further comparative analyses such as MSAs, phylogenetic trees, transfer of annotations, etc.

3.2 Small RNA Genomes Multiple Sequence Alignments

MSAs are the foundation of most comparative analyses and they have been widely used to help researchers to understand changes in biological sequences and evolutionary events. As is usual in bioinformatics, virologists have different tools and algorithms at their disposal for addressing this task. We briefly discuss progressive MSA algorithms and some specific approaches for virus genomes in *see* **Note 2**.

In this section, we will perform a MSA of whole small RNA genomes from flaviviruses in order to study macro genomic changes in the family. The steps of this approach may be summarized as follows: *Step 1*–Select similar genomes to be aligned, *Step 2*–Download and open VBRC's BBB tool, *Step 3*–Perform MSA, *Step 4*–Review MSA, and *Step 5*–Identify indels and misalignments.

3.2.1 Step 1: Select Similar Sequences to be Aligned

Zika virus (GB Accession NC_012532) and related genomes selected by the same procedures listed on Subheading 3.1 will be used for this example.

3.2.2 Step 2: Download and Open VBRC's BBB Tool

For organizing genomes and performing MSA, we will use the VBRC java tool BBB. Go to VBRC web platform (http://virol ogy.uvic.ca), download and open BBB java web start application.

3.2.3 Step 3: Perform Multiple Sequence Alignment

1. Use top menu "File" to import GenBank or FASTA files for the genomes. BBB loads the files and displays the unaligned nucleotide sequences in the main window. Rename genomes for easier identification, if necessary.

2. Using the mouse pointer and shift key, select all genome names in the left section. Type ctrl + w for a whole genome sequence selection.

3. Go to the top menu "Tools" and select "Align selection." Choose MAFFT to generate whole genome sequences alignment. BBB will prompt some warnings and start the alignment, which runs on the VBRC servers.

4. Once the process is finished, a window with the resulting alignment will appear for quick inspection. Select OK and sequences in the main window will be rearranged. The MSA can be exported in FASTA or any available format to be used in other tools, if required.

3.2.4 Step 4: Review Multiple Sequence Alignment

1. Users can inspect MSA directly in the tool, which shows a user-friendly display with easy-to-identify substitutions and indels. Additionally, BBB can generate a visual summary of the complete alignment: Click on the top menu "Report" -> "Visual summary." BBB will show a graphic representation of the MSA, as well as genes encoded by the genome and additional information if an annotated GenBank file was used.

2. Another piece of useful information is the percent of identity table. Click on "Report" -> "Percent identity table." This table provides information of similarity among the aligned genomes.

3. Under "Report" and "Tools" top menus, there are tools to perform several other analyses based on the MSA (e.g., plot similarity between sequences). We recommend users to explore and use them according to their requirements.

3.2.5 Step 5: Identify Indels and Misalignments

1. Figure 1a shows a portion of a whole genome MSA with selected flaviviruses where the user can clearly see two different indels events. Inspection of the flanking sequences shows that the region is poorly conserved. Such variable regions often mislead aligners to create unlikely events, as the two adjacent deletions (if compared against a consensus sequence) observed in Fig. 1a. Thus, it is prudent to inspect MSAs, and manually correct alignment errors. BBB has a tool to select and realign regions of MSAs. We have realigned the sequences and the alternative alignment shows a single indel event, which is

A

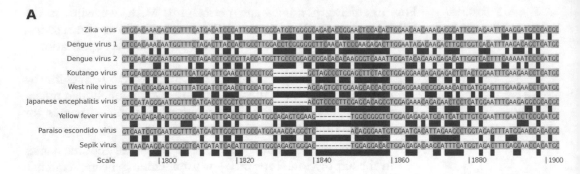

B

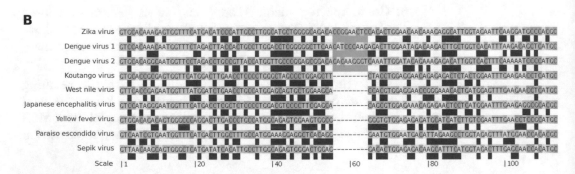

Fig. 1 (**a**) Portion of the genomic MSA for flaviviruses where it is possible to identify two misplaced adjacent indels in a very unconserved region (1830–1859 nt). (**b**) Alternative alignment for the same region, showing a single and more likely indel event. *Blue* rectangles mean substitutions, while *red* and *green* rectangles mean deletions and insertions, respectively. Display was generated by BBB and indels have a consensus sequence as a reference

more likely to have happened in the evolutionary history of the sequences (Fig. 1b).

2. This region of the flavivirus genomes encodes the central portion of the envelope protein E, which is responsible for binding to the host cell surface receptor (see Uniprot P06935 for West Nile virus record). Therefore, this highly variable region could be involved in host specificity.

3.3 Genome Analysis Using Ortholog Groups

In this section, we demonstrate the use of ortholog groups as important features in the comparative analysis of viruses. Sometimes, complete genome alignments are difficult or impossible due to common events of rearrangement and HGT. However, another approach is to compare the gene content of genomes, i.e., ask if genomes encode the same set of homologs genes. To illustrate this, we will use the VBRC Viral Orthologs Clusters (VOCs) database, which contains information about genomes and ortholog groups from several families of double-strand DNA viruses. For more information about other viral ortholog group databases, *see* **Note 3**.

Our goal in this section is to choose a marker gene present in all viruses from a group (conserved ortholog group) and proceed with the MSA of the proteins. Next, we will use MSA information to identify conserved sites in the protein and make a phylogenetic tree based on the marker gene. Procedures may be summarized as follows: *Step 1*–Download and open VOCs, *Step 2*–Access ortholog groups and genome information, *Step 3*–Perform protein MSA, *Step 4*–Identify conserved regions, and *Step 5*–Phylogenetic analysis.

3.3.1 Step 1: Download and Open VOCs

Go to VBRC web platform (http://virology.uvic.ca) and select "VOCs" under the "Tools" tab. Download the Java web start application and open it.

3.3.2 Step 2: Access Orthologs Groups and Genome Information

At the first window, VOCs will show a list of viral families available in the database. We will work with the tailed phages family *Myoviridae* in this example. Choose it and a new window will open. VOCs' main window shows information about viruses present in the database. For detailed explanation and tutorials, go to VBRC page http://virology.uvic.ca/help/tool-help/quick-start-pages/vocs-quick-start-page/.

1. Without selecting any particular genome in the list of genomes, click on the bottom button "OrtGrpView." A second window should open with a table of all existing ortholog groups for the *Myoviridae* family.

2. Click on the "no. of viruses" table header to order ortholog groups by the number of viruses with genes assigned to it. By looking at this table, the user can easily identify a set of genes with at least one representative for all the 35 species in the group. This set of genes is called core-genome and they are the basis for many comparative and phylogenetic analyses.

3.3.3 Step 3: Perform Protein Multiple Sequence Alignment

As an illustrative example, we have chosen the VOCs ortholog group 19406 (the Terminase large subunit (TerL) protein) as a case study. The TerL gene is thought as being a marker gene in the majority of tailed phages [6] and it is one of the 18 core-genes in T4-like viruses. It is important to mention that any of these genes could be considered for the analyses described in this section or even the entire set, as it is common in more complex studies.

1. Click on "OrtGrView" bottom button and select the large terminase protein (ID 19406) ortholog group.

2. Click on "align" and then select the MUSCLE tool. VOCs will open a new BBB window after process is completed.

3.3.4 Step 4: Identify Conserved Regions

1. BBB window shows the full amino acid alignment for all TerL proteins. Click on Report -> visual summary. BBB will open a new window containing a graphic representation of the MSA (Fig. 2).

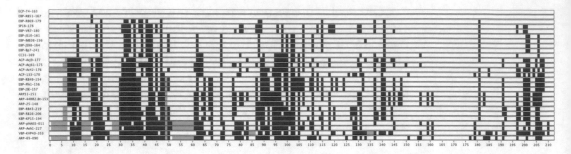

Fig. 2 Visual summary representing the N-terminus of the TerL protein MSA. Conserved regions are shown in *white*, while substitutions, deletions, and insertions are shown in *blue, red,* and *green*, respectively. Modifications in the sequences have T4 top sequence as a reference

2. By inspecting the figure, the user can clearly identify conserved and non-conserved regions in the protein. Non-conserved regions are shown with blue, red and light-green color, which means substitutions, deletions, and insertions, respectively. All modifications have the phage T4 top protein as reference. Our MSA example shows that TerL protein has N-terminus and C-terminus very variable and with frequent indels. On the other hand, a very conserved region can be spotted between the amino acid positions 140 and 180. Further investigation and searches against curated databases could provide more information about secondary/tertiary structures and active sites. For instance, phage lambda's active site is located at the amino acid in position 179, according to Uniprot curation (record P03708) [22]. However, deep and specific analyses strongly depend on researchers' particular interest and are out of the scope of this chapter.

3.3.5 Step 5: Phylogenetic Analysis

Different algorithms and tools are available to create phylogenetic trees. Creating robust phylogenetic trees for viruses is a difficult task; therefore, we briefly explore some of the methods and suitable tools, *see* **Note 4**. We recommend the maximum likelihood method for building trees, since it is a robust method and very efficient for viral genome phylogenies [23]. For illustrative purposes only, we will use an embedded function present in BBB to create a simple Neighbor-joining tree based on the TerL marker gene.

1. Inspect both the visual summary and alignment itself in BBB to make sure it is correct, i.e., that the sequences have enough similarity to be considered orthologous and that regions around gaps are correctly aligned. This remark is also valid for paralogous proteins, which can be a major source of errors in phylogenetic analyses.

2. Click on "Report" top menu and then on "Neighbor joining tree." BBB will generate the tree according to a distance matrix for the TerL MSA and display the result in a new window.

3.4 Viruses from Environmental Samples

Improvements in techniques of environmental communities sequencing, also known as metagenomics, have brought entire viral communities to the attention of virologists. Now, a large number of researchers are faced with the challenging task of analyzing thousands of extremely diverse viral sequences in a fast and accurate way.

Although we recognize the importance of contig assembly and its role as a major source of problems in downstream analysis, we will base this section on the assumption that readers already have a dataset of viral contigs recovered from environmental samples. For a brief discussion about the assembly of viral metagenomic data and software available, *see* **Note 5**.

Our goal in this section is to extract information from large amounts of sequences and compare viral communities in a broader perspective. For illustrative purposes, we will describe methods for analyzing a set of 51,960 contigs assembled with MIRA 4 [24] from *Illumina* paired-ends reads. Samples for sequencing were collected from a bacterial composting operation at the Sao Paulo Zoo Park, Brazil [25]. Steps may be summarized as follows: Step 1–Access the Metavir online platform, Step 2–Upload sequences to analysis, Step 3–Taxonomic composition, and Step 4–Virome comparisons.

3.4.1 Step 1: Access the Metavir Online Platform

1. Go to the Metavir web site (http://metavir-meb.univ-bpclermont.fr/). Sign in using login and password created according to explanations in the Materials' section.

2. The Metavir homepage presents several tutorial analyses that the user can perform with public viromes without uploading any data. Take a time to browsing it around.

3.4.2 Step 2: Upload Sequences to Analyze

1. Make sure contigs are in FASTA format with correct names, since some assemblers may repeat names or use inappropriate characters.

2. Click on "Upload new virome." Fill in requested metadata for the sample and upload the contigs FASTA file. Results are not computed immediately, and in fact, analyses may take days or weeks depending on the amount of data being analyzed and load on the servers.

3.4.3 Step 3: Taxonomic Composition

Metavir calculates taxonomic composition by running BLAST searches against the NCBI viral RefSeq database [26]. Relative abundance for each species is normalized by genome size using the GAAS tool [27]. Additionally, users can select different methods of taxonomic identification (best Blast hit, last common ancestor and predicted genes best hit) and thresholds of E-value or bit score.

Taxonomic composition is available under the "Taxonomy" tab. Set computational parameters to E-value = 10e-7 and

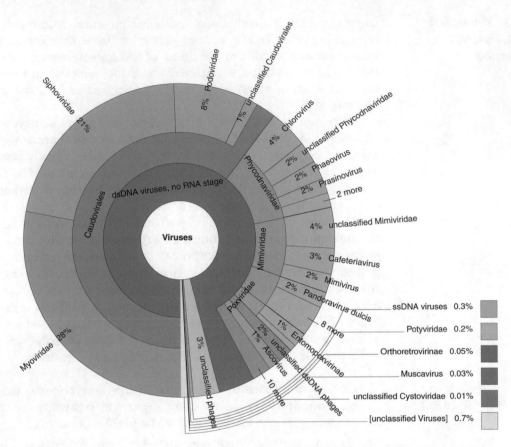

Fig. 3 Example of a taxonomic composition plot generated by the Metavir online platform. Results show relative abundance of taxa identified in the composting sample according to the methodology described in the platform

"Contigs lowest common ancestor (LCA)" as compositional type. Using low E-value (number of sequences expected to be found by chance in the database with score equal to or higher than the observed) matches assure that random hits are not used in taxonomic identification and LCA composition type will avoid imprecise identification of organisms at the species level when sufficient evidence is not found. Results are displayed with Krona tools [28] and an example can be seen in Fig. 3.

3.4.4 Step 4: Virome Comparisons

Metavir generates di, tri, and tetra nucleotide profiles from the virome being analyzed, as well as a BLAST composition profile. These profiles can be used to compare the private virome with other publicly available viromes. For illustrative purposes, we compare the profile of our composting contigs with other environmental viromes and determine the similarity among these viral communities.

1. Click on the tab "Virome comparison" and select "BLAST-based comparison" as the comparison method. Set visualization to "Cluster tree." Next, select public viromes to compare against, examples include: Seawater samples from Gulf of Mexico and British Columbia, fresh water viromes from Lake Pavin and Lake Bourget, an Antarctic open soil sample and a saltern medium sample. Click on "Compare these viromes" button.

2. Metavir generates a cluster tree based on a similarity score matrix computed for each virome pair as described in the Metavir online platform. Viromes with similar species composition or from similar environment (e.g., Gulf of Mexico and British Columbia coast) usually cluster together in cluster trees. For our example (ZC4day01), the thermophile composting virome was grouped with the Antarctic open soil sample and those were grouped with the saltern medium sample, as shown in Fig. 4. Comparisons and clusters become more informative as more samples are added to the analysis. Results shown in Fig. 4 indicate that BLAST composition for the composting

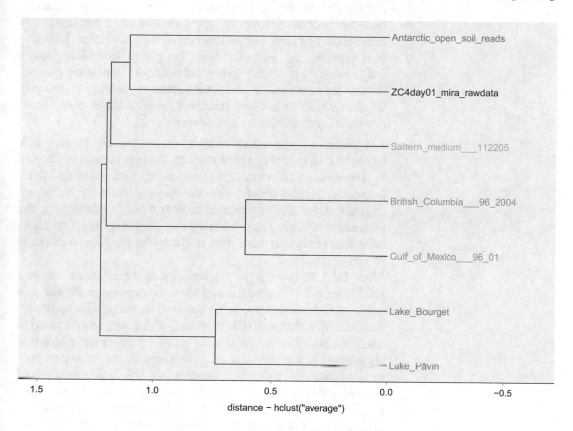

Type of virome   • Freshwater • Hyperarid_desert • Hypersaline • Private • Seawater

Fig. 4 Example of a cluster tree generated by Metavir virome comparison analyses. ZC4day01 refers to the composting virome being analyzed and other public viromes were used to show the similarity among the different BLAST composition profiles

viral community is more similar to Antarctic open soil and saline medium environments than the other viromes compared.

3. Profiles for the sample can be downloaded and used with statistical tools for generating charts and additional analyses, as required by the researcher's interest.

4   Notes

1. Viral genomes are known for having relatively high mutation rates (nucleotide exchange), and many also undergo genome rearrangements and HTG [19, 29]. These latter events cause serious problems for genomic analyses based on standard techniques, which assume nucleotide sequences have evolved in a Darwinian fashion with identifiable and discreet common ancestors. Amino acid sequences have the advantage of changing less frequently than their nucleotide counterparts and being less susceptible to big rearrangements events (genes are more discreet entities). However, even orthologous proteins may present change rates higher than usual for bacterial and eukaryotic proteins, as was observed for phage ortholog groups assignment [6]. Thus, many orthologous proteins present similarities beyond a threshold that standard techniques would be able to identify (the so-called "twilight zone") and the challenge remains to be addressed.

   For accurate comparative analyses based on alignments, it is important to ignore genome regions that are tainted by recombination events. Moreover, regions around insertion and deletion sites (indels) should also be checked carefully to ensure that the alignment algorithms have not made mistakes in the placement of such events. In any case, it is important to highlight that extra attention should always be paid for alignments of viral sequences.

2. Most MSA tools use a progressive algorithmic process, where a guide tree is first estimated and then sequences are aligned in a pairwise fashion according to the tree topology. These procedures are iterative, with the tree and MSA being re-estimated in each round. The score system used by pairwise alignment algorithms is arguably the most influential component in progressive multiple sequence aligners and this is where some of the available algorithms differ. For instance, some aligners such as ClustalW [30] and MUSCLE [16] use a matrix score system, giving a score for each modification observed. On the other hand, tools such as T-Coffee [31] and MAFFT [17] use a system based on consistency, which compiles a primary library of global and local alignments and then use the library as a

position-specific substitution matrix during a regular progressive alignment. Recent methods usually require more computer power and may produce more accurate MSA. For a survey about MSA tools, please consider [32].

Additionally, some specific tools help to address alignment issues associated with viral genomes; e.g., MAUVE [33] is a powerful tool that allows the user to create global alignments of sequences with inversions and rearrangements. A visual overview of the alignment shows all blocks aligned, facilitating identification of such occurrences (see methods for poxvirus analyses in [34]). The ALPHA aligner [8] is another tool that exploits functional co-linearity among related strains and uses a partial order MSA algorithm to capture mosaicism in a set of phage genomes. ALPHA's graphic visualization can be very useful to understand the mosaic structure of phage genomes.

3. Some research groups have been making efforts to create groups of viral orthologous proteins and, thus, facilitate retrieval of functional and evolutionary information about new genes being characterized. For instance, the Cluster of Orthologous Groups (COGs) database curates a special section for Nucleo-Cytoplasmic Large DNA Viruses (NCLDV) [35] and another for Phages Orthologous Groups (POGs) [6]. Unfortunately, a user-friendly display of information is not provided, and data can only be downloaded in a text format. Similarly, the eggNog database [36], which despite having a web interface and allowing online searches, has not yet implemented graphical displays for the viral orthologs groups division and data is only available in a text format (at the time of writing). Lastly, the VOCs database [14] stores genomic and ortholog groups information about the main families of large DNA viruses and provides a Java web start application for user-friendly retrieve of information. Nevertheless, the viral genomes present in VOCs comprise a small fraction of the existing diversity of viruses.

4. The most common methods for estimating phylogenies include distance matrix, Neighbor-joining, maximum parsimony, Bayesian inference, and maximum likelihood. Some of these methods use substitution models that try to predict how sequences have changed across their evolutionary history. Thus, there are several factors that researches should take into account before starting phylogenetic analysis.

As a brief suggestion, robust trees have been generated using the maximum likelihood method. Best fitting models will widely depend on the sequences being analyzed. There are programs capable of testing sequence data and suggesting the most suitable model. MEGA [37] is a complete software that includes packages for the main phylogeny estimation methods, as well as model testing packages. RAxML version 8 is another popular program for phylogenetic analyses of large datasets under maximum likelihood [38].

5. NGS metagenomic studies generate large amounts of short sequences that need to be assembled in longer contigs in order to allow the extraction of a broader set of information about the microbial community. Viral genomes, as we already explored in *see* **Note 1**, present features that make the assembly more complex. High mutation rates and HGT often mislead assembly software to create chimeric contigs or create none at all. Therefore, careful and thought-out assembly of NGS sequences is essential to avoid mistakes that would carry through to all downstream analyses.

   MIRA 4 [24] assembler is an out of the box assembler for practically any kind of NGS data that generates good results for viral genome assemblies. It also has the advantage of being highly customizable and having extensive documentation. Researchers interested in assembling viral data can change parameters for overlap and mismatches to produce better results. Additionally, Spades [39] and IDBA-UD [40] assemblers may also be useful for viral genomic data.

Acknowledgments

This work has been supported by grants #2014/16450-8 and #2015/14334-3, São Paulo Research Foundation (FAPESP) to D.A. and an NSERC Discovery grant to C.U.

References

1. Ureta-Vidal A, Ettwiller L, Birney E (2003) Comparative genomics: genome-wide analysis in metazoan eukaryotes. Nat Rev Genet 4:251–262

2. Edwards R, Rohwer F (2005) Viral metagenomics. Nat Rev Microbiol 3:801–805

3. Rosario K, Breitbart M (2011) Exploring the viral world through metagenomics. Curr Opin Virol 1:289–297

4. Domingo E, Escarmis C, Sevilla N et al (1996) Basic concepts in RNA virus evolution. FASEB J 10:859–864

5. Qin L, Upton C, Hazes B et al (2011) Genomic analysis of the vaccinia virus strain variants found in dryvax vaccine. J Virol 85:13049–13060

6. Kristensen DM, Waller AS, Yamada T et al (2013) Orthologous gene clusters and taxon signature genes for viruses of prokaryotes. J Bacteriol 195:941–950

7. Sharma D, Priyadarshini P, Vrati S (2015) Unraveling the web of viroinformatics: computational tools and databases in virus research. J Virol 89:1489–1501

8. Bérard S, Chateau A, Pompidor N et al (2016) Aligning the unalignable: bacteriophage whole genome alignments. BMC Bioinformatics 17:30

9. Pickett BE, Greer DS, Zhang Y et al (2012) Virus pathogen database and analysis resource (ViPR): a comprehensive bioinformatics database and analysis resource for the coronavirus research community. Viruses 4:3209–3226

10. Altschul SF, Gish W, Miller W et al (1990) Basic local alignment search tool. J Mol Biol 215:403–410

11. Marchler-Bauer A, Zheng C, Chitsaz F et al (2013) CDD: conserved domains and protein three-dimensional structure. Nucleic Acids Res 41:D348–D352

12. Brister JR, Ako-adjei D, Bao Y et al (2014) NCBI viral genomes resource. Nucleic Acids Res 43(Database issue):D571–D577

13. Roux S, Tournayre J, Mahul A et al (2014) Metavir 2: new tools for viral metagenome comparison and assembled virome analysis. BMC Bioinformatics 15:76

14. Ehlers A, Osborne J, Slack S et al (2002) Poxvirus orthologous clusters (POCs). Bioinformatics (Oxford, England) 18:1544–1545

15. Sievers F, Wilm A, Dineen D et al (2011) Fast, scalable generation of high-quality protein multiple sequence alignments using clustal omega. Mol Syst Biol 7:539

16. Edgar RC (2004) MUSCLE: multiple sequence alignment with high accuracy and high throughput. Nucleic Acids Res 32:1792–1797

17. Katoh K, Standley DM (2013) MAFFT multiple sequence alignment software version 7: improvements in performance and usability. Mol Biol Evol 30:772–780

18. Hillary W, Lin S-H, Upton C (2011) Base-by-base version 2: single nucleotide-level analysis of whole viral genome alignments. Microb Inform Exp 1:2

19. Hatfull GF, Jacobs-Sera D, Lawrence JG et al (2010) Comparative genomic analysis of 60 mycobacteriophage genomes: genome clustering, gene acquisition, and gene size. J Mol Biol 397:119–143

20. Goris J, Konstantinidis KT, Klappenbach JA et al (2007) DNA-DNA hybridization values and their relationship to whole-genome sequence similarities. Int J Syst Evol Microbiol 57:81–91

21. Hatfull GF (2008) Bacteriophage genomics. Curr Opin Microbiol 11:447–453

22. Bateman A, Martin MJ, O'Donovan C et al (2015) UniProt: a hub for protein information. Nucleic Acids Res 43:D204–D212

23. Hasegawa M, Fujiwara M (1993) Relative efficiencies of the maximum likelihood, maximum parsimony, and neighbor-joining methods for estimating protein phylogeny. Mol Phylogenet Evol 2(1):1–5

24. B. Chevreux (2005) MIRA: an automated genome and EST assembler, Duisburg, Heidelberg. pp 1–161

25. Martins LF, Antunes LP, Pascon RC et al (2013) Metagenomic analysis of a tropical composting operation at the São Paulo zoo park reveals diversity of biomass degradation functions and organisms. PLoS One 8:e61928

26. Tatusova T, Ciufo S, Fedorov B et al (2014) RefSeq microbial genomes database: new representation and annotation strategy. Nucleic Acids Res 42:553–559

27. Angly FE, Willner D, Prieto-Davó A et al (2009) The GAAS metagenomic tool and its estimations of viral and microbial average genome size in four major biomes. PLoS Comput Biol 5:e1000593

28. Ondov BD, Bergman NH, Phillippy AM (2011) Interactive metagenomic visualization in a web browser. BMC Bioinformatics 12:385

29. Duffy S, Shackelton LA, Holmes EC (2008) Rates of evolutionary change in viruses: patterns and determinants. Nat Rev Genet 9:267–276

30. Chenna R, Sugawara H, Koike T et al (2003) Multiple sequence alignment with the Clustal series of programs. Nucleic Acids Res 31:3497–3500

31. Di Tommaso P, Moretti S, Xenarios I et al (2011) T-coffee: a web server for the multiple sequence alignment of protein and RNA sequences using structural information and homology extension. Nucleic Acids Res 39:13–17

32. Notredame C (2007) Recent evolutions of multiple sequence alignment algorithms. PLoS Comput Biol 3(8):e123

33. Darling AE, Mau B, Perna NT (2010) Progressivemauve: multiple genome alignment with gene gain, loss and rearrangement. PLoS One 5(6):e11147

34. Da Silva M, Upton C (2012) Bioinformatics for analysis of poxvirus genomes. Methods Mol Biol 890:233–258

35. Yutin N, Wolf YI, Raoult D et al (2009) Eukaryotic large nucleo-cytoplasmic DNA viruses: clusters of orthologous genes and reconstruction of viral genome evolution. Virol J 6:223

36. Huerta-Cepas J, Szklarczyk D, Forslund K et al (2016) eggNOG 4.5: a hierarchical orthology framework with improved functional annotations for eukaryotic, prokaryotic and viral sequences. Nucleic Acids Res 44:D286–D293

37. Tamura K, Stecher G, Peterson D et al (2013) MEGA6: molecular evolutionary genetics analysis version 6.0. Mol Biol Evol 30:2725–2729

38. Stamatakis A (2014) RAxML version 8: a tool for phylogenetic analysis and post-analysis of large phylogenies. Bioinformatics 30:1312–1313

39. Bankevich A, Nurk S, Antipov D et al (2012) SPAdes: a new genome assembly algorithm and its applications to single-cell sequencing. J Comput Biol 19:455–477

40. Peng Y, Leung HCM, Yiu SM et al (2012) IDBA-UD: a de novo assembler for single-cell and metagenomic sequencing data with highly uneven depth. Bioinformatics 28:1420–1428

Chapter 16

Comparative Genomics of Gene Loss and Gain in *Caenorhabditis* and Other Nematodes

Christian Rödelsperger

Abstract

Nematodes, such as *Caenorhabditis elegans*, form one of the most species-rich animal phyla. By now more than 30 nematode genomes have been published allowing for comparative genomic analyses at various different time-scales. The majority of a nematode's gene repertoire is represented by either duplicated or so-called orphan genes of unknown origin. This indicates the importance of mechanisms that generate new genes during the course of evolution. While it is certain that nematodes have acquired genes by horizontal gene transfer from various donors, this process only explains a small portion of the nematode gene content. As evolutionary genomic analyses strongly support that most orphan genes are indeed protein-coding, future studies will have to decide, whether they are result from extreme divergence or evolved de novo from previously noncoding sequences. In this contribution, I summarize several studies investigating gene loss and gain in nematodes and discuss the strengths and weaknesses of individual approaches and datasets. These approaches can be used to ask nematode-specific questions such as associated with the evolution of parasitism or with switches in mating systems, but also can complement studies in other animal phyla like vertebrates and insects to broaden our general view on genome evolution.

Key words Duplication, Lateral gene transfer, Orphan genes, Parasite, Genome evolution

1 Introduction

Together with insects, nematodes are the most successful animal phyla. They have invaded almost all ecological niches and have developed parasitism multiple times independently [1].

The nematode *Caenorhabditis elegans* is one of the most widely studied model organisms and its genome was the first to be sequenced from a multicellular organism [2]. The sequencing of the related nematode *Caenorhabditis briggsae* initiated various comparative genomic studies on nematodes [3–6]. But also outside the *Caenorhabditis* genus, there is great potential for further comparisons such as with the necromenic species *Pristionchus pacificus*, which has been established as a satellite model for comparative studies in various aspects of biology involving developmental

João C. Setubal et al. (eds.), *Comparative Genomics: Methods and Protocols*, Methods in Molecular Biology, vol. 1704, https://doi.org/10.1007/978-1-4939-7463-4_16, © Springer Science+Business Media LLC 2018

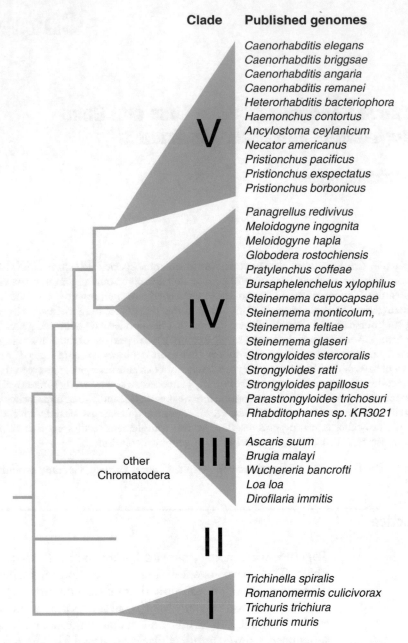

Fig. 1 Nematode phylogeny. The tree shows a schematic phylogeny of nematode clades [1] with names of species for which a draft genome assembly has been published

plasticity [7, 8], immunity [6, 9], but also population and comparative genomics [10, 11]. By now, more than thirty nematode genomes have been published (Fig. 1), which form a robust phylogenetic framework for evolutionary studies at many different levels and time-scales [5, 10, 12–15]. Their relatively small genome size [16] and species richness makes them a good system to ask various biological questions and enables sequencing of large numbers of individual strains for population genomic analysis [10, 13, 17, 18]. Furthermore, the establishment of various reverse genetic tools in multiple species [19–21] allows detailed functional characterizations of individual genes and gene families [4, 22]. Recent comparative and experimental studies in nematodes have shown that novel genes that have arisen either by duplication or are of unknown origin can control ecologically relevant traits in nematodes and play important roles in development [7, 8, 23]. Novel genes can be introduced into a genome by basically three mechanisms: duplication, horizontal gene transfer, and de novo gene formation. In this contribution, I will discuss several approaches to investigating patterns of gene gain and loss in nematodes. Please note that none of the described methods is nematode-specific, but I give numerous examples of their applications in nematode contexts.

2   Gene Duplications

Duplicated genes represent more than a third of typical multicellular genome [24] supporting a major role of duplication events during genome evolution. In his visionary book, Susumu Ohno outlined several alternative scenarios that could determine the fate of genes following duplication. Most prominent is the idea that duplication relaxes the sequence constraint on the ancestral gene and allows the two new copies to functionally diverge either to separate the ancestral functions (subfunctionalization) or even to develop novel functions (neofunctionalization) [25]. While empirical studies have shown accelerated evolution following duplication [26, 27], the most likely scenario for the largest part of duplicate genes is that one of the copies is lost [26, 28].

The long-term retention of duplicates suggests that there is a fitness cost associated with the loss of one of the duplicates [29] and multiple scenarios have been discussed in the literature that may explain the retention of duplicates with (e.g., subfunctionalization, neofunctionalization) or without (e.g., selection for higher gene dosage) diversification. There have been numerous studies revealing evidence for one or the other scenario [8, 22, 23, 26–28], but it is difficult to assess which one has the largest contribution, because different scenarios often result in similar predictions [29]. For example, asymmetry [30] in the rate of evolution between the two duplicates is consistent with neofunctionalization but also with subfunctionalization. One additional complication is that duplicate genes may diversify at many different levels. Thus, while selection for higher gene dosage might have maintained a set of initial duplicates, these duplicates may later specialize or gain new functions in certain tissues or stages. Thus, the most robust characterization of gene duplications can only be made by detailed functional studies on individual gene families [22]. However, comparative genomics approaches are still very useful in describing the general patterns of sequence and expression divergence without making any strong inferences about what processes have generated these patterns.

2.1 Detecting Gene Family Expansions by Comparing Protein Domain Counts

One simple way to screen for gene family expansions is to compare the distribution of protein domain counts (e.g., PFAM) for two genomes [5, 14, 31]. This may reveal very drastic changes in gene family sizes such as the expansion of BTB domain-containing proteins and of the cullin scaffold proteins in *Panagrellus redivivus* [5]. However, it has been shown that independent expansions and losses in both lineages can lead to an overall similar count and let a gene family appear as conserved, while in reality it undergoes substantial turnover. One very extreme case that demonstrates the missing resolution in the detection of duplications based on protein domain counts is the finding that the GST gene family has the same size ($N = 59$) in *C. elegans* and *P. pacificus* but only one of the genes is actually preserved as one-to-one ortholog between the two nematodes [32]. Furthermore, this approach has the limitation that visualization and interpretation of the data becomes increasingly difficult as soon as the comparison includes three or more species. In addition, at least three species are needed to distinguish expansions in one lineage from the deletions in the other lineage. Another disadvantage of using protein domains is that many nematode-specific gene families will be ignored if they have not yet been annotated in the PFAM database. As multiple methods for the detection of orthologs exist [33–36], similar comparisons can be done using gene family sizes as derived from orthologous clusters. This would overcome also the limitation that gene families defined by PFAM are often partially overlapping.

2.2 Phylogenetic Analysis

Reconstructing phylogenetic trees of individual gene families so far constitutes the gold standard for the detection of duplications and assigning orthology relationships. Such phylogenetic analyses usually start with homology searches by programs like BLAST to define the given gene family. This is followed by multiple sequence alignment [37, 38] with simultaneous hand curation of the obtained datasets taking into account all possible sources of errors in the data (*see* below). The next step is to find the best substitution model that explains the observed alignment [39], and finally the gene tree can be reconstructed [40]. Visual inspection of the phylogenetic trees might give some hints for which genes the initial BLAST searches might have missed orthologous sequences. This means that the whole process can be reiterated infinitely to continuously improve the dataset and final gene tree. This kind of work depends to a large extent on somewhat arbitrary decisions that have to be made by an experienced researcher. Thus, it is invaluable to talk to experienced people to check the data. For certain gene families such as

Cytochrome P450 there are even researchers such as David Nelson [41] who are willing to clean the data and to annotate Cytochrome P450 sequences for individual genome projects. Despite its labor-intensive nature and the need to deposit final data in public repositories to ensure reproducibility, detailed phylogenetic analysis on hand-curated datasets is still superior to any automated approach for ortholog detection and gene tree reconstruction. This is because the amount of error in current gene annotations is still substantial [23, 42] and actually multiplies with the number of investigated species.

2.3 Assembly Artifacts and Need for Manual Curation

The large number of published nematode genomes comes at the cost that the quality of published genomes is quite heterogeneous. While the genome of *C. elegans* is probably the best available assembly among all animals (it does not contain any gaps), a number of highly fragmented draft assemblies were recently published with N50 values of only around 10 kb [43–45]. For clarification, the N50 value is a measure of contiguity of a genome assembly and is typically defined as the size of the smallest contig in the set of largest contigs that together make up half of the total genome size. Furthermore, only few genomes are constantly improved by incorporating new sequencing data or novel annotation pipelines. Thus, it is very important to bear in mind that genomes and consequently also gene annotations may be incomplete [42]. Especially, gene absence calls are difficult because based on protein homology searches alone it is not clear whether the gene was not annotated, not assembled, or is truly not present in a given genome. Therefore, one should at least confirm by TBLASTN searches against the corresponding genome assembly and ideally also check raw sequence reads to confirm that there is really no evidence for homologous sequences in a given genome. Finally, additional support can be gained from closely related genomes of the same genus. By now, multiple nematode genera such as *Caenorhabditis, Pristionchus, Strongyloides,* and *Steinernema* have several published genomes and missing evidence in multiple independently assembled nematode genomes gives much more confidence that a gene is truly absent [46]. Furthermore, it has been shown that assembly artifacts and misannotation can generate inflated gene counts and lead to errors in automated orthology detection methods [23, 47]. Thus, I strongly recommend for studies involving just one or only a small number of gene families to hand curate the sequences, e.g., use conserved sequences from related nematodes to close gaps in multiple alignments [22, 32]. While evidence for large gene duplications is typically quite robust, for many nematode genomes, there is still the chance that heterozygosity can lead to independently assembled haplotypes and thus could potentially lead to false signals of duplications [48]. It is important to note that the importance of this problem is quite different across nematode genomes. While most nematodes are too small to get enough DNA material for sequencing from a single individual, with exception of a few studies [45, 49, 50], typically populations of inbred worms are sequenced. As some species are hermaphroditic and do not suffer from inbreeding depression, inbreeding can be much more effective in these species resulting in overall better assemblies. Thus, differences in genetic diversity together with different inbreeding schemes create another layer of heterogeneity across nematode assemblies. One way to investigate whether heterozygosity can lead to additional duplications is to examine coverage profiles and the general performance of the assembly program [31]. Most assemblers employ different heuristic strategies to generate haploid assemblies from diploid genomes. These strategies can lead to overcompression of repeats and also of recently duplicated sequences. If this were the trend, then this would indirectly support that the identified duplications are indeed true.

2.4 Micro-evolutionary Studies of Gene Loss and Gain

One advantage of nematodes as compared to vertebrates is their small genome size [16] which allows population genomic studies involving whole genome sequencing of large numbers of natural isolates [10, 13, 18]. As gene loss and gains are usually introduced in individual worms that are members of particular populations, it will take some time until they either become fixated or will be lost in a given population. As selection needs time to purge deleterious alleles, genome-wide patterns might differ a lot between intra-species comparisons and inter-species comparisons. Thus, we have recently seen that comparisons between the nematodes *C. elegans* and *P. pacificus* which shared a common ancestor in the order of 10^8 years ago [51], reveal strong evidence for the selection for higher gene dosage driving duplications of developmentally regulated genes [23]. In contrast, intra-species comparisons of different *P. pacificus* strains with divergence times in the order of 10^6 generations [12] showed that most duplication events do not seem to be functional in the sense that the cumulative gene dosage in strains with a given duplication is not higher than in strains carrying a single copy [28]. This was in strong contrast to deletions, which showed a strong impact on gene expression levels. In the mentioned study, we identified duplications and deletions based on differences in read coverage for Illumina resequencing data [52]. This is quite comparable to the previously employed microarray hybridization techniques [53–55]. Both the approaches have the disadvantages that the resolution is in the order of kilobases and breakpoints are just loosely defined, but in the case of resequencing data, other alignment-based approaches can be applied that identify breakpoints at nucleotide level resolution [56, 57]. As is the case in any pairwise comparison, in the absence of an outgroup species, it is not possible to correctly interpret a deletion or duplication event relative to a reference strain as a derived event. It may well be that a recent duplication in the reference strain will be detected as a deletion in the strain of interest [7]. Thus, exploiting the species richness of nematodes, it is possible to polarize a comparison between strains of the same species with the help of genomic data for a closely related outgroup [28]. However, even without a polarized comparison, it is possible to detect hotspots of structural variations in a given genome and to identify gene classes that are preferentially affected by such events [28, 54, 55].

3   Horizontal Gene Transfer

One particular specific feature of nematode genomes as opposed to most insects and vertebrates is the presence of various well-characterized cases of horizontal gene transfers (HGTs) that is the transmission of genes across species borders. The most prominent cases consist in cell wall degrading enzymes (cellulases) that have been acquired at least three times independently in nematodes. While cellulases in plant parasitic nematodes of the *Meloidogyne* lineage and in the necromenic *P. pacificus* belong to the GHF5 class [51, 58], other plant parasitic nematodes of the *Bursaphelenchelus* lineage have acquired cellulases of a different class (GHF45) [59]. However, even though *Pristionchus* and *Meloidogyne* cellulases are members of the same class, they are so distantly related that it is most parsimonious to assume that they have been acquired in both lineages independently [60]. More precisely, while cellulases in the *Meloidogyne* lineage have most likely been acquired from bacteria, the most similar sequences to the *Pristionchus* cellulases are found in algae and slime molds [11, 51, 60]. Furthermore, the GHF45 cellulases in the *Bursaphelenchelus* lineage have been shown to be of fungal origin [59]. While horizontally transferred genes are typically identified as genes that do not show homology in any other nematode but have database hits outside nematodes [51, 61], the first question to be answered is whether the identified candidates represent contamination during the sequencing process. Strong evidence for contamination is if the sequences resemble known bacterial at very high sequence identity (e.g., >98%). To further support that horizontally transferred genes are actually part of the nematode genomes, the assembly and raw reads can be checked to show that horizontally transferred and nematode DNA are actually physically linked and are sequenced at similar depth. This can also be validated by inverse PCR. Furthermore expression evidence in the form of RNA-seq [60], qPCR [62], in situ hybridization [51], or reporter constructs and in the case of cellulases, further functional assays [51, 60] are very helpful to show that the gene has been integrated into the biology of the host organism. In addition to cellulases, two other gene families, antimicrobial peptides most likely from beetles and insect transposons were identified as horizontally acquired in nematodes of the *Pristionchus* lineage [51, 61]. Furthermore, analysis of codon usage suggested that several unknown genes in *P. pacificus* could be of insect origin [61]. At that time, we hypothesized that the lack of homology was due to the absence of genomic data of a host for *Pristionchus* nematodes and that sequencing of a scarab beetle genome could potentially reveal further evidence for HGTs. However, sequencing the genome of the scarab beetle *Oryctes borbonicus* that is host of *P. pacificus* on la Réunion Island in the Indian Ocean did not reveal any additional HGT events [31]. Together with the relative small number of confirmed HGTs, this finding supports that HGT only explains a tiny portion of the nematode gene content.

4   Orphan Genes

Orphan genes have been generally defined as genes that are restricted to certain taxonomic groups [63]. Such taxonomically restricted genes have been frequently called orphan, pioneer, novel, or young genes. Depending on the definition and phylogenetic sampling up to one third of an animal's gene repertoire are frequently identified as orphan genes [63]. Three mechanisms have been suggested to explain the emergence of orphan genes, strong divergence beyond the level of identification as homologous sequence, de novo gene formation, and horizontal gene transfer [16, 63]. Based on extensive screens for horizontal gene transfers in nematodes which only confirmed a handful of cases [14, 16, 31, 51, 58, 59, 63], it seems unlikely that this explains a substantial part of orphan genes. While it is very difficult to distinguish the two remaining scenarios on a genome-wide scale, another alternative explanation results from the fact that fragmented assemblies can result in extensive error in gene numbers and consequently could result in artificial orphan genes [47]. In a recent study, we addressed the question whether orphan genes are really protein-coding, artifacts, or even represent noncoding RNAs [64]. We used a simple set of assumptions to test, which fraction of orphan genes belongs to each of these classes. First, considering every sequence that is supported by expression evidence as a real biological entity allowed us to get an upper bound for genomic artifacts. Second, every sequence that either shows direct evidence for translation based on available proteomic data or shows evidence of selection against nonsynonymous mutations can be considered a truly protein-coding gene. In the example of *P. pacificus* where 9885 orphan genes were defined based on the absence of homologs in any available genome outside the family Diplogastridae (for comparison, *C. elegans* has ~6000 orphans when defined at the genus level [16]), we could show that depending on the thresholds, 42–81% of orphan genes are transcribed and 40–77% of them are truly protein-coding. While *P. pacificus* has more than 14 published RNA-seq datasets [6, 8, 23], proteome evidence for *P. pacificus* is restricted to only two studies [65, 66] and directly supports only 4% of orphan genes. Thus, the strongest contribution toward assigning a gene as truly protein-coding came from comparative genomic analyses. We therefore exploited the genome assembly of a closely related sister species *P. exspectatus* [18] to calculate estimates of selection on protein-coding genes for orthologous clusters [33]. Similarly, we calculated the strength of selection on individual genes between two divergent lineages within *P. pacificus* [18], which allowed us to make a statement even for species-specific orphans. Finally, we used the idea that selection estimates can be calculated even from data of a single genome alone, if paralogous sequences are available [67]. This demonstrated that a single genome alone is enough to show negative selection in 8–10% of orphan genes, but adding population and comparative genomics data was able to increase this estimate to 40–77%. Once the validity of orphan genes has been demonstrated, further studies can ask how old are they and how they evolve.

5 Gene Loss

The large amount of duplicated genes in present genomes [23, 24] and high rates of observed duplications in experimental evolution studies [53, 68] are equalized by continuous gene loss. Thus, in a pioneering work of comparative genomics, Lynch and Connery have demonstrated that the number of duplicated genes in *C. elegans* and other genomes decreases with the age of genes as approximated by synonymous site divergence [26]. Interestingly, while duplications have frequently been assumed to be associated with adaptations to novel environments [5, 51, 69], there seems to be much less research on gene loss. However, one context, in which deletions are studied in nematodes, is the evolution of mating systems. In the genus *Caenorhabditis*, hermaphroditism has arisen three times independently from outcrossing ancestral species [70]. Similarly, in the *Pristionchus* genus there have been most likely five independent mating type switches [71]. With the limited genome sequencing data available, it seems that hermaphroditic genomes tend to be 20–40% smaller than the genomes of closely related outcrossing species [18, 70] and it has been found that an observed segregation bias favoring smaller chromosomes in hermaphroditic species predicts this trend [72]. This would also be consistent with the finding that while in plants different genome sizes can be explained by deletions in noncoding regions and transposons, in *Caenorhabditis* all classes of genomic segments have been reduced in similar proportions [70]. In addition to segregation bias favoring smaller chromosomes [71], mating type transitions to hermaphroditism predict a relaxed constraint and potential loss of certain sex-specific genes [73–75]. However, empirical studies on genome size evolution in nematodes are still in their infancy, because similar to the studies on independent evolution of parasitism, studying the impact of mating system transitions on genome evolution requires sequencing sets of genomes and transcriptomes in different parts of the phylogeny.

6 Conclusion

Nematode genomes offer a range of very interesting and nematode-specific questions to ask such as "What are the genomic footprints of evolution of parasitism or mating system transitions?". But even for more general questions, such as "What is the origin of orphan genes?" and "What drives the retention of duplicate genes?" studies in nematodes offer a complementary animal system to support genomic trends identified in vertebrates or insects. For example, similar to recent work in beetles [31], one could ask whether certain nematode lineages (e.g., parasites) exhibit accelerated rates of gene turnover. While most nematode studies did such analysis on specific datasets such as individual gene families [32] or a specific clade of nematode species [68], a comprehensive genome-wide study of the rates of gene gain and loss is still lacking. In addition, established genetic tools and short generation times make some species excellent models for functional investigation of selected candidate genes [4, 22] and experimental evolution studies [12, 15, 53]. Their species-richness together with their small genome size facilitates easy generation of novel comparative genomic datasets that are particularly suited to ask a specific question [69, 76]. However, working with nematode genomes comes with certain costs, for example that so far there are no reliable estimates of divergence times between species, as informative fossil records are extreme scarce and approaches based on extrapolating divergence times from the per generation mutation rates suffer from the fact that the number of generations per year might vary by two orders of magnitude [12, 77, 78]. Further, the small size of most nematode species makes tissue-specific transcriptome profiling extremely difficult. Thus, the number of tissue-specific transcriptome studies [6, 79, 80] is far less than in vertebrates. Together with the fact that strong functional divergence between species [4, 81, 82] makes Gene Ontology term assignments for biological processes relatively unreliable, this makes the interpretation of gene sets, identified by comparative genomics approaches, quite difficult. Nevertheless, I am convinced that existing and future nematode datasets form a powerful phylogenetic framework to extend our views on genome evolution.

Acknowledgments

I would like to thank Praveen Baskaran, Neel Prabh, and Gabriel Markov for helpful comments on the manuscript.

References

1. Blaxter ML, De Ley P, Garey JR, Liu LX, Scheldeman P et al (1998) A molecular evolutionary framework for the phylum Nematoda. Nature 392:71–75

2. C. elegans Sequencing Consortium (1998) Genome sequence of the nematode C. elegans: a platform for investigating biology. Science 282:2012–2018

3. Stein LD, Bao Z, Blasiar D, Blumenthal T, Brent MR et al (2003) The genome sequence of *Caenorhabditis briggsae*: a platform for comparative genomics. PLoS Biol 1:E45

4. Verster AJ, Ramani AK, McKay SJ, Fraser AG (2014) Comparative RNAi screens in C. elegans and C. briggsae reveal the impact of developmental system drift on gene function. PLoS Genet 10:e1004077

5. Srinivasan J, Dillman AR, Macchietto MG, Heikkinen L, Lakso M et al (2013) The draft genome and transcriptome of Panagrellus redivivus are shaped by the harsh demands of a free-living lifestyle. Genetics 193:1279–1295

6. Lightfoot JW, Chauhan VM, Aylott JW, Rödelsperger C (2016) Comparative transcriptomics of the nematode gut identifies global shifts in feeding mode and pathogen susceptibility. BMC Res Notes 9:142

7. Mayer MG, Rödelsperger C, Witte H, Riebesell M, Sommer RJ (2015) The orphan gene dauerless regulates dauer development and intraspecific competition in nematodes by copy number variation. PLoS Genet 11:e1005146

8. Ragsdale EJ, Muller MR, Rödelsperger C, Sommer RJ (2013) A developmental switch coupled to the evolution of plasticity acts through a sulfatase. Cell 155:922–933

9. Rae R, Witte H, Rödelsperger C, Sommer RJ (2012) The importance of being regular: *Caenorhabditis elegans* and *Pristionchus pacificus* defecation mutants are hypersusceptible to bacterial pathogens. Int J Parasitol 42:747–753

10. McGaughran A, Rödelsperger C, Grimm DG, Meyer JM, Moreno E et al (2016) Genomic profiles of diversification and genotype-phenotype association in island nematode lineages. Mol Biol Evol 33(9):2257–2272

11. Rödelsperger C, Dieterich C (2015) Comparative and functional genomics. In: Sommer RJ (ed) *Pristionchus pacificus* a nematode model for comparative and evolutionary biology. Brill, Leiden; Boston, pp 141–165

12. Weller AM, Rödelsperger C, Eberhardt G, Molnar RI, Sommer RJ (2014) Opposing forces of A/T-biased mutations and G/C-biased gene conversions shape the genome of the nematode *Pristionchus pacificus*. Genetics 196:1145–1152

13. Thomas CG, Wang W, Jovelin R, Ghosh R, Lomasko T et al (2015) Full-genome evolutionary histories of selfing, splitting, and selection in Caenorhabditis. Genome Res 25:667–678

14. Kikuchi T, Cotton JA, Dalzell JJ, Hasegawa K, Kanzaki N et al (2011) Genomic insights into the origin of parasitism in the emerging plant pathogen *Bursaphelenchus xylophilus*. PLoS Pathog 7:e1002219

15. Denver DR, Dolan PC, Wilhelm LJ, Sung W, Lucas-Lledo JI et al (2009) A genome-wide view of *Caenorhabditis elegans* base-substitution mutation processes. Proc Natl Acad Sci U S A 106:16310–16314

16. Rödelsperger C, Streit A, Sommer RJ (2013) Structure, function and evolution of the Nematode genome. eLS. John Wiley & Sons, Ltd, Chichester

17. Palomares-Rius JE, Tsai IJ, Karim N, Akiba M, Kato T et al (2015) Genome-wide variation in the pinewood nematode *Bursaphelenchus xylophilus* and its relationship with pathogenic traits. BMC Genomics 16:845

18. Rödelsperger C, Neher RA, Weller AM, Eberhardt G, Witte H et al (2014) Characterization of genetic diversity in the nematode *Pristionchus pacificus* from population-scale resequencing data. Genetics 196:1153–1165

19. Lu TW, Pickle CS, Lin S, Ralston EJ, Gurling M et al (2013) Precise and heritable genome editing in evolutionarily diverse nematodes using TALENs and CRISPR/Cas9 to engineer insertions and deletions. Genetics 195:331–348

20. Tabara H, Grishok A, Mello CC (1998) RNAi in C. elegans: soaking in the genome sequence. Science 282:430–431

21. Witte H, Moreno E, Rödelsperger C, Kim J, Kim JS et al (2015) Gene inactivation using the CRISPR/Cas9 system in the nematode *Pristionchus pacificus*. Dev Genes Evol 225:55–62

22. Markov GV, Meyer JM, Panda O, Artyukhin AB, Claassen M et al (2016) Functional conservation and divergence of daf-22 paralogs in *Pristionchus pacificus* dauer development. Mol Biol Evol 33(10):2506–2514

23. Baskaran P, Rödelsperger C, Prabh N, Serobyan V, Markov GV et al (2015) Ancient gene duplications have shaped developmental stage-specific expression in *Pristionchus pacificus*. BMC Evol Biol 15:185

24. Wagner A (2001) Birth and death of duplicated genes in completely sequenced eukaryotes. Trends Genet 17:237–239

25. Ohno S (1970) Evolution by gene duplication. Springer, Berlin

26. Lynch M, Conery JS (2000) The evolutionary fate and consequences of duplicate genes. Science 290:1151–1155

27. Pegueroles C, Laurie S, Alba MM (2013) Accelerated evolution after gene duplication: a time-dependent process affecting just one copy. Mol Biol Evol 30:1830–1842

28. Baskaran P, Rödelsperger C (2015) Microevolution of duplications and deletions and their impact on gene expression in the nematode pristionchus pacificus. PLoS One 10: e0131136

29. Hahn MW (2009) Distinguishing among evolutionary models for the maintenance of gene duplicates. J Hered 100:605–617

30. Katju V (2013) To the beat of a different drum: determinants implicated in the asymmetric sequence divergence of *Caenorhabditis elegans* paralogs. BMC Evol Biol 13:73

31. Meyer JM, Markov GV, Baskaran P, Herrmann M, Sommer RJ et al (2016) Draft genome of the scarab beetle *Oryctes borbonicus* on La Reunion Island. Genome Biol Evol 8 (7):2093–2105

32. Markov GV, Baskaran P, Sommer RJ (2015) The same or not the same: lineage-specific gene expansions and homology relationships in multigene families in nematodes. J Mol Evol 80:18–36

33. Li L, Stoeckert CJ Jr, Roos DS (2003) OrthoMCL: identification of ortholog groups for eukaryotic genomes. Genome Res 13:2178–2189

34. Remm M, Storm CE, Sonnhammer EL (2001) Automatic clustering of orthologs and in-paralogs from pairwise species comparisons. J Mol Biol 314:1041–1052

35. Rödelsperger C, Dieterich C (2008) Syntenator: multiple gene order alignments with a gene-specific scoring function. Algorithms Mol Biol 3:14

36. Tatusov RL, Koonin EV, Lipman DJ (1997) A genomic perspective on protein families. Science 278:631–637

37. Gouy M, Guindon S, Gascuel O (2010) SeaView version 4: a multiplatform graphical user interface for sequence alignment and phylogenetic tree building. Mol Biol Evol 27:221–224

38. Edgar RC (2004) MUSCLE: a multiple sequence alignment method with reduced time and space complexity. BMC Bioinformatics 5:113

39. Darriba D, Taboada GL, Doallo R, Posada D (2011) ProtTest 3: fast selection of best-fit models of protein evolution. Bioinformatics 27:1164–1165

40. Schliep KP (2011) Phangorn: phylogenetic analysis in R. Bioinformatics 27:592–593

41. Nelson DR (2009) The cytochrome p450 homepage. Hum Genomics 4:59–65

42. Gilabert A, Curran DM, Harvey SC, Wasmuth JD (2016) Expanding the view on the evolution of the nematode dauer signalling pathways: refinement through gene gain and pathway co-option. BMC Genomics 17:476

43. Godel C, Kumar S, Koutsovoulos G, Ludin P, Nilsson D et al (2012) The genome of the heartworm, *Dirofilaria immitis*, reveals drug and vaccine targets. FASEB J 26:4650–4661

44. Mortazavi A, Schwarz EM, Williams B, Schaeffer L, Antoshechkin I et al (2010) Scaffolding a Caenorhabditis nematode genome with RNA-seq. Genome Res 20:1740–1747

45. Susoy V, Herrmann M, Kanzaki N, Kruger M, Nguyen CN et al (2016) Large-scale diversification without genetic isolation in nematode symbionts of figs. Sci Adv 2:e1501031

46. Rödelsperger C, Menden K, Serobyan V, Witte H, Baskaran P (2016) First insights into the nature and evolution of antisense transcription in nematodes. BMC Evol Biol 16:165

47. Denton JF, Lugo-Martinez J, Tucker AE, Schrider DR, Warren WC et al (2014) Extensive error in the number of genes inferred from draft genome assemblies. PLoS Comput Biol 10:e1003998

48. Barriere A, Yang SP, Pekarek E, Thomas CG, Haag ES et al (2009) Detecting heterozygosity in shotgun genome assemblies: lessons from obligately outcrossing nematodes. Genome Res 19:470–480

49. Jex AR, Liu S, Li B, Young ND, Hall RS et al (2011) *Ascaris suum* draft genome. Nature 479:529–533

50. Tallon LJ, Liu X, Bennuru S, Chibucos MC, Godinez A et al (2014) Single molecule sequencing and genome assembly of a clinical specimen of *Loa loa*, the causative agent of loiasis. BMC Genomics 15:788

51. Dieterich C, Clifton SW, Schuster LN, Chinwalla A, Delehaunty K et al (2008) The *Pristionchus pacificus* genome provides a unique perspective on nematode lifestyle and parasitism. Nat Genet 40:1193–1198

52. Xie C, Tammi MT (2009) CNV-seq, a new method to detect copy number variation using high-throughput sequencing. BMC Bioinformatics 10:80

53. Farslow JC, Lipinski KJ, Packard LB, Edgley ML, Taylor J et al (2015) Rapid increase in frequency of gene copy-number variants during experimental evolution in Caenorhabditis elegans. BMC Genomics 16:1044

54. Maydan JS, Flibotte S, Edgley ML, Lau J, Selzer RR et al (2007) Efficient high-resolution deletion discovery in *Caenorhabditis elegans* by array comparative genomic hybridization. Genome Res 17:337–347

55. Maydan JS, Lorch A, Edgley ML, Flibotte S, Moerman DG (2010) Copy number variation in the genomes of twelve natural isolates of *Caenorhabditis elegans*. BMC Genomics 11:62

56. Ye K, Schulz MH, Long Q, Apweiler R, Ning Z (2009) Pindel: a pattern growth approach to detect break points of large deletions and medium sized insertions from paired-end short reads. Bioinformatics 25:2865–2871

57. Emde AK, Schulz MH, Weese D, Sun R, Vingron M et al (2012) Detecting genomic indel variants with exact breakpoints in single- and paired-end sequencing data using SplazerS. Bioinformatics 28:619–627

58. Kyndt T, Haegeman A, Gheysen G (2008) Evolution of GHF5 endoglucanase gene structure in plant-parasitic nematodes: no evidence for an early domain shuffling event. BMC Evol Biol 8:305

59. Kikuchi T, Jones JT, Aikawa T, Kosaka H, Ogura N (2004) A family of glycosyl hydrolase family 45 cellulases from the pine wood nematode *Bursaphelenchus xylophilus*. FEBS Lett 572:201–205

60. Mayer WE, Schuster LN, Bartelmes G, Dieterich C, Sommer RJ (2011) Horizontal gene transfer of microbial cellulases into nematode genomes is associated with functional assimilation and gene turnover. BMC Evol Biol 11:13

61. Rödelsperger C, Sommer RJ (2011) Computational archaeology of the Pristionchus

62. Schuster LN, Sommer RJ (2012) Expressional and functional variation of horizontally acquired cellulases in the nematode *Pristionchus pacificus*. Gene 506:274–282

63. Tautz D, Domazet-Loso T (2011) The evolutionary origin of orphan genes. Nat Rev Genet 12:692–702

64. Prabh N, Rödelsperger C (2016) Are orphan genes protein-coding, prediction artifacts, or non-coding RNAs? BMC Bioinformatics 17:226

65. Borchert N, Dieterich C, Krug K, Schutz W, Jung S et al (2010) Proteogenomics of *Pristionchus pacificus* reveals distinct proteome structure of nematode models. Genome Res 20:837–846

66. Borchert N, Krug K, Gnad F, Sinha A, Sommer RJ et al (2012) Phosphoproteome of *Pristionchus pacificus* provides insights into architecture of signaling networks in nematode models. Mol Cell Proteomics 11:1631–1639

67. Katju V, Lynch M (2003) The structure and early evolution of recently arisen gene duplicates in the *Caenorhabditis elegans* genome. Genetics 165:1793–1803

68. Lipinski KJ, Farslow JC, Fitzpatrick KA, Lynch M, Katju V et al (2011) High spontaneous rate of gene duplication in *Caenorhabditis elegans*. Curr Biol 21:306–310

69. Hunt VL, Tsai IJ, Coghlan A, Reid AJ, Holroyd N et al (2016) The genomic basis of parasitism in the Strongyloides clade of nematodes. Nat Genet 48:299–307

70. Fierst JL, Willis JH, Thomas CG, Wang W, Reynolds RM et al (2015) Reproductive mode and the evolution of genome size and structure in caenorhabditis nematodes. PLoS Genet 11:e1005323

71. Weadick CJ, Sommer RJ (2016) Mating system transitions drive life span evolution in Pristionchus nematodes. Am Nat 187:517–531

72. Wang J, Chen PJ, Wang GJ, Keller L (2010) Chromosome size differences may affect meiosis and genome size. Science 329:293

73. Wright AE, Mank JE (2013) The scope and strength of sex-specific selection in genome evolution. J Evol Biol 26:1841–1853

74. Cutter AD (2008) Reproductive evolution: symptom of a selfing syndrome. Curr Biol 18: R1056–R1058

75. Thomas CG, Woodruff GC, Haag ES (2012) Causes and consequences of the evolution of reproductive mode in Caenorhabditis nematodes. Trends Genet 28:213–220

76. Dillman AR, Macchietto M, Porter CF, Rogers A, Williams B et al (2015) Comparative genomics of Steinernema reveals deeply conserved gene regulatory networks. Genome Biol 16:200

77. Cutter AD (2008) Divergence times in Caenorhabditis and Drosophila inferred from direct estimates of the neutral mutation rate. Mol Biol Evol 25:778–786

78. Mayer MG, Sommer RJ (2011) Natural variation in *Pristionchus pacificus* dauer formation reveals cross-preference rather than self-preference of nematode dauer pheromones. Proc Biol Sci 278:2784–2790

79. Spencer WC, Zeller G, Watson JD, Henz SR, Watkins KL et al (2011) A spatial and temporal map of *C. elegans* gene expression. Genome Res 21:325–341

80. McGhee JD, Sleumer MC, Bilenky M, Wong K, McKay SJ et al (2007) The ELT-2 GATA-factor and the global regulation of transcription in the *C. elegans* intestine. Dev Biol 302:627–645

81. Sommer RJ (2012) Evolution of regulatory networks: nematode vulva induction as an example of developmental systems drift. Adv Exp Med Biol 751:79–91

82. Sinha A, Sommer RJ, Dieterich C (2012) Divergent gene expression in the conserved dauer stage of the nematodes *Pristionchus pacificus* and *Caenorhabditis elegans*. BMC Genomics 13:254

Chapter 17

Comparative Genomics in *Drosophila*

Martin Oti, Attilio Pane, and Michael Sammeth

Abstract

Since the pioneering studies of Thomas Hunt Morgan and coworkers at the dawn of the twentieth century, *Drosophila melanogaster* and its sister species have tremendously contributed to unveil the rules underlying animal genetics, development, behavior, evolution, and human disease. Recent advances in DNA sequencing technologies launched Drosophila into the post-genomic era and paved the way for unprecedented comparative genomics investigations. The complete sequencing and systematic comparison of the genomes from 12 Drosophila species represents a milestone achievement in modern biology, which allowed a plethora of different studies ranging from the annotation of known and novel genomic features to the evolution of chromosomes and, ultimately, of entire genomes. Despite the efforts of countless laboratories worldwide, the vast amount of data that were produced over the past 15 years is far from being fully explored.

In this chapter, we will review some of the bioinformatic approaches that were developed to interrogate the genomes of the 12 Drosophila species. Setting off from alignments of the entire genomic sequences, the degree of conservation can be separately evaluated for every region of the genome, providing already first hints about elements that are under purifying selection and therefore likely functional. Furthermore, the careful analysis of repeated sequences sheds light on the evolutionary dynamics of transposons, an enigmatic and fascinating class of mobile elements housed in the genomes of animals and plants. Comparative genomics also aids in the computational identification of the transcriptionally active part of the genome, first and foremost of protein-coding loci, but also of transcribed nevertheless apparently noncoding regions, which were once considered "junk" DNA. Eventually, the synergy between functional and comparative genomics also facilitates in silico and in vivo studies on *cis*-acting regulatory elements, like transcription factor binding sites, that due to the high degree of sequence variability usually impose increased challenges for bioinformatics approaches.

Key words Comparative genomics, Drosophila 12 genomes project, Multiple genome alignment, Evolutionary conservation, Homology-based prediction of protein-coding genes, Noncoding RNAs, miRNAs, Transcription factor binding sites

1 Introduction

Over the past two decades, comparative genomics was fueled by the complete sequencing of entire genomes and also *Drosophila melanogaster*, a primary model in genetics, developmental, and evolutionary biology, together with species from the same genus, highly

João C. Setubal et al. (eds.), *Comparative Genomics: Methods and Protocols*, Methods in Molecular Biology, vol. 1704, https://doi.org/10.1007/978-1-4939-7463-4_17, © Springer Science+Business Media LLC 2018

benefitted from novel DNA sequencing technologies. The beginning of the post-genomic era for the fruit flies starts in the year 2000 with the sequencing and assembly of the *D. melanogaster* genome [1]. This groundbreaking achievement stemmed from the combined efforts of two consortia, the Celera Genomics and the Berkeley Drosophila Genome Project (BDGP) and the use of whole genome shotgun sequencing (WGS), a DNA sequencing technology that was previously used only for small viral and bacterial genomes. WGS provided a stunning amount of information regarding the structure and complexity of the *D. melanogaster* genome, which contains approximately 14,000 protein-coding genes together with a broad variety of non-protein-coding loci, including 127 miRNA genes [2] and a diversity of transposable elements, a highly dynamic class of mobile sequences that is found both in plants and in animals. Five years after *D. melanogaster*, also the genome of *D. pseudobscura* was fully sequenced [3]. The evolutionary distance between *D. melanogaster* and *D. pseudobscura* estimated in 25–55 Mya was expected to permit the investigation of both protein-coding regions as well as *cis*-acting regulatory elements (CRE) [4]. The comparison between the genomes of these species represents one of the first examples of comparative genomics in metazoan Eukaryotes in the post-genomic era. The study unveiled an unexpected degree of gene synteny conservation between the two species, improved substantially gene annotation, and shed light on the mechanisms of chromosome rearrangement and evolution. However, it became soon apparent that the fine mapping of CRE could be only achieved by increasing the number of the sequenced genomes from species with intermediate phylogenetic distances from *D. melanogaster* [3, 5]. The 12 Drosophila genome project sequenced the genomes of 10 additional Drosophila species [6–8], which were selected based on their different behavioral, developmental, and ecological characteristics, to sample, at least in part, the extraordinary biodiversity of the Drosophila genus and thus allow to infer general principles underlying speciation, adaptation, and ultimately evolution. The interrogated species ranged from *D. sechellia* and *D. persimilis*, sibling species of *D. simulans* and *D. pseudobscura* respectively within the Sophophora radiation, to the distantly related *D. virilis*, *D. mojavensis*, and *D. grimshawi* from the Drosophila subgenus. Besides phylogenetic considerations, also behavioral habits were included in the criteria of selection by choosing for instance fruit flies like *D. sechellia*, which is endemic of the Seychelles Archipelago and feeds on plants that are generally toxic to other Drosophilids. The project achieved a more comprehensive understanding of gene structure and evolution, ncRNA conservation, and chromosome dynamics over a wide range of phylogenetic distances. Furthermore, the analysis of CRE and miRNAs prompted the development of new bioinformatics tools for the prediction of RNA structures and functional elements. Comparative genomics showed that the transposable element content between the genomes diverges from approximately 2.7% in *D. simulans* to ~25% in *D. ananassae*, and more detailed analyses about the distribution and abundance of ancestral transposon families, like Galileo and 1360 that appear to have been lost in certain Drosophila species, allowed elucidating the interspecies transmission of mobile elements during evolution. Over the past 10 years, the genomes of numerous additional Drosophila species have been sequenced in the context of larger studies, like the modENCODE (Model Organism Encyclopedia of DNA Elements) Project or complementary projects carried out by individual groups. With thousands of genome-wide assays modENCODE provided a striking amount of information regarding genome structure, chromosome organization, epigenetics, chromatin marks, binding sites for regulatory factors, noncoding RNAs, as well as origins of DNA replication and their role in the regulation of gene expression and RNA processing [9, 10].

The heavy datasets produced by the sequencing machines prompted the quest for novel bioinformatic tools to systematically analyze and compare the genomes in order to extract the relevant information. Such undertaking indeed still poses several challenges due to incomplete sequencing and assembly of some genomes and the lack of colinearity between genomes of even closely related species. Furthermore, the inherent repetitive nature and the abundance of sequences like transposable elements and satellite DNA, which make up a substantial proportion of animal genomes, still represents a major challenge for the field of bioinformatics. This chapter provides an overview of several types of comparative genomics analyses that were carried out by the Drosophila 12 Genomes Project. It illustrates the approaches and tools that can be used for comparing sets of genomes from related species [6], and the potential of such comparative analyses to improve the functional annotation of these genomes [7]. The techniques involved have been covered in earlier chapters, so the focus of this chapter is on demonstrating their practical application using the 12 Drosophila genomes. Wherever relevant, updated tools are presented instead of those used in the original project.

2   Materials

Throughout this chapter we employ comparative genomics approaches on the *Drosophila* genomes from the Drosophila 12 Genomes Project [6–8]. The project conducted studies on the earlier published genome assemblies of *D. melanogaster* (GCA_000001215.1) as well as *D. pseudobscura* (GCA_000001765.2) [3], and additionally produced scaffolds of the genomic sequence for *D. simulans* (GCA_000259055.1),

D.   sechellia   (GCA_000005215.1),   D.   yakuba
(GCA_000005975.1),   D.   erecta   (GCA_000005135.1),
D.   ananassae   (GCA_000005115.1),   D.   persimilis
(GCA_000005195.1),   D.   willistoni   (GCA_000005925.1),
D.   virilis   (GCA_000005245.1),   D.   mojavensis
(GCA_000005175.1), and D. grimshawi (GCA_000005155.1).
These genome sequences occupy approximatively 2 Gb of disk
space and can for instance be downloaded from Genbank employing former accession numbers given in parentheses (http://www.
ncbi.nlm.nih.gov/assembly), but they are also available from other
relevant databases such as Flybase (http://flybase.org) [11],
Ensembl (http://www.ensembl.org) [12], or from the UCSC
genome browser [13]. Note that since the conclusion of the Drosophila 12 Genomes Project some of the genome assemblies have
been updated (e.g., D. melanogaster is currently at Release 6), and
also genomes of several more Drosophila species have been added,
e.g., including D. biarmipes, D. suzukii, D. bipectinata,
D. eugracilis, D. elegans, D. kikkawai, D. takahashii, D. rhopaloa,
D. ficusphila, D. miranda, and D. albomicans.

Table 1 provides a summary of all software employed in this
chapter, along with the corresponding download links and

Table 1
Software tools relevant to comparative genomics in Drosophila species

Task	Software	Website	References
Whole genome alignment	Lastz & multiz	http://www.bx.psu.edu/miller_lab/	[14, 15]
Evolutionary conservation of genomic DNA	PhastCons, PhyloP	http://compgen.cshl.edu/phast/	[17]
Analysis of transposable element evolution	PILER	http://www.drive5.com/piler/	[19]
Annotating protein-coding genes	PhyloCSF	https://github.com/mlin/PhyloCSF/wiki	[25]
Orthology prediction	OrthoMCL	http://www.orthomcl.org/orthomcl/	[29]
Identifying protein evolutionary rates	PAML	http://abacus.gene.ucl.ac.uk/software/paml.html	[31]
Identifying (non-coding) genomic RNAs	EvoFold	http://moma.ki.au.dk/~jsp/software.html	[32]
	Vienna RNA package	http://www.tbi.univie.ac.at/RNA/	[33]
Annotating transcription factor binding motifs	BigFoot	https://sourceforge.net/projects/bigfoot/	[39]

Note that the table does not provide a comprehensive list of all tools that can be used to conduct the described analyses
but rather provides examples in accordance with the studies conducted by the 12 Drosophila Genomes Project

references. The spectrum of these programs ranges from whole genome sequence alignment to the identification of protein-coding genes, noncoding RNAs, and regulatory elements. Most of the tasks described herein can be run on a personal computer. However, comparative analyses of entire genome sequences from multiple species can be computationally intensive, especially in the case of genome-wide multiple sequence alignments. Therefore for some studies, such as the phylogeny-based gene orthology predictions (Subheading 3.4.2), it is more convenient to obtain pre-computed datasets from databases where available rather than to compute them oneself. For instance, the MULTIZ whole genome alignments computed by the original Drosophila 12 Genomes Project are available in the MAF format (*see* **Note 1**) at UCSC http://hgdownload.cse.ucsc.edu/goldenPath/dm3/multiz15way. In the remainder of this chapter, we aim to provide a guideline for the manifold different analyses employing comparative genomics of the 12 Drosophila genomes. Depending on the number of alternative approaches and the overhead of technical details for installing every single program in a multi-step analysis or in the case of multiple alternatives, we restrict command line examples where suitable.

3 Methods

3.1 Computing Whole Genome Alignments

Objective: Aligning the entire genomic sequences of multiple species.

Approach: Multiple alignment is a computationally hard problem, particularly when the sequences to be aligned extend to entire chromosomes. A practicable solution is to divide the creation of a multiple alignment into two heuristic steps. First, pairwise sequence alignments are constructed for all pairs of genomes using a local alignment algorithm. Subsequently, the pairwise alignments are coalesced into a multiple sequence alignment by iterating several layers of grouping steps, i.e., chaining, netting, etc. (http://genomewiki.ucsc.edu/index.php/Whole_genome_alignment_howto). Pairwise and multiple genome alignments are pre-required for many types of analyses in comparative genomics. One simple example is to assess the conservation level of genomic intervals based on the sequence similarity implied by pairwise alignments of multiple genomes to a reference genome, as illustrated in Fig. 1 (bottom panel).

Tools: The program LASTZ [14], an improved version replacing the earlier BLASTZ algorithm, can be employed for aligning (multiple) pairs of genomes, and subsequently MULTIZ [15] generates multiple genome sequence alignments from these pairwise alignments. Both the programs can be downloaded from http://www.bx.psu.edu/miller_lab/.

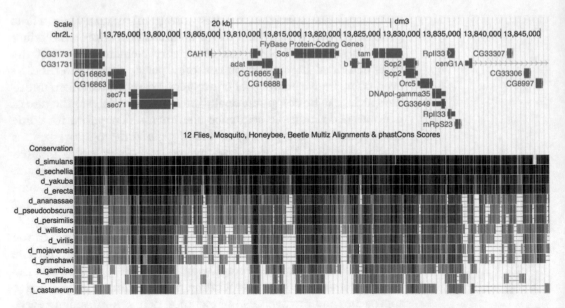

Fig. 1 Multiple sequence alignment and evolutionary conservation in a selected genomic region of the 12 Drosophila genomes, considering three non-Drosophila insect genomes as an outgroup. Genomic coordinates are based on the *Drosophila melanogaster* (dm3) genome, and the top track shows some protein-coding genes from the Flybase annotation in the region. The conservation track at the bottom visualizes the genome alignments between dm3 and all other species by *gray* boxes, i.e., darker shades are employed for intervals of higher similarity between the corresponding two genomes

Example: For instance, in order to align the chromosome 4 sequence of each *D. simulans* and *D. yakuba* with chromosome 4 of *D. melanogaster*, call:

```
lastz dm3.chr4.fa droSim1.chr4.fa --notransition --step=20 --nogapped --for-
mat=maf > dm3_4.droSim1_4.maf
    lastz dm3.chr4.fa droYak2.chr4.fa --notransition --step=20 --nogapped --format=maf >
dm3_4.droYak2_4.maf
```

The "--notransition," "--step=20," and "--nogapped" options lower the sensitivity but still provide good alignments, while greatly reducing the run time. More detailed information on the parameter control is provided by the LASTZ documentation (http://www.bx.psu.edu/miller_lab/dist/README.lastz-1.02.00/README.lastz-1.02.00a.html). Next, use the tba (i.e., the "Threaded Block Aligner") command from the MULTIZ package to combine these alignments:

```
tba "((dm3 droSim1) droYak2)" *.*.maf tba.dm3.droSim1.droYak2.
maf
```

3.2 Assessing the Evolutionary Conservation of Genomic DNA

Objective: Detecting the degree of genome-wide evolutionary conservation from genomic alignments.

Approach: The identification of nucleotide conservation in a multiple genome sequence alignment can be accomplished using a phylogenetic Hidden Markov Model (phylo-HMM), which estimates the probability that a given genomic site is in a conserved state [16]. Such an approach allows correlation between adjacent sites to be taken into account (i.e., by the order of the HMM) and bases on the reasonable assumption that evolutionary conservation usually occurs at the level of genomic elements (exons, protein-binding sites, etc.) rather than at single nucleotides. In this regard, a given site is more likely to be considered conserved if its neighboring sites show a high similarity across the set of species under analysis than if the site is flanked by variable nucleotides. Importantly, the model incorporates the phylogenetic information such that nucleotide similarity between closely related species is considered less informative than nucleotide similarity between more divergent species.

Tools: PhastCons and PhyloP, both from the PHAST software suite [17] (http://compgen.cshl.edu/phast/). PhastCons is based on a two-state phylo-HMM, and outputs the probability of a site being conserved. PhyloP is based on a model of neutral evolution and indicates both conservation and accelerated evolution.

Example: Run phastCons on a multiple sequence alignment to determine conservation scores by

```
phastCons --target-coverage 0.393 --expected-length 23.8 --rho
0.3 --msa-format MAF tba.dm3.droSim1.droYak2.maf noncons.mod >
conservation_scores.wig
```

This command requires a multiple sequence alignment input file ("tba.dm3.droSim1.droYak2.maf") and a phylogenetic model for non-conserved regions ("noncons.mod"), which can be produced using the "PhyloFit" program from the same PHAST software suite. PhastCons outputs a wiggle track with conservation scores, i.e., a long table of genomic positions/intervals and the conservation score they have been assigned (https://genome.ucsc.edu/goldenpath/help/wiggle.html). Refer to the phastCons documentation (http://compgen.cshl.edu/phast/help-pages/phastCons.txt) for more information about setting the program parameters.

3.3 Detecting Transposable Elements

Objective: Detecting and analyzing the dynamics of transposable element sequences.

Approach: Transposable elements are marked by repeats, which can be detected in a newly sequenced genome for instance by straightforwardly scanning for known repeat sequences, for instance from a related species. For the Drosophila genomes analyzed herein, this translates to scanning for known *D. melanogaster* repeat families in the other Drosophila species. However, such an approach certainly biases the results obtained toward the already known repeat families. Therefore, complementary software tools have been developed for detecting reads de novo, i.e., without relying on prior knowledge of specific repeat sequences or families.

Tools:

– ReAS [18]: The tool can be requested by email to ReAS@genomics.org.cn and performs ab initio repeat identification using an approach based on *k*-mers. In a nutshell, ReAS identifies *k*-mers that are statistically over-represented in the target genome and then merges these into consensus sequences that are employed for genome-wide scanning.

– PILER (http://www.drive5.com/piler/) [19]: The program identifies repeats from characteristic patterns of local alignments and provides the genomic locations of the identified repeats as well as consensus repeat sequences. These patterns can subsequently be employed to scan the relevant genomes with tools such as RepeatMasker [20] (http://www.repeatmasker.org/) or RepeatRunner [21] (http://www.yandell-lab.org/software/repeatrunner.html).

Example: PILER-DF (PILER Dispersed Family) is a search mode of the PILER program employing parameters that are designed for identifying transposable elements. It requires two other programs to be installed–PALS for aligning a genome with itself and MUSCLE for creating a multiple sequence alignment of the identified repeats. Running the PILER-DF pipeline involves three steps:

1. Find local alignments of the given genome with itself using the "pals" program.

2. Identify families of three or more intact, isolated copies of a repeat using the "piler" program.

3. Align repeat family sequences using the "muscle" program to create a consensus sequence.

The PILER user guide (http://www.drive5.com/piler/piler_userguide.html) describes in detail the use of the program.

3.4 Comparative Genomics of Protein-Coding Genes

Due to its immediate functional impact, the annotation of protein-coding genes in newly sequenced genomes traditionally receives special attention in the field of computational genomics. From the several ways to analyze coding genes, we will cover in this chapter particularly the ones that employ comparative genomics techniques in order to annotate genes on the genome, to map genes between species and to investigate the evolutionary rates of proteins. However, due to the strong bias in the availability of transcriptomic data between the different Drosophila species (*see* **Note 2**), we will not include the inter-species comparison of transcript structures and splicing patterns in our analyses.

3.4.1 Annotating Protein-Coding Genes

Objective: Identifying the genomic locations and the exon-intron structure of protein-coding genes.

Approach: There are two general approaches to finding genes in genomic sequences: ab initio methods that predict gene structure based on the given DNA sequence alone, and homology-based methods that employ additionally information from evolutionarily related genomes. Both the approaches were used by the 12 Drosophila Genomes Project, annotating genes by combining the results of multiple gene finding tools into a consensus set [6]. Based on identifying exons by exploiting GC content and DNA sequences of functional elements like splice site motifs, start codons and stop codons, results from ab initio methods rendered sometimes problematic in detecting the 5′- and 3′-boundaries of genes, and therefore eventually split or merged the open reading frames from known *D. melanogaster* genes into separate gene predictions. Homology-based methods are less prone to such artifacts (Fig. 2), and therefore were employed to improve the ab initio gene annotations. Latter approach is particularly effective if transcriptome data or high quality gene models are available for one or more species, as homology can be used to transfer such information to the less well-annotated genomes.

Another application of comparative genomics relevant to the analysis of protein-coding genes is the Codon Substitution Frequency (CSF) analysis [8]. This method looks for patterns of evolutionary conservation that are characteristic for protein-coding sequences: for instance, insertions and deletions occurring preferentially in distances that are a multiple of three, or patterns of conservation in triplet positions such that—by the degeneration of the genetic code—the variable positions do not change the encoded amino acid, or substitute amino acids by such with relatively unchanged biochemical properties.

Tools:

- Ab initio prediction of gene models: AUGUSTUS (http://bioinf.uni-greifswald.de/webaugustus/) [22]. The approach uses an advanced splicing model including intron length, GC-content, and exonic reading frame to annotate gene models. For more details, *see* Chapter 6, Comparative Genome Annotation (S. Konig, L. Romoth, M. Stanke) of this volume.

- Homology-based gene model prediction: N-SCAN (http://mblab.wustl.edu/software.html) [23], CONTRAST (http://contra.stanford.edu/contrast/) [24]. N-SCAN employs a hidden Markov model based on context-dependent substitution

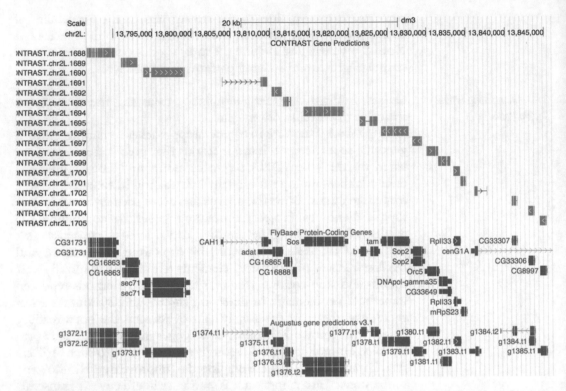

Fig. 2 Homology-based (CONTRAST, *top track*) and ab initio gene predictions (AUGUSTUS, *bottom track*) for *Drosophila melanogaster* compared to FlyBase annotation of protein-coding genes (*center track*). Although overall performing considerably well, particularly when considering the fact that no additional source of information is employed, the ab initio gene prediction merges the CG31731 & CG16863 genes (i.e., the g1372 fusion transcripts at the *bottom-left*), the CG16865 & Sos genes (the g1376.t3 transcript to the *bottom-center*), and the CG33306 & CG33307 genes (by the g1384.t2 transcript to the *bottom-right*). Gene prediction based on comparative genomics, in contrast, naturally keeps these loci separated. However, complex gene models like nested genes are difficult for both approaches (cf. the cenG1A locus to the *right*)

patterns in a phylogenetic model created from a multiple genome sequence alignment. CONTRAST uses a combination of machine learning techniques to predict protein-coding genes from a multiple genome sequence alignment.

– PhyloCSF   (https://github.com/mlin/PhyloCSF/wiki) [25]. PhyloCSF uses codon substitution frequencies in a phylogenetic model derived from a multiple sequence alignment to identify potential protein-coding regions. It is not designed to run on entire genome sequences, and regions with a potential gene content should be subset from the genome in the first place, using complementary gene prediction approaches.

Examples: N-SCAN is a gene prediction tool that takes advantage of homology information, which has been designed specifically for Drosophila and human genomes. After downloading and unpacking the Linux distribution from http://mblab.wustl.edu/

software/download/, the N-SCAN pipeline can be run for the provided example data by running the binary:

```
./bin/Nscan_driver.pl -d nscanOutput examples/example.fa
examples/nscandriver.config
```

where the input file "example.fa" contains the DNA sequence to be scanned, and "nscandriver.config" provides the configuration parameters. The corresponding results are placed in the "nscanOutput" folder. Note that, for proper operation, N-SCAN relies on other programs like RepeatMasker and LASTZ/MULTIZ (Subheading 3.1). More detailed instructions are available in the README file in the distribution release.

PhyloCSF works on pre-aligned genomic sequences for the locus being investigated, which can be extracted from a MAF file by using for instance the "msa_view" program from the PHAST software package (Subheading 3.2). Furthermore, also a phylogenetic model of the involved species involved is required, in order to execute the command

```
./PhyloCSF 12flies PhyloCSF_Examples/tal-AA.fa
```

where "PhyloCSF_Examples/tal-AA.fa" is a FASTA format file containing the DNA sequences from the different genomes involved, and "12flies" additionally provides the prefix for a set of files in the "PhyloCSF_Parameters" subfolder of the distribution, which describe the phylogeny of interest. More information on PhyloCSF can be found at https://github.com/mlin/PhyloCSF/wiki.

3.4.2 Orthology Prediction

Objective: Finding orthologous genes in two or more species.

Approach: Orthology inference—the identification of orthologous genes between species—is most readily performed using phylogenetic techniques that reconstruct the evolutionary relationships between genes across species [26]. However, exact phylogenetic reconstructions can become computationally intensive, especially when performed on a genome-wide scale. Consequently, often heuristic approaches are applied [26], which usually exploit sequence alignments between genes to identify reciprocal best hits, i.e., pairs of genes from different genomes that mutually show the highest similarity (i.e., the best hit) compared to all other genes in each species. Synteny maps describing the ordering of genes along each chromosome provide a further source of information to resolve ties, and permit distinguishing between multiple potential candidates for an orthologous gene pair. The Drosophila 12 Genomes Project employed a heuristic approach involving the combination of a reciprocal best hit algorithm ("fuzzy" reciprocal best hits) with synteny information (by the "Synpipe" pipeline developed within the project) in order to identify orthologous genes [6]. Orthology inference enables analysis of evolutionary dynamics in gene duplication, as observed in lineage-specific expansions of a gene family (*see* **Note 3**).

Tools:

– Phylogeny-based orthology inference: Some public databases provide pre-computed phylogeny-based gene orthology mappings for extensive collections of species. Examples are the Ensembl Compara database (http://www.ensembl.org/info/genome/compara/homology_method.html) [27] and PhylomeDB (http://phylomedb.org/) [28].

– Heuristic approaches to orthology inference: OrthoMCL (http://www.orthomcl.org/orthomcl/) [29]. OrthoMCL is a tool for constructing orthologous groups of genes across multiple species, using a Markov Cluster algorithm to group putative orthologs and paralogs.

Phylogeny-based orthology predictions use computationally intensive pipelines, for instance OrthoMCL comes as a suite of programs that need to be run sequentially. See the user guide for more information (http://www.orthomcl.org/common/downloads/software/v2.0/UserGuide.txt).

However, the databases with pre-computed sets of orthologous genes at hand are quite comprehensive. PhylomeDB, for example, contains proteome-wide orthology predictions for over 1000 species. For more information about the general topic of orthology prediction, *see* also Chapter 6, Comparative Genome Annotation (S. Konig, L. Romoth, M. Stanke) in this volume.

3.4.3 Estimating Protein Evolution Rates

Objective: Identifying protein sequences under particular selective constraints, either purifying (slower evolving) or positive (faster evolving) selection.

Approach: Natural selection on protein-coding sequences can be detected using the ratio of mutations that change the identity of the amino acid (non-synonymous mutations) to those that do not (synonymous mutations), referred to as the dN/dS ratio [30]. A ratio greater than one is indicative of positive selection, suggesting that mutations that change the amino acid being retained to a greater degree than silent mutations. In contrast, a ratio less than one indicates selection against mutations that change the identity of amino acids, or purifying selection.

Tool: PAML (http://abacus.gene.ucl.ac.uk/software/paml.html) [31]. PAML (Phylogenetic Analysis by Maximum Likelihood) is a software package for conducting phylogenetic analyzes on DNA or protein sequences. Among multiple other applications, the approach computes the dN/dS ratios of protein-coding genes.

Example: PAML is a collection of programs for various phylogenetic analyses. These tools generally require three input files: a multiple sequence alignment, a phylogenetic tree file modeling the evolutionary relationships between the species under analysis, and a configuration file (i.e., "control file") which lists the parameter configurations. Information about running the programs and example input files can be obtained from http://abacus.gene.ucl.ac.uk/ziheng/data.html and a detailed example is provided at http://abacus.gene.ucl.ac.uk/ziheng/data/pamlDEMO.pdf. Additionally, the program homepage (above) provides to download a graphical user interface for the PAML package.

3.5   Predicting Noncoding RNA Loci

Objective: Detecting loci that transcribe noncoding RNAs in genomic sequences.

Approach: Noncoding RNAs (ncRNAs) lack an open reading frame and therefore the strongest markers used to predict protein-coding genes. They are usually attempted to be localized by scanning genome sequences for potential RNAs that form specific secondary structures. This approach, employed by the Drosophila 12 Genomes Project, can obviously also produce a considerable number of false positives [6, 7]. Therefore, the Consortium in the first place focused on evolutionarily conserved regions in order to narrow down the search space when looking for ncRNAs. Subsequently, nucleotide sequences characteristic of RNA secondary structures (e.g., palindromic sequences that would fold into stem-loop structures) were investigated. However, RNA secondary structures can also commonly be found in protein-coding mRNAs, and to solve this issue predicted ncRNAs were removed if they exhibited protein-coding potential as determined by homology to known protein-coding genes or evolutionary patterns characteristic of protein-coding regions (*see* Subheading 3.4.1).

Tool: EvoFold (http://moma.ki.au.dk/~jsp/software.html) [32]. EvoFold predicts RNAs from genomic sequence using conservation information from genome-wide multiple sequence alignments. Note that EvoFold tends to over-predict and therefore requires a careful filtering for higher scoring sequences to achieve reliable results.

Example: EvoFold can be downloaded as a single runnable program from the URL above. It can be run with:

```
./EvoFold_static --configFilePath EvoFoldConfig.v7b --completeFile=allPred.tab test1.
ama dros12way.nwk
```

where "--configFilePath" points to a folder with configuration files (as provided by the downloaded program package), "--completeFile" provides the name of the output file, "dros12way.nwk" provides an evolutionary tree in Newick format containing the species in the multiple sequence alignment, and "test1.ama" is a proxy for the multiple sequence alignment in the AMA format, which differs from the MAF format (*see* **Note 1**) by employing dots for sequences absent from the alignment blocks.

3.6 Identifying Micro-RNAs

Objective: Detecting the location of micro-RNAs in genomic sequences.

Approach: Micro-RNAs (miRNAs) are a subclass of ncRNAs with very characteristic attributes, which can be exploited to detect them by scanning the genomic sequence for specific RNA secondary structures, in particular stem-loop forming complementary sequences. The Drosophila 12 Genomes Project used a complex pipeline based on the Vienna RNA Package [33] to compute secondary structures in a 120 nt sliding window across the genome for identifying such stem-loop structures, and subsequently filter them according to different criteria. Complementary programs like miRseeker [34] and miRscan [35] have been developed specifically to scan for miRNAs in genomic sequences using evolutionary conservation as a guide, but unfortunately are currently not publicly available.

Tool: The Vienna RNA package [33] (http://www.tbi.univie.ac.at/RNA/) is a set of programs for the prediction and comparison of RNA secondary structures.

Example: A tutorial on using the various programs in the Vienna RNA package can be found at: http://www.tbi.univie.ac.at/RNA/tutorial/.

3.7 Finding Transcription Factor Binding Site Motifs

Objective: Identifying transcription factor binding site motifs in the sequences of regulatory elements.

Approach: Phylogenetic footprinting is a technique that aims to identify conserved transcription factor binding motifs in orthologous DNA sequences from different species, such as the regions upstream of genes containing the promoter [36–38]. In order to reduce the number of false positives, additional information derived from the conservation of the motif orientation and of motif clustering can be included in the analyses.

Tool: BigFoot (https://sourceforge.net/projects/bigfoot/) [39].

Example: BigFoot is a Java program that comes with an integrated graphical user interface. It requires the Java Virtual Machine to be installed on the host machine, but the program itself does not require any installation procedure. After downloading the release from the URL given above and unpacking it, run the graphical interface with:

```
java -Xmx512M -server -jar BigFoot.jar
```

Alternatively, the program can also be executed from the Linux command line, providing a list of available options by

```
java -jar BigFoot.jar --help
```

Nicely formatted HTML help pages are provided within the downloaded package, which may be consulted for extended information on using the program.

4 Notes

1. MAF format. The Multiple Alignment Format (MAF) has been designed to provide a text-based visualization for the alignment of more than two sequences. The format can handle strand orientation as well as genomic rearrangements, which makes it suitable to also represent genomic sequence alignments. MAF files are line-based, starting with a defined header followed by alignment blocks represented by paragraphs separated by blank lines. The header consists of a mandatory line starting with the word "##maf" followed by white-space-separated "variable = value" pairs, and an optional parameters line starting with the comment symbol "#." The remainder of the file describes the alignment, with the first symbol of each line indicating the type of information provided. Each alignment block begins with a line starting with the letter "a" followed by attributes of the alignment in the subsequent block, such as its alignment score. Subsequent lines in the block begin with "s" and comprise the fields sequence name, start position, aligned block length, strand, total sequence length, and eventually the alignment block sequence of the corresponding genome. Optionally, MAF files can contain lines starting with an "i" (i.e., "information" lines providing additional context of the preceding sequence line), an "e" (i.e., "empty" lines to represent empty parts of the alignment block), or "q" (i.e., "quality" lines that show quality scores per aligned base). For a more detailed description of the MAF format, refer to https://genome.ucsc.edu/FAQ/FAQformat.html#format5. The following is an example block of the MAF file available at http://hgdownload.cse.ucsc.edu/goldenPath/dm3/multiz15way/chr4.maf.gz:

```
##maf version=1 scoring=autoMZ.v1
...
a score=-90546.000000
s dm3.chr4            3216 19 + 1351857 TCCTT--------------------GATCAGGCATTGC------G
s droSim1.chrU    13429381 31 - 15797150 tcctt-------tgcccgc-------caatgggcacttc-cgggtg
i droSim1.chrU       C 0 C 0
s droSec1.super_74    88019 29 +  162789 tcctc-------ttcttgc--g--aacaaaaagcactta------g
```

```
i droSec1.super_74            C O C O
s droYak2.chr4                   665704 34 -  1374474 TCCCCAGATCATTGCTTGAATG--GAGATTGGG
                                 AAT----------

i droYak2.chr4                C O C O
s droEre2.scaffold_4748          77341 44 +  111971 tcaccgggcgagagctggcacg--gtctccgagca
                                 ctgctcccatg

i droEre2.scaffold_4748       C O C O
s droAna3.scaffold_13043         255667 27 +  509009 TGTCC---------CTTTCACG--GATGCGACACA
                                 CT-------G

i droAna3.scaffold_13043      C O C O
s dp4.Unknown_group_449          18597 5 -  22890 --------------------------------------
                                 ---tcctg

i dp4.Unknown_group_449       I 11 C O
s droPer1.super_378              9586 4 +  18190 ---------------------------------------
                                 --TCCT-

i droPer1.super_378           n 10109 C O
s droWil1.scaffold_181148       214241 19 -   5435427 ------------TCCTTGCTAG--
                                 GGCACTTCG-------------

i droWil1.scaffold_181148     C O N O
s droVir3.scaffold_12734         3109 19 +  510240 -------------------acgttgacaatgcttc
                                 caa-------

i droVir3.scaffold_12734      N O I 8
s droMoj3.scaffold_6498          1426871 17 -  3408170 -------------------TCG--GATACGGCA
                                 TACTA-------

i droMoj3.scaffold_6498       I 6 C O
e triCas2.singleUn_1817          6011 389 +  22356 I
```

2. Noticeably, the gene models employed in the Drosophila 12 Genomes Project do not include information about exon-intron structures and alternative splicing. Instead, a single consensus model for each gene has been produced for the comparative studies of genes. While the comparison of splicing patterns in between the different Drosophila species can certainly provide more insights about the processing of transcribed loci, such undertaking might also produce artifacts in the case of unreliable gene models or poorly conserved splicing patterns. To date, extensive transcript annotation and high-quality gene models have been produced only for *D. melanogaster*, while they are not yet available for other Drosophila species. These limitations are likely to introduce a strong bias in the study, and evolutionary dynamics in (alternative) splicing additionally can hamper reliable analyses based on comparative transcriptomics.

3. During evolution, a gene can undergo duplication events, which after the speciation event of a certain lineage produce one or more redundant copies (i.e., paralogs) of the original locus. Consequently, all these paralogs of a gene are

orthologous to the ancestral gene preserved in other species. Under the scenario of such lineage-specific gene amplification events that occurred in one or both species under comparison, orthology cannot always be reduced to uniquely resolved one-to-one mappings between genes, and also entails one-to-many or many-to-many mappings.

References

1. Adams MD, Celniker SE, Holt RA et al (2000) The genome sequence of Drosophila melanogaster. Science 287:2185–2195

2. Misra S, Crosby MA, Mungall CJ et al (2002) Annotation of the Drosophila melanogaster euchromatic genome: a systematic review. Genome Biol 3(12): research0083.1–research083.22

3. Richards S, Liu Y, Bettencourt BR et al (2005) Comparative genome sequencing of Drosophila pseudoobscura: chromosomal, gene, and cis-element evolution. Genome Res 15:1–18

4. Bergman CM, Pfeiffer BD, Rincón-Limas DE et al (2002) Assessing the impact of comparative genomic sequence data on the functional annotation of the Drosophila genome. Genome Biol 3:RESEARCH0086

5. Kellis M, Patterson N, Endrizzi M et al (2003) Sequencing and comparison of yeast species to identify genes and regulatory elements. Nature 423:241–254

6. Clark AG, Eisen MB, Smith DR et al (2007) Evolution of genes and genomes on the Drosophila phylogeny. Nature 450:203–218

7. Stark A, Lin MF, Kheradpour P et al (2007) Discovery of functional elements in 12 Drosophila genomes using evolutionary signatures. Nature 450:219–232

8. Lin MF, Carlson JW, Crosby MA et al (2007) Revisiting the protein-coding gene catalog of Drosophila melanogaster using 12 fly genomes. Genome Res 17:1823–1836

9. Roy S, Ernst J, modENCODE Consortium et al (2010) Identification of functional elements and regulatory circuits by Drosophila modENCODE. Science 330:1787–1797

10. Nègre N, Brown CD, Ma L et al (2011) A cis-regulatory map of the Drosophila genome. Nature 471:527–531

11. Attrill H, Falls K, Goodman JL et al (2016) FlyBase: establishing a gene group resource for Drosophila melanogaster. Nucleic Acids Res 44:D786–D792

12. Herrero J, Muffato M, Beal K et al (2016) Ensembl comparative genomics resources. Database 2016:bav096. https://doi.org/10.1093/database/baw053

13. Speir ML, Zweig AS, Rosenbloom KR et al (2016) The UCSC genome browser database: 2016 update. Nucleic Acids Res 44: D717–D725

14. Harris RS (2007) Improved pairwise alignment of genomic DNA. Pennsylvania State University, State College, PA

15. Blanchette M, Kent WJ, Riemer C et al (2004) Aligning multiple genomic sequences with the threaded blockset aligner. Genome Res 14:708–715

16. Felsenstein J, Churchill GA (1996) A hidden markov model approach to variation among sites in rate of evolution. Mol Biol Evol 13:93–104

17. Siepel A, Bejerano G, Pedersen JS et al (2005) Evolutionarily conserved elements in vertebrate, insect, worm, and yeast genomes. Genome Res 15:1034–1050

18. Li R, Ye J, Li S et al (2005) ReAS: recovery of ancestral sequences for transposable elements from the unassembled reads of a whole genome shotgun. PLoS Comput Biol 1:e43

19. Edgar RC, Myers EW (2005) PILER: identification and classification of genomic repeats. Bioinformatics 21(Suppl 1):i152–i158

20. Tempel S (2012) Using and understanding RepeatMasker. Methods Mol Biol 859:29–51

21. Smith CD, Edgar RC, Yandell MD et al (2007) Improved repeat identification and masking in dipterans. Gene 389:1–9

22. Stanke M, Waack S (2003) Gene prediction with a hidden Markov model and a new intron submodel. Bioinformatics 19(Suppl 2): ii215–ii225

23. Gross SS, Brent MR (2006) Using multiple alignments to improve gene prediction. J Comput Biol 13:379–393

24. Gross SS, Do CB, Sirota M, Batzoglou S (2007) CONTRAST: a discriminative, phylogeny-free approach to multiple informant de novo gene prediction. Genome Biol 8:R269

25. Lin MF, Jungreis I, Kellis M (2011) PhyloCSF: a comparative genomics method to distinguish protein coding and non-coding regions. Bioinformatics 27:i275–i282

26. Kristensen DM, Wolf YI, Mushegian AR, Koonin EV (2011) Computational methods for gene Orthology inference. Brief Bioinform 12:379–391

27. Vilella AJ, Severin J, Ureta-Vidal A et al (2009) EnsemblCompara genetrees: complete, duplication-aware phylogenetic trees in vertebrates. Genome Res 19:327–335

28. Huerta-Cepas J, Capella-Gutiérrez S, Pryszcz LP et al (2014) PhylomeDB v4: zooming into the plurality of evolutionary histories of a genome. Nucleic Acids Res 42:D897–D902

29. Li L, Stoeckert CJ Jr, Roos DS (2003) OrthoMCL: identification of ortholog groups for eukaryotic genomes. Genome Res 13:2178–2189

30. Nielsen R (2005) Molecular signatures of natural selection. Annu Rev Genet 39:197–218

31. Yang Z (2007) PAML 4: phylogenetic analysis by maximum likelihood. Mol Biol Evol 24:1586–1591

32. Pedersen JS, Bejerano G, Siepel A et al (2006) Identification and classification of conserved RNA secondary structures in the human genome. PLoS Comput Biol 2:e33

33. Lorenz R, Bernhart SH, Höner Zu Siederdissen C et al (2011) ViennaRNA package 2.0. Algorithms Mol Biol 6:26

34. Lai EC, Tomancak P, Williams RW, Rubin GM (2003) Computational identification of drosophila microRNA genes. Genome Biol 4:R42

35. Lim LP, Lau NC, Weinstein EG et al (2003) The microRNAs of Caenorhabditis elegans. Genes Dev 17:991–1008

36. Blanchette M, Tompa M (2002) Discovery of regulatory elements by a computational method for phylogenetic footprinting. Genome Res 12:739–748

37. Zhang Z, Gerstein M (2003) Of mice and men: phylogenetic footprinting aids the discovery of regulatory elements. J Biol 2:11

38. Ganley ARD, Kobayashi T (2007) Phylogenetic footprinting to find functional DNA elements. Methods Mol Biol 395:367–380

39. Satija R, Novák A, Miklós I et al (2009) BigFoot: Bayesian alignment and phylogenetic footprinting with MCMC. BMC Evol Biol 9:217

Chapter 18

Comparative Genomics in *Homo sapiens*

Martin Oti and Michael Sammeth

Abstract

Genomes can be compared at different levels of divergence, either between species or within species. Within species genomes can be compared between different subpopulations, such as human subpopulations from different continents. Investigating the genomic differences between different human subpopulations is important when studying complex diseases that are affected by many genetic variants, as the variants involved can differ between populations. The 1000 Genomes Project collected genome-scale variation data for 2504 human individuals from 26 different populations, enabling a systematic comparison of variation between human subpopulations. In this chapter, we present step-by-step a basic protocol for the identification of population-specific variants employing the 1000 Genomes data. These variants are subsequently further investigated for those that affect the proteome or RNA splice sites, to investigate potentially biologically relevant differences between the populations.

Key words Comparative genomics, Population variation, Human genomics, Single-nucleotide polymorphisms

1 Introduction

Historically comparative genomics primarily involves the comparison of genomes from different species, employing one single sequence being used to represent each species [1]. However, genomic variation incurs at multiple levels, also between strains, populations, and individuals of the same species. Comparative genomics within a species can be used to investigate population dynamics and the evolutionary history since the speciation event when it diverged from other species. Such studies can also be applied to our own species, and in recent years there has been a surge of interest in investigating human evolution and tracing the migratory patterns of ancient human subpopulations using DNA recovered from fossil human remains [2]. Studies along these lines have shed light on our recent ancestry, including inter-breeding with other closely related hominins [3] and ancient migratory patterns [4].

Comparative population genomics can also be employed at an even more fine-grained level to determine how modern human

João C. Setubal et al. (eds.), *Comparative Genomics: Methods and Protocols*, Methods in Molecular Biology, vol. 1704,
https://doi.org/10.1007/978-1-4939-7463-4_18, © Springer Science+Business Media LLC 2018

subpopulations differ genetically from each other. This is important for biomedical and genetic research, as every individual's genome is unique and human genomes share a varying degree of similarity with each other depending on whether the corresponding donors are from the same or from different populations. Disparities between individuals from different populations can manifest in variations of the sequence of bases in the genome, so-called Single Nucleotide Polymorphisms (SNPs), insertions or deletions of short sequences ("indels"), and genomic rearrangements ("structural variants"). Such population differences imply that, instead of using a single reference genome [5, 6], it would be more appropriate to use population-specific reference genomes, for instance one based on African genomes for studies involving Africans, one for East Asians, one for Europeans, etc.

Considerations along these lines are particularly relevant for the investigation of complex diseases, which are influenced by several different genetic factors that each have a relatively small effect on the disease risk. To advance in identifying potential causal variants typically Genome-Wide Association Studies (GWAS) are employed, which employ oligonucleotide chips to determine individual genotypes at variable genomic sites (SNPs) for large numbers of individuals both with and without the disease in question [7]. Potential causal or protective variants then are identified by genetic variants that are over-represented in either cases or controls respectively. However, due to population-genetic differences, individuals from different populations certainly can have different such disease-relevant variants. Therefore, GWAS need to be carried out in genetically homogeneous populations, also in order to avoid the detection of spurious associations that are created by different population backgrounds between cases and controls. Failure to control for the population makeup can readily result in predicting false positives because–due to the multigenic nature of complex diseases–the disease-associated variants are usually only marginally enriched in one of the investigated groups.

The first large-scale population genomic study in humans, the international HapMap Project [8], focused particularly on investigating single-nucleotide polymorphisms (SNPs) in different human subpopulations. A major goal of this project was to facilitate GWAS by allowing expanding the number of observed genetic variants through imputation [9], a computational technique that takes advantage of correlations in the co-occurrence of SNPs. These correlations can be obtained from the extensive SNP data of the HapMap project and allow extrapolating the observations from the limited number of SNPs interrogated by a SNP array to other, uninterrogated SNPs. However, since the HapMap project has been limited to surveying common genetic variants, also imputation based on the respective SNP arrays cannot fail to provide a complete picture of an individual's genomic landscape.

In order to also assess rare variants systematically throughout the human genome, the 1000 Genomes project has been established with the objective of sequencing the genome sequences from more than a thousand individuals from different populations [10]. Data produced in this project provides an excellent resource for performing analyses on comparative genomics in human. In this chapter, we provide a protocol for comparing the genomes of individuals from three different populations that have been sequenced in the 1000 Genomes Project, i.e., Europeans, Chinese, and Yoruba from Western Africa. The presented analyses first identify genetic variants characteristic for each population and then further analyze their potential effects on protein-coding genes. The study we present is to provide an example of how comparative genomics can be employed to investigate variations between different populations of the human species.

2 Materials

2.1 Hardware and Operating System Requirements

The analyses explained herein can, in principle, be performed on any personal computer or laptop, but in practice the sizes of the analyzed datasets may require large amounts of disk space, e.g., tens or hundreds of gigabytes, and also of CPU processing time, like hours to days. Therefore, it is recommendable to execute the commands below on a workstation with at least 500 GB of available disk space, 4–8 GB of RAM, and 2–4 CPUs.

All the steps of the analyses are described as command lines that can be executed by *bash* or by a similar shell interpreter on a default UNIX-like operating system, such as Linux or Mac OSX. The installation of third-party software further requires the system to be set up for C/C++ compilation, to compile the corresponding programs from source code. Super-user privileges are not necessary to conduct the analyses, but can be used to install scripts or programs system-wide.

2.2 Installation of Required Programs

2.2.1 HTS Lib

HTS Lib (High Throughput Sequencing Library; http://www.htslib.org) is required by VCF Tools described in the next section. It contains the *bgzip* and *tabix* programs for compressing and indexing VCF files respectively.

Retrieve with:

```
wget https://github.com/samtools/htslib/releases/download/
1.3/htslib-1.3.tar.bz2
```

Compile with:

```
tar -xvjf htslib-1.3.tar.bz2
cd htslib-1.3/
```

```
./configure
make
```

Install system-wide with (requires root privileges):

```
sudo make install
```

Alternatively, a local installation can be performed by the command

```
make prefix=$HOME/.local install
```

Note that the installation location *$HOME/.local* can be arbitrarily changed, but the corresponding folder should be in the user's $PATH environment variable.

2.2.2 *VCF Tools*

Our examples employ VCF Tools [11], a program suite to analyze files formatted in the Variant Call Format (VCF) that has been designed to store information on genome variants (described below). Note that BCF Tools (https://samtools.github.io/bcftools) provide a faster alternative for most of the VCF Tools, but will not be covered here for reasons of simplicity.

Obtain VCF Tools with:

```
wget https://github.com/vcftools/vcftools/releases/download/
v0.1.14/vcftools-0.1.14.tar.gz
```

Compile with:

```
tar -xvzf vcftools-0.1.14.tar.gz
cd vcftools-0.1.14/
./configure
make
```

Install with (requires root privileges):

```
sudo make install
```

or perform a local install with (again, the installation location *$HOME/.local* can be changed as desired, but should be in the user's $PATH environment variable):

```
make prefix=$HOME/.local install
```

Most of the VCF Tools commands are Perl scripts that make use of modules provided with the VCF Tools installation. To ensure that the Perl interpreter is able to find them, the location of these modules needs to be added to the PERL5LIB environment variable, either by (in the case of a system-wide installation of VCF Tools):

```
export PERL5LIB=/usr/local/share/perl5
```

or with (replace *$HOME/.local* with installation location if different):

```
export PERL5LIB=$HOME/.local/share/perl5
```

The export command above should be added to the user's startup shell script (usually "~/.bashrc" or "~/.profile") to make it run automatically each time a new shell is started. Otherwise, the command will need to be run manually in every new shell before VCF Tools can be executed. If the environment variable PERL5-LIB is not set correctly, running one of the VCF Tools commands fails with an error message that starts with: "*Can't locate Vcf.pm in @INC (you may need to install the Vcf module)*"

<table>
<tr><td>*2.2.3 BED Tools*</td><td>In our toy study, we will employ Bedtools for arithmetic operations on genomic intervals, for instance when overlapping SNPs with coding exons (Subheading 3.2).</td></tr>
</table>

Retrieve Bedtools with

```
wget
https://github.com/arq5x/bedtools2/releases/download/v2.24.0/
bedtools-2.24.0.tar.gz
```

Compile with

```
tar -xvzf bedtools-2.24.0.tar.gz
cd bedtools2/
make
```

A system-wide installation is achieved by copying the programs to a default folder in the $PATH variable. For instance (requires root privileges):

```
sudo cp ./bin/* /usr/local/bin/
```

Alternatively, a local install can be performed with (the installation location *$HOME/.local/bin* can be changed as desired, but should be in the user's $PATH environment variable)

```
cp ./bin/* $HOME/.local/bin/
```

2.2.4 AStalavista

The AStalavista Scorer tool [12] can be employed to estimate the effect of genomic variants within splice sites on the corresponding splicing efficiency. In order to run AStalavista, Java (version>= 1.6) needs to be installed on the system and should be available in the user's $PATH environment variable. Java is available for most Linux distributions, and can be installed via their standard package management systems.

Retrieve AStalavista with:

```
wget
http://artifactory.sammeth.net/artifactory/barna/barna/barna.
astalavista/3.2/astalavista-3.2.tgz
```

Unpack with:

```
tar -xvzf astalavista-3.2.tgz
```

This will create a new folder called "astalavista-3.2" within the current directory. AStalavista does neither require compilation nor installation, and can be run directly from the "bin" subfolder of the unpacked tar archive. In order to run it from anywhere on the system simply by typing the "*astalavista*" command, add the full path of the "astalavista-3.2/bin" subfolder to the $PATH environment variable. This can be done once by modifying the "*.bashrc*" or "*.profile*" configuration files in the user's home folder, and the new $PATH will be available in every new shell session that is started.

2.3 Download the Human Reference Genome

As detailed in the next section, genomic variation data are generally stored as sets of variable positions relative to a reference genome. There are different reference assemblies of the human genome and different versions of the same assembly (*see* **Note 1**). It is important to choose the appropriate reference for each analysis, because the genomic coordinates and also the names of chromosomes can differ between them. As we will compare in this chapter the population variants obtained from the 1000 Genomes Project [10], it is intuitive to obtain the reference genome sequence directly provided at the FTP site of the 1000 Genomes Project, which is one large compressed FASTA file (file size: ~900 MB).

```
wget
ftp://ftp.1000genomes.ebi.ac.uk/vol1/ftp/technical/reference/
phase2_reference_assembly_sequence/hs37d5.fa.gz
```

However, in the subsequent sections, we focus with our analyses only on chromosome 19, one of the smallest, nevertheless rather gene-rich chromosomes in the human genome, mainly by motivations to reduce the computation time. The 1000 Genomes site provides exclusively the copy of the entire reference genome downloadable by the above command, but the Ensembl genome browser database provides a version of the reference human genome that is compatible with that of the 1000 Genomes Project and allows downloading each chromosome individually. We therefore can obtain the sequence of chromosome 19 only more rapidly by

```
wget ftp://ftp.ensembl.org/pub/grch37/release-83/fasta/
homo_sapiens/dna/Homo_sapiens.GRCh37.dna.chromosome.19.fa.gz
```

2.4 Download VCF Files of Individuals from Different Populations

The reference format called the "Variant Call Format" (VCF) developed by the 1000 Genomes Project and described by Table 1 (see also http://www.1000genomes.org/wiki/Analysis/vcf4.0) stores genetic variation data as sets of variable positions relative to a reference genome rather than providing the complete individual genome sequence. Such data structure allows, on the one hand, storing (potentially partial) variant data obtained using SNP microarrays rather than full genome sequencing. On the other hand, it also reduces the variation of individual genomes obtained by sequencing to the amount of information necessary to describe their differences based on a reference, avoiding the redundant storage of bases that are the same (~99.9% in the case of the human genome).

Table 1
Each line of a VCF file corresponds to a variant, and the fields (i.e., columns) are by specification tab-separated. Note that the INFO field (column 8) describes multiple attributes of the variant as *key = value* entries, for instance alternative allele frequencies (key "AF")

Field Number	Name	Brief description
1	CHROM	The name of the reference sequence (typically a chromosome) on which the variation has been called.
2	POS	The 1-based position of the variation in the given sequence.
3	ID	The identifier of the variation, e.g., a dbSNP *rs* identifier or just "." if unknown.
4	REF	The base(s) of the reference sequence at the position of the variant.
5	ALT	The sequences of alternative alleles at this position.
6	QUAL	A quality score associated with the inference of the given alleles.
7	FILTER	A flag indicating which of a given set of filters the variation has passed.
8	INFO	An extensible list of semicolon-separated key-value pairs describing extended information on the variation.
9	FORMAT	An (optional) extensible list of fields for describing the samples.
+	SAMPLES	For each (optional) sample described in the file, values are given for the fields listed in FORMAT.

The 1000 Genomes Project provides one VCF file per chromosome, and the variants of all 1000 Genomes individuals in chromosome 19 can be downloaded from the project's FTP site by the
command (file size: ~350 MB):

```
wget
ftp://ftp.1000genomes.ebi.ac.uk/vol1/ftp/release/20130502/
ALL.chr19.phase3_shapeit2_mvncall_integrated_v5a.20130502.
genotypes.vcf.gz
```

The VCF file provides the genotypes (SNPs and indels) of all
2504 individuals from the different populations that have been
investigated in the project (e.g., Chinese, Yoruba, . . .). The downloaded VCF file is *bgzip*compressed but needs not be inflated
because the VCF Tools program can operate directly on compressed VCF files. However, an index file is required to randomly
access different parts of the considerably large file, which can be
downloaded from the same source (file size: 55 KB):

```
wget
ftp://ftp.1000genomes.ebi.ac.uk/vol1/ftp/release/20130502/
ALL.chr19.phase3_shapeit2_mvncall_integrated_v5a.20130502.
genotypes.vcf.gz.tbi
```

The use of an index file significantly speeds up the processing of
the VCF file by the VCF Tools program used in the subsequent
steps. To further limit the computational resources and time, we
restrict our example to biallelic SNPs with one reference and one
alternative allele and exclude multi-allelic SNPs as well as insertion/
deletion variants by the following command:

```
vcftools --gzvcf
ALL.chr19.phase3_shapeit2_mvncall_integrated_v5a.20130502.
genotypes.vcf.gz --chr 19 --min-alleles 2 --max-alleles
2 --remove-indels --recode --recode-INFO-all --stdout | bgzip -c
> chr19_biallelicSNPs_ALL.vcf.gz
```

The above command stores the filtered SNPs in another compressed VCF file using the *bgzip*command, which is subsequently
again indexed by

```
tabix -p vcf chr19_biallelicSNPs_ALL.vcf.gz
```

Note that the indexing process should generally be carried out
every time a new VCF file is generated, and some of the VCF Tools
require the input VCF file(s) to be both bgzip-compressed and
tabix-indexed.

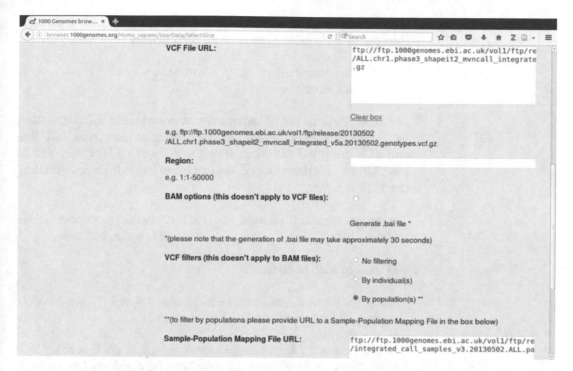

Fig. 1 Screenshot of the Data Slicer web page. The Data Slicer web tool of the 1000 Genomes Project allows downloading subsets of variants, filtering either by genomic location, by specific individuals, or by population groups to obtain population-specific VCF files. The page http:/www.1000genomes.org/data-slicer provides further instructions on the use of the program

2.4.2 Obtaining Genomic Variants per Population

The VCF file downloaded in the previous section contains the pooled genotypes of individuals from all populations. To facilitate our analysis of comparing individuals from different populations with each other, we would prefer to separate the variants into different files, one for each population. This task can be achieved manually through the *Data Slicer* web tool (http://browser. 1000genomes.org/Homo_sapiens/UserData/SelectSlice) of the 1000 Genomes Project (Fig. 1).

Note that downloading each population VCF file separately for every analyzed population by the data-slicer requires repeating the biallelic SNP filtering in each of the downloaded files (Subheading 2.4.1.). Alternatively, individuals can be segregated by population from the VCF file with all individuals obtained in the previous section. To do so, we require a file that provides the population for individual ID from the 1000 Genomes Project, which can be retrieved with

```
wget ftp://ftp.1000genomes.ebi.ac.uk/vol1/ftp/release/
20100804/20100804.ALL.panel
```

The first column of this file provides the individual IDs, and the second column correspondingly the population IDs. A list of individual IDs for a particular population (e.g., CEU = Central Europeans from Utah) can thus be obtained by

```
awk '$2=="CEU"{print $1}' 20100804.ALL.panel | sort -u >
individuals_CEU.txt
```

However, this list of individuals obtained from the population panel also contains IDs that are not present in the actual VCF file, and VCF Tools will fail when trying to retrieve an ID that is not in the VCF file. We therefore generate a list of individuals described by the VCF file using

```
zcat chr19_biallelicSNPs_ALL.vcf.gz | grep "^#CHROM" | cut
-f10- | tr '\t' '\n' | sort -u > individuals_VCF.txt
```

and then overlap both lists by

```
comm individuals_CEU.txt individuals_VCF.txt | awk '/\t\t/
{print $1}' > individuals_CEU_VCF.txt
```

The genotypes for a certain subset of individuals (specified by a list of IDs as we have just generated) can be obtained from a VCF file using the *vcf-subset* command from VCF Tools, using a list of individual IDs to be filtered from the VCF file. Employing the IDs of CEU individuals, their corresponding SNPs can be obtained by the *vcf-subset* command

```
vcf-subset -c individuals_CEU_VCF.txt chr19_biallelicSNPs_ALL.
vcf.gz | bgzip -c > chr19_biallelicSNPs_CEU.vcf.gz
```

This process then is repeated accordingly to obtain the variants of individuals from all other populations. Combining the commands described above in a little shell script, we can retrieve the population-specific individual genotypes for the CEU (European), CHB (Chinese), and YRI (African) populations.

```
for pop in CEU CHB YRI
do
    echo "Getting list of individual IDs for population ${pop}"
    awk -v pop=${pop} '$2==pop{print $1}' 20100804.ALL.panel |
    sort -u > individuals_${pop}.txt
    comm individuals_${pop}.txt individuals_VCF.txt | awk '/\t
    \t/{print $1}' > individuals_${pop}_VCF.txt
    echo "Filtering VCF file for population ${pop} SNPs"
    vcf-subset -r -t SNPs -c individuals_${pop}_VCF.txt
    chr19_biallelicSNPs_ALL.vcf.gz | bgzip -c > chr19_bial-
    lelicSNPs_${pop}.vcf.gz
```

```
        echo "Indexing SNPs VCF file for population ${pop}"
        tabix -p vcf chr19_biallelicSNPs_${pop}.vcf.gz
    done
```

The above script will generate three indexed and compressed VCF files that contain subsets of the individuals from the 1000 genomes project, one for each of the three populations, and the corresponding set of variants.

2.5 Download the Gencode Reference Annotation

In our example, we employ the Gencode genes as a reference transcriptome annotation for the human genome [13]. The entire Gencode transcriptome annotation dataset can be downloaded from the Gencode annotation FTP site with the command (file size: ~38 MB):

```
wget
ftp://ftp.sanger.ac.uk/pub/gencode/Gencode_human/re-
lease_19/gencode.v19.annotation.gtf.gz
```

Subsequently, the downloaded *gzip* archive is decompressed with

```
gunzip gencode.v19.annotation.gtf.gz
```

Table 2
GTF Files are tab-separated tables with nine columns. According to the specification, all but the final column must contain a value, and "empty" columns should be assigned a "." (dot)

Field Number	Name	Brief description
1	SEQNAME	The name of the chromosome, scaffold, or contig.
2	SOURCE	The name of the program that generated this feature, or the data source (database or project name).
3	FEATURE	The feature type name, e.g., gene, variation, similarity, etc.
4	START	The (1-based) start position of the feature in SEQNAME.
5	END	The (1-based) end position of the feature in SEQNAME.
6	SCORE	A floating point value representing the quality of the feature.
7	STRAND	The directionality of the feature with respect to the sequence of SEQNAME, defined as + (forward) or − (reverse).
8	FRAME	The reading frame ("0", "1," or "2") of a CDS overlapping the feature, where "0" indicates the first, "1" the second, and "2" the third base of a codon.
9	ATTRIBUTE	A semicolon-separated list of tag-value pairs (separated by a space), providing additional information about each feature (e.g., gene_id "ACTB")

The GTF format of the downloaded file is described in Table 2. Refer also to the pages http://mblab.wustl.edu/GTF22.htmland http://www.ensembl.org/info/website/upload/gff.htmlfor   a more detailed description of the GTF format. The Gencode annotation uses the GRCh37 assembly, but prefixes the chromosome names with "chr," whereas the 1000 Genomes Project VCF file uses the NCBI/Ensembl style of chromosome names that lack this prefix. To make the files compatible with each other, we shorthandy remove the "chr" prefix from the (smaller) GTF file with the command

```
sed 's/^chr//' gencode.v19.annotation.gtf > gencode.v19.GRCh37.
annotation.gtf
```

3 Methods

Genomes of individuals from different populations can differ in their composition by type and frequency of genomic variants, like SNPs and indels. These differences can emerge from variants being subject to positive selection in specific populations [14], although this is not necessarily always the case [15]. Genomic variants that have been sampled in large numbers from donors of different populations, like in the 1000 Genomes Project, provide the power to compare different populations and to identify variants that are common in a certain population but rare in others. We term these as population "marker" variants and in this section we will identify population marker variants for three different populations from the 1000 Genomes Project—a European population (CEU), an East Asian population (CHB), and an African population (YRI). It should be noted that the definition of a marker depends, to a high degree, on the reference panel of populations included in the comparison. In our case, we will naturally discover less markers when we increase the number of populations we compare to. In order to discover marker SNPs and to evaluate their functional impact, we employ a workflow with three main steps (Fig. 2).

1. Retrieve bi-allelic SNP variants for all available genotypes in the CEU, CHB, and YRI population.

2. Determine marker variants, i.e., SNPs with a high non-reference allele frequency in one of the populations but not in the others.

3. Investigate the functional impact of these markers in the proteome and in splice sites.

Step (1) has already been achieved when preprocessing the downloaded VCF file (Fig. 2a) and segregating individuals/SNPs from different populations as described in Subheading 2.4.2 (Fig. 2b). Step (2) consists in collecting from each population the

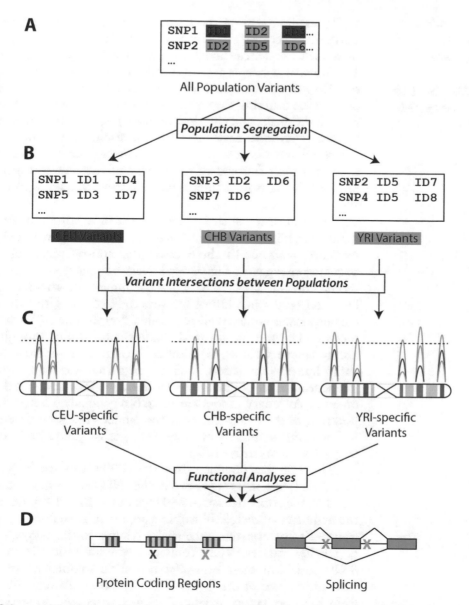

Fig. 2 Schema of the Analysis Workflow. (**a**) The file with all variants from the donors of the 1000 Genomes Project is segregated into individuals from the three populations CEU, CHB, and YRI (**b**). (**c**) Applying a threshold on the allele frequencies, population marker variants can be isolated. (**d**) The population markers then are submitted to functional analyses in order to estimate their impact on the proteome and splicing

SNPs with allele frequencies above a certain threshold (Subheading 3.1.1) and comparing them to SNPs correspondingly collected from other populations (Subheading 3.1.2). Step (3) then analyzes thus obtained marker SNPs to protein-coding regions (Subheading 3.2) and to splice sites (Subheading 3.3).

3.1 Determining Population "Marker" SNPs

3.1.1 Filter SNPs Based on Non-reference Allele Frequency

VCF files allow storing the frequency of the corresponding allele along with every variant, and the 1000 Genomes Project provides these allele frequencies across their entire dataset (Subheading 2.4). Two popular concepts are employed for measuring allele frequencies: the *non-reference allele frequency* that measures the proportion of the allele differing from the reference genome across all investigated individuals, and the *derived allele frequency* that attempts to impose an evolutionary model to determine which of the two (or more) variants at a genomic site corresponds to the ancestral allele that then (instead of the variant of the reference genome) provides the basis for computing the relative frequency of derived alleles.

As the ancestral allele is often also the most common allele of a variant site, it intrinsically has a high chance of being included in the reference genome. In these cases, the non-reference allele frequency converges to the derived allele frequency of a variant. It should however be noted here that the human reference sequence is based on only a handful of individuals [5, 6], and therefore also contains low-frequency alleles (called "minor alleles") that were present in the sequenced individuals even though the non-reference allele would actually be more representative for the entire human population. Such variants then show up with high frequencies in all populations. Allele frequencies computed based on an evolutionary model are therefore generally a better choice; however, as the evolutionary status cannot always be determined for each SNP, some variants may fail to get assigned a derived allele frequency value (*see* **Note 2**).

The VCF files obtained from the 1000 Genomes Project provide allele frequencies (encoded in the INFO column, see Table 1) based on the entire dataset of 2504 genomes. In order to determine the frequency of each SNP within a population, we re-compute the frequencies of non-reference alleles relative to the corresponding population dataset. VCF Tools can compute and directly filter SNPs based on their non-reference allele frequencies in a file, through the use of the "*--non-ref.-af*" option. To filter the SNPs from the population-specific VCF files based on three different minimum non-reference allele frequency thresholds of 0.5, 0.7, and 0.9, we can therefore employ a script

```
for t in 0.5 0.7 0.9
do
     for pop in CEU CHB YRI
     do
          echo "Getting marker SNPs at frequency threshold ${t}
          for population ${pop}"
          vcftools -non-ref-af ${t} --gzvcf
          chr19_biallelicSNPs_${pop}.vcf.gz --recode --stdout |
          bgzip -c >
```

```
chr19_biallelicSNPs_${pop}_marker_${t}.vcf.gz
        echo "Indexing VCF file"
        tabix -p vcf chr19_biallelicSNPs_${pop}_marker_${t}.
        vcf.gz
    done
done
```

The above command will generate nine indexed and compressed VCF files, containing exclusively SNPs passing the corresponding one of the three thresholds in each of the three populations.

3.1.2 Compare SNP Occurrences Between Populations

Next, we compare the SNPs frequently observed in a population–as determined by the previous step–with SNPs that are frequent in the other populations under consideration, to remove alleles with a ubiquitously high alternative allele frequency (i.e., cases where the human reference genome includes a minor allele, *see* Subheading 3.1.1). There are different possibilities of achieving this goal, one is provided by using the VCF Tool "*vcf-isec*" to intersect the VCF files with frequent SNPs from different populations. Accordingly, the command below subtracts from all SNPs that occur frequently (i.e., above threshold t = 0.5, 0.7, or 0.9) the SNPs with alternative frequencies >0.5 in one of the other populations:

```
for t in 0.5 0.7 0.9
do
    # CEU-specific marker SNPs
    vcf-isec --force --complement
chr19_biallelicSNPs_CEU_marker_${t}.vcf.gz
chr19_biallelicSNPs_CHB_marker_0.5.vcf.gz
chr19_biallelicSNPs_YRI_marker_0.5.vcf.gz | bgzip -c >
chr19_markers_CEU-only_${t}.vcf.gz
        tabix -p vcf chr19_markers_CEU-only_${t}.vcf.gz
        # CHB-specific marker SNPs
        vcf-isec --force --complement
chr19_biallelicSNPs_CHB_marker_${t}.vcf.gz
chr19_biallelicSNPs_CEU_marker_0.5.vcf.gz
chr19_biallelicSNPs_YRI_marker_0.5.vcf.gz | bgzip -c >
chr19_markers_CHB-only_${t}.vcf.gz
        tabix -p vcf chr19_markers_CHB-only_${t}.vcf.gz
        # YRI-specific marker SNPs
        vcf-isec --force --complement
chr19_biallelicSNPs_YRI_marker_${t}.vcf.gz
chr19_biallelicSNPs_CEU_marker_0.5.vcf.gz
chr19_biallelicSNPs_CHB_marker_0.5.vcf.gz | bgzip -c >
chr19_markers_YRI-only_${t}.vcf.gz
        tabix -p vcf chr19_markers_YRI-only_${t}.vcf.gz
done
```

As can be seen from the example above, the command "*vcf-isec*" operates directly on indexed bgzip-compressed VCF files. The "*–complement*" option returns the variants that are present in the first but absent from the subsequent VCF files passed to the command. The "*–force*" option is required to instruct the program to proceed with processing the files despite the nonoverlapping individual ID sets between the files. Alternatively, the *vcf-isec*tool can also be employed to obtain SNPs that are common to all VCF files (*see* **Note 3**).

The command line loop from above will generate nine indexed and compressed VCF files with population-specific marker SNPs— one for each of the three populations at each of the three thresholds. We then compare the number of marker SNPs in each population (and at each threshold) by counting the lines in these output files, disconsidering header lines that start with a "#" symbol:

```
for f in chr19_markers_???-only_0.?.vcf.gz
do
    echo "Marker SNP count for: ${f}"
    zcat $f | grep -v "^#" | wc -l
done
```

An alternative to the latter approach of intersecting VCF files and counting the number of nonoverlapping variants is to directly use the "*vcf-compare*" tool, which reports the number of variants present in all possible logical relations of the input VCF files. In the example below, we provide as an input to *vcf-compare*three files with frequent SNPs in each of the populations (cutoff at a certain frequency threshold). As output, we obtain the number of SNPs that are unique to each population, the number of SNPs present in every pairwise combination of populations, as well as the number of SNPs intersecting between all three of them. This can be done for each threshold level in one command with

```
for t in 0.5 0.7 0.9
do
    vcf-comparechr19_biallelicSNPs_CEU_marker_${t}.vcf.gz
chr19_biallelicSNPs_CHB_marker_${t}.vcf.gz
chr19_biallelicSNPs_YRI_marker_${t}.vcf.gz|grep"^VN"|cut-f
2->venn_numbers_population_markers_${t}.txt
done
```

The bash script above compares the populations for each threshold level *$t*, and the output of the *vcf-compare*program is parsed to retrieve the lines with the variant counts prefixed by "VN." For each of these lines, the count field (i.e., the second column) is followed by a list of SNP numbers for each possible overlap between the populations, which we store in a file "*venn_numbers_population_markers_${t}.txt*" for subsequent analyses. Note that, in contrast to the previous approach, the comparison here excludes SNPs that occur in the other populations with a frequency above the corresponding threshold $t (instead of >0.5 applied in the previous approach).

Analyzing the population marker SNPs identified in this section, we notice that only a minority of SNPs are specific to one population and that the proportion of marker SNPs also varies between different populations. Furthermore, results should be interpreted with caution as they are based on non-reference allele frequencies that might be biased by the variant composition of the human reference genome. A more thorough approach should employ derived alleles as determined by an evolutionary model (*see* Subheading 3.1.1).

3.2 Determine Population Marker SNPs that Affect Protein-Coding Regions

The BEDTools suite of programs can be used to perform many kinds of operations on genomic intervals. It can process files in BED, GTF, and VCF formats, either provided as plain text or as gzip-compressed files. In the example further below we employ the *intersect*tool that overlaps genomic intervals of two different files to intersect the SNPs in a VCF file with protein-coding exonic regions from the Gencode GTF annotation, in order to identify the SNPs that are located within exons. To speed up the intersection process by BEDtools (and to also reduce the memory requirements, *see* **Note 4**), we make sure that both of the intersected input files are sorted by chromosome names and genomic positions.

```
cat gencode.v19.GRCh37.annotation.gtf | awk '$3=="CDS"' | sort
-k1,1 -k4,4n > gencode.v19.GRCh37.CDS.sorted.gtf
```

The above command extracts the protein-coding regions from the entire Gencode annotation, sorting them by their chromosomal positions. As the indexed VCF files obtained in the previous step (Subheading 3.1.2) are already sorted, we can directly employ the *bedtools intersect*command, for instance to identify maker SNPs with a population allele frequency of >0.9 that fall into coding regions.

```
bedtools intersect -sorted -wa -a chr19_markers_common_0.9.
vcf.gz -b gencode.v19.GRCh37.CDS.sorted.gtf | sort -u >
chr19_markers_common_0.9_CDS.vct
```

In the above example, the "-*wa*" option tells bedtools to only keep the SNPs that overlap with the coding exons, discarding information about the exons that they intersect (*see* **Note 5**). Post-processing by the UNIX *sort*command with the "-*u*" option removes duplicate lines (i.e., SNPs), which are caused by different coding regions overlapping at the same genomic position (e.g., by alternatively spliced transcripts). To obtain the marker SNPs affecting protein-coding regions for all populations, we employ a (*bash*) shell loop based on the previous example code line:

```
for t in 0.5 0.7 0.9
do
    for pop in CEU CHB YRI
    do
        bedtools intersect -sorted -wa -a chr19_markers_${pop}-
        only_${t}.vcf.gz -b gencode.v19.GRCh37.CDS.sorted.gtf |
        sort -u | sort -k1,1 -k2,2n > chr19_markers_${pop}-only_
        ${t}_CDS.vcf
    done
done
```

The script generates nine chromosomal coordinate-sorted VCF files with the corresponding subsets of marker SNPs in protein-coding exons, one for each population at each marker SNP frequency threshold. Note that there are rather few population marker SNPs that affect protein-coding regions, especially at higher marker thresholds.

3.3 Determine Population Marker SNPs that Affect RNA Splicing

To score the effects of SNPs on splice sites, the "*AStalavista Scorer*" tool can be employed. As an input, the FASTA formatted chromosome sequences, a GTF file with the transcriptome information, an (uncompressed) VCF file with the SNPs, and a GeneID splice site model are required [16]. A description of the input file (and other) parameters is available by

```
astalavista -t scorer --help
```

The GeneID models for human splice sites can be downloaded from the CRG website

```
wget ftp://genome.crg.es/pub/software/geneid/human.070123.
param
```

The genome sequence is to be split into single FASTA files, each one containing the sequence of one chromosome. Note that due to a technical limitation, the current version of AStalavista requires the chromosome file names to be prefixed by "chr" (i.e., following the pattern "*chrID.fa*", where "*ID*" should be the same as the chromosome), also when the Ensembl GRCh37 assembly (without "chr" prefixes) is employed.

```
for chr in $(seq 1 22) X Y
do
    wget -O - ftp://ftp.ensembl.org/pub/grch37/release-
    83/fasta/homo_sapiens/dna/Homo_sapiens.GRCh37.dna.
    chromosome.${chr}.fa.gz | gunzip > ${chr}.fa
done
```

With these files, the *astalavista scorer* tool can now be run to calculate the effects of the population marker SNPs on the splice site sequence, considering the changes implied for the splicing efficiency.

```
for t in 0.5 0.7 0.9
do
     for pop in CEU CHB YRI
     do
         astalavista -t scorer --gid human.070123.param --
         chr .
         --in gencode.v19.annotation.gtf.gz --vcf
         chr19_markers_${pop}-
         only_${t}.vcf --so chr19_markers_${pop}-only_
         ${t}_sites.vcl
     done
done
```

The output (specified by the "*–so*" option) of the tool are VCL (VCF-like) formatted files, one per population-threshold combination, that contain the (reference) sequences of all splice donor and acceptor sites from the transcriptome described by the GTF file (in column 4) and their associated splicing scores (in column 6). For each splice site that is affected by one or more variants from the input VCF file additionally the variant splice site sequence (column 5) and splicing scores of all alternative alleles (a key-value pair in column 8) are provided (see http://sammeth.net/confluence/display/ASTA/.VCL+format). In order to filter the output files keeping exclusively known reference splice site sequences (i.e., column 7 is "PASS") that are affected by population marker SNPs, we employ

```
for f in chr19_markers_???-only_0.?_sites.vcl
do
     cat $f | awk '$5 != "." && $7 == "PASS"' > $(basename
     -s .vcl $f)_withSNPs.vcl
done
```

Notice that, as in protein-coding regions, there are relatively few splice sites that are affected by population-specific marker SNPs. Nevertheless, some of these SNPs change the splicing score of splice sites. For instance, marker SNP rs1974982 of the YRI population increases the splicing score of a splice donor site from 1.30 to 3.96, whereas the YRI-marker rs8101879 abolishes the activity of the harboring splice donor site.

4   Notes

1. The human reference genome sequence can be downloaded from several sources, such as the NCBI website, and the UCSC [17] and Ensembl [18] genome browsers. Although the human genome sequence has been declared "complete" already in 2004 [19], there are still gaps in the assembled sequence that are difficult either to sequence (e.g., due to biophysical properties such as [GC] content) or to assemble (e.g., in repetitive regions). Continued efforts to fill in these gaps resulted in a series of updated genome assemblies, which since 2009 are released by the Genome Reference Consortium (GRC) (http://www.ncbi.nlm.nih.gov/projects/genome/assembly/grc/) under the naming pattern GRCh.. (where h stands for human and ".." is the assembly version number). However, neither the GRC assembly names nor the names and composition of the chromosomes are necessarily conserved across the databases that provide a copy of the corresponding reference genome. For instance, the UCSC genome browser traditionally employs a hg.. version numbering (for "human genome"), which until recently was not synchronized with the corresponding GRC version numbering (https://genome.ucsc.edu/FAQ/FAQreleases.html). At the time of writing this chapter, the still widely used GRCh37 assembly from February 2009 corresponds to hg19 in the UCSC database, despite employing a different version of the mitochondrial genome. To enhance the synchronization with GRCh genomes, the UCSC database recently adapted their assembly numbering, and GRCh38 (the most recent human genome from December 2013) corresponds to hg38 in the UCSC database.

   In addition to these differences in the assembly nomenclature, the canonical names of chromosomes and other contigs are not necessarily constant across databases. The UCSC genome browser, for instance, prefixes chromosome numbers and letters with "chr." In contrast, databases associated with members of the GRC (e.g., the NCBI and Ensembl databases) do not employ such a prefix. As a bottom line, it is important to consider benefits of different assemblies and versions of the human genome before starting an analysis, and the consistent use of datasets compatible with a chosen reference is paramount. Additional information on the differences between heterogeneous versions of human reference assemblies is available at the site https://wiki.dnanexus.com/Scientific-Notes/human-genome.

2. MAF vs DAF vs NRAF: The Minor Allele Frequency (MAF) refers to the least frequent allele(s) at a genomic site. The Derived Allele Frequency (DAF) is based on an evolutionary model used to estimate which allele is ancestral and which has

been obtained through mutation (i.e., the "derived allele"). Derived variant alleles can also be more frequent than the ancestral allele, although in practice this scenario is quite exceptional. The ancestral allele is determined employing genomes of closely related species, and therefore DAFs cannot be determined for SNPs that fail to map to the corresponding genomes. Finally, a Non-Reference Allele Frequency (NRAF) is computed for all alleles that differ from the reference sequence (i.e., the alternative alleles).

3. To obtain non-reference alleles that are highly prevalent in all populations, *vcf-isec* can be instructed to return SNPs present in three VCF files using the "*–nfiles = 3*" argument, by using

```
for t in 0.5 0.7 0.9
do
        vcf-isec --force --nfiles =3
    chr19_biallelicSNPs_CEU_marker_${t}.vcf.gz
    chr19_biallelicSNPs_CHB_marker_${t}.vcf.gz
    chr19_biallelicSNPs_YRI_marker_${t}.vcf.gz | bgzip -c >
    chr19_markers_common_${t}.vcf.gz
  tabix -p vcf chr19_markers_common_${t}.vcf.gz
    done
```

4. When comparing two files, *bedtools* per default loads one of them completely into the computer's working memory (RAM). With large files this can use up a lot of RAM, however, we can run bedtools with the "*-sorted*" option if the intervals from both the input files are sorted by chromosomal coordinates. This makes bedtools use a different algorithm in which it reads in both files concurrently in small chunks. Especially for large files, this approach is *much* faster, and uses *much* less RAM than the default algorithm.

5. Some minor modifications to the "*bedtools intersect*" command can modify the elements provided in the output: using "*-wb*" instead of "*-wa*" obtains exons with SNPs instead of the SNPs, and using "*-wo*" instead of "*-wa*" obtains the mapping of the SNPs to the exons.

References

1. Miller W, Makova KD, Nekrutenko A, Hardison RC (2004) Comparative genomics. Annu Rev Genomics Hum Genet 5:15–56

2. Gibbons A (2015) Revolution in human evolution. Science 349:362–366

3. Pääbo S (2015) The diverse origins of the human gene pool. Nat Rev Genet 16:313–314

4. Allentoft ME, Sikora M, Sjögren K-G et al (2015) Population genomics of bronze age Eurasia. Nature 522:167–172

5. Lander ES, Linton LM, Birren B et al (2001) Initial sequencing and analysis of the human genome. Nature 409:860–921

6. Olivier M, Aggarwal A, Allen J et al (2001) A high-resolution radiation hybrid map of the human genome draft sequence. Science 291:1298–1302

7. McCarthy MI, Abecasis GR, Cardon LR et al (2008) Genome-wide association studies for complex traits: consensus, uncertainty and challenges. Nat Rev Genet 9:356–369

8. Gibbs RA, Belmont JW, Hardenbol P et al (2003) The international HapMap project. Nature 426:789–796

9. Manolio TA, Collins FS (2009) The HapMap and genome-wide association studies in diagnosis and therapy. Annu Rev Med 60:443–456

10. Abecasis GR, Auton A, Brooks LD et al (2012) An integrated map of genetic variation from 1,092 human genomes. Nature 135:0–9

11. Danecek P, Auton A, Abecasis G et al (2011) The variant call format and VCFtools. Bioinformatics 27:2156–2158

12. Foissac S, Sammeth M (2015) Analysis of alternative splicing events in custom gene datasets by AStalavista. Methods Mol Biol 1269:379–392

13. Harrow J, Frankish A, Gonzalez JM et al (2012) GENCODE: the reference human genome annotation for the ENCODE project. Genome Res 22:1760–1774

14. Sabeti PC, Reich DE, Higgins JM et al (2002) Detecting recent positive selection in the human genome from haplotype structure. Nature 419:832–837

15. Xue Y, Zhang X, Huang N et al (2009) Population differentiation as an indicator of recent positive selection in humans: an empirical evaluation. Genetics 183:1065–1077

16. Blanco E, Parra G, Guigó R (2007) Using geneid to identify genes. Curr Protoc Bioinformatics Chapter 4:Unit 4.3

17. Speir ML, Zweig AS, Rosenbloom KR et al (2016) The UCSC genome browser database: 2016 update. Nucleic Acids Res 44: D717–D725

18. Flicek P, Amode MR, Barrell D et al (2014) Ensembl 2014. Nucleic Acids Res 42: D749–D755

19. International Human Genome Sequencing Consortium (2004) Finishing the euchromatic sequence of the human genome. Nature 431:931–945

INDEX

Printed in the United States
By Bookmasters